MW00845182

Musculoskeletal Imaging

Rotations in Radiology

Published and Forthcoming Books in the **Rotations in Radiology** Series

Pediatric Radiology

Janet Reed, Edward Lee, Angelisa Paladin, Caroline Carrico, and William Davros

Cardiac Imaging

Charles White, Linda Haramati, Joseph J.S. Chen, and Jeffrey Levky

Chest Imaging

Melissa Rosado de Christensen, Sanjeev Bhalla, Gerald Abbott, and Santiago Martinez-Jiminez

Gastrointestinal Imaging

Angela Levy, Koenraad Mortele, and Benjamin Yeh

Emergency Radiology

Hani H. Abujudeh

Neuroradiology

Zoran Rumboldt, Giulio Zuccoli, Clifford Eskey, Timothy Amrhein, and Benjamin Huang

Breast Imaging

Christoph I. Lee, Constance D. Lehman, and Lawrence W. Bassett

Musculoskeletal Imaging

Mihra S. Taljanovic, Imran Omar, Kevin B. Hoover, and Tyson S. Chadaz

Rotations in Radiology

Volume 2

Musculoskeletal Imaging

Edited by

Mihra S. Taljanovic, MD, PhD, FACR

Professor, Radiology and Orthopaedic Surgery
Director of Musculoskeletal Imaging Research and Development
Department of Medical Imaging
The University of Arizona, College of Medicine
Banner University Medical Center
Tucson, Arizona

Imran M. Omar, MD

Associate Professor of Radiology
Chief, Musculoskeletal Radiology
Department of Radiology
Northwestern Memorial Hospital
Northwestern University Feinberg School of Medicine
Chicago, Illinois

Kevin B. Hoover, MD, PhD

Associate Professor
Director of Musculoskeletal Imaging and Intervention
Department of Radiology
Virginia Commonwealth University
Richmond, Virginia

Tyson S. Chadaz, MD

Assistant Professor of Radiology
Associate Program Director, Diagnostic Radiology Residency
Department of Medical Imaging
The University of Arizona, College of Medicine
Banner University Medical Center
Tucson, Arizona

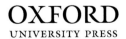

OXFORD
UNIVERSITY PRESS

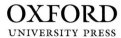

Oxford University Press is a department of the University of Oxford. It furthers
the University's objective of excellence in research, scholarship, and education
by publishing worldwide. Oxford is a registered trade mark of Oxford University
Press in the UK and certain other countries.

Published in the United States of America by Oxford University Press
198 Madison Avenue, New York, NY 10016, United States of America.

© Oxford University Press 2019

All rights reserved. No part of this publication may be reproduced, stored in
a retrieval system, or transmitted, in any form or by any means, without the
prior permission in writing of Oxford University Press, or as expressly permitted
by law, by license, or under terms agreed with the appropriate reproduction
rights organization. Inquiries concerning reproduction outside the scope of the
above should be sent to the Rights Department, Oxford University Press, at the
address above.

You must not circulate this work in any other form
and you must impose this same condition on any acquirer.

Library of Congress Control Number: 2018060177

ISBN 978-0-19-093817-8

9 8 7 6 5 4 3 2 1

Printed by Sheridan Books, Inc., United States of America

Foreword

Musculoskeletal radiology as a subspecialty encompasses all modalities and disease categories; it is difficult to master its many facets. Furthermore, it is challenging to create a text that succinctly yet comprehensively covers the subject. Rotations in Radiology, Musculoskeletal Imaging, edited by Drs. Taljanovic, Omar, Hoover and Chadaz achieves this goal. The contents accurately represent the series title: a clinical rotation in musculoskeletal radiology encompasses a vast array of diagnoses and techniques, with training led by a trusted mentor. Together the trainer and trainee embark on an educational adventure! The editors have captured this experience, organizing an amazing collection of authors, all internationally recognized experts in their field. Cutting-edge information is presented, along with the basics on all aspects of musculoskeletal radiology. Key points, bulleted lists and diagrams facilitate quick reference. Treatment options are included to provide additional insight. Each anatomic area is featured in a separate chapter with space dedicated to ultrasound techniques. Imaging features of trauma and sports injuries is presented as well as common and atypical infections, metabolic disease and hematopoietic disorders. A large section on musculoskeletal neoplasms is included. Techniques for common musculoskeletal procedures including arthrography of various joints are reviewed. Rounding out the text are chapters on relatively uncommon musculoskeletal diseases. This book is a must for the practitioner who would like to improve their musculoskeletal knowledge and skills—it is like sitting next to the experts.

—William B. Morrison, MD

Contents

Contributors

Sonia Airaldi, MD
Radiologia III—DISSAL
University of Genoa
Genoa, Italy

Nabeel Anwar, MD
Rush University Medical Center
Chicago, Illinois

Remide Arkun, MD
Professor of Radiology
Ege University Medical School
Bornova, Izmir, Turkey

Laura W. Bancroft, MD, FACR
Professor of Radiology and Educational Chair
of Radiology
University of Central Florida College of Medicine
Orlando, Florida
Chief of Musculoskeletal Radiology
Florida Hospital
Orlando, Florida

Noam Belkind, MD
Clinical Assistant Professor of Radiology
University of Arizona College of Medicine - Phoenix
Carl T Hayden VA Medical Center
Phoenix, Arizona

Eléonore Blondieux, MD, PhD
Associate Professor of Radiology
Faculté de Médecine, Sorbonne Université, Paris 06
Assistance Publique des Hôpitaux de Paris
Hôpital Armand-Trousseau
Paris, France

Kevin J. Blount, MD
Assistant Professor of Radiology
Northwestern University Feinberg School
of Medicine
Chicago, Illinois

David Brandel, MD
Department of Radiology
University of Michigan Health System
Ann Arbor, Michigan

Tyson S. Chadaz, MD
Assistant Professor of Radiology
Associate Program Director, Diagnostic
Radiology Residency
Department of Medical Imaging
The University of Arizona, College of Medicine
Banner University Medical Center
Tucson, Arizona

Andrew L. Chiang, MD
Assistant Professor of Radiology and Orthopedics
Medical Director, Musculoskeletal Imaging
Department of Radiology
Loyola University Medical Center
Maywood, Illinois

Abhijit Datir, MD, FRCR
Assistant Professor of Radiology
Emory University School of Medicine
Atlanta, Georgia

Matthew DelGiudice, MD
Musculoskeletal Radiologist
East Valley Diagnostic Imaging
Phoenix, Arizona

Vishal Desai, MD
Assistant Professor of Radiology
Musculoskeletal Division
Thomas Jefferson University
Philadelphia, Pennsylvania

Swati Deshmukh, MD
Assistant Professor of Radiology
Northwestern University Feinberg School of Medicine
Chicago, Illinois

Girish Gandikota, MBBS, FRCS, FRCR, RMSK
Professor of Radiology
Department of Radiology
University of Michigan Health System
Ann Arbor, Michigan

Ankur Garg, MD, MBA
Assistant Professor of Radiology
Northwestern University Feinberg School of Medicine
Chicago, Illinois

Dorothy L. Gilbertson-Dahdal, MD, MS
Professor of Radiology
Vice-Chair Education & Program Director, Diagnostic
Radiology Residency
Pediatrics Medical Director
Department of Medical Imaging
The University of Arizona, College of Medicine
Banner University Medical Center
Tucson, Arizona

Lana H. Gimber, MD, MPH
Adjunct Assistant Professor of Radiology
Department of Medical Imaging
The University of Arizona, College of Medicine
Banner-University Medical Center
Tucson, Arizona

James F. Griffith, MD, FRCR
Professor
Department of Imaging and Interventional Radiology
The Chinese University of Hong Kong
Hong Kong, China

Ali Guermazi, MD, PhD
Professor of Radiology & Medicine
Boston University School of Medicine
Boston, Massachusetts

Peter J. Haar, MD, PhD
Assistant Professor of Radiology
VCU Health
Virginia Commonwealth University
Richmond, Virginia

Daichi Hayashi, MD, PhD
Assistant Professor of Radiology
Stony Brook University School of Medicine
Stony Brook, New York
Research Assistant Professor of Radiology
Boston University School of Medicine
Boston, Massachusetts

Kevin B. Hoover, MD, PhD
Associate Professor of Radiology
Director of Musculoskeletal Imaging and Intervention
VCU Health
Virginia Commonwealth University
Richmond, Virginia

Tim B. Hunter, MD, MSc
Emeritus Professor of Radiology
Department of Medical Imaging
The University of Arizona, College of Medicine
Banner University Medical Center
Tucson, Arizona

Apostolos H. Karantanas, MD, PhD
Professor of Radiology
University of Crete
Heraklion, Greece
Chairman
Department of Medical Imaging
University Hospital of Heraklion
Heraklion, Greece

Kiran Khursid, MD
Research Associate
Department of Trauma and Emergency Radiology
Vancouver General Hospital
Vancouver, British Columbia, Canada

Benjamin D. Levine, MD
Associate Professor of Radiology
Department of Radiological Sciences
UCLA Health
Los Angeles, California

Laurie M. Lomasney, MD
Professor of Radiology and Orthopedics
Medical Director, Musculoskeletal Imaging
Department of Radiology
Loyola University Medical Center
Maywood, Illinois

Robert Lopez-Ben, MD
Clinical Adjunct Professor
University of North Carolina School of Medicine
Charlotte Radiology
Charlotte, North Carolina

Winnie A. Mar, MD
Associate Professor of Radiology
University of Illinois Hospital and Health Sciences Center
Chicago, Illinois

Carlo Martinoli, MD
Associate Professor of Radiology
Radiologia III—DISSAL
University of Genoa
Genoa, Italy

Stephanie McCann, MD
Radiology Resident, Class of 2017
Department of Radiology
University of Chicago School of Medicine
Chicago, Illinois

John Meyer, DO
Assistant Professor, Department of Diagnostic Radiology
and Nuclear Medicine, Rush Medical College
Vice Chair, Department of Radiology
Director, Division of Body Imaging, Department of
Diagnostic Radiology and Nuclear Medicine
Rush University Medical Center
Chicago, Illinois

Yoav Morag, MD
Associate Professor
Musculoskeletal Imaging Division
Department of Radiology
University of Michigan Health System
Ann Arbor, Michigan

Peter L. Munk, MDCM, FRCPC, FSIR
Professor of Radiology, Orthopedics and Palliative Care
University of British Columbia
Skeletal Imaging Section Head
Vancouver General Hospital
Vancouver, British Columbia, Canada

Michael O'Keeffe, MB Bch, BAO, MRCSI, FFRRCSI
Assistant Professor of Radiology
University of Toronto
Staff Radiologist Dept. of Emergency & Trauma Radiology
Sunnybrook Health Sciences Centre
Toronto, Ontario, Canada

Imran M. Omar, MD
Associate Professor of Radiology
Chief, Musculoskeletal Radiology
Department of Radiology
Northwestern Memorial Hospital
Northwestern University Feinberg School of Medicine
Chicago, Illinois

Pavan Parasu, MD
Radiology Resident
University of Illinois at Chicago
Department of Radiology
Chicago, Illinois

Wilfred C. G. Peh, MBBS, MD, FRCP (Glasg), FRCP (Edin), FRCR
Senior Consultant and Head
Department of Diagnostic Radiology
Khoo Teck Puat Hospital
Republic of Singapore
Clinical Professor
Yong Loo Lin School of Medicine
National University of Singapore
Republic of Singapore

Jack Porrino, MD
Associate Professor of Radiology
Yale School of Medicine
New Haven, Connecticut

Paul J. Read, MD
Clinical Assistant Professor of Radiology
Sidney Kimmel Medical College
Thomas Jefferson University Hospital
Philadelphia, Pennsylvania

Frank W. Roemer
Professor of Radiology
University of Erlangen-Nuremberg
Erlangen, Germany
Adjunct Associate Professor of Radiology
Boston University School of Medicine
Boston, Massachusetts

Jonathan D. Samet, MD
Assistant Professor of Radiology
Section Head, Musculoskeletal Imaging
Department of Medical Imaging
Ann & Robert H. Lurie Children's Hospital of Chicago
Northwestern University Feinberg School of Medicine
Chicago, Illinois

Leanne L. Seeger, MD, FACR
Professor of Radiology and Orthopedic Surgery
Chief, Musculoskeletal Radiology
Department of Radiological Sciences
UCLA Health
Los Angeles, California

Sumer N. Shikhare, MBBS, DNB, MMed, FRCR
Consultant
Department of Diagnostic Radiology
Khoo Teck Puat Hospital
Republic of Singapore

Albert Song, MD
Associate Professor of Musculoskeletal Imaging
Program Director Diagnostic Radiology Residency
Department of Radiology
Loyola University Medical Center
Maywood, Illinois

G. Scott Stacy, MD
Professor of Radiology
Section Chief, Musculoskeletal Radiology
Department of Radiology
The University of Chicago Medicine
Chicago, Illinois

Kathryn J. Stevens, MD
Associate Professor of Radiology and Orthopaedic
Surgery (by courtesy)
Stanford University Medical Center
Stanford, California

Mihra S. Taljanovic, MD, PhD, FACR
Professor, Radiology and Orthopaedic Surgery
Director of Musculoskeletal Imaging Research and
Development
Department of Medical Imaging
The University of Arizona, College of Medicine
Banner University Medical Center
Tucson, Arizona

Stephen Thomas, MD
Associate Professor of Radiology
University of Chicago School of Medicine
Chicago, Illinois

Josephina A. Vossen MD, PhD
Assistant Professor of Radiology
VCU Health
Virginia Commonwealth University
Richmond, Virginia

Alvin R. Wyatt II, MD
Department of Radiology
University of Washington
Seattle, Washington

Corrie M. Yablon, MD
Clinical Associate Professor of Radiology
Fellowship Director, Musculoskeletal Imaging
Department of Radiology
University of Michigan Health System
Ann Arbor, Michigan

Federico Zaottini, MD
Radiologia III—DISSAL
University of Genoa
Genoa, Italy

Adam C. Zoga, MD
Professor of Radiology
Vice Chair for Clinical Practice
Director of Musculoskeletal MRI
Musculoskeletal Fellowship Program Director
Thomas Jefferson University
Philadelphia, Pennsylvania

Section Four

Metabolic, Hematopoietic, Endocrine, and Deposition Diseases

Edited by Kevin B. Hoover

Metabolic Diseases

CHAPTER 71

Osteoporosis

Peter J. Haar

Introduction

Osteoporosis is the most common metabolic bone disorder, affecting approximately 200 million people worldwide. This is a systemic skeletal disease characterized by generalized loss of bone mass from otherwise normal bone. This loss of bone mass causes microarchitectural deterioration with a consequent increase in bone fragility and susceptibility to fracture.

Pathophysiology and Clinical Findings

Osteoporosis is described as primary, which is idiopathic, or secondary, due to a systemic cause. Primary osteoporosis, also called *involutional osteoporosis*, has 2 main clinical types: postmenopausal and senile. In postmenopausal osteoporosis, decreased estrogen levels result in accelerated bone resorption that is primarily trabecular. In senile osteoporosis, age-related changes in the bone formation–resorption balance result in slowly progressive bone loss that is primarily cortical. Rarely, primary osteoporosis can affect children, termed *idiopathic juvenile osteoporosis*. Risk factors for developing primary osteoporosis include advancing age, female gender, white or Asian ethnicity, thin body habitus, sedentary lifestyle, positive family history, poor dietary intake of calcium or vitamin D, and smoking.

Secondary osteoporosis refers to a loss of bone mass that can be attributed to a known cause. Some common causes of secondary osteoporosis include exogenous steroid use, alcoholism, multiple myeloma, heparin use, hyperthyroidism, hyperparathyroidism, malabsorption syndromes, chronic liver disease, Marfan syndrome, Ehlers-Danlos syndrome, leukemia, thalassemia, and multiple myeloma.

Although loss of bone mass in osteoporosis is asymptomatic, symptoms arise from complications, particularly fragility and insufficiency fractures. Fragility fractures result from minor trauma that would not fracture a normal bone, such as a fall from standing height. These are common in the proximal femur and distal radius. Insufficiency fractures result from normal stress on abnormal bone and are especially common in the vertebral bodies and pelvic bones. Approximately 1 in 3 postmenopausal women experience osteoporotic fractures, and 1 in 5 men older than the age of 50 experience osteoporotic fractures. These osteoporotic fractures can markedly decrease quality of life and reduce life expectancy. Although osteoporosis may be diagnosed radiographically after there is marked bone loss or fracture, quantitative bone mineral density (BMD) measurement methods, such as DXA, allow earlier diagnosis and treatment.

Imaging Strategy

The International Society for Clinical Densitometry (ISCD) recommends bone density testing for the following groups: all women aged 65 and older; all men aged 70 and older; anyone with a fragility fracture; anyone with a disease, condition, or medication associated with osteoporosis; anyone considering therapy for osteoporosis; women who have been on hormone replacement therapy for prolonged periods; and anyone being treated for osteoporosis, to monitor effects of therapy.

DXA is the current gold standard for osteoporosis diagnosis and fracture risk prediction. Other quantitative BMD measurement methods, such as quantitative ultrasound and quantitative computed tomography (QCT), can also be used, depending on availability. Because small variations in hardware can affect comparisons, follow-up quantitative BMD measurement studies should be done on the same machine for reliability.

In cases of suspected osteoporotic fractures, radiographs with at least 2 views should be performed. When there is a high clinical suspicion for a fracture, and where radiographs are inconclusive or negative, MRI should be performed.

Imaging Findings

Dual-Energy X-Ray Absorptiometry

- DXA is considered the current gold standard for osteoporosis diagnosis and fracture risk prediction.
- A comparison of the attenuations of x-ray beams of 2 different energies is used to measure BMD of the spine and hip (Figure 71.1).
- A T-score is reported for postmenopausal women and men age 50 years and older:
  - The T-score represents a standard deviation from the mean bone density (g/cm^2) of a healthy 30-year-old adult at peak bone mass, matched for gender and ethnic group.
    - A score of –1.0 or more is considered normal.
    - A score of –1.1 to –2.4 indicates osteopenia.
    - A score of –2.5 or less indicates osteoporosis.
- A Z-score is reported for premenopausal women and men age 50 years and younger.
  - The Z-score represents a standard deviation from the mean of individuals matched for gender, ethnic group, age, and body weight:
    - A score of less than or equal to –2.0 is below the expected range for age.

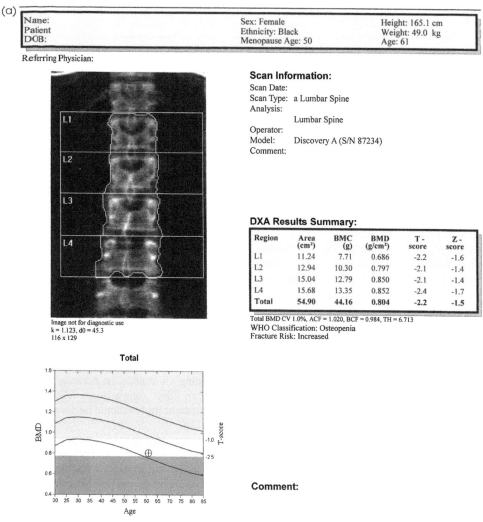

(a)

Name:			Sex: Female			Height: 165.1 cm
Patient			Ethnicity: Black			Weight: 49.0 kg
DOB:			Menopause Age: 50			Age: 61

Referring Physician:

Scan Information:
Scan Date:
Scan Type: a Lumbar Spine
Analysis:
            Lumbar Spine
Operator:
Model: Discovery A (S/N 87234)
Comment:

DXA Results Summary:

Region	Area (cm²)	BMC (g)	BMD (g/cm²)	T - score	Z - score
L1	11.24	7.71	0.686	-2.2	-1.6
L2	12.94	10.30	0.797	-2.1	-1.4
L3	15.04	12.79	0.850	-2.1	-1.4
L4	15.68	13.35	0.852	-2.4	-1.7
Total	54.90	44.16	0.804	-2.2	-1.5

Total BMD CV 1.0%, ACF = 1.020, BCF = 0.984, TH = 6.713
WHO Classification: Osteopenia
Fracture Risk: Increased

Image not for diagnostic use
k = 1.123, d0 = 45.3
116 x 129

Total

BMD / Age chart (BMD vs Age, T-score)

Comment:

Figure 71.1. Spine DXA report for a 61-year-old African American woman with osteoporosis. (*A*) The frontal image of the spine demonstrates absence of artifact and normal configuration of the vertebrae with regions of interest (ROI) over the vertebrae. The L1-L4 vertebrae demonstrate low bone mass (osteopenia) with T-scores between –1.1 and –2.4. (*B*) The hip image demonstrates normal orientation of the hip with ROI including the femoral neck and the trochanters. No fracture risk prediction by FRAX is provided because of the presence of osteoporosis (femoral neck T-score –2.5), and treatment is recommended.

- A score of more than –2.0 is within the expected range for age.
- The spine is positioned straight and centered in the field, including the lowest vertebra with ribs and the pelvic brim.
- The femur is positioned with 15 to 25 degrees of internal rotation, positioning the long axis of the femoral neck perpendicular to the x-ray beam.
- The distal third of the radius can be used if a patient is obese, if the spine and hip cannot be measured for other reasons, and in cases of hyperparathyroidism and anorexia.
- Vertebral fracture assessment (VFA) is a low-dose lateral image of the thoracic and lumbar spine that may be added to a standard DXA study to assess if there is a vertebral body fracture.

- The WHO Fracture Risk Assessment (FRAX) tool is a fracture risk assessment instrument developed at the University of Sheffield that accounts for risk factors such as height, weight, medication history, smoking history, and family history, in addition to DXA measurements at the femoral neck.
- The FRAX algorithms express fracture risk as a 10-year probability of hip fracture and a 10-year probability of major osteoporotic fracture (spine, hip, forearm, or shoulder). This more individualized fracture risk can affect decisions regarding medication changes, lifestyle modification, dietary measures, and future imaging.
- A DXA of the whole body may be used to measure total body composition and fat content with a high degree of accuracy.
- The following artifacts should be noted:

(b)

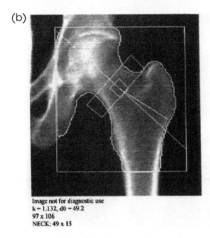

Image not for diagnostic use
k = 1.132, d0 = 49.2
97 x 106
NECK: 49 x 15

Scan Information:

Scan Date: January 17, 2017   ID: A0117170F
Scan Type: a Left Hip
Analysis: January 17, 2017 09:34 Version 13.5.3.1:3
             Left Hip
Operator: SLC
Model: Discovery A (S/N 87234)
Comment:

DXA Results Summary:

Region	Area (cm²)	BMC (g)	BMD (g/cm²)	T-score	Z-score
Neck	4.86	2.79	0.573	-2.5	-1.6
Troch	10.32	5.80	0.562	-1.4	-0.8
Total	32.59	21.98	0.674	-2.2	-1.5

Total BMD CV 1.0%, ACF = 1.020, BCF = 0.984, TH = 5.583
WHO Classification: Osteoporosis

Neck

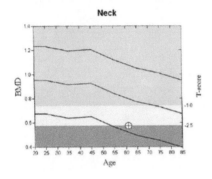

10-year Fracture Risk

FRAX not reported because:
Some T-score for Spine Total or Hip Total or Femoral Neck at
or below -2.5

Comment:

T-score vs. White Female. Source:BMDCS/NHANES White Female. Z-score vs. Black
Female. Source:BMDCS/NHANES

HOLOGIC

Figure 71.1. Continued.

- Sclerotic degenerative disease and vertebral compression fractures may falsely elevate BMD.
- Osteomalacia may underestimate bone mass.
- Obesity, metal hardware, soft tissue calcifications, scoliosis, and vertebral anomalies may also complicate BMD measurement with DXA.

Radiography
- To be detectable with radiographs, 30-50% of bone mineral has to be lost.
- A 10% loss of bone mass in the vertebrae can double the risk of vertebral fracture, and a 10% loss of bone mass of the hip can increase the risk of fracture by 2.5 times.
- Variations in technique alone can create the appearance of relative bone density or lucency.
- Radiographic signs of osteoporosis include decreased number of trabeculae, thinning of trabeculae, coarsened trabecular pattern, and thinning of the cortices (Figures 71.2 and 71.3).
- The width of both metacarpal cortices of the second digit should be more than half of the shaft diameter.
- Vertebral bodies show the earliest radiographic changes.

- Resorption of the horizontal trabeculae causes the *empty box vertebra* sign in which there is apparent increased density of the vertebral endplates (Figure 71.3C, D).
- In the femur, the Singh Index is based on the pattern of trabecular resorption (Figure 71.2B):
  - Mild is indicated by the loss of secondary trabeculae, along the medial portion of the intertrochanteric femur.
  - Intermediate is indicated by the loss of principal tensile trabeculae, curving approximately parallel to the femoral neck.
  - Severe is indicated by the loss of principal compressive trabeculae, oriented vertically in the femoral head.
- The following are common locations for osteoporotic fractures (Figure 71.3B):
  - With fragility, vertebral body compression fractures of the thoracic and lumbar spines, femoral neck, and distal radius are seen.
  - With insufficiency, fractures of the sacrum, pubic rami, superolateral femoral neck, and medial proximal tibia are seen.

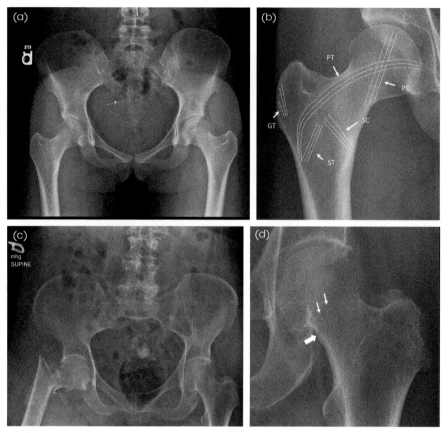

Figure 71.2. Radiographic appearance of normal BMD and osteoporosis. (*A*) AP pelvis radiograph of a healthy 32-year-old woman with normal BMD, shown for comparison. (*B*) Magnified image shows normal, continuous principal compressive (PC), principal tensile (PT), secondary compressive (SC), secondary tensile (ST), and greater trochanter (GT) trabeculae. ST and SC are more difficult to detect because of normal bone density, however, they crosshatch the bone lateral to the lesser trochanter. (*C*) AP pelvis radiograph of a 72-year-old woman with osteoporosis. There is a fragility fracture of the proximal right femur. (*D*) Magnified image shows cortical thinning along the medial portion of the left femoral neck (*thick arrow*). A coarsened trabecular pattern with discontinuity and holes in the trabeculae, including the PC trabeculae, are evident (*thin arrows*).

Quantitative Computed Tomography

- QCT is not commonly used.
- A calibration phantom is used to determine volumetric BMD (mg/cm^3) based on Hounsfield units.
- An advantage of QCT is that it can determine BMD of medullary bone independent from cortical bone.
- Disadvantages of QCT include higher cost and higher radiation dose than DXA, and it is not optimal for longitudinal measurements of treatment response.
- Using clinically acquired CT scans for QCT, or opportunistic QCT, is rapidly evolving:
  - Clinical CT scans obtained for other reasons either with a phantom during the scan (synchronous) or prior to the scan (asynchronous)
  - Benefit of no additional radiation dose

Magnetic Resonance Imaging

- MRI offers the highest sensitivity for detection of osteoporotic fractures (Figure 71.3).
- Cortical thinning is the key MRI finding of osteopenia and osteoporosis.
- MRI findings of disuse osteopenia include BME along subchondral bone, around intraosseous blood vessels, and at entheses of tendons and ligaments.

- Bone marrow T1 signal increases with osteoporosis, as trabeculae thin and are replaced by yellow (fatty) marrow.
- MRI at higher field strengths shows potential for visualizing and quantifying trabecular structure.

Quantitative Ultrasound

- US is used for the assessment of density of peripheral bones such as the calcaneus and phalanges.
- Advantages include low cost and no ionizing radiation.

Treatment Options

- Lifestyle modifications should be universally promoted in postmenopausal women to reduce bone loss including the following:
  - Adequate calcium and vitamin D intake
  - Exercise
  - Smoking cessation
  - Counseling on fall prevention
  - Avoidance of heavy alcohol use
  - Avoidance, if possible, of medications that increase bone loss, such as glucocorticoids
- The following groups should receive pharmacologic therapy:

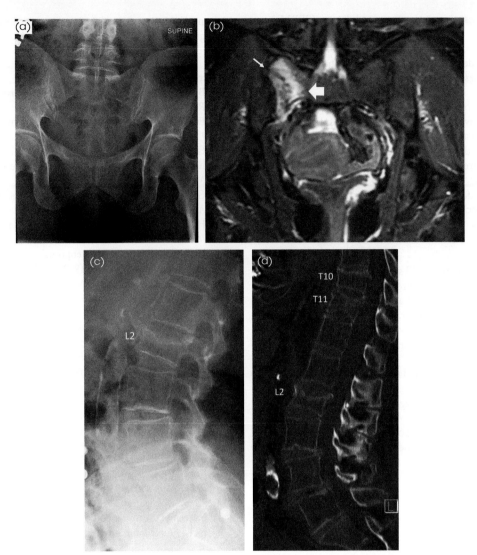

Figure 71.3. Insufficiency fractures. (*A*) On this AP radiograph of the pelvis, there is cortical thinning and a coarsened trabecular pattern, findings of bone mineral loss. The sacral fracture is radiographically occult. (*B*) On a coronal STIR MR image, there is abnormal high bone marrow signal of the right sacral ala (*thick arrow*), with a vertically oriented linear dark band, consistent with a fracture (*thin arrow*). The sacral ala is a common location for insufficiency fractures. (*C*) Lateral lumbar spine radiograph shows a moderate L2 superior endplate fracture. The adjacent vertebrae demonstrate an *empty box* appearance because of the thin cortical shell. (*D*) Sagittal reformatted CT image of the lumbar spine demonstrates additional fractures above L2, including a mild biconcave fracture deformity of T11, and a moderate superior endplate fracture of T10 vertebral bodies.

- Patients with a history of fragility fracture
- Patients with osteoporosis based on BMD measurement (T-score ≤ –2.5)
- Patients at high risk for fracture, calculated, for example, by the WHO FRAX.
  - Bisphosphonates are indicated:
    - Oral medication is often used as initial therapy because of favorable efficacy, cost, and long-term safety.
    - Bisphosphonates reduce resorption of bone by osteoclasts.
    - Chronic bisphosphonate use can lead to atypical femur fracture, such as transverse complete or incomplete fracture of the subtrochanteric proximal femur:
      - Originates at the lateral cortex, and often with endosteal or periosteal beaking or flaring

- Full-length parathyroid hormone and teriparatide (a recombinant form of the bioactive portion of parathyroid hormone) are indicated:
  - Anabolic agents that stimulate bone formation
  - Not considered initial therapy for most patients
  - Used in men and postmenopausal women with severe osteoporosis, patients with contraindications to bisphosphonates
- Denosumab can be offered:
  - Humanized monoclonal antibody against receptor activator of nuclear factor-kappa B (RANK) ligand that reduces osteoclastogenesis
  - Used in patients who have difficulty with dosing requirements of oral bisphosphonates, patients with impaired renal function, or patients who are unresponsive to other therapies

- Selective estrogen receptor modulators (SERMs) are indicated:
  - Can be used for treatment of osteoporosis when there is an independent need for breast cancer prophylaxis
  - Increases thromboembolic events and possibly hot flashes
- Combination therapy has only small benefits on BMD and no proven additional fracture prevention benefit.
- Surgical fixation of fractures in osteoporotic bone can be complicated by poor bone quality with inadequate fracture compression, implant anchorage, or screw pull-out or cut-out.
- Some risk factors for osteoporosis may also affect bone healing, such as smoking.

Key Points

- DXA is the current gold standard for osteoporosis diagnosis and fracture risk prediction.
- Bone density testing has been recommended in all women aged 65 and older, all men aged 70 and older, and younger patients who have risk factors for osteoporosis.
- Radiography alone is inadequate for detecting early bone loss.
- Detection of fragility and insufficiency fractures is highly important in patient care, often initiating lifestyle modification and pharmacologic therapy.
- MRI has a higher sensitivity for detecting nondisplaced fractures in osteopenic bone than does radiography, and should be considered when there is clinical suspicion for a radiographically occult fragility fracture.

Recommended Reading

Link TM. Radiology of osteoporosis. *Can Assoc Radiol J.* 2016;67(1):28–40.

Lorentzon M, Cummings SR. Osteoporosis: the evolution of a diagnosis. *J Intern Med.* 2015;277(6):650–61.

References

1. Bauer JS, Link TM. Advances in osteoporosis imaging. *Eur J Radiol.* 2009;71(3):440–49.
2. Eastell R. Treatment of postmenopausal osteoporosis. *N Engl J Med.* 1998;338(11):736–46.
3. Genant HK, Wu CY, van Kuijk C, Nevitt MC. Vertebral fracture assessment using a semiquantitative technique. *J Bone Miner Res.* 1993;8(9):1137–48.
4. Gillespy T 3rd, Gillespy MP. Osteoporosis. *Radiol Clin North Am.* 1991;29(1):77–84.
5. Honig S, Chang G. Osteoporosis: an update. *Bull NYU Hosp Jt Dis.* 2012;70(3):140–44.
6. Kanis JA. Diagnosis of osteoporosis and assessment of fracture risk. *Lancet.* 2002;359(9321):1929–36.
7. Kanis JA, McCloskey EV. Risk factors in osteoporosis. *Maturitas.* 1998;30(3):229–33.
8. Kaplan FS. Osteoporosis. pathophysiology and prevention. *Clin Symp.* 1987;39(1):1–32.
9. Krestan C, Hojreh A. Imaging of insufficiency fractures. *Eur J Radiol.* 2009;71(3):398–405.
10. Link TM. Radiology of osteoporosis. *Can Assoc Radiol J.* 2016;67(1):28–40.
11. Mayo-Smith W, Rosenthal DI. Radiographic appearance of osteopenia. *Radiol Clin North Am.* 1991;29(1):37–47.
12. Pisani P, Renna MD, Conversano F, et al. Screening and early diagnosis of osteoporosis through X-ray and ultrasound based techniques. *World J Radiol.* 2013;5(11):398–410.
13. Rosen CJ. Clinical practice. Postmenopausal osteoporosis. *N Engl J Med.* 2005;353(6):595–603.
14. Singh M, Nagrath AR, Maini PS. Changes in trabecular pattern of the upper end of the femur as an index of osteoporosis. *J Bone Joint Surg Am.* 1970;52(3):457–67.

CHAPTER 72

Rickets and Osteomalacia

Peter J. Haar

Introduction

Abnormal mineralization of cortical and trabecular bone is termed *osteomalacia* in adults and *rickets* in children. These conditions may be caused by a variety of different underlying systemic diseases in which there is lack of available calcium or phosphorus for mineralization of osteoid. In osteomalacia, this deficiency leads to abnormal remodeling of mature bone. In rickets, this deficiency leads to abnormalities at the sites of active bone growth.

Pathophysiology and Clinical Findings

Osteomalacia and rickets may be caused by a variety of different conditions that result in a lack of available calcium or phosphorus for mineralization of osteoid. Because vitamin D promotes gastrointestinal calcium absorption and calcium resorption in the renal proximal tubules, deficiency or abnormal metabolism of vitamin D can result in osteomalacia or rickets. In developed nations, a leading cause of osteomalacia and rickets is gastrointestinal malabsorption, which may be related to gastrointestinal surgery and short bowel syndrome, celiac disease, or biliary disease. Nutritional deficiencies of vitamin D, calcium, or phosphorus are relatively rare, but can be seen among strict vegetarians and vegans, and patients receiving total parenteral nutrition. Nutritional deficiency of vitamin D may be compounded by an inadequate exposure to sunlight, limiting vitamin D synthesis in the skin.

In adults, osteomalacia most commonly occurs with chronic renal failure, a condition termed *renal osteodystrophy*. Additional renal causes of osteomalacia and rickets include proximal tubular lesions, renal tubular acidosis, and dialysis-induced osteomalacia.

Abnormal vitamin D metabolism can be an underlying cause of osteomalacia or rickets, and may occur in liver disease and in specific hereditary disorders. Other causes of osteomalacia and rickets include anticonvulsant drugs such as phenytoin (Dilantin) and phenobarbital, and aluminum-containing antacids. Rarely, osteomalacia or rickets may occur as a paraneoplastic syndrome, termed *tumor-induced osteomalacia* or *oncogenic osteomalacia*, most commonly caused by small mesenchymal endocrine tumors.

As in osteoporosis, fragility fractures may be the presenting feature of osteomalacia. Other symptoms associated with osteomalacia include muscle weakness and diffuse bone pain. Hypocalcemia in patients with osteomalacia can cause numbness of the perioral area, hands, and feet, muscle spasms, and cardiac arrhythmia.

Children with rickets may present with growth retardation, bowing deformities, most commonly genu varum, joint pain and swelling, and metaphyseal fractures. SCFE can occur in association with rickets. Additionally, rickets may cause craniotabes, or softening of the bones of the skull, frontal bossing, and scoliosis. Children with rickets may present with seizures related to hypocalcemia.

Imaging Strategy

Because osteomalacia and rickets are disorders of bone mineralization, radiography is the most useful imaging modality in the diagnosis and evaluation of these conditions. CT provides cross-sectional detail of the mineralized portion of the bones, but because of its higher cost and radiation dose, CT is useful in evaluating these conditions in only rare, specific instances. Similarly, MRI is not generally useful in imaging osteomalacia or rickets, but may be valuable in specific instances, such as diagnosis of a nondisplaced insufficiency fracture. DXA has a higher sensitivity than radiographs for detection of bone demineralization, but no power to differentiate osteomalacia from osteoporosis.

Imaging Findings

Radiography
- Generalized osteopenia in osteomalacia and rickets (Figures 72.1-72.3)
  - Mild osteomalacia may be indistinguishable from osteoporosis.
  - Trabeculae may appear coarse and poorly defined.
- Deformities related to bone softening
  - Increased elasticity and decreased resistance to bending
  - Bowing of the weight-bearing long bones (Figures 72.1-72.3)
    - Saber shin, or anterior bowing of the tibia
    - Coxa vara–bending of the proximal femur (Figure 72.2A)
      - Severe varus angulation, termed *shepherd's crook deformity*
- Deformities of the spine
  - Basilar invagination
  - Vertebral endplate compression fractures
    - Biconcave vertebral bodies
  - Kyphosis and scoliosis
- Deformities of the pelvis

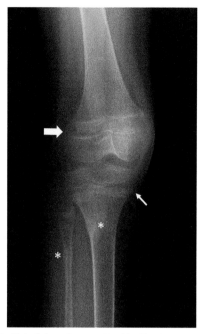

Figure 72.1. Rickets in a 9-year-old girl with vitamin D deficiency related to dietary aversions and psychiatric illness. AP radiograph of the knee shows diffuse bone demineralization with cortical thinning and a coarsened trabecular texture. The growth plates are widened (*thick arrow*), and there is metaphyseal cupping and fraying (*thin arrow*). There is a Looser zone of the lateral aspect of the proximal tibial metaphysis and a healing insufficiency fracture of the proximal shaft of the fibula (*asterisks*).

- Protrusio acetabuli
- Triradiate pelvis, with inward migration of the sacrum and acetabula
- Looser zones (pseudofractures) (Figures 72.1–72.3)
  - Transverse zones of lucency often along the concave (compressive) side of long bones
  - Also called *Milkman pseudofractures*
  - Lucencies filled with poorly mineralized osteoid tissue

- Commonly seen along the axillary margin of the scapula, inner margin of the femoral neck, ribs, pubic rami
- Osteomalacia with multiple Looser zones (*Milkman syndrome*)
- Growth plate deformities in rickets (Figure 72.1)
  - Widening of the growth plate
    - Ongoing cartilage growth without normal mineralization
  - Widening at the end of the metaphysis, with cupping at the margins
  - Irregularity or fraying along the metaphyseal margin
  - Physeal disruption
    - SCFE
    - Disruption of the physis of the proximal humerus
  - Costochondral junctions
    - Cupping and widening of the anterior rib ends
    - Knobs of bone at the costochondral joints, termed *rachitic rosary*

Computed Tomography
- Similar findings to those on radiography, with the advantages of cross-sectional imaging
- Not generally used because of high radiation dose and relative cost
- May be useful in specific situations, such as for detection of subtle insufficiency fractures or Looser zones

Magnetic Resonance Imaging
- Not generally used because of high cost and poor evaluation of bone mineralization
- Widening of the cartilaginous physes in rickets
- May be useful for detection of subtle insufficiency fractures or Looser zones

Nuclear Medicine
- Bone scan
  - Limited diagnostic value
  - Diffuse skeletal uptake with a superscan appearance
  - May reveal Looser zones

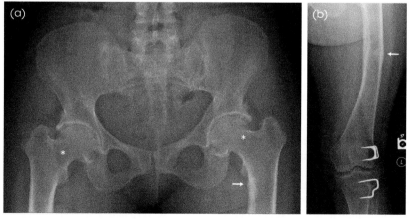

Figure 72.2. Osteomalacia in a 63-year-old woman treated for hypophosphatemia. (*A*) AP radiograph of the pelvis shows bilateral coxa vara (*asterisks*) and healed Looser zone at the compressive, medial side of the proximal left femur (*thin arrow*). (*B*) AP radiograph of the left femur shows lateral bowing. There is a healed Looser zone of the lateral midshaft of the left femur (*arrow*). Note metal staples related to remote surgical stabilization of the distal femoral and proximal tibial growth plates.

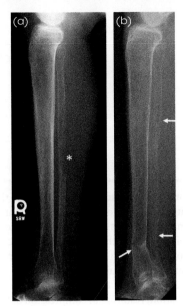

Figure 72.3. Osteomalacia in a middle-aged woman with Crohn disease, celiac disease, and malabsorption. (*A*) Lateral radiograph of the tibia and fibula at age 45 demonstrates diffuse bone demineralization and replacement of fibular bone by demineralized fibrous tissue (*asterisk*, biopsy proven). (*B*) Lateral radiograph of the tibia and fibula at age 51 shows further progression of bone demineralization, an atypical insufficiency fracture with bowing of the distal tibial shaft and extensive irregularity and fracture of the fibular shaft (*thin arrows*).

Dual-Energy X-Ray Absorptiometry
■ Detects low bone mineral density
■ Density depending on severity and duration of the disease

Treatment Options
■ Treatment depends on underlying cause of osteomalacia or rickets.
■ Oral, subcutaneous, or IV supplementation can be offered:
  ■ Vitamin D
  ■ Calcium
  ■ Phosphate
■ Behavioral modifications are indicated:
  ■ Dietary changes
  ■ Increased exposure to sunlight
■ Rickets is treated with the following:
  ■ Braces to stabilize bowing of bones
  ■ Surgical correction of severe bone deformations

Key Points
■ Abnormal mineralization of bone is termed osteomalacia in adults and rickets in children and may be caused by a variety of conditions in which there is a lack of available calcium or phosphorus.
■ Osteomalacia and rickets are often diagnosed with blood analysis.

■ Osteomalacia and rickets are best imaged with radiography, which detects osteopenia, and may be distinguished from osteoporosis by the presence of bowing deformities, Looser zones, or growth plate abnormalities.
■ CT and MRI have limited roles, but have a higher sensitivity for detecting subtle Looser zones and insufficiency fractures.
■ Treatment of osteomalacia and rickets depends on the underlying cause and involves supplementation of vitamin D, calcium, and/or phosphate.

Recommended Reading
Sundaram M. Founders lecture 2007: Metabolic bone disease: what has changed in 30 years? *Skeletal Radiol.* 2009;38(9):841–53.

Reginato AJ, Coquia JA. Musculoskeletal manifestations of osteomalacia and rickets. *Best Pract Res Clin Rheumatol.* 2003;17(6):1063–80.

References
1. Guglielmi G, Muscarella S, Leone A, Peh WC. Imaging of metabolic bone diseases. *Radiol Clin North Am.* 2008;46(4):735–54, vi.
2. Elder CJ, Bishop NJ. Rickets. *Lancet.* 2014;383(9929):1665–76.
3. Chapman T, Sugar N, Done S, Marasigan J, Wambold N, Feldman K. Fractures in infants and toddlers with rickets. *Pediatr Radiol.* 2010;40(7):1184–89.
4. Sundaram M. Founders lecture 2007: Metabolic bone disease: what has changed in 30 years? *Skeletal Radiol.* 2009;38(9):841–53.
5. Reginato AJ, Coquia JA. Musculoskeletal manifestations of osteomalacia and rickets. *Best Pract Res Clin Rheumatol.* 2003;17(6):1063–80.
6. Calder AD. Radiology of osteogenesis imperfecta, rickets and other bony fragility states. *Endocr Dev.* 2015;28:56–71.
7. Dadoniene J, Miglinas M, Miltiniene D, et al. Tumour-induced osteomalacia: a literature review and a case report. *World J Surg Oncol.* 2016;14(1):4.
8. Jevtic V. Imaging of renal osteodystrophy. *Eur J Radiol.* 2003;46(2):85–95.
9. Lawson J. Drug-induced metabolic bone disorders. *Semin Musculoskelet Radiol.* 2002;6(4):285–97.
10. Lenchik L, Sartoris DJ. Orthopedic aspects of metabolic bone disease. *Orthop Clin North Am.* 1998;29(1):103–34.
11. Phan CM, Guglielmi G. Metabolic bone disease in patients with malabsorption. *Semin Musculoskelet Radiol.* 2016;20(4):369–75.
12. Lim CY, Ong KO. Various musculoskeletal manifestations of chronic renal insufficiency. *Clin Radiol.* 2013;68(7):e397–411.
13. Krestan CR, Nemec U, Nemec S. Imaging of insufficiency fractures. *Semin Musculoskelet Radiol.* 2011;15(3):198–207.
14. Buckley O, Brien JO, Ward E, Doody O, Govender P, Torreggiani WC. The imaging of coeliac disease and its complications. *Eur J Radiol.* 2008;65(3):483–90.
15. Mankin HJ, Mankin CJ. Metabolic bone disease: a review and update. *Instr Course Lect.* 2008;57:575–93.

CHAPTER 73

Paget Disease

Peter J. Haar

Introduction

Paget disease is a chronic, progressive disease that results in excessive bone turnover and abnormal, disordered bone remodeling. Paget disease is usually asymptomatic and relatively common in the adult population, affecting approximately 3% of adults older than age 40. The disease has an active lytic phase that progresses to an inactive quiescent phase. Treatment of Paget disease includes therapies that decrease osteolysis and the surgical correction of osseous deformities.

Pathophysiology and Clinical Findings

Paget disease is often polyostotic and can involve any bone, though it most commonly involves the pelvis, femur, skull, tibia, vertebra, clavicle, and humerus. The disease begins with an active, lytic phase in which there is focal osteolysis, often in the subchondral region of a proximal long bone. In this phase, there is aggressive osteoclastic activity, and yellow bone marrow is replaced by hyperemic fibrovascular tissue. There is usually a sharp margin between the area of osteolysis and normal bone with the margin progressing at a rate of a few millimeters per year. Layers of disorganized woven bone then fill in the area of osteolysis as the margin progresses. In the inactive, quiescent phase, osteoclastic activity stops, osteoblastic activity predominates, and focal areas of woven bone are replaced by lamellar bone in a disorganized fashion. Endosteal and periosteal apposition bone formation continues, which can cause cortical thickening and bone enlargement in all dimensions.

Paget disease generally affects older patients, with a median age of 64 years. Only 4% of Paget cases occur in patients younger than age 40 years. Paget disease is slightly more common in men and patients of white ethnicity. Though the etiology of Paget disease is incompletely understood, there is some evidence of a relationship to measles, and other paramyxovirus infections, and an autosomal dominant genetic predisposition.

Although Paget disease is often asymptomatic for many years, patients may have deep bone pain or warmth of the overlying skin related to hyperemia. Common bone deformities in Paget disease include bowing of long bones, especially the weight-bearing femur and tibia. Deformity involving the joints, for example protrusio acetabuli, can cause secondary OA. Enlargement of the bones of the skull can cause increasing hat size, a classic sign of the disease.

Bone strength is weakened in Paget disease, and involved bones are at risk for pathologic fracture, particularly weight-bearing bones with the subtrochanteric femur being the most common site of fracture. Involvement of the skull and spine can cause impingement of neural structures. Paget disease involving the petrous temporal bone can cause hearing loss, and impingement of the optic nerve may cause changes in vision. Compression of the spinal cord or nerve roots may cause pain, paresis, gait abnormalities, or incontinence. Involvement of the base of the skull can cause platybasia and basilar invagination, resulting in compression of the brainstem or hydrocephalus.

The most devastating potential complication of Paget disease is malignant transformation to Paget sarcoma, which occurs in approximately 1% of cases of Paget disease, usually in patients with widespread disease. Sarcomatous degeneration is likely secondary to a high rate of bone turnover. Paget sarcomas are most often histologically osteosarcomas, but any type of bone or soft tissue sarcoma is possible.

A superimposed GCT may arise from bone with Paget disease, often in patients who develop Paget disease at a younger age, with extensive disease and a positive family history. Rarely, a benign soft tissue mass with rapid growth may arise adjacent to bone with Paget disease, termed a *Paget pseudosarcoma*.

Indications for medical treatment of Paget disease include symptoms of bone pain; risk of brain stem, cranial nerve, or spinal cord compromise; involvement of weight-bearing bones with risk of fracture; and optimization of bone turnover to reduce bone vascularity in patients undergoing surgery, to reduce intraoperative blood loss. Patients may be monitored clinically by measuring serum alkaline phosphatase and urinary hydroxyproline levels, which are increased with osteoclastic activity.

Imaging Strategy

Radiographs are usually sufficient to make the initial diagnosis of Paget disease; however, because Paget disease typically advances a few millimeters per year, radiographic changes alone are too slow to monitor the disease. Radiography may be useful in diagnosing complications such as pathologic fractures. Cross-sectional imaging is valuable for early diagnosis, particularly in the skull and spine. CT and MRI are often obtained for evaluation of complications of Paget disease, such as evaluation of neurologic symptoms related to nerve impingement, preoperative planning for arthroplasty, and diagnosis of sarcomatous degeneration. IV contrast is not usually required, except in the context of sarcomatous degeneration. A nuclear medicine bone scan can be useful to determine disease distribution and extent.

Imaging Findings

Radiography

- Active phase
  - Osteolysis, characteristically starting near a proximal epiphysis, and progressing distally along the shaft, which can involve entire bone
  - Sharp borders between normal bone and the area of osteolysis
  - Lytic border described as "candle flame" or "blade of grass"
- Inactive phase
  - New bone formation and sclerosis
  - Thickening of cortex
  - Coarsening or coalescence of trabeculations (Figure 73.1A)
  - Picture-frame vertebra
  - Bone deformities
    - Bowing, especially of weight-bearing bones
    - Expansion of the bone in all dimensions (Figure 73.2B)

- Protrusio acetabuli (Figure 73.1B)
- Basilar invagination
- Insufficiency fractures (Figure 73.1)
  - Often incomplete horizontal lucencies through the lateral cortex of long bones

Computed Tomography

- Similar findings to radiography (Figures 73.1B and 73.2B)
- Most useful for diagnosis in the skull and spine
  - Active phase round lytic lesion, often in the frontal bone, termed *osteoporosis circumscripta*
  - Widening of the diploic space of the skull
  - Inactive phase sclerosis of the skull with a *cotton wool* appearance

Magnetic Resonance Imaging

- Paget disease often discovered incidentally on MRI for unrelated symptoms
- Nearly any pattern of marrow signal alteration possible, including normal
  - Active phase
    - Reactive marrow changes and hypervascularity
    - Increased T2 signal and decreased T1 signal compared to adjacent normal marrow
    - Cortex may also have increased T2 signal
  - Inactive phase (Figure 73.2C)
    - Trabecular thickening and coarsening
    - Fatty replacement of marrow
    - May appear heterogeneous and speckled on both T1W and T2W imaging
    - Inhomogeneous enhancement
- Useful for diagnosing and evaluating complications of Paget disease
  - Superimposed GCT
    - Lytic, bubbly lesion with a narrow zone of transition
    - Mass with heterogeneous central low signal on T2W imaging
  - Sarcomatous degeneration
    - Cortical destruction
    - Marrow replacement
    - Possible associated soft tissue mass
    - Fatty marrow signal can differentiate focal aggressive osteolysis from sarcomatous degeneration
    - May be useful for biopsy planning
  - Neural impingement
    - Effects of basilar invagination on the posterior fossa and brainstem
    - Effects of osseous deformation or pathologic fracture of the spine on the spinal cord and nerve roots
  - Evaluation of joints
    - Cartilage destruction
    - Ligamentous injury
    - Arthroplasty planning
  - Pathologic fractures (Figure 73.1)
    - Low signal linear fracture
    - Adjacent BME

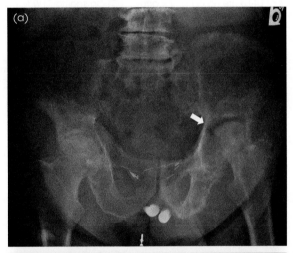
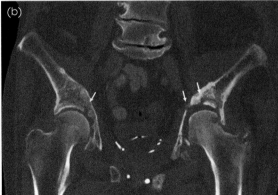

Figure 73.1. Paget disease of the pelvis in a 64-year-old man. (*A*) AP radiograph of the pelvis shows enlargement, cortical thickening, and trabecular coarsening of the bilateral innominate bones. There is left-sided protrusio acetabuli with secondary OA (*thick arrow*). A penile prosthesis is incidentally imaged. (*B*) A coronal, reformatted CT image demonstrates pathologic fractures of the superior acetabuli (*thin arrows*) with depression of the left acetabulum.

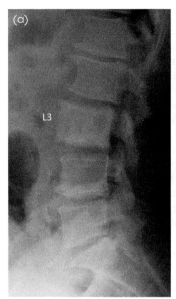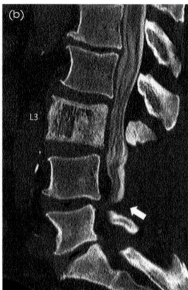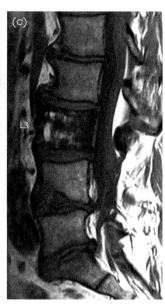

Figure 73.2. Paget disease of the L3 vertebra in a 68-year-old man. (*A*) Lateral radiograph of the lumbar spine shows enlargement of the L3 vertebral body in all dimensions with sclerosis and cortical thickening, giving a *picture-frame* appearance. (*B*) On the sagittal CT myelogram image, there is thickening and coarsening of the bony trabeculae. The vertebral body enlargement causes mild narrowing of the spinal canal. L4 laminectomy and severe canal stenosis at L4-L5 are noted (*thick arrow*). (*C*) On sagittal T1W MR image, note cortical thickening and abnormal trabeculae of L3 vertebral body of low signal, whereas focal nonossified intramedullary areas anteriorly demonstrate high signal consistent with fat.

Nuclear Medicine
- Technetium 99m methylene diphosphonate (^{99m}Tc-MDP) bone scan
  - High uptake with active disease
  - Useful to determine disease distribution and extent
  - Can be negative in the early osteolytic phase of the disease

Treatment Options
- Medical therapies that decrease osteolysis
  - Bisphosphonates suppress osteoclast-mediated bone resorption and are the mainstay medical treatment for Paget disease.
  - Calcitonin has a lower potency and shorter duration compared to bisphosphonates and is an adjunct or second-line treatment.
- Surgical treatment of pathologic fracture or prophylactic fixation of an impending fracture, arthroplasty in severe secondary arthritis, spinal or skull base decompression and osteotomy to correct severe deformity

Key Points
- Paget disease is a bone disorder of older patients in which there is increased bone turnover and disorganized bone remodeling.
- It most commonly occurs in the spine, pelvis, skull, femur, and tibia.
- It has an active lytic phase with a sharply demarcated angular blade-of-grass or flame-shaped border.
- An inactive quiescent phase is characterized by bone enlargement in all dimensions, weakening, trabecular coarsening, and cortical thickening.

- Complications include pathologic fracture, nerve impingement in the skull base and spine, associated GCT, and sarcomatous degeneration.

Recommended Reading

Theodorou DJ, Theodorou SJ, Kakitsubata Y. Imaging of Paget disease of bone and its musculoskeletal complications: review. *AJR Am J Roentgenol.* 2011;196(6 suppl):S64–75.

Lalam RK, Cassar-Pullicino VN, Winn N. Paget disease of bone. *Semin Musculoskelet Radiol.* 2016;20(3):287–99.

References

1. Bolland MJ, Cundy T. Paget's disease of bone: clinical review and update. *J Clin Pathol.* 2013;66(11):924–27.
2. Galson DL, Roodman GD. Pathobiology of Paget's disease of bone. *J Bone Metab.* 2014;21(2):85–98.
3. Smith SE, Murphey MD, Motamedi K, Mulligan ME, Resnik CS, Gannon FH. From the archives of the AFIP. Radiologic spectrum of Paget disease of bone and its complications with pathologic correlation. *Radiographics.* 2002;22(5):1191–1216.
4. Boutin RD, Spitz DJ, Newman JS, Lenchik L, Steinbach LS. Complications in Paget disease at MR imaging. *Radiology.* 1998;209(3):641–51.
5. Melton LJ 3rd, Tiegs RD, Atkinson EJ, O'Fallon WM. Fracture risk among patients with Paget's disease: a population-based cohort study. *J Bone Miner Res.* 2000;15(11):2123–28.
6. Cooper C, Harvey NC, Dennison EM, van Staa TP. Update on the epidemiology of Paget's disease of bone. *J Bone Miner Res.* 2006;21(suppl 2):P3–8.
7. Mangham DC, Davie MW, Grimer RJ. Sarcoma arising in Paget's disease of bone: declining incidence and increasing age at presentation. *Bone.* 2009;44(3):431–36.

8. Singer FR, Bone HG 3rd, Hosking DJ, et al. Paget's disease of bone: an endocrine society clinical practice guideline. *J Clin Endocrinol Metab.* 2014;99(12):4408–22.

9. Lyles KW, Siris ES, Singer FR, Meunier PJ. A clinical approach to diagnosis and management of Paget's disease of bone. *J Bone Miner Res.* 2001;16(8):1379–87.

10. Silverman SL. Paget disease of bone: therapeutic options. *J Clin Rheumatol.* 2008;14(5):299–305.

11. Al-Rashid M, Ramkumar DB, Raskin K, Schwab J, Hornicek FJ, Lozano-Calderon SA. Paget disease of bone. *Orthop Clin North Am.* 2015;46(4):577–85.

12. Theodorou DJ, Theodorou SJ, Kakitsubata Y. Imaging of Paget disease of bone and its musculoskeletal complications: review. *AJR Am J Roentgenol.* 2011;196(6 suppl):S64–75.

13. Lalam RK, Cassar-Pullicino VN, Winn N. Paget disease of bone. *Semin Musculoskelet Radiol.* 2016;20(3):287–99.

14. Kaufmann GA, Sundaram M, McDonald DJ. Magnetic resonance imaging in symptomatic Paget's disease. *Skeletal Radiol.* 1991;20(6):413–18.

Hematopoietic Diseases

CHAPTER 74

Anemias

Kevin B. Hoover

Introduction

Anemia is a very common clinical condition that may be incidentally detected on blood tests or on imaging studies. Imaging is not routinely used for diagnosis, however, it is used in evaluating the various sequelae of anemia. Radiographs and MRI are the most important imaging modalities for monitoring of disease, especially the hemoglobinopathies. Sickle cell anemia and thalassemia are common hemoglobinopathies and have both overlapping and specific imaging characteristics (Table 74.1).

Pathophysiology and Clinical Findings

Anemia is characterized by the decrease in functional hemoglobin (Hb) or red blood cell (RBC) mass that impairs oxygen delivery to tissues and the return of carbon dioxide to the lungs for elimination. The hypoxia of anemia stimulates erythropoiesis and the reconversion of quiescent yellow marrow to active red marrow (discussed in detail in Chapter 75, "Bone Marrow Conversion and Reconversion"). In adults, Hb concentrations below 13.5 g/dL in men and 12.0 g/dL in women are considered anemic, and there is an associated low hematocrit. Symptoms of anemia are primarily related to impaired oxygen delivery: weakness, fatigue, difficulty concentrating, and poor work productivity. In 2013, 27% of the world's population was anemic, affecting more than 10% of the population of every country in the world.

In general, anemia can result from acute high-volume or chronic low-volume blood loss, RBC destruction, or impaired production. Iron deficiency anemia is by far the most common cause, accounting for more than 60% of anemias worldwide. It is a clinical, not imaging, diagnosis that results in impaired RBC production. Aplastic anemia is an uncommon type that results in pancytopenia from RBC destruction. It is idiopathic in approximately 50% of cases, but is associated with a number of etiologies including drugs, radiation, paroxysmal nocturnal hemoglobinuria, Fanconi anemia, viral hepatitis, pregnancy, and thymoma. Hemoglobinopathy, specifically that caused by sickle cell disease (SCD) and thalassemia, is the second most common cause of anemia, accounting for approximately 10% of patients. Hemoglobinopathy results from mutations in either the α or β chains of Hb, and is diagnosed using DNA analysis. There is increased RBC destruction caused by hemolysis and osteoporosis because of trabecular bone destruction, medullary compartment expansion, and cortical thinning. Osteoporosis is often more severe in male patients because of hypogonadism.

Sickle Cell Disease

SCD is caused by mutations in the β-globin (HbS) gene resulting in Hb polymerization when deoxygenated. This can block blood flow resulting in painful ischemic crises commonly affecting the bone and soft tissues. There is also hemolysis of the deformed RBC. The most severe form of SCD is sickle cell anemia (SCA) in patients who are homozygous for HbS. SCA has the most characteristic imaging findings. Bone ischemia results in ON in approximately 50% of SCA patients by age 35. SCA patients are also more prone to infections caused by ischemia-related spleen loss, ON, and multiple hospital admissions. Approximately 18% of SCA patients develop osteomyelitis, which is clinically difficult to distinguish from ON. Septic arthritis occurs in approximately 7% of patients most commonly in the hip joint and in areas affected by ON.

Thalassemia

Both α- and β-thalassemia are caused by mutations in the respective Hb chains. The disease severity is related to the total number of mutated chains (of 4 α chains and 2 β chains). Hemolytic anemia, splenomegaly, and bone marrow space expansion occur. Because of treatment with repeated blood transfusions, iron is deposited, causing damage to such tissues as the heart, liver, and pancreas. This can be prevented by using iron-chelating agents (eg, deferiprone or deferoxamine), which also affect the musculoskeletal system. The imaging findings are similar for the thalassemia subtypes.

Imaging Strategy

Anemia is not routinely imaged except for the hemoglobinopathies. SCA and thalassemia patients with musculoskeletal symptoms are first evaluated with radiographs. If the findings are negative, or repeat imaging is indicated, especially in young patients, MRI is useful in determining the presence of red marrow reconversion and ON. When there is a concern for infection, contrast-enhanced MRI is useful to detect rim-enhancing fluid collections, which can be aspirated for diagnostic purposes. In thalassemia, MRI may detect evidence of transfusion-related iron overload in the abdominal viscera and bone marrow.

Imaging Findings

Chronic Anemia
Radiography
- Insufficiency fractures, such as vertebral fractures

Table 74.1. Comparison of Imaging Findings in Sickle Cell Anemia and Thalassemia

FINDINGS	SICKLE CELL ANEMIA	THALASSEMIA
Osteoporosis with vertebral fractures	+	++
Coarse bone appearance	+	+
Medullary expansion	+	+
Hair-on-end appearance	+	+
Limb length discrepancy	+	+
Osteonecrosis	+	–
Osteomyelitis	+	–
Extramedullary hematopoiesis	+ (Less commonly musculoskeletal)	+ (Commonly musculoskeletal)

- Biconcave vertebral endplates and fish-mouth appearance
- Coarse appearance of the trabecular bone
- Calvarium expansion with *hair-on-end* appearance
- Premature growth plate fusion with bone shortening in both SCA and thalassemia
  - May be asymmetric

Magnetic Resonance Imaging
- MRI is the most sensitive modality to detect the bone and marrow changes.
- Anemia results in compensatory hyperplasia of hematopoietic or red marrow, bone marrow reconversion (Figure 74.1).
  - Discussed in detail in Chapter 75, "Bone Marrow Conversion and Reconversion"
  - Vertebral fish-mouth vertebral deformity

Nuclear Medicine
- Much less commonly used than MRI in evaluating anemia
  - Marrow imaging targets (tracers)
    - Reticuloendothelial system (eg, technetium 99m [^{99m}Tc]-sulfur colloid, ^{99m}Tc-microaggregated human serum albumin)
    - Erythropoietic marrow (eg, iron 52 [^{52}Fe] citrate-labeled RBCs)
    - Myeloid marrow (eg, ^{99m}Tc- or ^{111}indium-labeled white blood cells [WBCs], ^{99m}Tc-labeled antigranulocyte antibody)
  - In general, uptake present in red marrow and low in yellow marrow
    - Decreased uptake in marrow replacing or destructive processes
  - Fluorodeoxyglucose (FDG)-PET for detecting increased activity in areas of red marrow reconversion

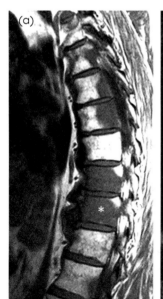
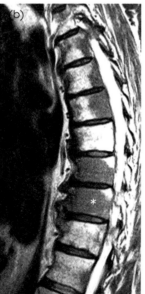
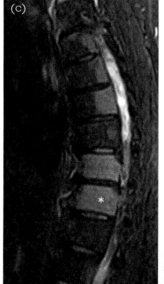
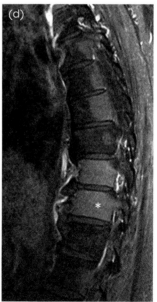

Figure 74.1. Idiopathic aplastic anemia in a 25-year-old man on immunosuppression (cyclosporine) with masslike areas of red marrow reconversion. (*A*) Sagittal T1W and (*B*) T2W MR images of the thoracic spine demonstrate multiple areas of masslike, biopsy-proven marrow reconversion (*asterisks*), which are isointense to muscle. (*C*) A STIR MR image demonstrates these areas of red marrow are hyperintense, and a (*D*) T1W image postcontrast MR image with fat saturation demonstrates enhancement.

Ultrasound

- Not used to evaluate anemia

Aplastic Anemia
Radiography and Computed Tomography

- Not sensitive for detecting aplastic anemia

Magnetic Resonance Imaging

- Fatty replacement of marrow results in homogeneous high signal on T1W and T2W images and low signal on STIR.
- Treatment response may result in diffuse red marrow or islands of red marrow, which are hyperintense on STIR and hypointense on T1W images.

Nuclear Medicine

- Marrow imaging and FDG-PET show diffuse absence in aplastic anemia:
  - Increased uptake with treatment including granulocyte-macrophage colony-stimulating factor (GM-CSF), stem cell transplantation, immunosuppression

Sickle Cell Anemia
Radiography

- ON more commonly diffuse than focal
  - Heterogeneous pattern of bone sclerosis, especially in the pelvis, ribs, and spine (Figure 74.2A)
  - Focal ON
    - Often of the epiphyses, especially femoral and humeral (also called *avascular necrosis*)
    - Indistinguishable from ON due to other causes, except more often bilateral and diffuse
    - H-shaped vertebrae caused by endplate ON (Figure 74.3)
  - ON of the small tubular bones of hands and feet resulting in sickle cell dactylitis or *hand-foot* syndrome from persistent red marrow in children younger than 6 years
  - Features of ON discussed in detail in Chapter 115, "Osteonecroses and Osteochondroses" (Figure 74.4)
- Osteomyelitis
  - Often normal radiographs
  - Imaging findings nonspecific; may also be seen in ON
    - Periostitis, osteopenia (acute) and sclerosis (chronic) (Figure 74.4A)

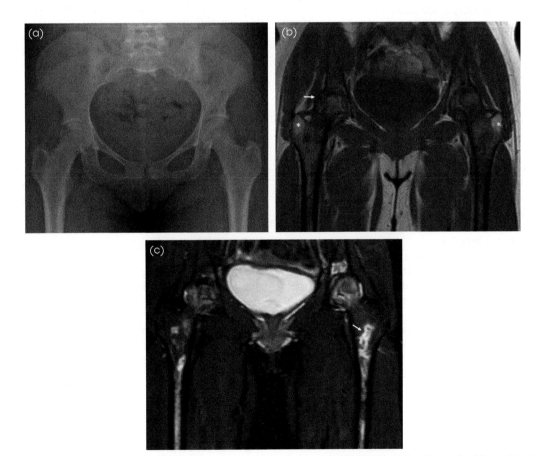

Figure 74.2. SCA in a 19-year-old woman with right hip pain and femoral head ON. (*A*) A frontal radiograph of the pelvis shows diffuse heterogeneous bone density without definite evidence of ON. (*B*) Coronal T1W MR image demonstrates diffuse replacement of yellow marrow by heterogeneous low signal with sparing of the greater trochanters (*asterisks*). A somewhat flattened right femoral head suggests subacute, partial subchondral collapse (*thin arrow*). (*C*) A coronal STIR image shows diffuse areas of marrow fluid signal that best demonstrate the characteristic serpentine contour of ON in the left femoral shaft (*thin arrow*).

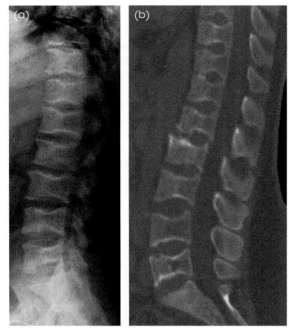

Figure 74.3. Vertebral SCA involvement. (*A*) Lateral radiograph of the lumbar and lower thoracic spine in a 44-year-old patient shows a heterogeneous bone density and H-shaped vertebral bodies because of endplate ON. (*B*) Reformatted sagittal CT image shows multiple H-shaped vertebral bodies and spondylosis in a different 42-year-old patient.

- Discussed in detail in Chapter 86, "Osteomyelitis of the Long and Flat Bones"
- Septic arthritis—may be occult on radiographs
  - Periarticular osteopenia, erosions, and asymmetric joint-space narrowing are characteristic.
  - Septic arthritis is discussed in detail in Chapter 87, "Septic Arthritis."

Computed Tomography
- May be useful for ON treatment planning
- Less sensitive than scintigraphy or MRI in detecting the early stages of ON

Magnetic Resonance Imaging
- Vertebral compression fractures with fish-mouth vertebral deformity and H-shaped vertebrae can be detected.
- MRI is the most sensitive and specific modality for the identification of ON with a 97-100% accuracy (Figure 74.2*B, C*).
  - Discussed in detail in Chapter 115
- MRI is sensitive for detection of acute bone marrow ischemia:
  - Reversible high signal on fluid-sensitive sequences (T2W FS and STIR)
  - May progress to ON
- Changes of osteomyelitis can be detected on MRI prior to radiographs:
  - Difficult to detect or distinguish from ON
    - Increased fluid signal caused by red marrow reconversion can obscure edema.
    - BME; fluid collections in the adjacent soft tissue; periostitis; and abnormal enhancement of

periosteum, muscle, fascia, and fat may be seen in osteomyelitis and ON (Figure 74.4*B-E*).
  - IV contrast can help target rim-enhancing fluid signal collections for diagnostic aspiration (Figure 74.4*E*).
  - Chapter 86 has a detailed discussion of osteomyelitis of the flat and long bones.
- Aseptic and septic joint effusions can be detected:
  - Aseptic joint effusions are common in SCA.
  - Septic arthritis is associated with periarticular edema and diffuse synovial enhancement.
  - Difficult to distinguish especially if there is ON.
  - Joint aspiration is often required to determine the cause.
  - A detailed discussion can be found in Chapter 87.
- Extramedullary hematopoiesis not common and usually identified in the abdominal viscera (eg, liver, spleen).

Nuclear Medicine
- Marrow imaging shows increased uptake present in areas of red marrow reconversion:
  - Focal decreases in ON
- Three phase ^{99m}Tc-methylene diphosphonate (MDP) bone scan of ON typically shows uptake in all 3 phases, except in very early ischemia, in which it can have normal or decreased uptake.
- Labeled WBC scans have been used to distinguish osteomyelitis from ON.
  - ON has characteristically low uptake, whereas osteomyelitis typically exhibits high uptake. However, uptake in reconverted red marrow can complicate interpretation.
  - Concurrent use of sulfur colloid radiotracer can increase specificity of diagnosis. Uptake is decreased in ON, but not osteomyelitis.

Ultrasound
- Not routinely used
- Can be used, especially in children, to identify fluid collections and guide fluid sampling to help distinguish ON from infection

Thalassemia
Radiography
- Medullary bone expansion (Figure 75.5*E*) is seen:
  - Diploic space widening of the inner and outer tables of the skull
  - Maxillary bones displacing the orbits and the teeth
  - Ribs, especially at the costovertebral joints
    - May be difficult to see on radiographs
    - Can also extend beneath the periosteum and create a *bone-within-a-bone* appearance
  - Vertebrae may also have a bone-within-a-bone appearance
- Extramedullary hematopoiesis is seen, especially near the costovertebral joint.
- High serum iron levels from frequent transfusions result in joint abnormalities:
  - Symmetrical loss of joint space, cystic lesions of the periarticular bone, collapse and flattening of subchondral bone, and osteophyte formation

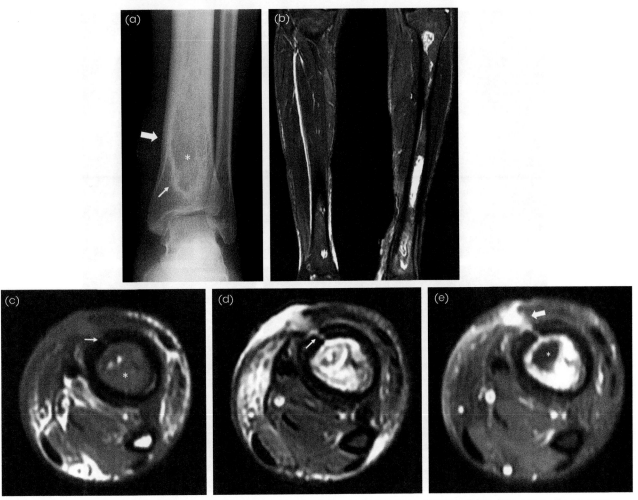

Figure 74.4. SCA in a 25-year-old man with chronic ulcer of the lower leg and chronic methicillin-sensitive *Staphylococcus aureus* (MSSA) osteomyelitis. (*A*) AP radiograph of the distal tibia and fibula shows a well-circumscribed lucency in the left distal tibia (*asterisk*) with surrounding sclerosis (*thin arrow*) and chronic-appearing periostitis (*thick arrow*). Medial soft tissue swelling is also demonstrated. (*B*) A coronal STIR MR image of the bilateral legs demonstrates bilateral areas of circumscribed medullary fluid signal consistent with ON. (*C*) Axial T1W MR image through the left leg demonstrates circumferential cortical irregularity involving the tibia with a cloaca extending through the medial cortex to a soft tissue ulcer (*thin arrow*), with replacement of much of marrow fat signal (*asterisk*). (*D*) Axial T2W FS MR image demonstrates hyperintense fluid signal within the tibial marrow extending through the cloaca and into the soft tissues (*thin arrow*). (*E*) Axial T1W FS postcontrast MR image shows enhancement in the infected tissue (*thick arrow*) with an area of nonenhancement (*asterisk*) consistent with devitalized marrow.

- Chondrocalcinosis
- Chelation treatment results in bone abnormalities
  - Premature growth plate fusion, but less common than in patients who are not transfused
  - Diffuse vertebral flattening (platyspondyly)

Computed Tomography
- Rib changes better visualized, including:
  - Expansion with erosion of the inner cortex
  - Extrinsic erosions with paraspinal soft tissue masses caused by extramedullary hematopoiesis

Magnetic Resonance Imaging
- Vertebral insufficiency fractures and chelation-related platyspondyly (thalassemia) can be identified.
- MRI detects iron deposition.
  - Repeated transfusions result in a darkened marrow appearance especially on GRE pulse sequences despite chelation therapy (Figure 75.5*A-C*).

- Characteristic signal loss is used to detect evidence of iron overload on liver MRI.
- Extramedullary hematopoiesis is detected with high sensitivity:
  - Paravertebral, mediastinal, or presacral masses (Figure 74.5*D*)
    - Also in the abdominal viscera, skin, and breasts
  - Identical signal characteristics to the vertebral marrow

Nuclear Medicine and Ultrasound
- Not routinely used in evaluation

Treatment Options
- Iron deficiency anemia is treated with iron supplementation.
- Aplastic anemia is treated by removal of inciting agent (if known), transfusions, bone marrow transplant, or immunosuppression.

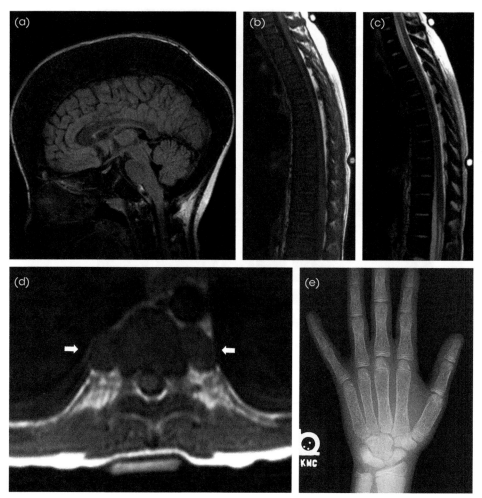

Figure 74.5. β-Thalassemia in a 14-year-old boy on iron chelation therapy. (*A*) Sagittal fluid attenuated inversion recovery (FLAIR) MR image of the brain demonstrates yellow marrow replacement and diploic space enlargement. (*B*) Sagittal T1W MR image of the thoracic spine demonstrates diffuse yellow marrow replacement with signal isointense to muscle and hypointense to the intervertebral discs. (*C*) Sagittal T2W MR image demonstrates extensive low signal throughout the imaged vertebrae related to iron deposition caused by repeated blood transfusions. (*D*) An axial T1W MR image demonstrates symmetric areas of extramedullary hematopoiesis at the costovertebral junctions (*thick arrows*). (*E*) Bone age PA hand radiograph of the same patient at age 16 demonstrates delayed skeletal maturity with diffuse marrow expansion causing undertubulation of the metacarpals and phalanges, osteopenia with a heterogeneous bone density and cortical thinning.

- Painful crises of SCA are treated symptomatically.
- Surgical treatment of ON is used, especially of the epiphyses, most frequently using core decompression and arthroplasty.
- Osteomyelitis and septic arthritis in SCA are treated with IV antibiotics and often with incision and drainage.
- Blood transfusions with iron chelation are used to treat thalassemia.
- Vitamin D and bisphosphonates are given for osteoporosis.

Key Points

- Anemia has a wide variety of causes with iron deficiency and hemoglobinopathy, especially SCA and thalassemia, most common.
- Anemia is a clinical diagnosis that may be incidentally detected on imaging, especially by MRI.

- Radiographs are a standard initial imaging study, especially in patients with pain, and can detect osteoporotic fractures, ON, and chronic osteomyelitis.
- MRI is the most sensitive imaging study for the sequelae of anemia, such as red marrow reconversion, ON, and osteomyelitis.

Recommended Reading

Martinoli C, Bacigalupo L, Forni GL, Balocco M, Garlaschi G, Tagliafico A. Musculoskeletal manifestations of chronic anemias. *Semin Musculoskelet Radiol.* 2011;15: 269–80.

References

1. Camaschella C. Iron-deficiency anemia. *N Engl J Med.* 2015;372:1832–1843.

2. Ejindu VC, Hine AL, Mashayekhi M, Shorvon PJ, Misra RR. Musculoskeletal manifestations of sickle cell disease. *Radiographics*. 2007;27:1005–21.

3. Hanrahan CJ, Shah LM. MRI of spinal bone marrow: part 2, T1-weighted imaging-based differential diagnosis. *AJR Am J Roentgenol*. 2011;197:1309–21.

4. Hughes M, Akram Q, Rees DC, Jones AK. Haemoglobinopathies and the rheumatologist. *Rheumatology (Oxford)*. 2016;55(12):2109–18.

5. Kassebaum NJ, GBD 2013 Anemia Collaborators. The global burden of anemia. *Hematol Oncol Clin North Am*. 2016;30(2):247–308.

6. Levin TL, Sheth SS, Ruzal-Shapiro C, Abramson S, Piomelli S, Berdon WE. MRI marrow observations in thalassemia: the effects of the primary disease, transfusional therapy, and chelation. *Pediatr Radiol*. 1995;25:607–13.

7. Martinoli C, Bacigalupo L, Forni GL, Balocco M, Garlaschi G, Tagliafico A. Musculoskeletal manifestations of chronic anemias. *Semin Musculoskelet Radiol*. 2011;15:269–80.

8. Murphey MD, Foreman KL, Klassen-Fischer MK, Fox MG, Chung EM, Kransdorf MJ. From the radiologic pathology archives imaging of osteonecrosis: radiologic-pathologic correlation. *Radiographics*. 2014;34:1003–28.

9. Powers JM, Buchanan GR. Diagnosis and management of iron deficiency anemia. *Hematol Oncol Clin North Am*. 2014;28:729–45, vi-vii.

10. Steinberg ME, Steinberg DR. Classification systems for osteonecrosis: an overview. *Orthop Clin North Am*. 2004;35:273–83, vii-viii.

11. Tunaci M, Tunaci A, Engin G, et al. Imaging features of thalassemia. *Eur Radiol*. 1999;9(9):1804–809.

12. Tyler PA, Madani G, Chaudhuri R, Wilson LF, Dick EA. The radiological appearances of thalassaemia. *Clin Radiol*. 2006;61:40–52.

CHAPTER 75

Bone Marrow Conversion and Reconversion

Kevin B. Hoover

Introduction

The bone marrow is one of the largest organs in the body and it changes in composition throughout life. With skeletal maturation large areas of hematopoietic, (red) marrow convert to primarily fatty (yellow) marrow. Conversely, stress and underlying disease can reverse the process, resulting in reconversion of yellow to red marrow. Rather than a disease itself, red marrow conversion is a secondary, and often incidental, finding in a wide variety of disease processes. It is detected by marrow-sensitive imaging modalities, especially MRI.

Pathophysiology and Clinical Findings

Hematopoiesis begins in the fetal yolk sac. In the second trimester, this process transfers to the liver and spleen and begins transfer to bone marrow. By term, the medullary cavity of long bones is the primary site of hematopoiesis. Hematopoietic, red marrow consists of approximately 40% fat, 40% water, and 20% protein with 60% fat cells and 40% hematopoietic cells. Fatty, yellow marrow consists of 80% fat, 15% water, and 5% protein with 95% fat cells and 5% nonfat cells (hematopoietic or reticuloendothelial cells). The normal process of conversion from red to yellow marrow is centripetal with the distal bones converting more rapidly than the proximal bones. Conversion begins with the phalanges prior to birth. By age 25 years, the adult pattern is reached with red marrow residing in the axial skeleton (skull, vertebrae, ribs, sternum, pelvis) and proximal, peripheral skeleton (humeri, femora). The specific pattern of conversion in the long bones begins with the epiphyses and apophyses and sequentially progresses to the diaphyses, the distal metaphyses and, finally, the proximal metaphyses. In the vertebral bodies, conversion starts around the central basivertebral plexus with red marrow persisting through mid adulthood. In the pelvis, red marrow persists around the SI and hip joints and the symphysis pubis in adulthood.

Reconversion of yellow to red marrow follows a reverse, centrifugal pattern, and is caused by a number of conditions (Table 75.1). For example, in the long bones, reconversion starts in the proximal metaphysis then involves the distal metaphysis and finally the diaphysis. Only in severe stress is there epiphyseal reconversion. The reconversion process varies by bone with the spine and flat bones converting most quickly. Knowledge of the pattern of conversion and reconversion is useful in distinguishing benign from malignant causes.

This can be a challenge, however, because malignant causes of marrow infiltration often follow the blood supply, which is greatest in areas of red marrow. A definitive diagnosis may require bone biopsy.

Imaging Strategy

Bone marrow conversion and reconversion are routinely and incidentally detected on MRI obtained for other reasons. T1W MR images are most useful in distinguishing red marrow from yellow marrow. Fluid-sensitive sequences (STIR, T2W FS) and postcontrast T1W FS can help distinguish benign from malignant causes of marrow signal abnormality, but are not as useful because red marrow demonstrates both fluid signal and enhancement. T2W MR images without FS are not as useful because red and yellow marrow and marrow replacing processes are all relatively hyperintense. Chemical shift MRI with in- and out-of-phase sequences is not commonly used, but it is helpful because it is sensitive to the presence of microscopic fat in red marrow. Radiographs may be useful to identify the cause of marrow conversion and nuclear medicine studies when there are contraindications to MRI.

Imaging Findings

Radiography and Computed Tomography
- Cannot detect marrow conversion or reconversion
- Can sometimes identify characteristic bone changes of underlying cause if pathologic (eg, sickle cell anemia)

Magnetic Resonance Imaging
- MRI is highly sensitive in detection of marrow elements:
  - Characteristic signals of red and yellow marrow (Table 75.2) (Figures 75.1-75.3)
    - Yellow marrow is hyperintense on T1W images relative to muscle.
    - Red marrow typically maintains some intermixed fat and T1W hyperintensity relative to muscle.
      - Islands of red marrow may have *bullseye* appearance on T1W images:
      - Central focus of hyperintense signal surrounded by isointense to hypointense signal
      - Highly sensitive and specific for an island of red marrow

Table 75.1. Causes of Red Marrow Reconversion

CATEGORY	REPRESENTATIVE CONDITIONS
Anemia	Chronic anemia: sickle cell disease, thalassemia, iron deficiency, athletes (hemolysis), pregnancy
Hypoxemia	Smoking (obese, female), high altitude
Increased demand	Athletes
Nutritional	Vitamin C deficiency (scurvy)
Chemotherapy	GM-CSF
Marrow replacement/ infiltration	Lymphoma, leukemia, myelofibrosis, metastatic disease, multiple myeloma, osteonecrosis

Abbreviation: GM-CSF, granulocyte-macrophage colony-stimulating factor.

- Yellow marrow is hypointense and red marrow hyperintense relative to muscle on T2W FS and STIR MR images.
- On T1W postcontrast MR imaging, red marrow enhances and yellow marrow does not:
  - Addition of fat saturation makes enhancement more apparent because of the suppression of the otherwise high background signal of yellow marrow.
- The following are characteristic marrow reconversion locations:
  - Flame-shaped appearance in the proximal humeral or femoral metaphyses
  - Subchondral proximal epiphyses (Figure 75.1*A,B*)
  - Vertebral endplates
  - Endosteum of long bones (Figure 75.3*C,D*)
- Distinguishing marrow replacement by tumor from reconversion can be a challenge on MRI (Table 75.2):
  - Marrow replacement by tumor may also involve the characteristic locations of red marrow reconversion:
    - This is especially true of bone marrow tumors (discussed in detail in Chapters 58, "Normal Bone Marrow and Benign Bone Marrow Lesions" and Chapter 59, "Malignant Marrow Bone Tumors").
  - Tumor characteristically obliterates fat resulting in hypointense T1 signal (Figure 75.3*C,D*):
    - Highly sensitive and specific finding on high field strength magnets ($\geq$1.5 T) is seen.
    - Diffuse multiple myeloma and leukemia are exceptions, which can contain focal or microscopic fat.
  - The "halo sign" is highly specific for metastasis, showing a rim of hyperintensity on fluid-sensitive images.
- Chemical shift MRI demonstrates signal cancellation in red marrow on out-of-phase sequences because of the presence of both fat and water in the same voxel (Figure 75.2):
  - Look for 20% or more signal loss on out-of-phase sequences.
  - Tumor rarely has signal loss.
  - Myelofibrosis, sclerotic metastases and hematoma may also lack signal loss.
  - Renal cell cancer metastases and infiltrative multiple myeloma may show signal loss (false negative) if macroscopic or microscopic fat are present.
- Infection can also involve characteristic areas of marrow reconversion:
  - Metaphyseal areas have the greatest blood flow and the greatest number of infections.

Table 75.2. MRI Characteristics of Reconverted Red Marrow and Tumor

RED MARROW	TUMOR
Hyperintense T1 signal relative to muscle	Hypointense T1 signal relative tomuscle
Hyperintense T1 signal relative to normal intervertebral discs	Hypointense T1 signal relative to normal intervertebral discs
Feathery margins[a]	Sharp margins[a]
No mass effect[a]	Mass effect[a]
No bone destruction[a]	Bone destruction[a]
Extraosseous soft tissue mass (extramedullary hematopoiesis)[a]	Extraosseous soft tissue mass
Metaphyseal	Epiphyseal
Symmetric	Asymmetric
Follows pattern of reconversion	Does not follow pattern of reconversion
Bullseye sign	Halo sign

[a] Less sensitive.

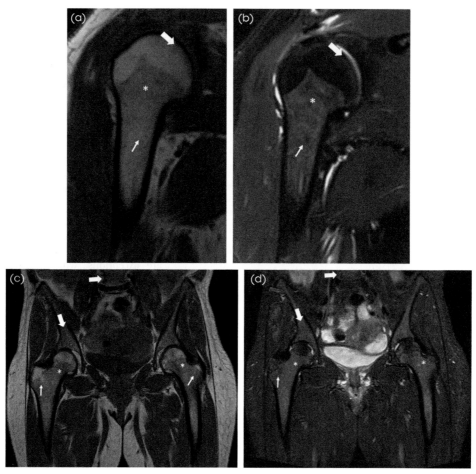

Figure 75.1. Normal red marrow. (*A*) Coronal T1W and (*B*) T2W FS MR images of the shoulder in a 46-year-old woman show normal red marrow within the proximal humeral diametaphysis (*asterisks*). The red marrow is hyperintense relative to muscle and hypointense relative to the fat seen in the humeral head proximal to the physeal scar. Islands of interspersed fat signal are also seen (*thin arrows*). Normal, subarticular red marrow signal is present in the medial humeral head (*thick arrows*). (*C, D*) In a different patient, a similar distribution of red marrow is seen on (*C*) coronal T1W and (*D*) STIR MR images within the proximal femora (*asterisks*) sparing the femoral heads and greater trochanters. Islands of interspersed fat marrow signal (*thin arrows*) and red marrow within the pelvis and lower lumbar spine are present (*thick arrows*).

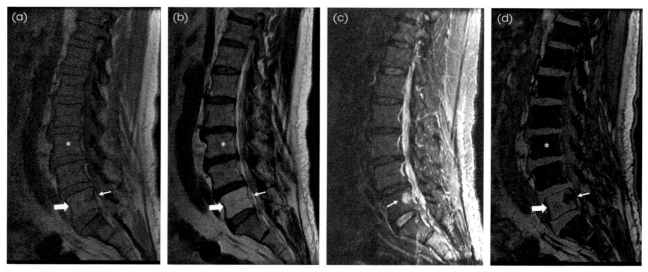

Figure 75.2. Microscopic and macroscopic fat evaluation in a 70-year-old man with a renal mass and possible metastasis. (*A*) Sagittal T1W in-phase and (*B*) T2W MR images show heterogeneous marrow signal (*asterisks*) with relatively hyperintense signal in the L5 vertebra (*thick arrow*) containing an area of relatively hypointense signal in the posterior vertebral body near the Batson plexus in (*A*) that is hyperintense in (*B*) (*thin arrows*). (*C*) A sagittal STIR MR image demonstrates diffuse low bone marrow signal with a focus of high signal in the posterior L5 vertebral body (*thin arrow*). (*D*) A sagittal T1W out-of-phase MR image demonstrates hyperintense signal in the L5 vertebra from macroscopic fat (*thick arrow*) with focal hypointense signal from microscopic fat in the posterior L5 vertebral body (*thin arrow*). This appearance is consistent with a large hemangioma with a more focal vascular dorsal component. Note signal drop in the reminder of the imaged spine compared with (*A*) consistent with normal red marrow.

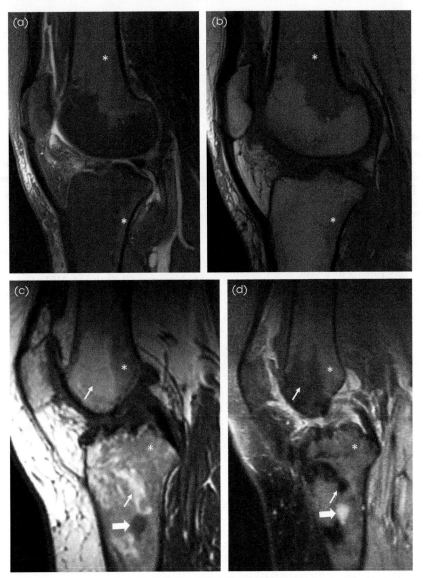

Figure 75.3. Marrow reconversion about the knee. (*A, B*) Sagittal T2W FS and PDW MR images of the knee demonstrate a typical pattern of replacement of yellow marrow with red marrow extending to, but not past, the physeal scar of the distal femur and along the posterior margin of the proximal tibia (*asterisks*). (*C*) Sagittal T1W and (*D*) STIR MR images of the knee in a different patient demonstrate heterogeneous fat replacement involving the epiphyses (*asterisks*) with interspersed areas of fat signal (*thin arrows*). In (*C*), a focus of hypointense and isointense (T1W) and hyperintense (STIR) signal in (*D*) relative to muscle in the proximal tibial diaphysis (*thick arrows*) was a biopsy-proven metastatic breast carcinoma lesion.

- Diffuse, polyostotic involvement in infection is infrequent, especially in adults.
- This is discussed in detail in Chapter 86, "Osteomyelitis of the Long and Flat Bones."
- Medical treatments can alter the marrow pattern.
  - With chemotherapy, a diffusely increased marrow fluid signal intensity is seen in the first week from edema, followed by yellow marrow conversion, and then multifocal red marrow reconversion after 3-4 weeks:
    - May eventually normalize
- Granulocyte-macrophage colony-stimulating factor (GM-CSF) shows diffuse, patchy red marrow reconversion peaks at 2 weeks and normalizes 6 weeks after treatment.

Nuclear Imaging
- Nuclear imaging is less commonly used than MRI in marrow imaging largely because of lower signal-to-noise ratio, specificity, and expense in the case of fluorodeoxyglucose (FDG)-PET.
- Bone marrow imaging with sulfur colloid and labeled red blood cells, white blood cells, and antibodies shows uptake in reconverted marrow:
  - Marrow replacing or destructive processes, including ON, neoplasm, aplastic anemia, show decreased uptake.
  - Increased uptake with GM-CSF is seen.
- FDG-PET is useful for distinguishing areas of reconversion from replacement by tumor:

- Tumors and myelodysplastic syndromes have elevated signal relative to liver and elevated standardized uptake values (SUVs).
- Red marrow signal and SUV are also increased after GM-CSF; scanning should optimally wait up to 4-6 weeks after treatment.

Treatment Options
- Specific to the underlying disorder(s)

Key Points
- Physiologic conversion of marrow from red to yellow with aging occurs in a predictable, centripetal manner from the peripheral skeleton to the axial skeleton.
- Pathologic marrow reconversion from yellow to red marrow reverses this pattern in a centrifugal manner secondary to primary or secondary anemia.
- MRI, and less commonly nuclear imaging, can identify marrow reconversion and help distinguish it from marrow replacement processes, such as tumor.
- Characteristic locations of marrow reconversion and the presence of focal or microscopic fat on MRI are useful features, but biopsy may still be required to exclude malignancy.

Recommended Reading

Kricun ME. Red-yellow marrow conversion: its effect on the location of some solitary bone lesions. *Skeletal Radiol.* 1985;14:10–19.

Shah LM, Hanrahan CJ. MRI of spinal bone marrow: part I, techniques and normal age-related appearances. *AJR Am J Roentgenol.* 2011;197:1298–308.

References

1. Agool A, Glaudemans AW, Boersma HH, Dierckx RA, Vellenga E, Slart RH. Radionuclide imaging of bone marrow disorders. *Eur J Nucl Med Mol Imaging.* 2011;38:166–78.
2. Blebea JS, Houseni M, Torigian DA, et al. Structural and functional imaging of normal bone marrow and evaluation of its age-related changes. *Semin Nucl Med.* 2007;37:185–94.
3. Chan BY, Gill KG, Rebsamen SL, Nguyen JC. MR imaging of pediatric bone marrow. *Radiographics.* 2016;36:1911–30.
4. Hanrahan CJ, Shah LM. MRI of spinal bone marrow: part 2, T1-weighted imaging-based differential diagnosis. *AJR Am J Roentgenol.* 2011;197:1309–21.
5. Kricun ME. Red-yellow marrow conversion: its effect on the location of some solitary bone lesions. *Skeletal Radiol.* 1985;14:10–19.
6. Poulton TB, Murphy WD, Duerk JL, Chapek CC, Feiglin DH. Bone marrow reconversion in adults who are smokers: MR imaging findings. *AJR Am J Roentgenol.* 1993;161:1217–21.
7. Shah LM, Hanrahan CJ. MRI of spinal bone marrow: part I, techniques and normal age-related appearances. *AJR Am J Roentgenol.* 2011;197:1298–308.

CHAPTER 76

Plasma Cell Dyscrasias

Kevin B. Hoover

Introduction

The plasma cell dyscrasias are diseases without cure with ongoing clinical trials and evolving diagnostic criteria. Blood and urine testing, bone marrow biopsy, and radiography are the primary tests used for diagnosis. Familiarity with advanced imaging findings is important, because MRI and PET/CT are often used to evaluate symptomatic patients prior to and after treatment.

Pathophysiology and Clinical Findings

The plasma cell dyscrasias are neoplasms arising from the clonal proliferation of plasma cells in the bone marrow. In general, these diseases are more common in men than women and more common in African Americans than whites. They are associated with the secretion of monoclonal immunoglobulins (heavy or light chain) or their fragments, which are referred to as *M protein, myeloma protein*, or *paraprotein*. End-organ damage is graded using the CRAB (elevated calcium level, renal failure, anemia, bone lesions) criteria (Table 76.1). The plasma cell dyscrasias are classified primarily by the quantity of serum M protein, the proportion of plasma cells in the bone marrow, and the presence of end-organ damage (Table 76.2). Monoclonal gammopathy of undetermined significance (MGUS) and asymptomatic or smoldering multiple myeloma (SMM) are not detectable on imaging. Waldenström macroglobulinemia (WM) is a type of non-Hodgkin lymphoma, which can transform to high-grade lymphoma and requires biopsy to be distinguished from multiple myeloma (MM). Amyloid deposition is associated with MM and WM (see Chapter 51, "Amyloidosis"). MGUS, SMM, WM,

and amyloid deposition are referred to in Table 76.2. MM, plasmacytoma, and POEMS will be the focus of discussion in the remainder of this chapter.

Imaging Strategy

The metastatic bone survey (MBS) is standard for the staging of plasma cell dyscrasias and part of the CRAB criteria. The MBS often includes radiographs of the entire axial skeleton including the skull and the peripheral skeleton proximal to the elbows and the ankles. In MGUS, the MBS is commonly acquired only if the M protein level is 1.5 g/dL or higher and there is concern for bone lesions or myeloma. An annual MBS is used for surveillance of SMM. In general, MRI or PET/CT are used when a patient complains of neurologic symptoms or bone pain and has a negative MBS (10-20% of MM patients). MRI of the symptomatic region or bone may be acquired using the appropriate FOV and coil with T1W and fluid-sensitive (STIR and T2W FS) imaging. As discussed further, whole body or axial skeleton MRI using the appropriate FOV and coil selection, is useful in diagnosis and evaluating treatment response. DXA is often acquired to determine the need for osteoporosis treatment (see Chapter 71, "Osteoporosis").

Imaging Findings

Radiography

- In MM, there are characteristic lytic, *punched-out* holes in the bone that may result in endosteal scalloping (Figure 76.1A,B):
  - Absent surrounding sclerosis
  - Often uniform in size
  - More sensitive than MRI in detecting skull and rib lesions
  - Sclerotic lesions rare (~3%) and associated with POEMS (Table 76.2)
- Osteopenia, especially of spine, may be seen in diffuse MM (Figure 76.1C).
- Imaging detects pathologic fractures (Figure 76.1A,C):
  - Vertebral fracture may result in severe compression (vertebra plana).
- Lytic lesions do not heal, therefore resolution is not sensitive for response to therapy.
- WM rarely has focal lytic lesions and more commonly appears normal or osteopenic.

Table 76.1. CRAB[a] Criteria for End-Organ Damage

TEST	ABNORMAL VALUE
Serum calcium	>11 mg/dL
Creatinine	>2.0 mg/dL
Hemoglobin	<10 mg/dL
Bone lesions (metastatic bone survey)	Lytic bone lesion ≥5 mm

[a] Elevated calcium level, renal failure, anemia, bone lesions.

Table 76.2. World Health Organization Classification of Plasma Cell Neoplasm

NAME	CLINICAL	PROGRESSION TO MM	DESCRIPTION
MGUS	■ Asymptomatic ■ 3% of adults >50 years	■ Heavy-chain 1-1.5% per year ■ Light-chain 0.3% per year	■ M protein <3 g/dL ■ <10% clonal marrow plasma cells ■ No CRAB criteria, amyloidosis, lymphoproliferative disorder
SMM	■ Asymptomatic	■ First 5 years 10% ■ Next 5 years 3% ■ Next 10 years 1-2%	■ M protein >3 g/dL *AND/OR* ■ >10% <60% clonal marrow plasma cells ■ Negative CRAB criteria or amyloidosis
SPB or solitary extraosseous plasmacytoma	■ Bone pain ■ Pathologic fracture ■ Extraosseous (~80% upper airway) ■ <5% plasma cell dyscrasias ■ Men > women	■ ~50% in 10 years	■ Single biopsy proven bone or soft tissue deposit ■ No serum or urine M protein ■ <10% plasma cells ■ Negative CRAB criteria (serologic)
MM	■ Bone pain ■ Pathologic fracture ■ Anemia (most common) ■ Fatigue ■ Weight loss ■ 1.3% of all cancers ■ 10-15% of all hematologic malignancies	■ 5-year survival 45%	■ ≥10% plasma cells in bone marrow *OR* ■ Extraosseous plasmacytoma *AND* ■ Positive CRAB criteria *OR 1 of following:* ■ >60% clonal marrow cells ■ >1 focal lesion >5 mm on MRI study ■ Abnormal serum-free light-chain ratios
POEMS	■ Rare (3:10^7 in Japan) ■ Symptomatic (description)		■ Monoclonal plasma disorder ■ Peripheral neuropathy *AND 1 of following:* ■ Osteosclerotic myeloma (87% patients) ■ Castleman disease ■ Elevated vascular endothelial growth factor ■ Organomegaly ■ Endocrinopathy ■ Typical skin changes ■ Volume overload ■ Papilledema ■ Thrombocytosis/polycythemia
WM	■ Lymph-adenopathy, organomegaly, hyperviscosity, syndrome 20% familial ■ Rare (3:10^6)		■ Lymphoplasmacytic lymphoma in bone marrow *AND* ■ +IgM monoclonal gammopathy
AL^a	■ Symptoms secondary to deposition (multisystem)		■ Light-chain deposition ■ De novo (primary) ■ Secondary in MM and WM

Abbreviations: AL, amyloidosis; CRAB, elevated calcium level, renal failure, anemia, bone lesions; IgM, immunoglobin M; MGUS, monoclonal gammopathy of uncertain significance; MM, multiple myeloma; MRI, magnetic resonance imaging; POEMS, polyneuropathy, organomegaly, endocrinopathy, monoclonal protein, skin changes; SMM, asymptomatic (smoldering) multiple myeloma; SPB, solitary plasmacytoma of bone; WM, Waldenström macroglobulinemia.

^{a} Discussed in Chapter 51, "Amyloidosis."

- Plasmacytoma is a solitary, expansile lesion arising from plasma cells:
  - Most commonly arising in the axial skeleton, sternum, and proximal extremities

Computed Tomography
- CT has similar findings to radiographs with greater detection sensitivity.

- This modality offers lower sensitivity than MRI for diffuse marrow replacement and extraosseous lesions.
- Vertebral plasmacytomas may have characteristic bony struts extending into lytic lesions, which are called a *mini-brain* appearance as they may resemble sulci of the brain (Figure 76.2*A,B*).

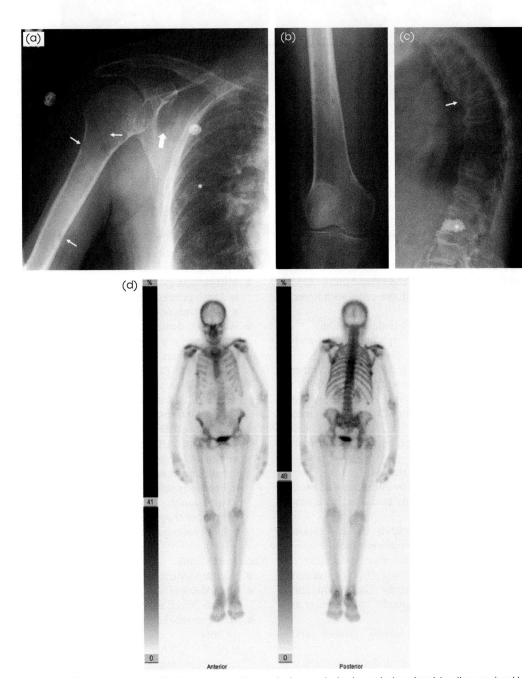

Figure 76.1. MM in an 81-year-old man. (*A*) AP shoulder radiograph demonstrates bone lesions involving the proximal humerus (*thin arrows*) including areas of endosteal scalloping, a large lesion of the scapula (*thick arrow*), and diffuse involvement of the clavicle and ribs. A pathologic fracture is identified in the seventh posterolateral sixth rib (*asterisk*). Note diffuse osteopenia. (*B*) On the AP radiograph, innumerable punched-out, lytic lesions of the right femur are noted. (*C*) On the lateral radiograph of the thoracic spine, multiple pathologic vertebral body compression fractures of the thoracic and lumbar spine are identified with varying degrees of height lost (greatest at T6, *thin arrow*). An area of vertebral augmentation is seen at L1 (*asterisk*). (*D*) A technetium bone scan shows punctate areas of rib uptake that are consistent with fractures, including the right seventh rib. However, innumerable osseous lesions of the axial and peripheral skeleton are not apparent.

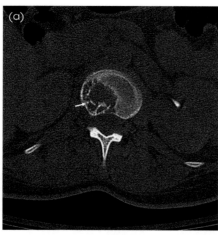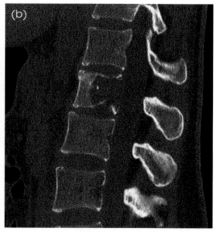

Figure 76.2. MM of the spine in a 30-year-old man with back pain. (*A*) Axial and (*B*) sagittal reformatted CT images demonstrate a well-circumscribed, solitary lytic lesion of the upper lumbar vertebral body with areas of intact trabeculae best seen on the axial image (*thin arrow*) resulting in an appearance said to resemble a brain (ie, mini-brain). A left ureteral calculus is incidentally noted.

Magnetic Resonance Imaging

- Marrow involvement in MM exhibits hypointense signal on T1W and hyperintense signal on fluid-sensitive MR sequences.
- There are 5 patterns of MM marrow involvement on MRI:
  1. Normal (~28% patients)
  2. Focal with a solitary lesion of larger than 5 mm (~30%)
  3. Diffuse, homogeneous (~28%); associated with lowest survival (Figure 76.3*A,B*)
  4. Diffuse and multifocal (~11%) (Figure 76.3*C-E*)
  5. Variegated (micronodular, speckled, "salt-and-pepper") (~3%) (Figure 76.3*F-H*)
- Prognosis is worsened with increase in lesion number and the extent the marrow is involved:
  - More than 7 focal lesions on whole body MRI (most sensitive imaging technique for MM) associated with decreased survival
- In general, postcontrast imaging is not recommended in the initial evaluation of MM:
  - No increase in sensitivity to detect MM
  - Elevated reaction risk caused by disease-related renal insufficiency and coagulopathy associated with thalidomide treatment
  - However, can detect incompletely treated disease, which may diffusely or peripherally enhance
- Multiple posttreatment appearances may be visualized:
  - Marrow reconversion followed by conversion (see Chapter 75, "Bone Marrow Conversion and Reconversion"); may take 9 months up to 5 years to return to normal
  - Unchanged, even if successfully treated and nonviable
  - Lesions changed to fat signal or decreased in size (unlike radiographs)
  - Partial treatment when a diffuse homogeneous pattern converts to variegated or focal diffuse
  - ON detected in approximately 9% of treated patients
  - Complicated by stem cell transplantation (SCT)

- MRI is superior to radiography, CT, and PET/CT in detecting fractures and cord compression:
  - Distinguishing pathologic versus osteoporotic fractures
    - Epidural mass is diagnostic of pathologic fracture.
    - Replacement of pedicle fat with hyperintense fluid signal suggests pathologic fracture.
- MRI detects extraosseous myeloma unlike radiography and with greater sensitivity than CT:
  - Most common after SCT
- WM often demonstrates diffuse homogeneous or variegated marrow pattern with lymphadenopathy.
- Plasmacytomas are hypointense on T1W and hyperintense T2W MR images:
  - Homogeneous enhancement on T1W postcontrast images is seen, which is commonly used to evaluate single lesions.
  - Single vertebra involvement may result in collapse or endplate fracture.
  - Cancellous bone involvement with sometimes sclerotic cortex is seen.
  - Predominantly lytic: Vertebrae may have a mini-brain appearance.
  - Because they are indistinguishable from metastases, biopsy is required.

Nuclear Medicine

- Nuclear medicine is primarily used in clinical trials.
- Fluorodeoxyglucose (FDG)-PET/CT has greater sensitivity to detect osseous and extraosseous MM than MBS.
- Management is changed in approximately 50% of patients.
- FDG-PET/CT has greater sensitivity than MRI to detect response to treatment:
  - Decreased metabolic activity occurs within hours.
  - Continued activity decline after 3-4 weeks indicates ongoing treatment response.
  - Survival rate is decreased if
    - Persistent, diffusely elevated marrow activity (likely relapse in ≤6 months)

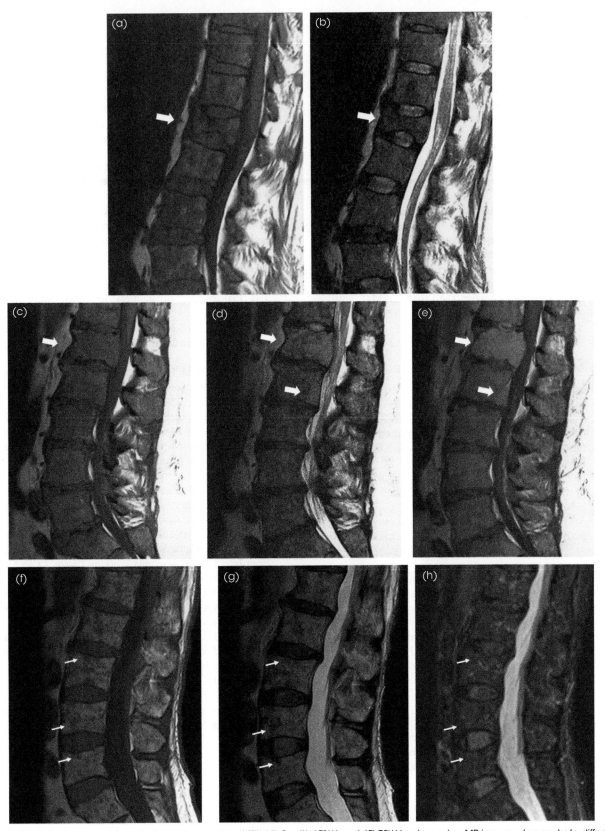

Figure 76.3. Patterns of vertebral MM involvement on MRI. (*A*) Sagittal T1W and (*B*) T2W lumbar spine MR images demonstrate diffuse bony involvement with pathologic fracture of L2 (*thick arrow*) and replacement of normal marrow fat by densely packed signal tumor cells. (*C-E*) In a different patient, diffuse and multifocal marrow involvement is demonstrated on T1W (*C*), T2W (*D*), and T1W postcontrast (*E*) sagittal MR images of the lumbar spine with more discrete lesions (*thick arrows*) demonstrated on a background of diffusely abnormal and enhancing marrow constituents. (*F-H*) In another patient, note a variegated pattern of marrow involvement with a diffusely speckled appearance that is predominantly dark on T1W (*F*) and T2W (*G*) sagittal MR images of the lumbar spine and more heterogeneous on STIR image (*H*) (*thin arrows*).

- Extramedullary disease after SCT
- Elevated overall baseline (pretreatment) marrow standardized uptake value (SUV) (>4.0-4.2)
- More than 3 bone lesions detected
- False positives include steroid treatment, infarct, hemangiomas, sites of bone marrow biopsy, SCT, and granulocyte-macrophage colony-stimulating factor.
- Nuclear scintigraphy is not indicated in assessing MM (Figure 76.1D):
    - MM inhibits osteoblastic activity.

Treatment Options

- SMM or MGUS are not treated, only monitored for progression.
- Plasmacytomas may be treated with radiation and may require surgical stabilization.
- MM is not curable with current therapies, and many patients are enrolled in clinical trials using age-adjusted chemotherapy (eg, thalidomide) with or sometimes without SCT, often with maintenance chemotherapy.
- POEMS and WM are treated similar to MM.

Key Points

- MM is the most common of the plasma cell dyscrasias, which are diseases caused by the proliferation of plasma cells and the abnormal secretion of immunoglobulins.
- Diagnosis is made by the testing of serum and urine, bone marrow biopsy, and radiographs.
- The MBS is routinely used for the staging and monitoring of disease, which commonly detects lytic, punched-out lesions that are often similar in size.
- MRI, but also PET/CT, is used to evaluate symptomatic patients with negative radiographs and in clinical trials.

Recommended Reading

Angtuaco EJ, Fassas AB, Walker R, Sethi R, Barlogie B. Multiple myeloma: clinical review and diagnostic imaging. *Radiology.* 2004;231:11–23.

Ferraro R, Agarwal A, Martin-Macintosh EL, Peller PJ, Subramaniam RM. MR imaging and PET/CT in diagnosis and management of multiple myeloma. *Radiographics.* 2015;35:438–54.

References

1. Agarwal A, Chirindel A, Shah BA, Subramaniam RM. Evolving role of FDG PET/CT in multiple myeloma imaging and management. *AJR Am J Roentgenol.* 2013;200:884–90.
2. Amini B, Yellapragada S, Shah S, Rohren E, Vikram R. State-of-the-art imaging and staging of plasma cell dyscrasias. *Radiol Clin North Am.* 2016;54:581–96.
3. Angtuaco EJ, Fassas AB, Walker R, Sethi R, Barlogie B. Multiple myeloma: clinical review and diagnostic imaging. *Radiology.* 2004;231:11–23.
4. Dimopoulos MA, Hillengass J, Usmani S, et al. Role of magnetic resonance imaging in the management of patients with multiple myeloma: a consensus statement. *J Clin Oncol.* 2015;33:657–64.
5. Durie BG. The role of anatomic and functional staging in myeloma: description of Durie/Salmon plus staging system. *Eur J Cancer.* 2006;42:1539–43.
6. Fechtner K, Hillengass J, Delorme S, et al. Staging monoclonal plasma cell disease: comparison of the Durie-Salmon and the Durie-Salmon PLUS staging systems. *Radiology.* 2010;257:195–204.
7. Ferraro R, Agarwal A, Martin-Macintosh EL, Peller PJ, Subramaniam RM. MR imaging and PET/CT in diagnosis and management of multiple myeloma. *Radiographics.* 2015;35:438–54.
8. Galieni P, Cavo M, Pulsoni A, et al. Clinical outcome of extramedullary plasmacytoma. *Haematologica.* 2000;85:47–51.
9. Hanrahan CJ, Shah LM. MRI of spinal bone marrow: part 2, T1-weighted imaging-based differential diagnosis. *AJR Am J Roentgenol.* 2011;197:1309–21.
10. Kuwabara S, Dispenzieri A, Arimura K, Misawa S, Nakaseko C. Treatment for POEMS (polyneuropathy, organomegaly, endocrinopathy, M-protein, and skin changes) syndrome. *Cochrane Database Syst Rev.* 2012;(6):CD006828. doi:CD006828.
11. Marti-Bonmati L, Ramirez-Fuentes C, Alberich-Bayarri A, Ruiz-Llorca C. State-of-the-art of bone marrow imaging in multiple myeloma. *Curr Opin Oncol.* 2015;27:540–50.
12. Palumbo A, Avet-Loiseau H, Oliva S, et al. Revised International Staging System for Multiple Myeloma: a report from International Myeloma Working Group. *J Clin Oncol.* 2015;33:2863–69.
13. Rajkumar SV, Dimopoulos MA, Palumbo A, et al. International Myeloma Working Group updated criteria for the diagnosis of multiple myeloma. *Lancet Oncol.* 2014;15:e538–48.
14. Regelink JC, Minnema MC, Terpos E, et al. Comparison of modern and conventional imaging techniques in establishing multiple myeloma-related bone disease: a systematic review. *Br J Haematol.* 2013;162:50–61.
15. Walker R, Barlogie B, Haessler J, et al. Magnetic resonance imaging in multiple myeloma: diagnostic and clinical implications. *J Clin Oncol.* 2007;25:1121–28.

CHAPTER 77

Histiocytoses

Kevin B. Hoover

Introduction

The histiocytoses are myeloid cell disorders arising from dendritic cells and macrophages. Langerhans cell histiocytosis (LCH) is the most common dendritic cell disorder with Erdheim-Chester disease (ECD) and juvenile xanthogranuloma being less common. Juvenile xanthogranuloma is a disease of early childhood and will not be discussed further. The macrophage disorders include Rosai-Dorfman disease (RDD) and hemophagocytic lymphohistiocytosis. Hemophagocytic lymphohistiocytosis is not associated with musculoskeletal disease and will not be discussed further. The histiocytoses primarily involve children, but can affect adults.

Langerhans Cell Histiocytosis

Pathophysiology and Clinical Findings

Tiny intracellular Birbeck granules detected by electron microscopy and Langerhans cell type markers detected on immunostaining distinguish LCH from the other histiocytoses. The 3 major types are unifocal (or localized), multifocal unisystem (or chronic recurring), and multifocal multisystem (or fulminant). Approximately 70% of LCH cases are unifocal involving the bones and lungs. Approximately 20% of cases are multifocal unisystem involving bones and the reticuloendothelial system: liver, spleen, lymph nodes, and skin. Approximately 10% of cases are multifocal multisystem involving the reticuloendothelial system with anemia and thrombocytopenia. Bones are involved in approximately 80% of LCH patients. Pulmonary nodular and cystic involvement, diabetes insipidus (DI), and liver and spleen enlargement are associated with LCH because of tissue infiltration. The number of organs involved determines the disease severity. Multifocal multisystem disease often results in fatality during childhood.

Imaging Strategy

Radiographs are standard for the initial assessment of suspected bone lesions. A metastatic bone survey with radiographs of the axial and peripheral skeleton is standard to look for polyostotic disease. MRI is used to confirm a solid neoplasm, narrow the differential diagnosis, evaluate for risk of pathologic fracture, and guide biopsy. Routine MRI sequences for mass imaging are acquired including T1W, fluid-sensitive (STIR, T2W FS) and T1W FS pre- and postcontrast. In suspected disease of the spine and skull, MRI is indicated to characterize extraosseous extension and involvement of the pituitary gland in patients with DI. Similar sequences to those used for bone masses are routinely used to evaluate the spine,

and specific neuroradiology protocols are used to evaluate the brain, skull, and sella turcica. CT is an alternative if MRI is unavailable or contraindicated.

Imaging Findings
Radiography

- Flat bone involvement, especially in adults
  - Skull most commonly with characteristic lesions that lack periostitis
    - *Punched-out* lytic lesions
    - Beveled edge caused by differential inner and outer table destruction
    - *Geographic skull* with large maplike lytic lesions
    - Temporal bone and orbit involvement
  - Mandible destruction with *floating teeth*
  - Innominate bone lesions sometime not purely lytic; may have sclerotic margins and surrounding sclerosis
- Lytic vertebral body lesions
  - May result in complete collapse especially in children (vertebral plana) (Figure 77.1A)
  - Posterior elements and discs spared
- Lytic long bone lesions
  - They may be expansile with endosteal scalloping, cortical thinning, and septations.
  - They can have a *budding* appearance caused by endosteal scalloping.
  - Less common is an aggressive appearance with a permeative pattern and periostitis.
  - Chronic lesions have more sclerotic margins and may eventually resolve and heal.
  - In children, this is most common in metaphyses and diaphyses, and rarely involves the epiphyses.
  - Femur, tibia, and humerus are the most commonly involved sites.
- Lesions containing central bone fragment or sequestrum
  - Can resemble osteomyelitis, especially if there is an aggressive lesion appearance, or other less common lesions with sequestra (eg, lymphoma, osteoblastoma)

Computed Tomography

- Similar lytic appearance to radiography
- Soft tissue involvement more conspicuous than radiographs

Magnetic Resonance Imaging

- Nonspecific appearance resembles other solid neoplasms:
  - Imaging is hyperintense on T2W, isointense T1W, and hyperintense on T1W postcontrast (Figure 77.1B-D).

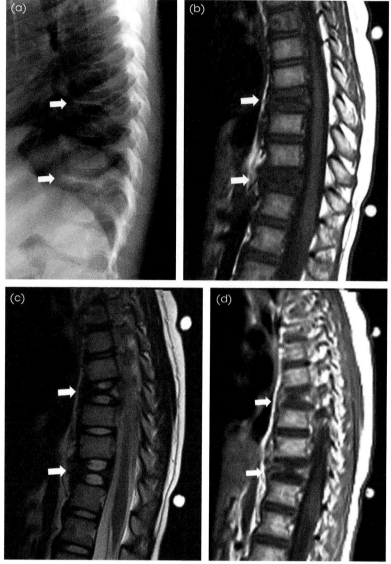

Figure 77.1. LCH of the spine in a 5-year-old patient. (*A*) Lateral radiograph of the thoracic spine demonstrates pathologic fractures with severe compression (vertebra plana) at the T8 and T11 levels. (*B*) Sagittal T1W, (*C*) STIR, and (*D*) T1W postcontrast MR images demonstrate both pathologic fractures without associated soft tissue masses.

- Spine lesions may show early heterogeneous enhancement.
- Acute long bone lesions may less commonly appear aggressive with periostitis, BME, and adjacent soft tissue edema:
  - Soft tissue extension of long bone lesions is uncommon.
- Chronic lesions have lower signal intensity on T2W sequences.
- Anemia may result in marrow reconversion (discussed in Chapter 75, "Bone Marrow Conversion and Reconversion").

Ultrasound
- Soft tissue extension appears isoechoic to muscle.

Nuclear Medicine
- Nuclear scintigraphy may show uptake, but may be negative in more chronic and treated lesions.

- Fluorodeoxyglucose (FDG)-PET and FDG-PET/CT are the most sensitive modalities in detection of disease.

Treatment Options
- Skull and long bone LCH is treated with curettage and packing, curettage with intralesional steroid, or radiation.
- Chemotherapy (eg, vinblastine) and/or steroids is used if there are multiple lesions.
- Spine lesions are treated with radiation, especially with risk of vertebra plana.

Erdheim-Chester Disease

Pathophysiology and Clinical Findings
ECD is a rare disease typically diagnosed in adulthood by the presence of cells that lack Birbeck granules and Langerhans' cell markers. Nearly all patients have long bone involvement

and periarticular pain. Central nervous system involvement is common and includes extraaxial masses resembling meningiomas, retroorbital infiltration resulting in exophthalmos, and DI caused by sellar involvement. The retroperitoneum may also be involved, which is rarely symptomatic.

Imaging Strategy
Radiographs for evaluation of symptomatic periarticular pain are routinely acquired. MRI may be useful in excluding other causes of osseous sclerosis (eg, chronic osteomyelitis, CRMO)

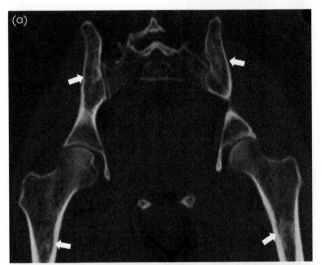

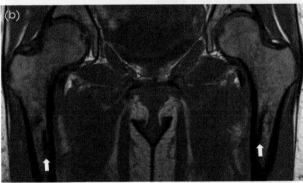

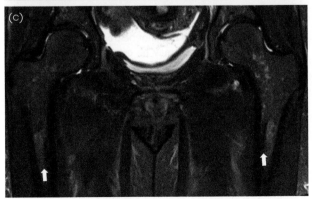

Figure 77.2. ECD of the pelvis and proximal femurs in a 53-year-old woman. (*A*) Oblique coronal reformatted CT image demonstrates areas of symmetric, patchy bone sclerosis in the proximal femora and iliac wings (*thick arrows*). (*B*) Coronal T1W and (*C*) STIR MR images show areas of low signal corresponding to sclerotic bone with patchy areas of signal hyperintensity, in (*C*), within the proximal femoral shafts (*thick arrows*).

using a mass protocol like LCH. MRI of the brain, sella, and orbits is also acquired in symptomatic patients similar to LCH patients, with CT as an alternative.

Imaging Findings
Radiography and Computed Tomography
- Patchy medullary sclerosis of long bones (Figure 77.2*A*)
  - Involving the metadiaphysis with sparing of the epiphysis
- Often bilateral and symmetrical
- Lower extremity long bones more commonly involved than the upper extremities

Magnetic Resonance Imaging
- Imaging shows patchy areas of T2 hyperintensity in areas of long bone involvement and areas of low signal on all sequences corresponding to bone sclerosis (Figure 77.2*B,C*).
- Retroperitoneal and perirenal tissue may be detected incidentally on spine MRI, which may resemble lymphoma.

Nuclear Medicine
- Nuclear scintigraphy shows diffuse, symmetric uptake toward the end of the lower extremity long bones.
- Disease in bones with negative radiographs is detected.

Treatment Options
- Observation in mild disease
- Interferon or chemotherapy

Rosai-Dorfman Disease

Pathophysiology and Clinical Findings
RDD is also known as *sinus histiocytosis with massive lymphadenopathy*. It is a rare disorder more common in males, children, young adults, and those of African descent. The cells lack Birbeck granules, but do show dendritic cell markers as in LCH. An extensive inflammatory cellular component is seen on biopsy, which includes characteristic engulfment of lymphocytes or plasma cells by dendritic cells. The number of inflammatory cells may obscure dendritic cells and result in a misdiagnosis of infection. Clinically, lymphadenopathy, which is often massive, fever, mild anemia, and elevated ESR are characteristic manifestations. Musculoskeletal involvement is uncommon in patients (~7%) and rare in the absence of lymphadenopathy (<1% all reported cases). The clinical course is variable, but most patients have a favorable prognosis with little or no pain.

Imaging Strategy
CT is usually performed in areas with lymphadenopathy and may detect incidental bone lesions. Given the rarity of RDD, staging of disease is not standardized, but may involve CT scanning of the chest, abdomen, and pelvis, or nuclear medicine including nuclear scintigraphy and PET/CT scans.

Imaging Findings
Radiography and Computed Tomography
- Monostotic or polyostotic lytic lesions most commonly involving the skull, tibia, and femur (Figure 77.3)
  - Medullary with multiloculated or serpentine margin

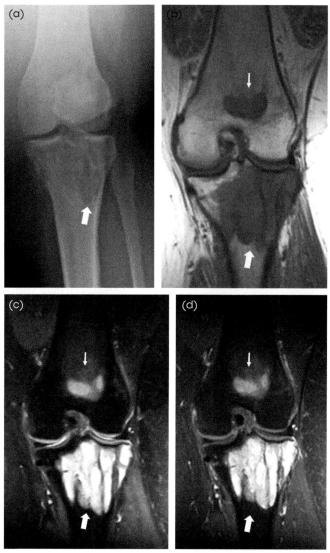

Figure 77.3. RDD involving the knee in an 18-year-old patient. (*A*) AP radiograph of the knee demonstrates a large, lytic lesion of the proximal tibia with a multiloculated appearance (*thick arrow*). (*B*) Coronal PDW and (*C*) PDW FS MR images demonstrate the large lesion of the proximal tibia (*thin arrow*) and an additional distal femoral lesion (*thick arrow*) with fluid signal characteristics: isointense on PDW image and hyperintense on PDW FS image. (*D*) A coronal T1W FS postcontrast MR image demonstrates diffuse enhancement consistent with solid lesions requiring biopsy for diagnosis.

- May have sclerotic margins
- May resemble LCH and metastatic disease
- Not associated with an aggressive appearance (eg, soft tissue mass, cortical destruction)
- Sclerotic lesions rare

Magnetic Resonance Imaging
- Infiltrative with marrow replacement with T1W signal iso- or hypointense to muscle and high signal on fluid-sensitive sequences (Figure 77.3*B-D*)
- Soft tissue mass and cortical destruction rare

Nuclear Medicine
- Intense uptake of bone lesions with nuclear scintigraphy and FDG-PET
- Detects asymptomatic disease

Treatment Options
- Good prognosis and may not be treated.
- Symptomatic lesions may be curettaged and less commonly packed.

Key Points
- Histiocytoses are uncommon diseases that commonly involve the bones in LCH and ECD.
- In adults, LCH often involves the flat bones, especially the skull, with geographic, punched-out lesions that have beveled edges.
- ECD results in a symmetric sclerotic appearance of the metadiaphyses of long bones, especially the lower extremities.

- Although bone involvement by the histiocytoses is not routinely aggressive in appearance or behavior, biopsy is often obtained for diagnosis and to exclude malignancy.
- Treatment is limited to symptomatic lesions or those at risk for pathologic fracture.

Recommended Reading
Zaveri J, La Q, Yarmish G, Neuman J. More than just Langerhans cell histiocytosis: a radiologic review of histiocytic disorders. *Radiographics*. 2014;34:2008–24.

References
1. Baker JC, Kyriakos M, McDonald DJ, Rubin DA. Primary Rosai-Dorfman disease of the femur. *Skeletal Radiol*. 2017;46:129–35.
2. Haupt R, Minkov M, Astigarraga I, et al. Langerhans cell histiocytosis (LCH): guidelines for diagnosis, clinical work-up, and treatment for patients till the age of 18 years. *Pediatr Blood Cancer*. 2013;60:175–84.
3. Hoover KB, Rosenthal DI, Mankin H. Langerhans cell histiocytosis. *Skeletal Radiol*. 2007;36:95–104.
4. Khung S, Budzik JF, Amzallag-Bellenger E, et al. Skeletal involvement in Langerhans cell histiocytosis. *Insights Imaging*. 2013;4:569–79.
5. Mantilla JG, Goldberg-Stein S, Wang Y. Extranodal Rosai-Dorfman disease: clinicopathologic series of 10 patients with radiologic correlation and review of the literature. *Am J Clin Pathol*. 2016;145:211–21.
6. Song YS, Lee IS, Yi JH, Cho KH, Kim DK, Song JW. Radiologic findings of adult pelvis and appendicular skeletal Langerhans cell histiocytosis in nine patients. *Skeletal Radiol*. 2011;40:1421–26.
7. Veyssier-Belot C, Cacoub P, Caparros-Lefebvre D, et al. Erdheim-Chester disease. Clinical and radiologic characteristics of 59 cases. *Medicine (Baltimore)*. 1996;75:157–69.
8. Zaveri J, La Q, Yarmish G, Neuman J. More than just Langerhans cell histiocytosis: a radiologic review of histiocytic disorders. *Radiographics*. 2014;34:2008–24.

CHAPTER 78

Lymphoproliferative and Myeloproliferative Disorders

Kevin B. Hoover

Introduction

WHO classification includes 13 types of tumors of hematopoietic and lymphoid tissues (Table 78.1). These include tumors discussed in other chapters (see Chapter 76, "Plasma Cell Dyscrasias" and Chapter 77, "Histiocytoses"). In this chapter, examples of the myeloproliferative neoplasms (primary myelofibrosis, mastocytosis), leukemia (leukemia and preleukemic disorders), and lymphomas (primary and secondary lymphoma of bone, Waldenström macroglobulinemia) will be discussed with a focus on distinguishing features and the role of imaging in diagnosis and management.

Imaging Strategy

Bone marrow is the primary site of involvement in lymphoproliferative and myeloproliferative disorders and, therefore, radiography is an insensitive modality in their evaluation. Although disease may be detected on radiography, the findings are rarely specific. CT is more sensitive than radiography in detecting the fractures, bone lesions, and periosteal reaction that may occur; however, it is still much less sensitive than MRI and nuclear imaging in detecting marrow involvement. MRI using T1W, fluid-sensitive (T2W FS or STIR) and T1W postcontrast sequences is commonly used for bone and bone marrow imaging. These sequences are sensitive in detecting disease; however, differentiating disease from red marrow, especially in younger patients, distinguishing the type of disease, and discerning viable from nonviable disease after treatment can be difficult. All of these diseases routinely show replacement of fat with low T1 signal intensity with the exception of diffuse multiple myeloma (see Chapter 76, "Plasma Cell Dyscrasias"), however, T2 signal intensity varies by disease. Two useful MRI techniques not as widely used are whole body (WB) MRI and diffusion-weighted imaging (DWI). WB MRI is optimal in evaluating disease without the use of radiation, especially in children and pregnant individuals, however, it is not available at all institutions. DWI depicts restricted water movement (diffusion) as hyperintensity, which occurs in tumors more than normal marrow. Nuclear scintigraphy is often useful for confirming disease and its distribution; however, it is insensitive to lytic disease. Fluorodeoxyglucose (FDG)-PET/CT is the most sensitive and specific technique to identify the presence of viable disease before and after treatment, but is also a significant source of radiation. It is commonly a combination of the different modalities that is used in patients with lymphoproliferative and myeloproliferative disorders because of the need to evaluate symptoms that arise and to determine disease remission and recurrence.

Myelofibrosis

Pathophysiology and Clinical Findings

Primary myelofibrosis is a myeloproliferative disorder that replaces bone marrow with fibrotic connective tissue. Approximately 20% of patients progress to leukemia. Secondary myelofibrosis is associated with multiple causes including polycythemia vera, radiation, or medical therapy for malignancy. Symptoms associated with primary myelofibrosis include hepatosplenomegaly, extramedullary hematopoiesis (EMH), severe anemia, bone pain, pruritus, thrombosis, and bleeding. Diagnosis of myelofibrosis, both primary and secondary, is based on bone marrow results including the presence of specific genetic mutations, evidence of marrow reticulin, and/or fibrosis, and serology. The median age at diagnosis is 60 years with equal numbers of men and women. After diagnosis, the mean life span is 2-3 years, with less than 10% of patients surviving more than 8 years. Mortality is largely caused by leukemia, cardiovascular events, infection, or bleeding.

Imaging Findings
Radiography

- Osteosclerosis present in 30-70% patients
  - Especially axial skeleton and metaphyses of femora, tibiae, and humeri
  - May be uniform or contain small areas of lucency
  - Long bone cortical thickening with endosteal sclerosis
  - *Sandwich vertebrae* with sclerotic endplates
  - Needs to be distinguished from metastasis, Paget disease, fluorosis, osteomalacia, renal osteodystrophy
- Periostitis uncommon
- Joint effusion secondary to hemarthrosis
  - Soft tissue tophi or articular gout in 5-20% patients.

Computed Tomography
- Can detect EMH usually in spleen, liver, and lymph nodes, sometimes paraspinal, rarely epidural
  - Iso- or hyperdense tissue with homogeneous enhancement
- Osteosclerosis (Figure 78.1A)

Table 78.1. World Health Organization (WHO) Classification of Tumors of Hematopoietic and Lymphoid Tissues

WHO CLASSIFICATION	EXAMPLES
Myeloproliferative neoplasms	Polycythemia vera Primary myelofibrosis Essential thrombocythemia Mastocytosis Chronic leukemias
Myeloid and lymphoid neoplasms with eosinophilia and abnormalities of PDGF-A, PDGF-B, or FGFR1	
Myelodysplastic/myeloproliferative neoplasms	Chronic leukemias
Myelodysplastic syndromes	Myelodysplastic syndrome Refractory anemias
AML and related precursor neoplasms	
Acute leukemias of ambiguous lineage	
Precursor lymphoid neoplasms	Lymphoblastic leukemia/lymphoma
Mature B-cell neoplasms	Plasma cell dyscrasias Burkitt lymphoma
Mature T- and NK-cell neoplasms	Leukemias and lymphomas
Hodgkin lymphoma	
Immunodeficiency-associated lymphoproliferative disorders	Posttransplant lymphoproliferative disorder Lymphomas associated with HIV infection
Histiocytic and dendritic cell neoplasms	Langerhans cell histiocytosis Erdheim-Chester disease

Abbreviations: AML, acute myeloid leukemia; FGFR1, fibroblast growth factor receptor 1; HIV, human immunodeficiency virus; NK, natural killer; PDGF-A, platelet derived growth factor receptor alpha; PDGF-B, platelet derived growth factor receptor beta.

Magnetic Resonance Imaging
- Fat replacement by fibrous tissue results in homogeneous low T1 and T2 signal relative to muscle (Figure 78.1B-D)
- Diaphyses and metaphyses of long bones may be involved with epiphyseal fat replaced in more severe disease
- Paraspinal EMH hypointense signal on T1WI, heterogeneous signal intensity on T2WI, and homogeneous postcontrast enhancement

Nuclear Medicine
- Nuclear scintigraphy showing diffuse radiotracer deposition with decreased or absent renal activity caused by increased cortical blood flow (superscan)
- Diffusely increased marrow uptake on FDG-PET/CT

Treatment Options
- Current drug therapies are not curative or been shown to prolong survival.
- Stem cell transplantation (SCT) is dangerous, resulting in mortality or significant morbidity in approximately 50% of patients.
- Many patients are observed or treated with conventional drugs (eg, hydroxyurea for splenomegaly).

Key Points
- Myelofibrosis is a premalignant condition with patients expecting a 2-3 year average life expectancy after diagnosis.
- It is most commonly associated with diffuse osteosclerosis.
- It is associated with EMH.

Mastocytosis

Pathophysiology and Clinical Findings

Systemic mastocytosis is a group of disorders arising from a clonal population of mast cells or their progenitors. This usually results in increased mast cell number in skin and other tissues. The bone and bone marrow are involved in approximately 90% of cases, and bone marrow may be the only tissue involved in some types of mastocytosis (eg, mast cell leukemia, aggressive systemic mastocytosis). The differential secretion of factors by mast cells is associated with different imaging findings including the release of histamine, which stimulates osteosclerosis, and heparin, prostaglandins, and proteases, which are associated with lytic bone lesions and osteopenia. Systemic mastocytosis may be associated with other hematologic disorders including myelodysplastic syndrome and acute myelogenous leukemia (AML). Symptoms and complications are related to mast cell infiltration, including organ dysfunction

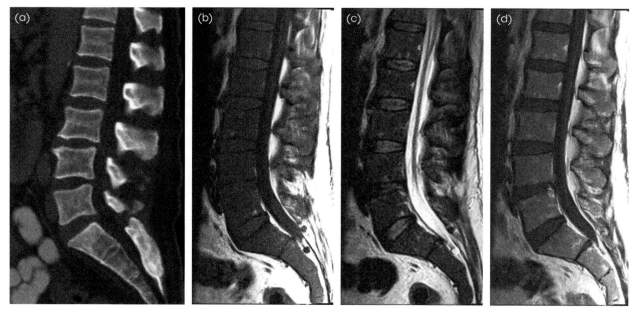

Figure 78.1. Myelofibrosis bone changes on CT and MRI. (*A*) Sagittal reformatted CT image of the lumbar spine in a 67-year-old man with biopsy proven myelofibrosis demonstrates diffuse sclerosis of the vertebral bodies. (*B-D*) Spine MRI of a 49-year-old patient with biopsy proven myelofibrosis. (*B*) Sagittal T1W, (*C*) T2W, and (*D*) Sagittal T1W postcontrast MR images of the lumbar spine demonstrate diffuse replacement of marrow fat by cellular infiltrate with resultant hypointensity compared to muscle and mild enhancement (compare *B* to *D*).

and fractures. Systemic mastocytosis is typically detected in the fifth through eighth decades of life in men and women, equally. The major criterion in diagnosis is the detection of mast cell aggregates on biopsy with minor criteria including cellular atypia and different serologic markers. There is a variable prognosis that worsens with the age at diagnosis.

Imaging Findings
Radiography

- Radiography has low sensitivity for detection of systemic mastocytosis.
- Osteopenia and osteoporosis are the most common and may be the first finding.
- Diffuse form primarily affects the axial skeleton, but focal forms may affect the axial or appendicular skeleton.
- Lesions may be lytic, especially in the axial skeleton, and similar in appearance to osteoporosis or multiple myeloma:
  - Lesions may be large and measure up to 5 cm in diameter.
  - Margins vary, including some with a *halo* of sclerosis.
- Sclerosis (osteosclerosis) can be diffuse with thickened cortex and narrowing of the medullary space, or focal and multiple, resembling metastatic disease (Figure 78.2*A*):
  - Associated with a poorer prognosis

Computed Tomography
- Higher sensitivity than radiography for bone marrow abnormalities with high attenuation in medullary bone relative to fat on nonenhanced CT
- Detects the cortical thickening and medullary compartment narrowing related to osteosclerosis (Figure 78.2B).

Dual-Energy X-Ray Absorptiometry
- DXA is used for diagnosis of osteoporosis and response to osteoporosis treatment.
- Normalization of bone density can be useful indicating response to mastocytosis therapy.

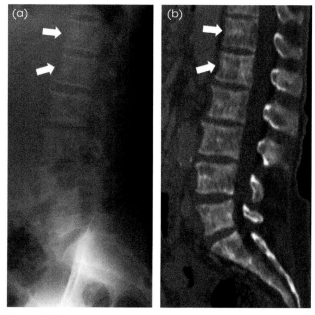

Figure 78.2. Mastocytosis in a 63-year-old woman. (*A*) Lateral radiograph of the lumbar spine demonstrates overall osteopenia with areas of patchy sclerosis (*thick arrows*). (*B*) Corresponding sagittal reformatted CT image shows patchy sclerosis throughout the visualized bones (*thick arrows*).

Magnetic Resonance Imaging

- Mastocytosis signal on fluid-sensitive sequences is often hyperintense, but may be hypointense depending on degree of fibrosis.
- Infiltrated marrow enhances on T1W postcontrast sequences.
- Sclerotic lesions and osteosclerosis are hypointense on T1W and fluid-sensitive sequences.
- Increase in marrow intensity on T1W images and decrease signal intensity on fluid-sensitive sequences seen in response to treatment.

Nuclear Medicine

- Nuclear scintigraphy identifies extent and progression of skeletal involvement with greater sensitivity than radiographs and lesser sensitivity than MRI or FDG-PET/CT.

Treatment Options

- The primary objective is to control symptoms by avoiding dietary and environmental triggers and with medication, such as antihistamines and steroids.
- More aggressive disease may require interferon or chemotherapeutic agents, such as kinase inhibitors (eg, imatinib).
- Bisphosphonates are given for osteoporosis.

Key Points

- Mastocytosis commonly involves the bone.
- Osteopenia and osteoporosis are common findings, especially in early disease.
- Osteosclerosis is associated with a worse prognosis.
- Bone lesions are commonly lytic, with variable margins and can be up to 5 cm in diameter.

Leukemia

Pathophysiology and Clinical Findings

The leukemias are the most common malignancies in children and the ninth most common in adults. These are broadly classified into AML, acute lymphoblastic leukemia (ALL), chronic myelocytic leukemia (CML), and chronic lymphocytic leukemia (CLL). Most leukemias infiltrate the bone marrow and lymphoid tissues, rather than forming masses. However, the myeloid leukemias, especially AML, can form focal masses called *chloromas* (myeloid or granulocytic sarcoma). These are also associated with myelodysplastic syndrome, myeloproliferative neoplasm, essential thrombocythemia, and polycythemia vera (PV). PV, a low-grade proliferative disorder of stem cells typically resulting in erythrocytosis, transforms into AML in approximately 15% of patients. Chloromas may precede diffuse disease and are usually solitary. Bone or bone marrow involvement is detected in approximately 50% of patients. Symptoms include those related to anemia, lymphadenopathy, and organomegaly. Arthritis and bone pain are uncommon in adults and more common in children. Diagnosis and follow-up assessment is primarily based on blood serology and bone marrow biopsy analysis, rather than imaging.

Imaging Findings
Radiography and Computed Tomography

- Often normal or with diffuse osteopenia, but variable
  - May be diffuse or regional
  - Permeative or mottled
  - Osteosclerosis
  - Periostitis
  - Lucent metaphyseal bands in skeletally immature patients, resolve after treatment
  - Compression and pathologic fractures common, but vertebra plana uncommon
  - Chloromas appearing as focal lytic lesions with soft tissue extension, seen better on CT
  - ON
  - Joint effusions

Magnetic Resonance Imaging

- Approximately 10% of patients have normal imaging, especially early in disease, and because of red marrow, leukemias can be hard to detect in younger or anemic patients.
- Diffuse, speckled, or regional T1 hypointensity and hyperintensity on fluid-sensitive sequences with variable enhancement (Figure 78.3) is seen.
- Chloromas are T1 isointense and mildly hyperintense on fluid-sensitive sequences with homogeneous enhancement, except if necrotic (Figure 78.3):
  - Usually epidural in the spine
- Intraarticular or periarticular hemorrhage can be detected, especially in younger patients
- PV is indistinguishable from AML and may also demonstrate a chloroma.

Nuclear Medicine

- FDG-PET/CT detects sites of clinically occult disease for staging and monitoring the response to treatment.

Key Points

- Leukemia may not be detectable on all imaging studies.
- Bone lesions may be aggressive in appearance with periostitis and a permeative pattern of bone destruction.
- Chloromas are discrete masses that are less common than diffuse marrow involvement, but can precede diffuse disease involvement or be associated with recurrent disease.
- MRI and FDG-PET/CT are the most sensitive techniques to detect marrow involvement and response to treatment.

Lymphoma

Pathophysiology and Clinical Findings

Primary lymphoma of the bone is seen in 10-25% of adult lymphoma patients. Secondary osseous involvement (metastases) is common and more common in non-Hodgkin lymphoma (NHL) than Hodgkin disease (HD). Approximately 40% of NHL patients have osseous involvement with an associated poor prognosis. Clinical findings of lymphoma are typically

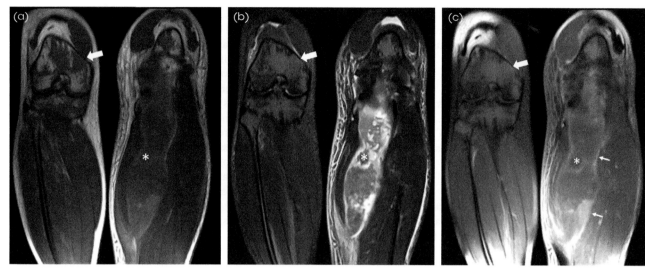

Figure 78.3. Acute myeloid leukemia in a 20-year-old man. (A) T1W, (B) STIR, and (C) T1W post contrast MR images of the bilateral legs demonstrate fatty marrow replacement (*thick arrow*) with enhancing tumor cells and a large soft tissue mass (*asterisk,* chloroma) that shows primarily rim enhancement (*thin arrows*).

fever, lymphadenopathy, and hepatosplenomegaly. Arthritis is rare in adults. In general, imaging is central in the staging of primary and secondary disease and follow-up.

Imaging Findings
Radiography
- Primary lymphoma of the bone includes the following findings:
  - Aggressive permeative or moth-eaten appearance is seen.
  - Patient may have focal lytic (70%), sclerotic, or mixed (28%) lesions.
  - Sclerotic appearance is more common in HD than NHL.
  - *Ivory vertebra* is characteristic, but uncommon, and seen in other diseases, including Paget disease, hemangioma, and blastic metastases.
  - Lamellated periostitis may be seen especially in HD.
  - There is a relative absence of cortical destruction.
  - Sequestra are identified in approximately 10% of primary lymphoma of the bone.
- Secondary osseous lymphoma includes the following findings:
  - Lytic lesions are most common.
  - Vertebral lesions usually involve the thoracic and lumbar spine.
  - Sclerotic lesions or ivory vertebra are less frequent.
  - Soft tissue masses and vertebral collapse are common.

Computed Tomography
- Primary lymphoma of the bone
  - CT is superior to radiography in detecting destruction, periostitis, sequestrum, extraosseous extension
- Secondary osseous lymphoma
  - Greater sensitivity than radiography, but less than MRI and PET/CT

Magnetic Resonance Imaging
- Primary lymphoma of the bone
  - Focal disease more common than in leukemia
  - Heterogeneous on T2 signal because of hypercellularity; isointense to hypointense relative to muscle (Figure 78.4B,D)
  - Homogeneous enhancement on T1W FS postcontrast MR sequences (Figure 78.4E)
  - Vertebral disease
    - *Wrap-around* sign is seen where there is vertebral and perivertebral disease sparing the cortex.
    - Epidural extension may cause spinal canal or neural foraminal stenosis.
- Secondary osseous lymphoma
  - Multifocal or diffuse
  - Typically low T1 signal and hyperintense on fluid-sensitive sequences
  - Moderate to high enhancement
  - Hyperintensity on DWI because of restricted diffusion caused by hypercellularity

Nuclear Medicine
- FDG-PET/CT is superior to nuclear scintigraphy, PET, contrast-enhanced CT, and MRI:
  - HD and NHL metastatic or primary involvement are hypermetabolic relative to the mediastinum and liver.
  - NHL bone marrow involvement is often diffuse.
  - False-positive activity at biopsy sites is detected by characteristic CT changes.
  - FDG-PET/CT has replaced gallium 67.
- FDG-PET/CT can sometimes replace bone marrow biopsy (eg, early HD, early diffuse large B-cell).
- FDG-PET/CT is useful in evaluating for residual, posttreatment disease; persistent metabolic activity is associated with relapse in 62-100% cases:
  - Optimal to scan 4-6 weeks after treatment
  - Superior sensitivity to residual disease compared to CT and MRI

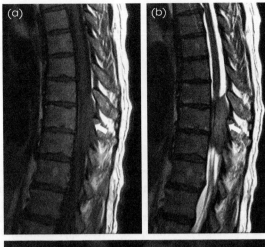
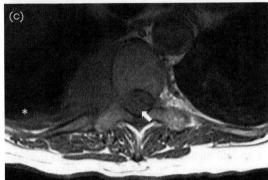
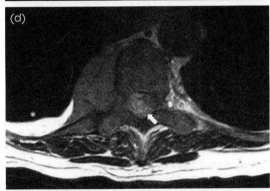
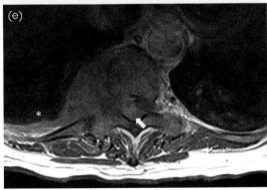

Figure 78.4. B-cell lymphoma in a 69-year-old patient.
(*A*) Sagittal T1W and (*B*) T2W MR images of the thoracic spine demonstrate a mass within the spinal canal without apparent vertebral involvement that is relatively hypointense on T2W imaging because of hypercellularity (*thick arrow*). (*C*) Axial T1W, (*D*) T2W, and (*E*) T1W postcontrast MR images identify the intra- and paraspinal mass with severe canal stenosis (*thick arrows*). The mass is hypointense on T2W imaging relative to the small right pleural effusion (*asterisk*).

Key Points

- Metastatic or secondary lymphoma of the bone is much more common than primary lymphoma of the bone.
- Osteolysis is more common than mixed lytic and sclerotic disease.
- The wrap-around sign of soft tissue extension from the bone with sparing of the cortex is a characteristic sign.
- The sclerotic ivory vertebra is a sensitive, but nonspecific, finding in lymphoma.
- Lymphoma may be hypointense or isointense on T2W sequences because of hypercellularity of lesions.
- MRI and FDG-PET/CT are the most sensitive techniques to detect marrow involvement and response to treatment.

Treatment Options

- These diseases have specific treatment regimens involving chemotherapy with or without SCT.
- Surgery is limited to treating pathologic fractures.
- Osteoporosis can be detected by DXA and managed using standard medical treatments.

Recommended Reading

Keraliya AR, Krajewski KM, Jagannathan JP, et al. Multimodality imaging of osseous involvement in haematological malignancies. *Br J Radiol.* 2016;89:20150980.

Morais SA, du Preez HE, Akhtar MR, Cross S, Isenberg DA. Musculoskeletal complications of haematological disease. *Rheumatology (Oxford).* 2016;55:968–81.

References

1. Fritz J, Fishman EK, Carrino JA, Horger MS. Advanced imaging of skeletal manifestations of systemic mastocytosis. *Skeletal Radiol.* 2012;41:887–97.
2. Guermazi A, de Kerviler E, Cazals-Hatem D, Zagdanski AM, Frija J. Imaging findings in patients with myelofibrosis. *Eur Radiol.* 1999;9:1366–75.
3. Hwang S, Panicek DM. Magnetic resonance imaging of bone marrow in oncology, Part 2. *Skeletal Radiol.* 2007;36:1017–27.
4. Keraliya AR, Krajewski KM, Jagannathan JP, et al. Multimodality imaging of osseous involvement in haematological malignancies. *Br J Radiol.* 2016;89:20150980.
5. Morais SA, du Preez HE, Akhtar MR, Cross S, Isenberg DA. Musculoskeletal complications of haematological disease. *Rheumatology (Oxford).* 2016;55:968–81.
6. Pawha PS, Chokshi FH. Imaging of spinal manifestations of hematological disorders. *Hematol Oncol Clin North Am.* 2016;30:921–44.
7. Tefferi A. Primary myelofibrosis: 2013 update on diagnosis, risk-stratification, and management. *Am J Hematol.* 2013;88:141–50.
8. Valls L, Badve C, Avril S, et al. FDG-PET imaging in hematological malignancies. *Blood Rev.* 2016;30:317–31.
9. Wadleigh M, Tefferi A. Classification and diagnosis of myeloproliferative neoplasms according to the 2008 World Health Organization criteria. *Int J Hematol.* 2010;91:174–79.

CHAPTER 79

Bleeding Diseases

Kevin B. Hoover

Introduction

Bleeding diseases disrupt the normal blood clotting process primarily by affecting platelet function or the clotting cascade. Genetic diseases that cause reduction or dysfunction of clotting factors (hemophilia A and B) and less commonly platelets (von Willebrand disease [vWD]) are the major bleeding diseases of the musculoskeletal system. Both acute and chronic joint diseases have characteristic imaging findings that can be detected on most imaging modalities, but are most optimally evaluated by MRI. Early intervention has resulted in less severe disease and imaging findings than in the past.

Pathophysiology and Clinical Findings

Normal hemostasis is maintained by a normal endothelial lining of blood vessels that produces anticoagulants (eg, nitric oxide, prostacyclin) and inhibits factors that stimulate coagulation (eg, von Willebrand factor [vWF]). In addition to trauma, medications, autoimmune diseases, and genetic mutations can alter this hemostasis and result in bleeding (Table 79.1). In general, the disruption of platelet function results in mucocutaneous bleeding (eg, easy bruising, skin bleeding, and prolonged bleeding from oropharyngeal, gastrointestinal, uterine mucosal surfaces) and factor deficiency results in musculoskeletal system bleeding. Tests to evaluate bleeding include a complete blood count (CBC) and coagulation studies (eg, prothrombin time [PT], activated partial thromboplastin time [aPTT]), mixing studies of normal and patient plasma, tests to evaluate specific platelet disorders, and genetic studies.

Hemophilia A and B

Hemophilia is an inherited, autosomal recessive X-linked disease affecting males associated with deficiency of factor VIII (hemophilia A) or factor IX (hemophilia B, Christmas disease) deficiency. Hemophilia A affects between 1 in 5,000 and 1 in 10,000 births. It is approximately fivefold more common than hemophilia B (1 in 30,000 births). Rarely, patients may develop hemophilia (acquired hemophilia) because of antibodies to factor VIII (FVIII). Acquired hemophilia primarily occurs in older patients (68-80 years of age), but is also seen less frequently in younger, postpartum females. Severe disease is defined when the plasma factor concentrations are less than 1% of normal. Factor XI (FXI) deficiency (hemophilia C) is autosomal and common in the Ashkenazi Jewish population (1:10), but has variable bleeding risk. The other factor deficiencies are very rare.

More than 80% of hemorrhages in hemophilia involve the musculoskeletal system. In severe disease, this occurs spontaneously and in milder disease after minor and major trauma (eg, surgery). Arthropathy affects approximately 90% of patients with severe hemophilia and is most common between the second and fourth decades. This commonly begins in the first decade of life with hemorrhage into larger joints, most commonly the ankle, but also the knee or elbow. In acute hemarthrosis, an inflammatory cycle is initiated by blood breakdown products, including iron, which are taken up by synovial cells lining the joint and macrophages. A chronic proliferative synovitis then develops because of the release of hydrolytic enzymes, related to synovial hemorrhage. Chronic hemophiliac arthropathy often results in fibrosis. Hemophiliacs have a 40-fold higher incidence of septic joints than the general population and a 10-fold higher incidence of infected arthroplasty. Pseudotumors are rare, encapsulated hematomas usually associated with direct trauma. Extraskeletal sequelae of hemophilia include intracranial hemorrhage (2-12% patients) and complications of blood product administration including hepatitis B and C and human immunodeficiency virus (HIV) infection.

A successful long-term outcome in patients with hemophilia depends on the prevention (prophylaxis) of bleeding with the administration of concentrated FVIII or factor IX (FIX). Of hemophilia patients, 20-30% of hemophilia A patients and 1-5% of hemophilia B patients develop antibodies (inhibitors) with an increased risk of uncontrollable bleeding, disability, and premature death. The incidence of inhibitors is decreased by initiating prophylaxis at a young age.

Von Willebrand Disease

vWD is the most common genetic bleeding disorder and occurs in up to 1% of the population. Acquired disease can be present in patients with aortic stenosis, left ventricular assist devices, essential thrombocytopenia, and polycythemia vera. It commonly presents with mucocutaneous bleeding, however, rare variants present similar to hemophilia A and B with musculoskeletal system involvement (type 2N) or both mucocutaneous and musculoskeletal system involvement (type 3). Type 2N can be misdiagnosed as hemophilia A with an associated delay in treatment.

Imaging Strategy

MRI is the imaging method of choice to detect abnormalities of hemophiliac arthropathy, the staging of severity, and the effect of treatment. GRE sequences are especially useful to

Table 79.1. Example Causes of Abnormal Bleeding

CAUSE	EXAMPLES
Medications	Warfarin; apixaban (and other Xa inhibitors); antiplatelet medications including clopidogrel, aspirin, nonsteroidal antiinflammatory drugs (NSAIDs)
Autoimmune diseases	Lupus anticoagulant, autoantibodies to factor VIII (acquired hemophilia), immune thrombocytopenic purpura
Genetic mutations	Platelet disorders (Bernard-Soulier disease), von Willebrand disease (multiple subtypes), common factor deficiencies (factor VIII or hemophilia A, factor IX or hemophilia B), factor XI, rare factor deficiencies (factor II, factor V, factor VII, factor X, factor XIII)

detect the susceptibility artifact because of hemosiderin deposition from hemorrhage. Cartilage is optimally assessed using PD FS and 3D spoiled gradient recalled acquisition in the steady state (SPGR) sequences. IV contrast is not usually necessary. Muscle involvement is also optimally assessed by MRI. US is limited in its evaluation of joints because of suboptimal assessment of cartilage and subchondral bone. However, it can be used to evaluate for the presence or resolution of joint effusions and hematomas. Conventional radiography is useful to monitor advanced cartilage and bone damage in a joint, but is insensitive to the early joint or soft tissue changes.

Imaging Findings

Radiography

- Early disease presents with pauciarticular involvement, periarticular osteopenia, joint effusion, and epiphyseal overgrowth most commonly of ankle, knee, and elbow.
  - Knee joint shows squaring of the patella and widening of intercondylar notch.
- Late disease presents with polyarticular involvement, subchondral bone irregularity including cystlike changes, joint-space narrowing from cartilage destruction, osteopenia, and ankyloses (Figures 79.1 and 79.2).
- Once radiographic changes are present, the course is usually progressive and irreversible.
- Improved prophylaxis with decreased disease severity limits usefulness of radiography and radiographic staging systems of hemophilia (eg, Pettersson scale).
- Pseudotumors of the soft tissues, especially of the pelvis and lower limbs can cause pressure erosions on bone and rarely calcify.
- Subperiosteal hemorrhage results in expansile, lobulated lytic lesions, especially in the pelvis, femur, tibia, and bones of hand.

Ultrasound

- Hemarthrosis appears as anechoic or heterogeneously hypoechoic joint fluid.
- Synovitis appears similar to inflammatory arthritis with thickened, nodular synovium with increased flow using color and power Doppler US.
- Intramuscular hemorrhage appears typically heterogeneous or hyperechoic in less than 3 days and progressively anechoic for more than 3 days (Figure 79.3):
  - Hemorrhage can be small and difficult to detect; consider repeating after first 24 hours.
  - Increase in echogenicity suggests new hemorrhage.
  - Iliopsoas, quadriceps, and gastrocnemius muscles are commonly involved.
- Evaluate the size of pseudotumors and change over time to exclude underlying hemorrhagic neoplasm.

Computed Tomography

- May be useful to evaluate pseudotumor for size stability, mass effect and complications, such as pathologic fracture
  - May be hyperdense in acute to subacute phase of hemorrhage
- Same articular changes detected as with radiography

Magnetic Resonance Imaging

- MRI is sensitive to early signal changes of arthropathy:
  - Effusions and hemorrhage are detected on T1W and fluid-sensitive sequences (Figure 79.4)
    - Hemorrhage gives variable signal from time of bleed (Table 79.2).
    - Hemosiderin gives low signal especially on GRE, which commonly *blooms* with involvement of multiple pixels because of susceptibility artifact (Figures 79.2 and 79.4).
      - Low signal also on T1W, T2W and STIR sequences
  - Synovial hypertrophy is indicated by T1 isointense and T2 iso- to hyperintense signal.
  - T1W postcontrast sequences help distinguish hypertrophic synovium from cartilage and fluid.
  - MRI is highly sensitive in detecting changes despite absence of patient-reported bleeding episodes.
- MRI detects later changes of arthropathy, including cartilage loss and erosions:
  - Subchondral cystlike changes are often hyperintense on T2W, but presence of hemosiderin-laden synovium may cause hypointense T2W signal (Figures 79.1–79.3)
- Intramuscular hemorrhage commonly demonstrates heterogeneous signal with age-dependent signal evolution (Table 79.2).
  - *Concentric ring* sign
    - Thin peripheral low signal intensity on all pulse sequences (hemosiderin)

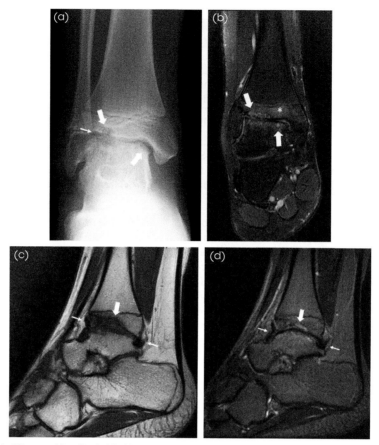

Figure 79.1. Hemophilia B in 15-year-old patient. (*A*) AP ankle radiograph demonstrates joint-space narrowing (*thin arrow*) and cystlike changes of the tibiotalar joint (*thick arrows*). (*B*) A coronal T2W FS MR image demonstrates fluid signal cystlike changes of the tibiotalar joint (*thick arrows*) and periarticular BME (*asterisk*). (*C*) Sagittal T1W and (*D*) STIR MR images demonstrate cystlike changes of the tibiotalar joint (*thick arrows*) and thickening and low signal of the anterior and posterior joint capsule (*thin arrows*).

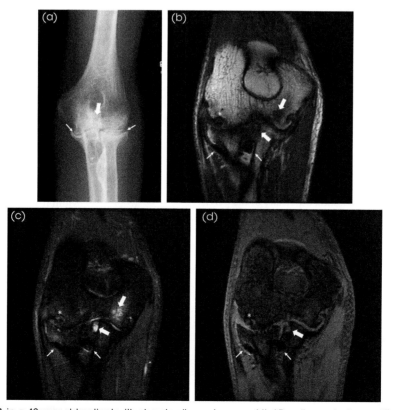

Figure 79.2. Hemophilia A in a 42-year-old patient with chronic elbow changes. (*A*) AP radiograph shows diffuse joint- space narrowing (*thin arrows*) with cystlike change (*thick arrow*), (*B*) Coronal T1W, (*C*) PDW FS, and (*D*) 3D gradient echo (GE) MR images demonstrate cystlike changes (*thick arrows*), erosion (*asterisk*) and low signal at the joint margin (*thin arrows*). Blooming of the low signal is seen on 3D GRE image consistent with hemosiderin.

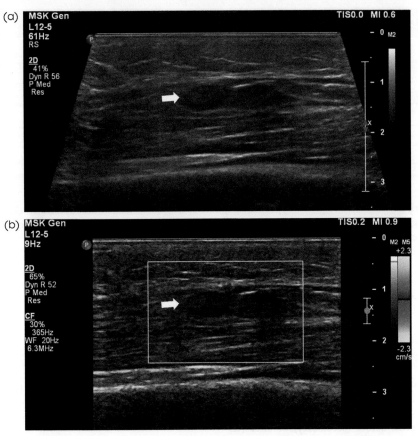

Figure 79.3. Hemophilia B in a 10-year-old boy with a triceps brachii hematoma. (*A*) Long-axis grayscale and (*B*) color Doppler US images shows a bilobed intramuscular mass (*thick arrow*) of mixed echogenicity without internal Doppler flow consistent with a subacute hematoma.

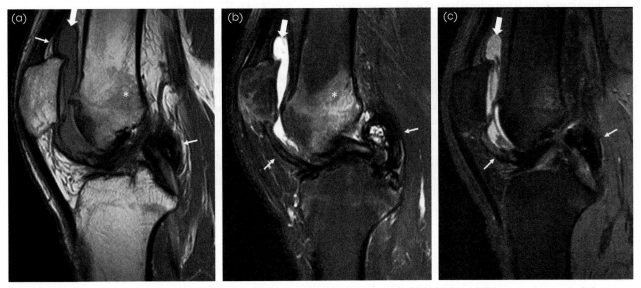

Figure 79.4. Hemophilia A in a 22-year-old patient. (*A*) Sagittal PDW, (*B*) T2W, and (*C*) 3D SPGR knee MR images demonstrate low signal of the joint capsule (*thin arrows*), a joint effusion (*thick arrows*), and BME of the subarticular bone (*asterisk*). Note blooming of the low signal of the joint capsule and intraarticular hemosiderin (*thin arrows*).

Table 79.2. Time-Dependent Magnetic Resonance Imaging Signal of Hemorrhage

TIME (DAYS)	HEMOGLOBIN STATE	T1W	T2W
Acute: 1-3	Deoxyhemoglobin	Isointense	Hypointense
Early subacute: 3-7	IntracellularMethemoglobin	Hyperintense	Hypointense
Late subacute: 7-14	ExtracellularMethemoglobin	Hyperintense	Hyperintense
Chronic	Hemosiderin	Hypointense	Hypointense

Abbreviations: T1W, T1 weighted; T2W, T2 weighted.

- Inner peripheral T1W signal hyperintensity (methemoglobin)
- Central intensity varying, depending on the amount of seroma, deoxyhemoglobin, and methemoglobin

Treatment Options
- Weight-based administration of factor VIII and factor IX concentrate for prophylaxis of hemophilia A and B, respectively, is often given on a weekly basis.
  - Primary prophylaxis (optimal) begins before the age of 3 years in absence of joint disease, before the second clinically evident joint bleed and may prevent arthropathy.
  - Secondary or tertiary prophylaxis begins after 2 or more joint bleeds, before (secondary) or after (tertiary) the onset of joint disease on physical examination and/or imaging and may slow disease progression and improve symptoms.
- Immune suppression, factor VIII concentrate, factor VIIa, or activated prothrombin complex concentrate is used for patients with acquired hemophilia.
- Desmopressin and vWF administration are used for vWD under guidance of a hematologist.
- Chronic synovitis is sometimes treated with synovectomy (radiation, open or arthroscopic surgery).
- End-stage arthritis is treated with arthroplasty and arthrodesis, especially in the ankle.

Key Points
- Bleeding diseases are commonly related to platelet dysfunction, which causes mucocutaneous hemorrhage, and clotting factor dysfunction, which causes musculoskeletal system hemorrhage.
- Hemophilia A and B and rare vWD subtypes commonly result in intraarticular hemorrhage, most commonly of the ankle joint.

- Joint changes are optimally evaluated using MRI especially with GRE sequences, which demonstrate hypointense *blooming* signal caused by the presence of hemosiderin.
- Soft tissue hemorrhage is optimally evaluated with MRI, which may demonstrate the concentric ring sign, but US and CT are also useful to exclude enlargement over time that can be seen in hemorrhagic neoplasms.

Recommended Reading
Maclachlan J, Gough-Palmer A, Hargunani R, Farrant J, Holloway B. Haemophilia imaging: a review. *Skeletal Radiol.* 2009;38:949–57.

References
1. Bush CH. The magnetic resonance imaging of musculoskeletal hemorrhage. *Skeletal Radiol.* 2000;29:1–9.
2. Jelbert A, Vaidya S, Fotiadis N. Imaging and staging of haemophilic arthropathy. *Clin Radiol.* 2009;64:1119–28.
3. Maclachlan J, Gough-Palmer A, Hargunani R, Farrant J, Holloway B. Haemophilia imaging: a review. *Skeletal Radiol.* 2009;38:949–57.
4. Morais SA, du Preez HE, Akhtar MR, Cross S, Isenberg DA. Musculoskeletal complications of haematological disease. *Rheumatology (Oxford).* 2016;55:968–81.
5. Oldenburg J. Optimal treatment strategies for hemophilia: achievements and limitations of current prophylactic regimens. *Blood.* 2015;125:2038–44.
6. Paddock M, Chapin J. Bleeding diatheses: approach to the patient who bleeds or has abnormal coagulation. *Prim Care.* 2016;43:637–50.
7. Rick M. Clinical presentation and diagnosis of von Willebrand disease. *UpToDate.* Updated March 20, 2017. www.uptodate.com/contents/clinical-presentation-and-diagnosis-of-von-willebrand-disease.

Endocrine Diseases

Pituitary Diseases

Kevin B. Hoover

Introduction

The pituitary gland is part of the hypothalamic-pituitary axis, which coordinates the endocrine system via the secretion of hormones. Thus, pituitary dysfunction can be related to hypothalamic or intrinsic pituitary disease (Box 80.1). Pituitary adenomas are the main cause of primary pituitary disease. Most patients with pituitary adenomas (70-75%) present with signs and symptoms of hormone hypersecretion, especially excess prolactin, excess growth hormone, and hypercortisolism. Hyperprolactinemia's primary effect on the musculoskeletal system is a decrease in bone density caused by amenorrhea. Excess growth hormone (acromegaly in adults) and hypercortisolism (Cushing disease) have a wide variety of musculoskeletal effects. Clinically nonfunctioning or *silent* adenomas (25-30%) are most often asymptomatic and incidentally identified on imaging, but may present with neurologic symptoms (eg, diplopia).

Acromegaly

Pathophysiology and Clinical Findings

Excess growth hormone (GH) results in gigantism in skeletally immature patients and acromegaly if excess GH persists, or starts, after skeletal maturity. Gigantism results from stimulation of the endochondral ossification at the physes by GH with increased longitudinal bone growth. Hypersecretion of GH after physeal closure reactivates bone formation especially at the chondroosseous junctions and the periosteum. Acromegaly is rare with a prevalence of 36-60 cases per million people.

GH production is regulated by the hypothalamic-pituitary axis. The somatotropic cells of the anterior lobe of the pituitary gland produce somatotropin, or GH. The hypothalamus stimulates the secretion of GH by producing GH-releasing hormone (GHRH) and inhibits it by producing somatostatin. Insulinlike growth factor 1 (IGF-1) production is stimulated by GH and, in turn, it inhibits GH secretion. Most cases of GH hypersecretion (~90%) are caused by benign pituitary adenomas, of which the majority are macroadenomas (73%). The remainder are caused by excess GHRH production by a hypothalamic adenoma and extrapituitary secretion of GH or GHRH (eg, pancreatic islet cell tumors, carcinoid tumors). The initial diagnostic test of acromegaly is serum IGF-1. Although a normal level usually excludes acromegaly, suppression of serum GH following oral glucose is the gold standard. MRI of the pituitary gland is performed after biochemical confirmation of acromegaly.

Acromegaly is characterized by disproportionate skeletal, tissue, and organ growth. Musculoskeletal changes develop approximately 10 years after the onset of GH hypersecretion with slow changes in facial features including prognathism and frontal bossing, hand and foot growth, and soft tissue hypertrophy. Arthropathy is detected in approximately 70% of patients, typically of the small joints of the hands and feet. Trigger finger can result from pulley thickening. Neuropathies caused by ulnar or median nerve enlargement are common. Carpal tunnel syndrome is diagnosed at presentation in approximately 64% cases of acromegaly.

Imaging Strategy

Contrast-enhanced MRI of the sella turcica is the first-line imaging test to diagnose acromegaly. GH-secreting macroadenomas are usually evident on MRI. If there is contraindication to MRI, or if unavailable, contrast-enhanced CT of the brain is performed. Radiographs are routinely obtained in the evaluation of musculoskeletal symptoms. US is optimal in evaluation of patients with peripheral neuropathy.

Imaging Findings
Radiography

- In general, there is joint-space widening from cartilage hypertrophy.
- Hands and feet show early widening of the MCP, MTP and interphalangeal (IP) joints.
  - Later findings include:
    - OA, may be premature, with joint-space narrowing and osteophytosis, capsular ossification
    - Tubular bone widening
    - Distal phalangeal *spade-shaped* tufts (Figure 80.1)
    - Exostoses
    - Sesamoid bone enlargement
    - Thickened plantar heel pad (>25 mm men; >23 mm women)
    - Skin thickening
- Skull findings include:
  - Enlarged, anteriorly protruding mandible (prognathism)
  - Enlarged supraorbital ridges, facial bones, calvarium, prominence of frontal and maxillary sinuses (frontal bossing)
  - Enlarged sella turcica from macroadenoma
- Spine findings include:
  - Widened intervertebral disc heights
  - Posterior vertebral scalloping, seen in multiple conditions (Table 80.1)
  - Paravertebral ossification

Box 80.1. Major Causes of Pituitary Disease

Hypothalamic disease

Tumors: craniopharyngiomas, metastases
Radiation therapy: central nervous system (CNS) and naso-
    pharyngeal malignancies
Infiltrative lesions: sarcoidosis, Langerhans cell histiocytosis
Infections: Tuberculous meningitis
Traumatic brain injury
Cerebrovascular accident (CVA)

Pituitary disease

Tumors: adenomas, cysts
Pituitary surgery: adenoma resection
Pituitary radiation: adenoma treatment
Infiltrative lesions: hypophysitis, hemochromatosis
Infection/abscess
Infarction: Sheehan syndrome
CVA
Genetic disease
Empty sella

Table 80.1. Conditions Associated with Posterior Vertebral Scalloping Sign

CONDITIONS	CAUSES
Acromegaly	Soft tissue hypertrophy, bone remodeling
Intraspinal tumor	Increased intraspinal pressure
Communicating hydrocephalus	
Marfan syndrome	Dural ectasia
Ehlers-Danlos syndrome	
Neurofibromatosis	
Ankylosing spondylitis	
Achondroplasia	Small spinal canal
Morquio syndrome	Congenital skeletal disorders
Hurler syndrome	

Ultrasound
- Increased nerve size with normal architecture except at sites of entrapment where echogenicity may be decreased and fascicles poorly visualized
  - Median nerve enlargement in carpal tunnel syndrome is frequently symptomatic.
- Can detect pulley thickening in patients with trigger finger

Computed Tomography
- Superior detection of skull changes including enlargement of the sella turcica and sinus enlargement

Magnetic Resonance Imaging
- Peripheral nerve enlargement and increased T2 signal (edema)

Treatment Options
- Treatment of acromegaly typically starts with surgical resection of the pituitary adenoma, often using a transsphenoidal approach.
- Medical treatment with or without adjunctive RT is used in patients with unsuccessful surgical resection or unresectable disease.
- In acromegaly, normal IGF-1 and undetectable GH levels indicate remission, however, treatment may not result in changes in musculoskeletal disease.

Key Points
- Acromegaly is usually caused by a pituitary macroadenoma that slowly causes bone, joint, and soft tissue overgrowth.
- Radiography can typically detect the bone and articular changes of acromegaly.
- US can diagnose median nerve enlargement in acromegaly patients with carpal tunnel syndrome.

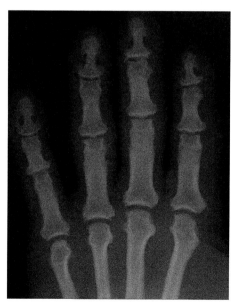

Figure 80.1. Acromegaly. PA radiograph of the fingers shows widening of the joint spaces, bone and soft tissue overgrowth, and splaying of the distal tufts.

Cushing Disease

Pathophysiology and Clinical Findings
Excess cortisol (hypercortisolism) results in a variety of signs and symptoms, called *Cushing syndrome* (Box 80.2).

Box 80.2. Signs and Symptoms of Cushing Syndrome

Truncal obesity
Rounded face (moon facies)
Buffalo hump
Striae
Myopathy
Fatigue
Lethargy
Bone pain
Osteoporosis and fracture
Hypertension
Hirsutism
Acne
Skin thinning
Easy bruising

The most common cause of hypercortisolism is exogenous steroid taken for medical reasons (eg, inflammatory arthritis, asthma, transplantation). The most common cause of endogenous hypercortisolism is Cushing disease (70-80% of cases). Less common causes of endogenous hypercortisolism are adrenal adenoma (approximately 8%), adrenal hyperplasia (approximately 1%), small cell lung cancer, and carcinoid.

Cushing disease is caused by an adrenocorticotropic hormone (ACTH)-producing pituitary adenoma. Cortisol regulation is primarily via the hypothalamic-pituitary axis. Corticotropin-releasing hormone (CRH) from the hypothalamus acts on the corticotroph cells of the pituitary gland, which in turn release ACTH. ACTH stimulates the adrenal cortex to secrete cortisol.

Important consequences of hypercortisolism are hypertension and osteoporosis, which are common indications for the initial clinical workup, especially in younger patients. Osteoporosis affects approximately 50% of patients with hypercortisolism of which 30-50% develop fractures. After exclusion of exogenous steroid intake, 2 separate screening tests are used, including late-night salivary cortisol, 24-hour urine free cortisol, or low-dose dexamethasone suppression testing. Serum ACTH measurement helps to confirm a pituitary adenoma. High-resolution MRI is used to identify the adenoma. When imaging is negative, petrosal sinus sampling for ACTH is sometimes required for diagnosis after CRH or desmopressin stimulation.

Imaging Strategy
The primary modality in the imaging diagnosis of Cushing disease is MRI of the sella turcica. Because greater than 90% of Cushing disease is caused by microadenomas less than 1 cm in diameter, high-resolution imaging, including thin 1.0-1.5 mm slices and pre- and postcontrast spoiled gradient recalled acquisition in the steady state (SPGR) sequences, is needed to overcome artifact at the sphenoid sinus-sella turcica interface. Contrast-enhanced CT

has a lower sensitivity than MRI in diagnosis of pituitary adenomas. Evaluation of the musculoskeletal system primarily starts with radiographs to evaluate symptomatic bones and joints. MRI is highly sensitive to the osseous and muscular effects of chronic steroid and is frequently used to evaluate ON and secondary articular surface collapse. DXA is routinely used to evaluate bone density and response to treatment.

Radiography
- Osteopenia with radiolucency, cortical thinning, loss of vertebral trabecular pattern with endplate prominence (*empty box* appearance) (Figure 80.2C,D)
  - Insufficiency fractures especially of vertebral bodies (Figure 80.2C,D)
  - Acetabular protrusio
  - Described in Chapter 71, "Osteoporosis"
- ON commonly of the femoral or humeral heads and shafts
  - Mixed lucent and sclerotic appearance of bone
  - Collapse of the articular surfaces with *crescent sign* and loss of curved surface
  - Described in Chapter 115, "Osteonecroses and Osteochondroses"

Dual-Energy X-Ray Absorptiometry
- The diagnosis of osteoporosis is discussed in Chapter 71, "Osteoporosis."

Computed Tomography
- Accurate detection of ON
- Muscle atrophy and fatty infiltration, which slowly resolves with treatment

Magnetic Resonance Imaging
- Most sensitive imaging technique to detect ON and articular surface collapse (see Chapter 115, "Osteonecroses and Osteochondroses")
- Muscle atrophy with loss of muscle volume, fatty replacement with increased T1 signal and loss of fascicular architecture, reversible with treatment

Nuclear Medicine
- In cases of nonpituitary Cushing disease, indium-111 (^{111}In)-pentetreotide scintigraphy or PET to detect ectopic ACTH-producing neoplasm (eg, carcinoid tumor) (Figure 80.2A)

Treatment Options
- Treatment of pituitary adenomas in Cushing disease typically starts with transsphenoidal surgical resection.
- Medical treatment with or without adjunctive RT is reserved for patients with unsuccessful surgical resection or unresectable disease.
- Sella turcica imaging is used to detect recurrence with low serum morning cortisol the best predictor of remission.

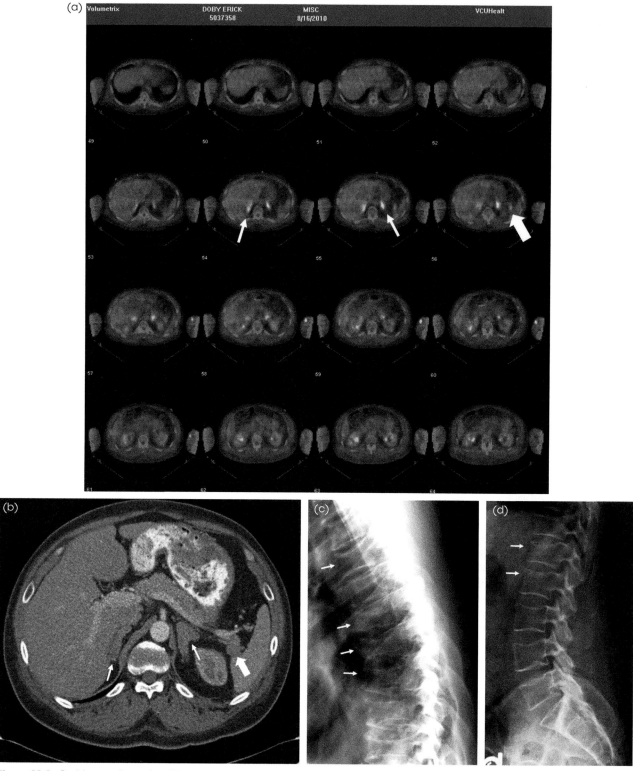

Figure 80.2. Cushing syndrome in a 37-year-old patient caused by ACTH-secreting pancreatic tumor. (*A*) Fused axial PET/CT images demonstrate increased metabolic activity within the adrenal glands (*thin arrows*) and less intense, but elevated uptake within the tail of the pancreas (*thick arrow*). (*B*) Axial postcontrast CT image demonstrates adrenal gland hyperplasia (*thin arrows*) and a tumor in the tail of the pancreas, as well as a fatty liver. Lateral radiographs of the (*C*) thoracic and (*D*) lumbar spine demonstrate multiple insufficiency fractures (*thin arrows*) with radiolucent, osteoporotic vertebrae.

Key Points

- Cushing disease caused by a pituitary microadenoma is the most common cause of endogenous hypercortisolism, but exogenous steroid is the most common cause overall.
- Osteoporosis and ON are common sequelae of Cushing disease that can often be detected radiographically, but DXA and MRI are often used for confirmation and treatment planning.

Recommended Reading

Boswell SB, Patel DB, White EA, et al. Musculoskeletal manifestations of endocrine disorders. *Clin Imaging*. 2014;38:384–96.

References

1. Bluestone R, Bywaters EG, Hartog M, Holt PJ, Hyde S. Acromegalic arthropathy. *Ann Rheum Dis*. 1971;30:243–58.
2. Boswell SB, Patel DB, White EA, et al. Musculoskeletal manifestations of endocrine disorders. *Clin Imaging*. 2014;38:384–96.
3. Chang CY, Rosenthal DI, Mitchell DM, Handa A, Kattapuram SV, Huang AJ. Imaging findings of metabolic bone disease. *Radiographics*. 2016;36:1871–87.
4. Dineen R, Stewart PM, Sherlock M. Acromegaly. *QJM*. 2017;110(7):411–20.
5. Lonser RR, Nieman L, Oldfield EH. Cushing's disease: pathobiology, diagnosis, and management. *J Neurosurg*. 2017;126:404–17.
6. Markenson JA. Rheumatic manifestations of endocrine diseases. *Curr Opin Rheumatol*. 2010;22:64–71.
7. Snyder P. Causes of hypopituitarism. *UpToDate*. Updated October 4, 2017. www.uptodate.com/contents/causes-of-hypopituitarism.
8. Wakely SL. The posterior vertebral scalloping sign. *Radiology*. 2006;239(2):607–609.

CHAPTER 81

Thyroid Diseases

Kevin B. Hoover

Introduction

High levels of thyroid hormone (hyperthyroidism) or low hormone levels (hypothyroidism) are associated with a variety of musculoskeletal manifestations. Two of the most clinically significant are development of low bone mass in hyperthyroidism and myopathy in both hyperthyroidism and hypothyroidism, both of which may reverse or improve with treatment. Other changes caused by thyroid disease, such as thyroid acropachy, are irreversible.

Pathophysiology and Clinical Findings

Thyroid hormone (TH) is a product of the follicular cells of the thyroid gland regulated via the hypothalamic-pituitary axis. TH production is regulated by thyroid-hormone-releasing hormone produced by the hypothalamus, which stimulates the pituitary gland to secrete thyroid-stimulating hormone (TSH). TSH stimulates the production of TH by the thyroid gland. Two forms of TH are triiodothyronine (T3, more active) and thyroxine (T4, less active) with T4 converted to T3 after secretion. A variety of conditions that disrupt the hypothalamic-pituitary axis are associated with abnormal TH levels (Table 81.1). Because of its central role in metabolism, TH dysregulation affects nearly every organ in the body. Serum T3, T4, and TSH are measured to detect dysregulation.

Hyperthyroidism

Excess osteoclast activity in hyperthyroidism causes osteopenia and osteoporosis. This preferentially involves cortical bone. Myopathy is found in up to 67% patients especially involving the proximal extremities, which are similar to hypothyroidism and resolves with treatment. Clinical evidence of adhesive capsulitis is also common, which also resolves with treatment. Thyroid acropachy is a rare manifestation of Graves disease (~0.5-1%) patients with treated or healing hyperthyroidism, which is typically irreversible. It is associated with periostitis primarily of the metacarpals, clubbing, nail changes, swelling of digits, arthralgia, exophthalmos (thyroid ophthalmopathy), and pretibial nodules (myxedema). In hyperthyroid patients, antithyroglobulin testing is performed in addition to testing TSH and TH levels, to exclude Graves disease, which is the most common cause of hyperthyroidism (Table 81.1).

Hypothyroidism

Iodine deficiency is the most common cause of hypothyroidism worldwide, but autoimmune Hashimoto thyroiditis is most common in the United States (Table 81.1). Hypothyroidism often presents with stiffness of the joints of the hands and knees. There are often noninflammatory joint effusions containing calcium pyrophosphate crystals. In adults, proximal muscle myopathy is common (25-79% patients) with proximal muscle weakness and delayed reflexes. Carpal tunnel syndrome (CTS) is a presenting condition in approximately 7% of patients. Diagnosis is made by serum TSH and free T4 concentration. The TSH value is commonly high and T4 low in primary hypothyroidism because of underlying thyroid glandular disease.

Imaging Strategy

Thyroid imaging using nuclear medicine and US are the primary imaging modalities used in the diagnosis and management of thyroid diseases. A radioactive iodine uptake (RAIU) scan with I-123, or I-131 with technetium-99m pertechnetate, is used to generate a thyroid image and determine iodine uptake. Thyroid US can detect nodules that may be secretory and hypervascular in some diseases (eg, Graves disease). DXA is important to diagnose and manage hyperthyroidism-related osteoporosis. Radiographs are a first-line modality to evaluate bone and joint symptoms. CT and MRI of the musculoskeletal system are not standard in the evaluation of thyroid disease, however, myopathic changes can be detected.

Imaging Findings

Hyperthyroidism
Radiography
- Findings include osteopenia associated with osteoporosis:
  - Fractures including vertebrae, femoral neck, and distal radius
- Thyroid acropachy results in periosteal new bone formation in the hands more often than feet (Figure 81.1):
  - Metacarpals and metatarsals more than phalanges
  - Often asymmetric

Dual-Energy X-Ray Absorptiometry
- Central and peripheral DXA are used to diagnose and monitor response to treatment with bisphosphonates or parathyroid hormone agonists.
  - See Chapter 71, "Osteoporosis" for a detailed discussion.

Table 81.1. Causes of Thyroid Disease

HYPERTHYROIDISM	HYPOTHYROIDISM
Toxic multinodular goiter	Autoimmune Hashimoto thyroiditis
Graves disease	Pituitary adenoma
Toxic thyroid adenoma	Sheehan syndrome
Subacute thyroiditis (de Quervain thyroiditis)	Postpartum thyroiditis
Thyroid-stimulating hormone (TSH)-secreting pituitary adenoma	Drug induced (lithium)
Metastatic thyroid carcinoma	Iodine deficiency
Gestational trophoblastic disease	Surgery
Struma ovarii	
Exogenous (factitious) hyperthyroidism from dietary and/or medical supplementation	

Computed Tomography and Magnetic Resonance Imaging
- Myopathy with decreased muscle size and fatty infiltration with low attenuation (CT) or increased T1 signal (MRI)

Hypothyroidism
Radiography
- Delayed skeletal maturation and decreased growth
  - Delayed epiphyseal ossification as a child continuing into adulthood with open physes, shortened bones, small epiphyses
  - Abnormal, *stippled* epiphyses with multiple ossification centers

- Shortened AP diameter of calvarium (brachycephaly) caused by premature coronal suture fusion
- Hypoplastic paranasal sinuses and mastoid air cells
- CPPD
  - See Chapter 36, "Calcium Pyrophosphate Dihydrate Deposition Disease"

Treatment Options
- Hyperthyroidism caused by Graves disease, toxic multinodular goiter, or toxic adenoma are most commonly treated with radioactive iodine ablation in the United States, but medical therapy and surgery are also used.
- Surgical treatment of hyperthyroidism has lower rate of treatment failure and risk of hypothyroidism.
- Synthetic T4 (levothyroxine) is standard for treatment of hypothyroidism with dose adjustments based on serum TSH levels.

Key Points
- Muscle weakness is a common musculoskeletal complaint in both hyperthyroidism and hypothyroidism. On cross-sectional imaging, this can be accompanied by fatty muscle atrophy that usually reverses with treatment.
- The arthralgia of hypothyroidism is associated with CPPD.
- Hyperthyroidism is associated with osteopenia and in patients with Graves disease, thyroid acropachy, with characteristic hyperostosis involving the metacarpals and metatarsals.

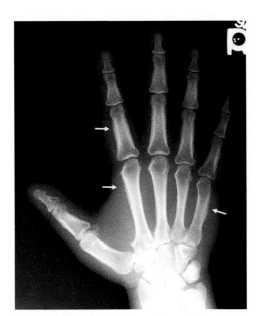

Figure 81.1. Thyroid acropachy in a 44-year-old man with a history of treated Graves disease. A PA hand radiograph demonstrates diffuse cortical thickening with aggressive asymmetric periostitis (*thin arrows*).

Recommended Reading
Boswell SB, Patel DB, White EA, et al. Musculoskeletal manifestations of endocrine disorders. *Clin Imaging.* 2014;38:384–96.

References

1. Anwar S, Gibofsky A. Musculoskeletal manifestations of thyroid disease. *Rheum Dis Clin North Am.* 2010;36:637–46.
2. Boswell SB, Patel DB, White EA, et al. Musculoskeletal manifestations of endocrine disorders. *Clin Imaging.* 2014;38:384–96.
3. Cakir M, Samanci N, Balci N, Balci MK. Musculoskeletal manifestations in patients with thyroid disease. *Clin Endocrinol (Oxf).* 2003;59:162–67.
4. Chang CY, Rosenthal DI, Mitchell DM, Handa A, Kattapuram SV, Huang AJ. Imaging findings of metabolic bone disease. *Radiographics.* 2016;36:1871–87.
5. Hoang JK, Sosa JA, Nguyen XV, Galvin PL, Oldan JD. Imaging thyroid disease: updates, imaging approach, and management pearls. *Radiol Clin North Am.* 2015;53:145–61.
6. Vanhoenacker FM, Pelckmans MC, De Beuckeleer LH, Colpaert CG, De Schepper AM. Thyroid acropachy: correlation of imaging and pathology. *Eur Radiol.* 2001;11:1058–62.
7. Yap FY, Skalski MR, Patel DB, et al. Hypertrophic osteoarthropathy: clinical and imaging features. *Radiographics.* 2017;37:157–95.

CHAPTER 82

Parathyroid Diseases and Renal Osteodystrophy

Kevin B. Hoover

Introduction

Parathyroid hormone (PTH) regulates serum calcium homeostasis along with vitamin D and calcitonin. Low PTH levels (hypoparathyroidism) result in low serum calcium, and elevated PTH levels (hyperparathyroidism) result in increased serum calcium and phosphate. Detection of parathyroid disease is often incidental with abnormal calcium levels detected on basic metabolic blood tests. DXA is routinely used to evaluate bone density in parathyroid diseases, and in the detection of parathyroid adenomas or ectopic sources of PTH in hyperparathyroidism using US and technetium 99m (^{99m}Tc)-sestamibi. Many of the characteristic changes of parathyroid disease can be seen on radiographs.

Hypoparathyroidism

Pathophysiology and Clinical Findings

The most common cause of hypoparathyroidism is parathyroid gland removal during thyroidectomy, radical neck dissection, or parathyroidectomy. Other causes include agenesis of the parathyroid glands, autoimmune-mediated disease, and genetic defects (eg, DiGeorge syndrome). Chronic kidney disease (CKD) is a common sequela. Pseudohypoparathyroidism is caused by end-organ insensitivity to PTH. There are 2 main types (types 1 and 2) with variable PTH levels and heritability. Pseudohypoparathyroidism, termed *Albright hereditary osteodystrophy*, is associated with a spectrum of findings that includes short stature, rounded facies, central obesity, subcutaneous calcifications, and mild intellectual disability. In hypoparathyroidism, the PTH level is normal or low in the setting of hypocalcemia. In pseudohypoparathyroidism, the findings are similar, except for elevated PTH levels.

Imaging Strategy

Imaging is not routinely acquired or needed for the diagnosis or management of hypoparathyroidism.

Imaging Findings

Hypoparathyroidism
Radiography
- Primary hypoparathyroidism causes an increase in bone mass:
  - Osteosclerosis and thickening of calvaria, narrowed diploic space
  - Spinal ossification similar to psoriatic arthritis is less common
  - Incidental soft tissue calcifications of shoulder joints, subcutaneous tissues of the hands (also basal ganglia, lenses with cataracts)
  - Crystal deposition (secondary to renal disease) including CPPD, monosodium urate, calcium hydroxyapatite
- Secondary hypoparathyroidism (Albright hereditary osteodystrophy) has the following findings:
  - Metatarsal and metacarpal shortening, usually of the fourth or fifth digits
  - Short middle and distal phalanges
  - Coned epiphyses of the phalanges, metacarpals, and metatarsals
  - Widening of the metacarpals and metatarsals
  - Occasionally spinal ossifications are present.

Dual-Energy X-Ray Absorptiometry
- Primary hypoparathyroidism associated with elevated bone mineral density (BMD) on DXA
- Spine more than hip

Hyperparathyroidism

Pathophysiology and Clinical Findings

Primary, secondary, and tertiary hyperparathyroidism are the 3 general categories of disease. Primary hyperparathyroidism is caused by excess secretion of PTH from the parathyroid glands most often by a parathyroid adenoma that is not regulated by serum calcium levels (Table 82.1). Up to 80% of patients with primary hyperparathyroidism are asymptomatic with hypercalcemia and elevated PTH levels. Secondary hyperparathyroidism is more common than primary disease with an increase in PTH levels caused by sustained serum hypocalcemia. Laboratory findings of secondary hyperparathyroidism include decreased serum calcium, decreased vitamin D levels, and either increased (in chronic renal disease) or decreased serum phosphate (in disorders of phosphate absorption) levels. Tertiary hyperparathyroidism occurs when patients with chronic secondary hyperparathyroidism acquire secondary parathyroid hyperplasia. These patients

Table 82.1. Causes of Hyperparathyroidism

PRIMARY	SECONDARY	TERTIARY
Parathyroid adenoma (80-85% of primary disease)	Chronic kidney disease (most common overall)	Chronic kidney disease
Glandular hyperplasia (10-15%)	Dietary calcium deficiency	
Parathyroid carcinoma (<1%)	Vitamin D disorders	
Multiple endocrine neoplasiatypes 1 and 2A	Conditions with disrupted phosphate metabolism	
Familial hypocalciuric hypercalcemia		
Familialisolated hyperparathyroidism		

have similar elevated calcium and phosphate levels to primary hyperparathyroidism.

Imaging Strategy
Radiography of symptomatic bones and joints is the first-line imaging study. Because of osteopenia, however, cross-sectional imaging may be valuable to detect subtle insufficiency-type fractures. Cross-sectional imaging is also used in characterization of brown tumors and possible pathologic fractures. A DXA scan is acquired every 12 months in conservatively treated hyperparathyroid patients (who do not undergo parathyroidectomy) to manage bone mass.

Imaging Findings

Hyperparathyroidism
Radiography
- Bone resorption is the earliest abnormality:

- Subperiosteal resorption is pathognomonic for hyperparathyroidism and one of the earliest findings that may resolve with treatment:
    - Characteristic phalangeal involvement
        - Tufts with eventual acroosteolysis
        - Radial aspect of the middle phalanges, especially the index and middle fingers (Figure 82.1)
        - Scalloping and cortical destruction
    - Medial tibia, humerus, femur
- Cortical resorption is seen, especially in the hands with cortical tunneling, endosteal scalloping, and cortical thinning:
- Trabecular resorption with osteopenia is seen:
    - Granular *salt-and-pepper* appearance, especially in the calvarium, resembling multiple myeloma
    - *Smudgy* trabecular appearance
- Imaging shows subchondral resorption:
    - Most commonly seen in the SI, sternoclavicular, AC, and symphysis pubis joints as well as the intervertebral disc margins.

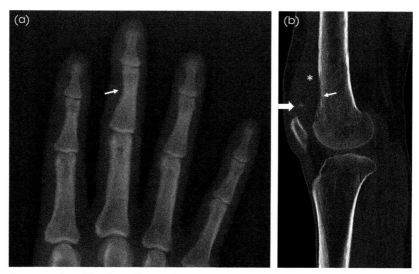

Figure 82.1. Secondary hyperparathyroidism in a 49-year-old man with CKD on dialysis. (*A*) Magnified PA radiograph of the fingers shows severe osteopenia with characteristic subperiosteal resorption of the radial margin of the middle phalanges (*thin arrow*). (*B*) Sagittal reformatted CT image from the left knee demonstrates an avulsion fracture of the quadriceps tendon (*thick arrow*) with associated joint effusion (*asterisk*). Subperiosteal resorption of the anterior aspect of the distal femoral metadiaphysis is also evident (*thin arrow*).

- Joint-space widening or *pseudowidening* is seen, especially at the SI joints, with iliac greater than sacral joint margin resorption:
  - Mimics seronegative spondyloarthropathies (SpA)
  - In the hands, starts at DIP and moves proximally to PIP and MCP joints.
  - The AC joint involves the clavicle more than the acromion.
  - Imaging shows subligamentous and subtendinous resorption:
    - Ischial tuberosities, femoral trochanters, coracoclavicular ligament insertions
    - Smooth scalloping or irregular margins, may mimic SpA
- Brown tumor (osteoclastoma, osteitis fibrosa cystica) is caused by excess osteoclastic resorption because of elevated PTH (Figure 82.2):
  - Lytic, sharply demarcated
  - Central or eccentric
  - Pelvis, ribs, femora, facial bones, long bone metaphyses
  - More often solitary than multiple
  - Occur in approximately 3% of primary hyperparathyroid patients and 2% of secondary hyperparathyroid patients, but more common in secondary disease because of its overall higher prevalence
  - May resolve with treatment
- Chondrocalcinosis is seen, particularly involving the menisci of the knee and the TFC of the wrist:
  - Also articular cartilage, ligaments, tendons, and synovium
  - Population similar to brown tumor and more common in primary hyperparathyroidism, but overall more prevalent in secondary disease
- Weakened tendons are caused by decreased collagen synthesis:
  - Especially rupture of quadriceps, patellar, and triceps tendons (Figure 82.1)

Computed Tomography
- Useful to exclude pathologic fractures arising from large brown tumors

Magnetic Resonance Imaging
- MRI is sometimes used to evaluate brown tumors, especially solitary lesions, which can have overlapping features with other solid lesions:
  - Cystic appearance is imaged; hyperintense on fluid-sensitive sequences, hypointense on T1W images with rim enhancement on T1W FS postcontrast images (Figure 82.2).
  - Tumors contain fibrous tissue, necrosis, and liquefaction.
- MRI is highly sensitive in detecting insufficiency and fragility fractures caused by osteoporosis.
- Torn tendons are often detected by fluid signal coursing through or along tendons (acute), or tendon attenuation or thickening (chronic).

Renal Osteodystrophy

Pathophysiology and Clinical Findings
The complex metabolic alterations resulting from chronic renal failure and its treatment by dialysis and renal transplant are currently described as chronic kidney disease mineral and bone-related disorder (CKD-MBD). The term *renal osteodystrophy* is applied specifically to the bone changes of CKD-MBD. Decreased renal function results in hypocalcemia because of retention of phosphate, which binds to serum calcium resulting in low active (ionized) calcium, and decreased activation of vitamin D with lower gastrointestinal absorption of calcium. Hypocalcemia, in turn, causes hyperparathyroidism with the release of calcium from bone, decreasing bone mineralization and altering bone turnover and volume. This is exacerbated by the development of resistance to the effects of PTH, further increasing PTH levels. Dialysis-associated changes may also be present in this patient population, which are associated with serum β_2 microglobulin elevation and considered part of the CKD-MBD.

Renal osteodystrophy results in a 2- to 14-fold increase in fracture risk, which remains elevated in patients treated with hemodialysis and, even more so, renal transplant. *Adynamic bone disease* (ABD) is the term used to describe low bone turnover. Its causes are multifactorial including aluminum toxicity, hypoparathyroidism caused by overtreatment with calcium and vitamin D, PTH resistance, uremia, and diabetes mellitus resulting in low collagen synthesis and mineralization. Other musculoskeletal changes of CKD-MBD include erosive osteoarthropathy and destructive spondyloarthropathy, which are also multifactorial related to amyloidosis, hyperparathyroidism, CPPD, metabolic bone disease, and ligamentous laxity. Infections frequently arise because of chronic disease, immunosuppression (eg, transplantation), recurrent arteriovenous (AV) fistula and graft access, and secondary infection of areas of ON. The soft tissue calcifications associated with CKD-MBD are precipitates of crystalline calcium-phosphate salts and CPPD.

Imaging Strategy
The imaging strategy is similar to hyperparathyroidism. DXA is used to evaluate any patient who may benefit from osteoporosis treatment. Radiography is the primary modality in evaluating symptomatic patients. MRI and nuclear scintigraphy are used primarily to evaluate for radiographically occult fracture or infection in osteopenic or osteoporotic patients.

Imaging Findings
Radiography
- Findings of primary hyperparathyroidism are detected including bone resorption, brown tumors, and chondrocalcinosis.
- Renal osteodystrophy also results in other findings because of abnormal bone mineralization and volume:
  - Hypocalcemia results in rickets in children or osteomalacia in adults.
    - Osteomalacia results in coarsened bony trabeculae and pseudofractures (Looser zones).

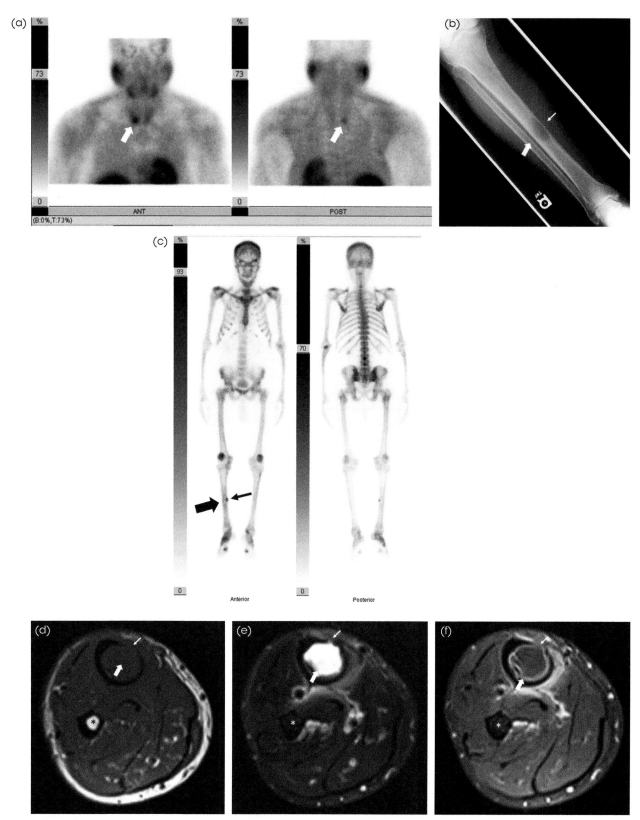

Figure 82.2. Primary hyperparathyroidism in a 58-year-old man with a parathyroid adenoma and a brown tumor. (*A*) A sestamibi scan demonstrates focal uptake superimposed on the lower pole of the right lobe of the thyroid gland (*thick arrow*) on anterior (*left*) and posterior (*right*) images consistent with a solitary parathyroid adenoma. (*B*) An AP radiograph of the tibia and fibula shows a solitary well-circumscribed, lytic bone lesion involving the tibial shaft (*thick arrow*) with a faint area of increased density (*thin arrow*) consistent with callus about the occult pathologic fracture. (*C*) A methylene diphosphonate (MDP) bone scan demonstrates a focus of hyperintense uptake in the cortex of the right tibia (*thin arrow*) adjacent to an area of subtle photopenia (*thick arrow*), corresponding to the lesion seen in (*B*). (*D*) Axial T1W, (*E*) T2W FS, and (*F*) T1W FS postcontrast MR images show bone marrow replacing lesion in the tibial diaphysis of low signal in (*D*), high signal in (*E*), and peripheral enhancement in (*F*) consistent with pathologically proven fibrous tissue representative of a brown tumor (*thick arrows*). Note cortical breakthrough of the medial tibial cortex with surrounding edema (*thin arrows*) consistent with a pathologic fracture. On all MR sequences, note normal bone marrow signal in the fibular diaphysis at the same level (*asterisks*).

- Loss of bone density (osteopenia), loss of cortical bone definition, bone resorption, and ABD can occur.
  - ABD is low bone turnover without osteoid accumulation associated with cortical and trabecular thinning.
- New bone formation with osteosclerosis can also occur more commonly in the axial (skull, pelvis, vertebrae) than the appendicular skeleton.
  - Vertebral endplate sclerosis called *rugger jersey spine*
  - Does not resolve with treatment
  - Uncommon in primary hyperparathyroidism
  - See Chapter 71, "Osteoporosis" and Chapter 72, "Rickets and Osteomalacia" for further discussion.
- Soft tissue calcifications are seen in up to 27% of CKD-MBD patients:
  - Primary locations include ocular, arterial, cartilaginous, periarticular, and visceral
  - Arterial *pipe stem* appearance, commonly seen with the dorsalis pedis artery of the foot and radial artery of the wrist
  - Chondrocalcinosis similar to primary hyperparathyroidism
  - Periarticular cloudlike calcifications
    - Multifocal, symmetrical, and can extend into joint
    - Also involve the bursae, tendons, and ligaments
    - May appear tumoral as lobulated masses indistinguishable from hereditary tumoral calcinosis
    - Mixed salt deposition, hydroxyapatite crystal deposition disease (HADD), CPPD, calcium hydroxyapatite, monosodium urate, especially around large joints
- Dialysis-related changes of CKD-MBD include amyloid deposition, destructive spondyloarthropathy, erosive osteoarthropathy, ON, infection, and tendinopathy and tendon tearing:
  - Amyloid deposition results in CTS in up to 31% of patients.
  - Destructive spondyloarthropathy simulates spondylodiscitis.
    - Osteolytic areas near endplates
    - Bone sclerosis of vertebral endplates with minimal osteophytosis
    - Narrowed or absent disc spaces
    - Cervical or craniocervical joints often involved
  - Erosive arthropathy of hands mimics both OA and RA.
    - Transplantation halts progression, but does not reverse arthropathy.
  - See the detailed discussion in Chapter 51, "Amyloidosis."
  - ON is also associated with long-term dialysis and renal transplantation.
  - Infection manifests most commonly as septic arthritis and osteomyelitis.
  - Extensor tendon pathology can result in abnormal patellar positioning, especially patella baja with quadriceps tendon rupture.

Computed Tomography
- Can be useful in evaluating for fracture including those associated with destructive spondyloarthropathy (Figure 82.3B), brown tumors, and osteomalacia

Dual-Energy X-Ray Absorptiometry
- Measures bone mass or quantity and predicts fracture risk in CKD-MBD
  - Central and distal radius measurements associated with fracture risk
  - Same T-score cut-offs for osteoporosis and osteopenia as for general population
  - WHO Fracture Risk Assessment (FRAX) tool not yet been shown to be predictive of fractures in CKD patients (see Chapter 71 on osteoporosis for a discussion on FRAX)

Magnetic Resonance Imaging
- Detects changes of destructive spondyloarthropathy (see Chapter 51)
- Detects tendinosis and tendon ruptures, especially the Achilles, quadriceps, and rotator cuff tendons
- Highly sensitive in detecting chronic hemodialysis-related ON

Nuclear Medicine
- Nuclear scintigraphic bone scan not routinely used in diagnosis, but may be used in evaluating for insufficiency fractures (Figure 82.2).
  - May show diffuse uptake in the skeleton with absent renal uptake- superscan

Treatment Options
- Hypoparathyroidism is treated with IV calcium in severely symptomatic cases with oral calcium and vitamin D treatment used for long-term management.
- Parathyroidectomy is the standard treatment for hyperparathyroidism.

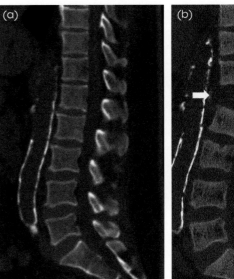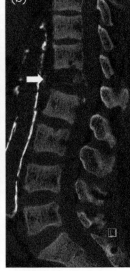

Figure 82.3. CKD-MBD in a patient with polycystic kidney disease. (*A*) Sagittal reformatted CT image of the lumbar spine demonstrates normal bony structures. Note atherosclerotic calcifications. (*B*) Three years later after the development of renal failure and beginning dialysis, diffuse bony sclerosis developed with destructive spondyloarthropathy of the L1 vertebra (*thick arrow*).

- For CKD-MBD and renal osteodystrophy, renal replacement therapy by dialysis or transplantation are standard.
- Dialysis (peritoneal or hemodialysis) improves bone changes of hyperparathyroidism, but ABD is more resistant.
- Renal transplantation improves renal osteodystrophy and soft tissue calcifications.
- Vitamin D and calcium replacement are used.
- Antiresorptive agents (eg, bisphosphonates) and osteoanabolic agents (eg, teriparatide) have been used, however, without support of randomized controlled trials.

Key Points
- CKD-MBD is the most common cause of parathyroid disease.
- Renal osteodystrophy is defined as the bone changes of CKD-MBD, including changes caused by primary hyperparathyroidism and kidney disease treatment.
- Resorption of bone is the most important radiographic finding in primary hyperparathyroidism.
- Increase in bone density is the most specific radiographic and DXA finding in hypoparathyroidism.

Recommended Reading
Chang CY, Rosenthal DI, Mitchell DM, Handa A, Kattapuram SV, Huang AJ. Imaging findings of metabolic bone disease. *Radiographics*. 2016;36:1871–87.

Lim CY, Ong KO. Various musculoskeletal manifestations of chronic renal insufficiency. *Clin Radiol*. 2013;68:e397–411.

References
1. Babayev R, Nickolas TL. Bone disorders in chronic kidney disease: an update in diagnosis and management. *Semin Dial*. 2015;28:645–53.
2. Chang CY, Rosenthal DI, Mitchell DM, Handa A, Kattapuram SV, Huang AJ. Imaging findings of metabolic bone disease. *Radiographics*. 2016;36:1871–87.
3. Lim CY, Ong KO. Various musculoskeletal manifestations of chronic renal insufficiency. *Clin Radiol*. 2013;68:e397–411.
4. Markenson JA. Rheumatic manifestations of endocrine diseases. *Curr Opin Rheumatol*. 2010;22:64–71.
5. Mitchell DM, Regan S, Cooley MR, et al. Long-term follow-up of patients with hypoparathyroidism. *J Clin Endocrinol Metab*. 2012;97:4507–14.
6. Moe S, Drueke T, Cunningham J, et al. Definition, evaluation, and classification of renal osteodystrophy: a position statement from Kidney Disease: Improving Global Outcomes (KDIGO). *Kidney Int*. 2006;69:1945–53.
7. West SL, Lok CE, Langsetmo L, et al. Bone mineral density predicts fractures in chronic kidney disease. *J Bone Miner Res*. 2015;30:913–19.

Lysosomal Storage Diseases

CHAPTER 83

Lipidoses

Kevin B. Hoover

Introduction

Lysosomal storage diseases (LSDs) are caused by the accumulation of proteins, polysaccharides, and lipids in the lysosomes of cells because of a genetic failure of enzymes needed for their breakdown. The progressive accumulation of substrates frequently affects the skeleton. The pathophysiology is not completely understood and likely involves a complicated interplay of substrate storage, tissue inflammation, and epigenetic factors. LSDs can be categorized as sphingolipidoses and mucolipidoses, and mucopolysaccharidoses (discussed in Chapter 84, "Mucopolysaccharidoses"). Table 83.1 summarizes the incidence and musculoskeletal findings of the sphingolipidoses and mucolipidoses, which are groups of diseases that share musculoskeletal imaging findings. Diagnosis relies primarily on peripheral blood lysosomal enzyme activity, but DNA testing is the most reliable technique for definitive diagnosis and detecting disease transmission.

Gaucher Disease

Pathophysiology and Clinical Findings

Gaucher disease (GD) is an autosomal recessive disorder caused by deficient β-glucocerebrosidase activity and accumulation of the lipid glucosylceramide. Macrophages, when filled with glucosylceramide, are referred to as *Gaucher cells*, which have a characteristic *crumpled silk appearance* of the cytoplasm. GD is the most common LSD and is classically subdivided into 3 different phenotypes. Type I GD is by far the most frequent with a particularly high frequency in the Ashkenazi Jewish population (1 in 850). There is no central nervous system involvement, although Parkinson disease has been described in these patients. Type 1 GD has a highly variable presentation, even among twins, which most often involves the bone (80%), but also results in cytopenia and hepatosplenomegaly. Types 2 and 3 GD are much less frequent and have either acute (type 2) or chronic (type 3) neurologic disease. Patients with type 2 GD die in infancy, and patients with type 3 GD present in childhood with a less severe phenotype.

Bone complications can be a first symptom of disease, presenting as bone crises, which are episodes of excruciating pain, possibly necessitating hospitalization for pain management. Patients also suffer from a chronic inflammatory state that is exacerbated during these crises, which are often accompanied by localized warmth and swelling, leukocytosis, raised ESR and fever, similar in presentation to juvenile idiopathic arthritis (JIA) and RA. Up to 43% of patients have a history of ON with up to 22% undergoing joint replacement. Osteoporosis is common in patients with GD, possibly related to chronic inflammation, in a similar fashion to the osteoporosis of JIA and RA. Both longer disease duration and history of splenectomy are associated with ON and osteoporosis.

Imaging Strategy

MRI is the imaging modality of choice. Sagittal T1W and STIR sequences of the lumbar spine, coronal T1W and STIR imaging of the pelvis, and coronal T1W and STIR sequences of both femora are optimal to evaluate disease status. In younger patients, T1W and STIR images of the tibias are useful, because the presence of red marrow in the femurs can make the detection of involvement difficult. Patients should have follow-up imaging every 12-24 months and/or at times of enzyme replacement therapy or substrate removal therapy (ERT and SRT, respectively). At the same sitting, axial T1W and T2W images are acquired through the upper abdomen to assess severity of spleen and liver involvement. DXA scanning is generally recommended for the evaluation and follow-up of bone density at 1-2 year intervals. The use of radiography is limited to evaluation of acute pain (eg, exclude fractures). Nuclear medicine, especially technetium 99m sestamibi (^{99m}Tc-sestamibi), is a useful alternative in evaluating disease status in patients with GD who are unable to undergo MRI or when MRI is unavailable.

Imaging Findings
Radiography

- Radiography is insensitive to marrow infiltration:
  - Detects changes in 30-40% of patients with GD
- Characteristic features include Erlenmeyer flask deformity of the femora, osteopenia, and sclerosis:
  - Cortical thinning and expansion of the distal metaphysis and metadiaphysis are seen with Erlenmeyer flask deformity (Figures 83.1 and 83.2):
    - An early clue to the diagnosis of GD, but neither sensitive or specific
    - Also detected in Niemann-Pick disease (NPD) and other conditions (Box 83.1)
  - Osteopenia is nearly universal in both children and adults:
    - Localized or diffuse
    - Associated with an increased risk of fragility fracture and reported in up to 28% of patients with GD
  - Areas of sclerosis caused by ON may be detected, especially involving the spine, pelvis, and proximal long bones (Figure 83.2):

Table 83.1. Musculoskeletal Characteristics of the Sphingolipidoses and Mucolipidoses

CONDITION	INCIDENCE	MUSCULOSKELETAL FINDINGS
SPHINGOLIPIDOSES		
Fabry disease	1:40,000–60,000 (males)	Short stature, crises of burning and aching pain in hands and feet, arthralgia, exercise intolerance, osteonecrosis with or without secondary osteoarthritis osteopenia/osteoporosis
Gaucher disease type I (nonneuropathic type)	1:40,000–60,000	Short stature, chronic bone pain and/or acute bone crises, osteonecrosis with or without secondary osteoarthritis, osteopenia/osteoporosis, recurrent fractures, Erlenmeyer flask deformities
Niemann-Pick disease (types A-C)	A-B: 1:250,000; C: 1:150,000	Erlenmeyer flask deformities, osteonecrosis
MUCOLIPIDOSES		
Mucolipidosis (ML) I (sialidosis syndrome)	1:5,000,000	Dysostosis multiplex (Table 83.2), myoclonic epilepsy
ML II (I-cell disease)	1:640,000	Disproportional short stature, joint stiffness/contractures, hip dysplasia, genu valgum, carpal tunnel syndrome, trigger fingers, dysostosis multiplex
ML III (pseudo-Hurler polydystrophy)	1:315,000	Disproportional short stature, joint stiffness/contractures, scoliosis, carpal tunnel syndrome, trigger fingers, dysostosis multiplex
α-Mannosidosis	1-1.6:500,000	Dysostosis multiplex

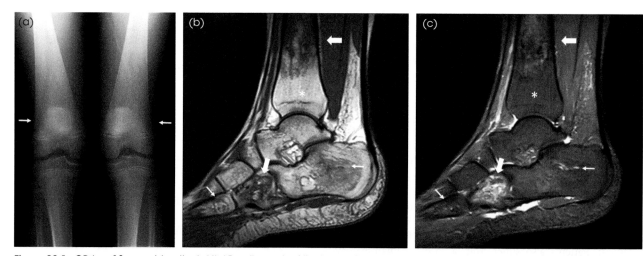

Figure 83.1. GD in a 13-year-old patient. (*A*) AP radiograph of the knees demonstrates the characteristic Erlenmeyer flask deformity of both distal femurs (*thin arrows*) with thin cortices consistent with osteopenia. (*B*) T1W and (*C*) STIR sagittal MR images of the ankle demonstrate areas of heterogeneous signal in the distal tibia and cuboid bone consistent with areas of ON (*thick arrows*). Heterogeneous signal within the calcaneus and proximal fifth metatarsal is abnormal (*thin arrows*), which may represent ON. Areas of normal fatty marrow (*asterisk*) caused by ERT are present.

Dual-Energy X-ray Absorptiometry

- Bone marrow density (BMD) in GD is significantly lower than expected for age and sex:
  - BMD is decreased centrally (lumbar spine, femoral neck) and peripherally (distal radius).

Magnetic Resonance Imaging

- Imaging shows infiltrated bone marrow in GD (relative to subcutaneous fat):
  - Decreased bone marrow signal on T1 and T2W sequences without fat saturation and relatively hyperintense fluid sensitive sequences is related to infiltration by Gaucher cells.
  - MRI may show a *salt-and-pepper pattern* because of scattered involvement.
  - Diffusely homogeneous or heterogenous patterns are seen.
  - Abnormal signal may persist after treatment.
  - Degree of bone involvement is unrelated to visceral involvement.
  - Treatment with ERT or SRT may lead to rapid recurrence of bright T1 fatty marrow signal within 1 year.
  - ON with characteristic signal changes may be present (Figure 83.1*B,C*).
- Extraosseous extension of Gaucher cells is rare and resembles malignancy, usually requiring biopsy.
- Assessment of GD burden is primarily qualitative (descriptive), but other methods are used at specialty centers:
  - Bone marrow burden (BMB) scores severity of disease by degree of signal intensity loss relative to subcutaneous fat on T1W and T2W imaging and by how diffuse replacement is (eg, basivertebral fat replacement, epiphyseal involvement) (Figure 83.3).
    - Stabilizes 5 years after ERT treatment
  - Quantitation of GD burden using T1 relaxation, chemical shift imaging and spectroscopy is used primarily in research.
  - Marrow signal changes of ON in GD is similar to other causes (see Chapter 115, "Osteonecroses and Osteochondroses").
  - ON is detected in GD even without a history of bone crisis.
  - Focal areas of increased T2 signal may represent bone crisis and represent a precursor to ON.

Nuclear Medicine

- In GD, ^{99m}Tc-sestamibi accumulates in areas of infiltration and is direct evidence of disease burden:
  - This is particularly useful in children in differentiating residual normal red marrow from pathologically infiltrated marrow.
  - ^{99m}Tc-sulfur colloid is taken up by normal bone marrow with reduced or abnormally distributed tracer uptake seen with GD infiltration.
  - The main disadvantages are poor spatial resolution and high radiation dose.

Treatment Options

- ERT with purified glucocerebrosidase is the most effective treatment for GD, which can prevent bone disease, reduce organomegaly, and improve anemia.

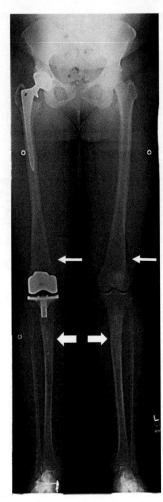

Figure 83.2. GD in a 42-year-old patient. A stitched leg length series demonstrates Erlenmeyer flask deformities (*thin arrows*) and patchy osteosclerosis of the tibial shafts caused by ON (*thick arrows*). Right hip and knee joint replacements were caused by secondary OA from ON.

- Femoral and humeral epiphyseal involvement can be complicated by articular collapse and secondary OA.

Box 83.1. Example Conditions with Erlenmeyer Flask Deformity of the Femurs

Marrow infiltration disorders
Gaucher disease
Niemann-Pick disease
Thalassemia
Lead poisoning
Craniotubular bone dysplasias
Frontometaphyseal dysplasia
Otopalatodigital syndrome
Craniometaphyseal dysplasia
Pyle disease
Engelmann disease (diaphyseal dysplasia)
Osteopetrosis

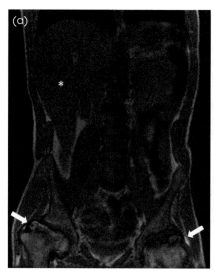 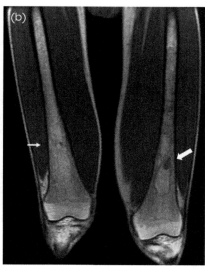 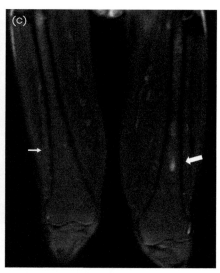

Figure 83.3. MRI of GD in a 45-year-old man. (A) Large field-of-view (FOV) T1W image demonstrates diffusely abnormal marrow signal with femoral head ON with articular surface collapse (thick arrows) and hepatomegaly (*asterisk*). Coronal T1W (B) and T2W with FS (C) images demonstrate diffuse marrow heterogeneity from ON (thick arrow) with asymmetric Erlenmeyer flask deformity on the right (thin arrow). Images courtesy of Jonathan Samet, MD, Lurie Children's Hospital, Chicago IL.

- Oral SRT with miglustat can give some benefit in mild- to moderately affected patients with GD with improvement in bone pain, improvement in BMD, and stabilization of MRI findings.
- Treatment for osteoporosis, such as bisphosphonates, calcium, and vitamin D, is given.
- Arthroplasty is recommended for treatment of ON-related OA.

Fabry Disease

Pathophysiology and Clinical Findings

Fabry disease (FD) is an X-linked recessive disease resulting in deficient galactosidase A. Together, GD and FD account for 20% of LSDs with a combined prevalence of 1 in 38,400 (live) births. Attacks of pain (Fabry crisis) in the extremities, similar to the bone crisis of GD, begin during adulthood or adolescence, decreasing in frequency and severity with age. Like GD, the Fabry crisis may be accompanied by systemic inflammation resulting in a misdiagnosis of inflammatory arthritis (eg, JIA, RA). The mean delay in diagnosis is approximately 14 years for male patients and 16 years in female heterozygotes from symptom onset. Similar to GD, osteopenia and osteoporosis are reported in patients with FD. More specific signs of FD include skin papules (angiokeratoma) and cornea color changes (cornea verticillata) with hypohidrosis or anhidrosis. Patients also experience gastrointestinal symptoms. Renal, cardiac, and cerebrovascular complications result in major morbidity if untreated.

Imaging Strategy

Although not as well-defined as for GD, a similar approach to evaluate the severity of disease involvement and response to treatment using MRI is practical. Nuclear medicine techniques are not well described for FD.

Imaging Findings
Radiography

- Loss of bone mass with osteopenia or osteoporosis is nearly universal in both children and adults with FD.
- ON may be detected, especially involving the spine, pelvis, and proximal long bones.
  - As in GD, this can be complicated by articular collapse and secondary OA.

Magnetic Resonance Imaging

- Assessment of marrow infiltration in FD has not been well described.
- Marrow signal changes of ON in FD is similar to other causes.

Treatment Options

- ERT is used for FD, but with a less consistent clinical response than GD.
- Bisphosphonates, calcium, and vitamin D are recommended for osteoporosis.
- Arthroplasty is used for severe joint disease.

Niemann-Pick Disease

Pathophysiology and Clinical Findings

NPD is an autosomal recessive disorder caused by deficiency of acid sphingomyelinase composed of 3 subtypes (A-C). The infiltration of bone marrow and spleen by lipid-engorged cells with a *soap bubble* appearance results in anemia and thrombocytopenia (also seen in GD). Neurologic involvement is common.

Imaging Strategy

A similar approach to evaluate the severity of musculoskeletal disease involvement and response to treatment using MRI is practical. Nuclear medicine techniques are not well described for NPD.

Imaging Findings
Radiography

- Erlenmeyer flask deformity is seen on imaging, which is neither sensitive or specific (Box 83.1).
- ON may be detected, which may be complicated by secondary OA.

Magnetic Resonance Imaging
- Assessment of marrow infiltration in NPD has not been well described.
- ON is similar in appearance to other causes.

Treatment Options
- Oral SRT with miglustat for NPD (type C)
- Bisphosphonates, calcium, and vitamin D for osteoporosis
- Arthroplasty

Mucolipidoses

Pathophysiology and Clinical Findings

Mucolipidosis (ML)—ML I, ML II, ML III, ML IV—and α-mannosidosis are rare, autosomal recessive genetic disorders caused by a deficiency in enzymes that metabolize glycoproteins. ML I-III result in musculoskeletal deformities resembling mucopolysaccharidosis (MPS) I. ML IV is not associated with skeletal disease. ML II rarely presents in adults because of death during childhood. There is a similar presentation of ML and MPS patients, described in Chapter 84, "Mucopolysaccharidoses." The treatment options are limited to treating symptoms as there are no medical treatments. These include surgery for cervical stenosis, kyphoscoliosis and hip dysplasia.

Imaging Strategy

The imaging strategy mirrors that of the MPS (see Chapter 84). The spectrum of findings seen in ML and MPS called *dysostosis multiplex* (Table 83.2) is evaluated using a baseline skeletal survey, typically acquired during childhood. Lateral flexion and extension radiographs of the cervical spine, a scoliosis series, and an AP pelvis radiograph should be obtained until skeletal maturity to evaluate for instability, gibbus deformity, and hip dysplasia. An annual cervical spine MRI may also be valuable given the frequency of cervical stenosis and its insidious onset.

Imaging Findings
Radiography

- Dysostosis multiplex is detected on radiographs (Table 83.2).
- Radiography is the primary technique to evaluate symptomatic patients.
- Atlantoaxial instability is detected on flexion-extension radiographs.
- Gibbus deformity with kyphosis is centered at the thoracolumbar junction:
  - Caused by L1 and L2 vertebral wedging deformity (see Chapter 84)

Magnetic Resonance Imaging
- Craniocervical stenosis caused by odontoid dysplasia and glycoprotein deposition (see Chapter 84)

Treatment Options
- Treatment is symptomatic.

Table 83.2. Radiology Manifestations of Dysostosis Multiplex Seen in the Mucolipidoses and Mucopolysaccharidoses	
Head	Macrocephaly; thickened skull; J-shaped sella turcica
Thorax	Short, wide clavicles; wide oar-shaped ribs;
Spine	Odontoid hypoplasia; anterior beaking of the lower thoracic and upper lumbar vertebral bodies; thoracolumbar kyphosis
Legs/arms	Shortened long bones; wide diaphysis; irregular metaphyses; narrow epiphyses
Hands/feet	Bullet-shaped phalanges; proximal pointing of metacarpals and metatarsals
Hips	Flattened acetabula; flaring of iliac wings; coxa valga deformity; dysplastic femoral heads; secondary osteoarthritis
Knees	Genu valgum; secondary subtalar varus

Key Points

- GD is the most common LSD and lipidosis with bone marrow replacement resulting in ON and osteoporosis. The other sphingolipidoses, FD and NPD, demonstrate similar findings.
- MRI of the spine, pelvis, and femurs is the primary imaging modality to evaluate disease and monitor treatment.
- Erlenmeyer flask deformity of the femurs is characteristic of GD and NPD, but is neither sensitive nor specific for disease.
- ML is a rare condition without effective treatments that results in bone changes similar to mucopolysaccharidoses.
- ERT is the primary treatment for GD with frequent joint replacements secondary to ON.

Recommended Reading

Katz R, Booth T, Hargunani R, Wylie P, Holloway B. Radiological aspects of Gaucher disease. *Skeletal Radiol.* 2011;40: 1505–13.

References

1. Aldenhoven M, Sakkers RJ, Boelens J, de Koning TJ, Wulffraat NM. Musculoskeletal manifestations of lysosomal storage disorders. *Ann Rheum Dis.* 2009;68:1659–65.
2. Clarke LA, Hollak CE. The clinical spectrum and pathophysiology of skeletal complications in lysosomal storage disorders. *Best Pract Res Clin Endocrinol Metab.* 2015;29:219–35.
3. Fedida B, Touraine S, Stirnemann J, Belmatoug N, Laredo JD, Petrover D. Bone marrow involvement in Gaucher disease at MRI : what long-term evolution can we expect under enzyme replacement therapy? *Eur Radiol.* 2015;25:2969–75.
4. Katz R, Booth T, Hargunani R, Wylie P, Holloway B. Radiological aspects of Gaucher disease. *Skeletal Radiol.* 2011;40:1505–13.
5. Mikosch P. Miscellaneous non-inflammatory musculoskeletal conditions. Gaucher disease and bone. *Best Pract Res Clin Rheumatol.* 2011;25:665–81.
6. Parker EI, Xing M, Moreno-De-Luca A, Harmouche E, Terk MR. Radiological and clinical characterization of the lysosomal storage disorders: non-lipid disorders. *Br J Radiol.* 2014;87:20130467.
7. Pastores GM. Musculoskeletal complications encountered in the lysosomal storage disorders. *Best Pract Res Clin Rheumatol.* 2008;22:937–47.

CHAPTER 84

Mucopolysaccharidoses

Kevin B. Hoover

Introduction

The mucopolysaccharidoses (Table 84.1) are autosomally inherited disorders, except for mucopolysaccharidosis (MPS) II, which is X-linked recessive. Together, these represent approximately 35% of all lysosomal storage diseases. In general, there is a spectrum in clinical presentation from less to more severe, which is related to the effect of the underlying mutation.

Pathophysiology and Clinical Findings

Although the exact pathogenesis of MPS has not been elucidated, the accumulation of glycosaminoglycans (GAGs) in connective tissue cells, chondrocyte apoptosis, and tissue inflammation are thought to give rise to musculoskeletal disease. One of the most important causes of morbidity in MPS is atlantoaxial instability, caused by abnormal odontoid development (odontoid dysplasia) and supporting ligament infiltration. Insidious development of myelopathy and spastic quadriparesis may result, especially in (untreated) MPS I, MPS IV, and MPS VI patients. These patients also have significant problems related to intubation. Delayed development of the axial skeleton more so than the peripheral skeleton results in a shorter trunk and longer limbs. Periarticular and soft tissue GAG deposition results in joint stiffness, contractures, trigger finger, and CTS, which may mimic RA. This also results in a characteristic *claw hand* clinical presentation reported in up to 58% of pediatric MPS patients. Because patients often lack intellectual impairment, severe growth retardation, or a grossly abnormal physical appearance, diagnosis is often delayed. Nonmusculoskeletal manifestations include hepatosplenomegaly, cardiac valve and myocardial abnormalities, respiratory infections, cervical cord compression, and deafness. Diagnosis is made by detection of elevated urinary GAG concentration (less sensitive), decreased peripheral blood lysosomal enzyme activity (more sensitive), and DNA mutation detection (most specific).

Imaging Strategy

Radiographs of the axial and appendicular skeleton (skeletal survey) are used for the baseline assessment of MPS disease, even in patients without musculoskeletal symptoms. Progression of skeletal abnormalities is monitored with annual cervical spine MRI, AP and lateral standing scoliosis radiographs, and AP pelvis radiography at least until complete skeletal maturity. The cervical spine MRI should use standard sagittal and axial T1W and T2W and sagittal STIR sequences without IV contrast. Lower extremity alignment (stitched leg length) radiographs should be considered when evaluating genu valgum. At baseline and every 3-5 years, lateral flexion and extension cervical spine radiographs under the voluntary control of the patient should be obtained. Flexion-extension CT can be helpful in equivocal cases. MRI evaluation of the thoracolumbar spine is most useful with the development of neurologic changes of lower extremity, bowel, or bladder.

Imaging Findings

Radiographs

- Radiography is used to evaluate the spectrum of skeletal deformities termed *dysostosis multiplex* (see Table 83.2 in Chapter 83, "Lipidoses"; also seen in mucolipidoses), including:
  - Symmetric lower extremity abnormalities are common (Figure 84.1):
    - Coxa valga with a femoral neck-shaft angle of greater than 140 degrees
    - Acetabular and femoral head dysplasia with joint subluxation and eventual secondary OA
    - Genu valgum
  - Gibbus deformity with angular kyphosis at the thoracolumbar junction is seen:
    - At the apex of the kyphosis, there is flattening (platyspondyly), anterior wedging, retrolisthesis of the vertebrae, and herniation of the intervertebral discs.
    - Beaked, bullet-shaped L1 and L2 vertebrae are pathognomonic for MPS (Figure 84.2A).
- Atlantoaxial instability can be detected on flexion-extension radiographs:
  - More than 5-8 mm change between views is consistent with instability.
  - Dynamic fluoroscopy and flexion-extension CT scans can be useful if radiographs are equivocal.

Magnetic Resonance Imaging

- Cervical spine MRI findings resulting in canal stenosis and spinal cord compression at the occipitocervical junction include:
  - A mass of GAG deposition posterior to the odontoid process, which is iso- or hypointense on T1W and hypointense on T2W MR images (Figure 84.2)
  - Dural and ligamenta flava thickening
  - C1 ring hypoplasia

Table 84.1. Summary of Mucopolysaccharidoses

CONDITION	INCIDENCE (100,00 LIVE BIRTHS)	PROGNOSIS	MUSCULOSKELETAL FINDINGS
MPS I Hurler syndrome (severe phenotype), Hurler-Scheie syndrome (intermediate), Scheie syndrome (mild)	0.11–1.67 (varies by country)	Untreated Hurler syndrome 50% mortality by age 5 years caused by cardiac or pulmonary disease; speech delay, subsequent cognitive, visual, and auditory decline	Disproportional short stature, joint stiffness/contractures, claw hands, odontoid hypoplasia, thoracolumbar kyphosis, scoliosis, hip dysplasia, genu valgum,CTS, trigger fingers, dysostosis multiplex
MPS II Hunter syndrome A (severe) and B (mild)	0.10–1.07	A: Death typically in the first or the second decade of life B: Patients live into early adult years	Disproportional short stature, joint stiffness/contractures thoracolumbar kyphosis, hip dysplasia, CTS, trigger fingers, dysostosis multiplex
MPS III Sanfilippo syndrome A-D	0.29–1.89	Normal development until ages 2–6 years; subsequent rapid neurologic deterioration	Short stature, mild joint stiffness/contractures, genu valgum, dysostosis multiplex
MPS IV Morquio syndrome A-B	0.15–1.31	Typically normal intelligence, longer lifespan than MPS	Disproportional short stature, hypermobile joints, odontoid dysplasia, thoracolumbar kyphosis, scoliosis, pectus carinatum, coxa valga, genu valgum, pes planus, dysostosis multiplex
MPS VI Maroteaux-Lamy syndrome	0.14–0.38	Typically normal intelligence	Disproportional short stature, joint stiffness/contractures (mainly hips), kyphoscoliosis, hip dysplasia, genu valgum, odontoid hypoplasia, CTS, trigger fingers, dysostosis multiplex
MPS VII Sly syndrome	0.02–0.29	Mild phenotype to lethal hydrops fetalis	Disproportional short stature, joint stiffness/contractures, odontoid hypoplasia, thoracolumbar kyphosis, dysostosis multiplex
MPS IX	Rare (case reports)		Periarticular nodular soft tissue masses (extremities) with episodes of painful swelling, short stature

Abbreviations: CTS, carpal tunnel syndrome; MPS, mucopolysaccharidosis.

- Absent, hypoplastic or fragmented odontoid process (odontoid dysplasia)
- Posterior intervertebral disc bulging
- Described mostly in patients with MPS I (untreated), MPS IV, and MPS VI
- Gibbus deformity of the upper lumbar spine demonstrates:
- Platyspondyly and vertebral beaking at apex (Figure 84.2B)
- Desiccated intervertebral discs with preserved height
- Conus often at or superior to kyphosis
- Stenosis of the thoracic and lumbar spine is less common, but may occur because of intervertebral disc herniations (Figure 84.2).

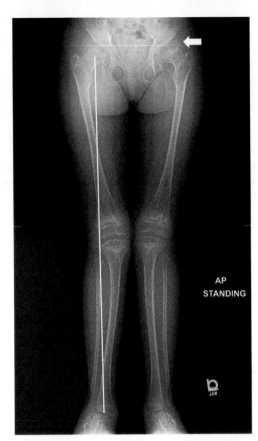

Figure 84.1. Morquio syndrome in a 10-year-old patient. A stitched leg length radiographic series demonstrates genu valgum with the mechanical axis (equivalent, *white line*) lateral to the knee joint. Left (*thick arrow*) and right hip dysplasia is evident with angulated acetabulums with acetabular under coverage of the femoral heads.

Treatment Options

- Stem cell transplantation (SCT) is the treatment of choice in MPS I (Hurler syndrome) with improved life span and slowed neurocognitive decline, but without musculoskeletal disease improvement (eg, gibbus deformity, hip dysplasia).
- Enzyme replacement therapy (ERT) is the treatment of choice in MPS I Hurler-Scheie and Scheie syndromes, MPS II, and MPS VI with improvement in patient movement, but no improvement in musculoskeletal disease. Adjuvant ERT is commonly used initially in MPS I (Hurler syndrome) because of the 9-month delay in enzyme activity after SCT. ERT does not cross the blood-brain barrier to address neurologic complications.
- Surgical stabilization and decompression may be warranted in patients with atlantoaxial instability, evidence of spinal cord impingement, and a deteriorating neurologic condition.
- Surgery is also used in patients with OA secondary to hip dysplasia, CTS, and kyphoscoliosis correction.

Key Points

- MPS is associated with multiple skeletal findings termed dysostosis multiplex.
- Cervical spine involvement with atlantoaxial instability and spinal stenosis require monitoring by flexion-extension radiographs and MRI to evaluate for progression.
- Beaked or bullet-shaped L1 and L2 vertebrae are pathognomonic for MPS and are associated with an angular kyphotic or gibbus deformity.
- Surgical treatment is usually required for correction of musculoskeletal disease complications (eg, spinal stenosis and instability, hip OA).

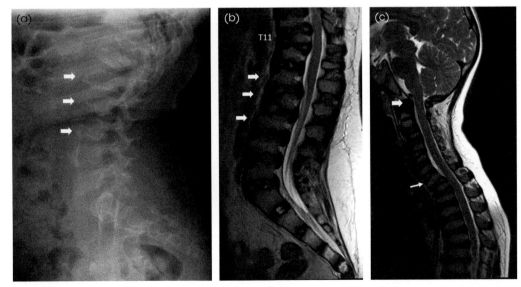

Figure 84.2. Morquio syndrome in a 12-year-old patient. (*A*) Lateral lumbar spine radiograph demonstrates multilevel vertebral flattening (platyspondyly) with anterior vertebral beaking most conspicuous at L1-L3 (*thick arrows*). (*B*) Sagittal T2W MR image of the lumbar spine demonstrates platyspondyly (*thick arrows*) with diffuse intervertebral disc bulges narrowing the spinal canal. A thoracic kyphosis and mild gibbus deformity centered at the T11 level is associated with mild spinal canal stenosis. (*C*) Sagittal T2W MR image of the cervical spine demonstrates narrowing of the foramen magnum by a hypertrophic dens (*thick arrow*). There is also anterolisthesis of C7 relative to T1 with multilevel platyspondyly and mild spinal canal stenosis (*thin arrow*).

Recommended Reading

White KK, Sousa T. Mucopolysaccharide disorders in orthopaedic surgery. *J Am Acad Orthop Surg.* 2013;21:12–22.

References

1. Aldenhoven M, Sakkers RJ, Boelens J, de Koning TJ, Wulffraat NM. Musculoskeletal manifestations of lysosomal storage disorders. *Ann Rheum Dis.* 2009;68:1659–65.
2. Clarke LA, Hollak CE. The clinical spectrum and pathophysiology of skeletal complications in lysosomal storage disorders. *Best Pract Res Clin Endocrinol Metab.* 2015;29:219–35.
3. Parker EI, Xing M, Moreno-De-Luca A, Harmouche E, Terk MR. Radiological and clinical characterization of the lysosomal storage disorders: non-lipid disorders. *Br J Radiol.* 2014;87:20130467.
4. Pastores GM. Musculoskeletal complications encountered in the lysosomal storage disorders. *Best Pract Res Clin Rheumatol.* 2008;22:937–47.
5. Rasalkar DD, Chu WC, Hui J, Chu CM, Paunipagar BK, Li CK. Pictorial review of mucopolysaccharidosis with emphasis on MRI features of brain and spine. *Br J Radiol.* 2011;84:469–77.
6. White KK. Orthopaedic aspects of mucopolysaccharidoses. *Rheumatology (Oxford).* 2011;50(suppl 5):v26–33.
7. White KK, Sousa T. Mucopolysaccharide disorders in orthopaedic surgery. *J Am Acad Orthop Surg.* 2013;21:12–22.
8. Zafeiriou DI, Batzios SP. Brain and spinal MR imaging findings in mucopolysaccharidoses: a review. *AJNR Am J Neuroradiol.* 2013;34:5–13.

Section Five

Infectious Diseases

Edited by Mihra S. Taljanovic and Tyson S. Chadaz

Pyogenic Infections

CHAPTER 85

Pyogenic Spondylodiscitis

Sumer N. Shikhare and Wilfred C. G. Peh

Introduction

Spondylodiscitis is defined as infection of the intervertebral disc and adjacent vertebrae. Pyogenic spondylodiscitis is not common and comprises only 2-5% of all cases of osteomyelitis. It has a bimodal age distribution, with first peak occurring in patients younger than 20 years and the second peak occurring in patients older than 50 years. It is slightly more prevalent in male patients. Pyogenic spondylodiscitis commonly affects the lumbar spine (50%), followed by the thoracic (35%) and cervical spine (15%). The common causative organisms are *Staphylococcus aureus* and streptococci, which are responsible for more than 50% of the cases. Other organisms causing pyogenic spondylodiscitis are *Escherichia coli*, *Klebsiella* spp., *Proteus* spp., *Enterobacter* spp., *Salmonella*, and *Pseudomonas aeruginosa*. The incidence of pyogenic spondylodiscitis has been on the rise in recent years because of aging populations with chronic debilitating diseases, an increase in the prevalence of diabetes mellitus, chronic liver or renal disease, human immunodeficiency virus infection, long-term steroid use, IV drug use, and spinal surgeries.

Pathophysiology

Spinal infection can spread by 2 main routes: hematogenous and nonhematogenous. Hematogenous arterial seeding is by far the most common route because of the rich arterial supply of the vertebral body. The spinal arteries bifurcate to supply 2 adjacent vertebral bodies. The arterioles enter the vertebral body through central nutrient foramina, undergo ramification, and are in abundance at the endplates, particularly in the anterior subchondral region. As a result, the infective process usually commences at the anterior subchondral region of the adjacent vertebral bodies. The intervertebral disc is avascular in adults, hence it is usually not initially infected by hematogenous spread of infection.

With disease progression, the infective process causes bone infarction, followed by vertebral body and endplate destruction, and resultant direct spread of infection to the adjacent disc space. Children, on the contrary, primarily develop discitis because of extensive intradiscal vascular anastomoses. In advanced cases, infection may spread into surrounding soft tissues and the spinal canal, causing paravertebral or psoas abscesses and epidural or subdural abscesses, respectively. The posterior elements of the vertebrae are rarely involved because of their poor blood supply. The venous spread of infection through the Batson paravertebral plexus is less common. This is a network of valveless veins that allow retrograde spread of infection to vertebrae secondary to increased intraabdominal pressure. The infection commonly arises from pelvic organs such as the female pelvis and urinary bladder. The less common nonhematogenous route includes infection by direct inoculation, postoperative infection, and from contiguous infected tissue. Unlike tuberculosis (TB), disc involvement occurs early in pyogenic spondylodiscitis because of production of the proteolytic enzymes.

Clinical Findings

The symptoms and signs of pyogenic spondylodiscitis are nonspecific. The most common presenting symptom is unremitting back or neck pain. Fever is less common and occurs in only approximately half of patients. Symptoms such as leg weakness, sensory deficit, paralysis, and incontinence are related to neurologic compromise and usually present late in the disease process. Laboratory investigations such as leukocyte count, ESR, and CRP level are often raised, but are nonspecific. Blood cultures, serology, and image-guided biopsy are important in supporting the imaging features of infection and for reaching a diagnosis.

Imaging Strategy and Findings

The imaging modalities frequently employed to diagnose pyogenic spondylodiscitis are conventional radiography, CT, and MRI. As patients commonly present with neck or back pain, the initial imaging study performed is often radiography of the spine. Figures 85.1 through 85.3 demonstrate radiographic, CT, and MRI findings of pyogenic spondylodiscitis.

Imaging Findings
Radiography

- Radiographs usually reveal no abnormality until 2 to 8 weeks after onset of symptoms.
- The earliest radiographic feature is erosion of the anterior aspect of the adjacent vertebral body endplates. This is followed by reduced disc height and vertebral osteolysis (Figure 85.1A,B).
- The disease progression is characterized by vertebral collapse and wedging, leading to gibbus deformity (Figure 85.2).
- The posterior elements of the vertebral body are uncommonly involved.
- In advanced cases, radiographs may reveal effacement of the paraspinal soft tissues suggesting paraspinal abscess (Figure 85.1A).
- The healing phase is characterized by increased bone density caused by sclerosis, obliteration of the disc space,

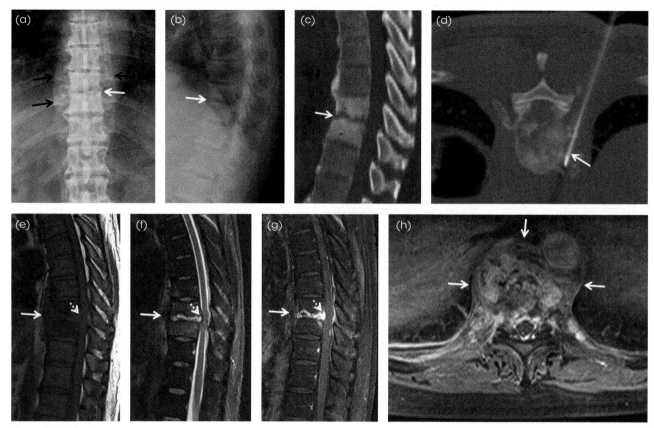

Figure 85.1. Acute pyogenic spondylodiscitis in a 60-year-old man. (*A*) AP and (*B*) lateral radiographs of the thoracic spine show eroded endplates at T9 and T10 vertebral bodies with reduced disc height (*white arrow*) and paravertebral soft tissue fullness on both sides (*black arrows*). (*C*) Sagittal reformatted CT image shows T9 and T10 endplate erosions with reactive sclerosis in the adjacent marrow and disc space narrowing (*arrow*). (*D*) A CT-guided percutaneous biopsy was performed at T9-10 level. Note biopsy needle (*arrow*). Sagittal (*E*) T1W, (*F*) STIR, and (*G*) contrast-enhanced T1W FS MR images show changes of pyogenic spondylitis with discitis involving the T9 and T10 vertebral bodies, seen as T1 hypointensity, T2 hyperintensity, and mild marrow enhancement. The intervening disc demonstrates increased signal intensity on STIR image with heterogeneous avid postcontrast enhancement in (*G*). Note thickening of the anterior paravertebral soft tissues (*arrows*) and epidural extension with spinal cord compression (*dashed arrows*). (*H*) Axial contrast-enhanced T1W FS MR image shows pre- and paravertebral abscess (*arrows*).

followed by ankylosis of the vertebral bodies and kyphotic and scoliotic deformity.

Computed Tomography

- Although, CT is not the initial modality of choice, it is superior to radiographs in the early detection of endplate erosions, bone destruction, and paraspinal and epidural space involvement (Figure 85.1*C*).
- Abscesses in the psoas muscle, paravertebral space, and epidural space characteristically demonstrate peripheral rim enhancement on postcontrast images.
- CT is the preferred imaging modality to assess spinal deformity and pathologic calcifications.
- Another major application of CT is in guiding percutaneous needle biopsy and drainage of abscess (Figure 85.1*D*).

Magnetic Resonance Imaging

MRI is the modality of choice in pyogenic spondylodiscitis because of its high sensitivity (96%) and specificity (94%) to detect early infection, as well as its high-contrast resolution and multiplanar imaging capability. The protocol must include fluid-sensitive fat-saturated (T2W FS or STIR) sequences, as

these are highly sensitive in demonstrating BME, before erosive bone changes appear. MRI is the best modality to evaluate the spinal canal, particularly the epidural space and spinal cord, as epidural abscess and cord compression are both considered surgical emergencies.

- BME is visible as an area of increased signal intensity on fluid-sensitive images with corresponding low signal intensity on T1W images and enhancement on postcontrast T1W FS images (Figure 85.1*E-G*).
- The intervening disc demonstrates increased signal intensity on fluid-sensitive images with postcontrast enhancement (Figure 85.1*F-G*).
- The finding of disc space involvement helps differentiate infection from neoplasm, as the disc is usually not affected in the latter.
- Postcontrast T1W FS sequences are also useful in assessing paravertebral space involvement (Figures 85.1*G,H* and 85.3*C*).
- Intraosseous, paravertebral, and epidural abscesses and phlegmonous tissues show low signal on T1W images and high signal on fluid-sensitive sequences (Figure 85.3*A,B*). On the postcontrast T1W FS images,

remains narrowed, but the initially increased fluid-sensitive signal intensity decreases with progressive increase in marrow signal on T1W images, consistent with fatty deposition in previously involved areas.

Imaging features of pyogenic spondylodiscitis may be similar to TB spondylodiscitis in approximately 75% of cases.

- MRI may be helpful in differentiating pyogenic spondylodiscitis from TB spondylodiscitis.
- Imaging features that favor TB spondylodiscitis include subligamentous spread of infection to 3 or more vertebral levels, multiple vertebral body involvement, skip lesions, and posterior element involvement.
- In pyogenic spondylodiscitis, paraspinal masses are usually smaller than in TB spondylodiscitis.

Nuclear Imaging

Radionuclide studies are more sensitive in detecting early infectious process compared to radiographs. Technetium-99m-labeled methylene diphosphonate (^{99m}Tc-MDP) and gallium-67 citrate bone scans are sensitive but lack specificity for spinal infections, as they may show increased activity in other conditions, such as degenerative disc disease, osteoporotic fractures, and neoplasms. Poor anatomical detail is another disadvantage of radionuclide studies. Indium-111–labeled leukocyte radionuclide study has high specificity but is very low in sensitivity (17%), with resultant high rate of false-negative results in chronic pyogenic spondylodiscitis in which there is relative scarcity of leukocytes.

Differential Diagnosis

- Degenerative disc disease
- Noninfective inflammatory disc disease

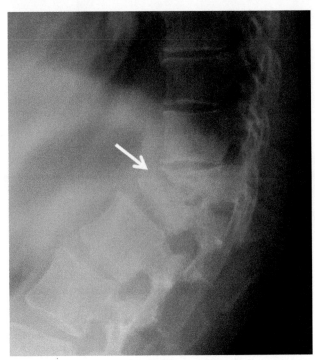

Figure 85.2. Chronic spondylodiscitis in a 65-year-old patient. Lateral radiograph of the thoracic spine shows collapse and wedging of the 2 adjacent vertebral bodies, leading to gibbus deformity (*arrow*).

intradiscal (Figure 85.3*C*), intraosseous, paravertebral, and epidural abscesses show rim enhancement, whereas the phlegmonous tissues typically show diffuse enhancement (Figures 85.1*G,H* and 85.3*C*).

- MRI may also be used as a tool in assessing treatment response. In the healing phase, the disc space usually

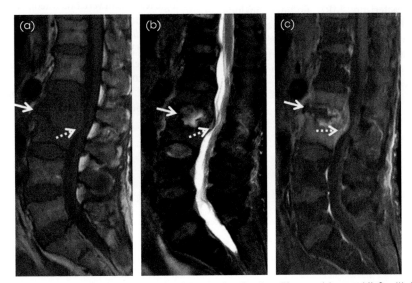

Figure 85.3. Pyogenic spondylodiscitis with phlegmonous epidural extension in a 71-year-old man. (*A*) Sagittal T1W MR image shows low signal intensity in the L2-L3 intervertebral disc and in the adjacent vertebral bodies with erosive changes of the endplates (*arrow*) and epidural extension (*dashed arrow*). (*B*) Sagittal T2W FS MR image shows high signal at the L2-L3 intervertebral disc (*arrow*). Note mild increased signal in the adjacent vertebral bodies and epidural space (*dashed arrow*). In (*C*), postcontrast T1W FS sagittal MR image, note marked enhancement of the vertebral bodies and prevertebral phlegmon, enhancement of the epidural phlegmon (*dashed arrow*) with rim-enhancing intradiscal abscess (*arrow*).

- Tuberculous spondylodiscitis
- Spinal neoplasm

Treatment Options

- Pyogenic spondylodiscitis is usually treated conservatively using antimicrobial therapy and nonpharmacological treatments such as bed rest and physiotherapy.
- Recommended duration of antimicrobial therapy is 6 to 8 weeks of IV antibiotics to reduce failure and recurrence rate. While awaiting microbiological results, empirical therapy should be started, covering *S. aureus*, gram-negative organisms and anaerobes. Once an organism has been identified, the specific antibiotic can be continued intravenously.
- In the early phase, immobilization is recommended until acute pain subsides, followed by ambulation in an appropriate cast or brace.
- Indications for surgical intervention include failure of medical management, intractable pain, neurologic complications, and extensive bony destruction causing spinal instability or severe kyphotic deformity.
- The aim of surgical management is to attain optimum healing while preserving the neurologic function and is achieved with aggressive radical debridement and decompression, along with anterior fusion for spinal stabilization.

Key Points

- The most common mode of spread of pyogenic spondylodiscitis is hematogenous arterial seeding.
- The earliest radiographic features are reduced disc height and endplate erosions.
- MRI is the modality of choice for early diagnosis because of high sensitivity.
- Earliest and characteristic MRI findings include increased T2 signal involving the disc and adjacent vertebral endplates with corresponding low T1 signal and post gadolinium-based contrast enhancement (Gd).
- The intervertebral disc involvement is early in pyogenic spondylodiscitis because of proteolytic enzymes.

Recommended Reading

Varma R, Lander P, Assaf A. Imaging of pyogenic infectious spondylodiskitis. *Radiol Clin North Am.* 2001;39:203–13.

References

1. An HS, Seldomridge JA. Spinal infections: diagnostic tests and imaging studies. *Clin Orthop Relat Res.* 2006;444:27–33.
2. Carragee EJ. Pyogenic vertebral osteomyelitis. *J Bone Joint Surg Am.* 1997;79:874–80.
3. Cheung WY, Luk KDK. Pyogenic spondylitis. *Int Orthop.* 2012;36:397–404.
4. Fantoni M, Trecarichi EM, Rossi B, et al. Epidemiological and clinical features of pyogenic spondylodiscitis. *Eur Rev Med Pharmacol Sci.* 2012;16(suppl 2):2–7.
5. Gouliouris T, Aliyu SH, Brown NM. Spondylodiscitis: update on diagnosis and management. *J Antimicrob Chemother.* 2010;65(suppl 3):11–24.
6. Hong SH, Choi JY, Lee JW, Kim NR, Choi JA, Kang HS. MR imaging assessment of the spine: infection or an imitation? *Radiographics.* 2009;29:599–612.
7. Kaya S, Ercan S, Kaya S, et al. Spondylodiscitis: evaluation of patients in a tertiary hospital. *J Infect Dev Ctries.* 2014;8:1272–76.
8. Leone A, Dell'Atti C, Magarelli N, et al. Imaging of spondylodiscitis. *Eur Rev Med Pharmacol Sci.* 2012;16(suppl 2):8–19.
9. Mylona E, Samarkos M, Kakalou E, Fanourgiakis P, Skoutelis A. Pyogenic vertebral osteomyelitis: a systematic review of clinical characteristics. *Semin Arthritis Rheum.* 2009;39:10–17.
10. Pola E, Logroscino CA, Gentiempo M, et al. Medical and surgical treatment of pyogenic spondylodiscitis. *Eur Rev Med Pharmacol Sci.* 2012;16(suppl 2):35–49.
11. Wiley AM, Trueta J. The vascular anatomy of the spine and its relationship to pyogenic vertebral osteomyelitis. *J Bone Joint Surg.* 1959;41B:796–809.
12. Ratcliffe JF. Anatomic basis for the pathogenesis and radiologic features of vertebral osteomyelitis and its differentiation from childhood discitis. A microarteriographic investigation. *Acta Radiol Diagn.* 1985;26:137–43.
13. Shikhare SN, Singh DR, Shimpi TR, Peh WCG. Tuberculous osteomyelitis and spondylodiscitis. *Semin Musculoskelet Radiol.* 2011;15:446–58.
14. Varma R, Lander P, Assaf A. Imaging of pyogenic infectious spondylodiskitis. *Radiol Clin North Am.* 2001;39:203–13.

CHAPTER 86

Osteomyelitis of the Long and Flat Bones

Sumer N. Shikhare and Wilfred C. G. Peh

Introduction

Osteomyelitis (OM) is defined as inflammation of the bone and bone marrow as a result of bacterial infection. Other less common causative agents include fungi, parasites, and viruses.

Pathophysiology

Long bone OM can occur secondary to hematogenous spread, direct inoculation into bone, or from a contiguous source of infection. Hematogenous spread is more common in children and elderly people. In adults, hematogenous OM commonly affects the spine, pelvis, and small bones. Direct inoculation usually occurs secondary to surgery or trauma. OM caused by adjacent soft tissue infection is commonly seen in patients with diabetes mellitus or in bedridden patients.

The hematogenous form is usually caused by a single pathogen, the commonest organism being *Staphylococcus aureus (S. aureus)* in children and adults. A new gram-negative coccobacillus organism, *Kingella kingae,* is now isolated with greater frequency in children. Children with sickle cell disease may be infected with *Salmonella.* The commonest organisms isolated in infants are *S. aureus, Streptococcus agalactiae,* and *Escherichia coli.* Increasingly, methicillin-resistant *S. aureus* (MRSA) is being isolated from patients with OM. In OM secondary to direct inoculation or contiguous spread, multiple organisms may be isolated.

Hematogenous OM has a predilection for the metaphyses of long bones and is attributed to the peculiar vascular pattern in this region, where terminal branches of the nutrient artery form a mesh of hairpin bends before draining into a large network of sinusoidal veins. This arrangement causes blood to flow slowly in the metaphysis, favoring bacterial colonization. In infants and adults, the metaphyseal and epiphyseal vessels communicate with each other, hence the metaphyseal infection can pass to the epiphysis. In children, however, very few vessels cross the epiphyseal plate, which act as a relative barrier to the spread of infection. A recent study has shown a higher incidence of transphyseal spread of infection than previously thought.

The acute stage of OM is characterized by BME caused by inflammatory exudates. As the infective process progresses across the medullary cavity, the increased intraosseous pressure causes pus to track within Volkmann canals and spread subsequently into the subperiosteal space, causing periosteal stripping. If untreated, the infected bone undergoes devascularization secondary to vascular stasis and small-vessel thrombosis, resulting in a necrotic bone fragment known as *sequestrum.* If the infective process is aborted at this stage by appropriate treatment, resolution and healing occurs. If the infection persists beyond 6 weeks, chronic OM is established, characterized by an *involucrum,* which is an area of periosteal new bone encasing the sequestrum. The involucrum may develop perforations, termed *cloaca,* through which the pus may track into the surrounding soft tissue and eventually to the skin surface via a sinus tract.

Clinical Findings

A high index of clinical suspicion, together with laboratory and imaging findings, is required to diagnose OM. The clinical symptoms are usually nonspecific and include fever, chills, swelling, erythema, and pain over the involved bone. Children are usually irritable and lethargic. In cases of direct inoculation or contiguous spread of disease, patients may present with focal bone pain, erythema, swelling, and pus drainage around the area of surgery, trauma, or wound infection. Laboratory investigations should include complete blood count, ESR, CRP, cultures, and Gram stain. Cultures of blood and material obtained by needle aspiration of the involved bone are necessary to identify the causative organism and yield positive findings in up to 87% of cases. Bone biopsies usually taken at the time of debridement should undergo histopathologic examination and culture and sensitivity.

Imaging Strategy

The imaging modalities frequently employed to diagnose OM are conventional radiography, radionuclide scanning, CT, and MRI. In all patients with suspected OM, evaluation usually begins with radiographs. Figures 86.1–86.5 demonstrate radiographic, CT, MRI, and radionuclide imaging findings of acute and chronic OM.

MRI is the modality of choice in imaging OM because of its high spatial resolution, multiplanar ability, and better soft tissue contrast. In OM, the specificity and sensitivity of MRI ranges from 50% to 90% and 60% to 100%, respectively. MRI can detect changes as early as 3 to 5 days after the infective process begins. MRI protocol should include T1W and T2W sequences supplemented by T2W FS or STIR sequences. IV Gd-based T1W FS postcontrast sequences are helpful in depicting nonenhancing intraosseous, subperiosteal, and soft tissue fluid collections and areas of tissue necrosis, rim-enhancing abscesses, and enhancing phlegmons.

In the acute stage, when the radiographs are not of much help, radionuclide imaging may be useful for the early detection of OM. It can detect OM as early as 48 hours after

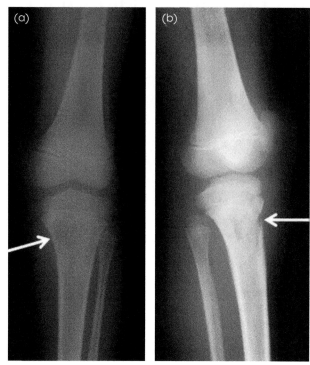

Figure 86.1. Acute OM of the left tibia in an 18-year-old man. (*A*) AP and (*B*) oblique radiographs of the tibia and fibula show permeative bone destruction (*arrows*) involving the proximal metaphysis of the left tibia. The lesion has wide zone of transition. There is cortical break noted anteriorly with adjacent soft tissue edema.

the onset of infection. Additionally, bone scan is helpful in detecting multifocal OM.

Imaging Findings

Radiography
- In the early stages of OM, radiographs may be normal and changes are usually visible approximately 2 to 3 weeks after the onset of infection.
- Early radiographic findings include soft tissue swelling, subcutaneous edema, and blurring of the soft tissue planes.
- In OM caused by contiguous spread of infection, the earliest radiographic finding is usually soft tissue edema and periosteal reaction that closely resembles posttraumatic periosteal reaction and periosteal reaction caused by chronic venous stasis.
- As disease progresses, osseous findings such as osteoporosis, permeative bone erosion, and trabecular destruction caused by infection in the medullary space are seen (Figure 86.1).
- As infection spreads outward across the haversian and Volkmann canals, there is increased osteolysis and cortical erosion (Figure 86.1). This is followed by periostitis, caused by lifting of the periosteum by the subperiosteal abscess.
- In adults, the periosteum is attached firmly to the cortex, ensuring good cortical blood supply and resisting periosteal elevation and new bone formation.

- In late stage or chronic stage of OM, radiographs usually reveal bone expansion and remodeling, cortical thickening, and may show sequestrum, involucrum, and cloaca (Figure 86.2*A*).
  - A sequestrum is seen as a sclerotic bone fragment within a lucent lesion.
  - An involucrum is thick periosteal new bone surrounding the sequestrum.
  - Cloaca appears as a lucent defect within the cortical bone.
  - Sequestrum and involucrum are unusual findings in adults compared to the pediatric population.
- Some patients, particularly children, may develop an intraosseous abscess known as a *Brodie abscess* in the subacute or chronic stages of OM (duration of at least 6 weeks). These are seen as well-defined round to oval lucent lesions with dense surrounding sclerosis and associated periosteal reaction (Figure 86.3*A*). *Brodie abscess* commonly involves the metaphysis of the long bones, particularly the distal or proximal portions of the tibia.

Computed Tomography
- Although CT is not the modality of choice in OM, it is superior to radiographs in demonstrating the amount of bone destruction, periosteal reaction, intraosseous gas, and soft tissue extension (Figure 86.4*A,B*).
- CT is more useful in cases with chronic OM, for identifying sequestra, involucra, and cloacae, features that are important in deciding surgical management.
- Another advantage of CT is its usefulness in image-guided biopsy.

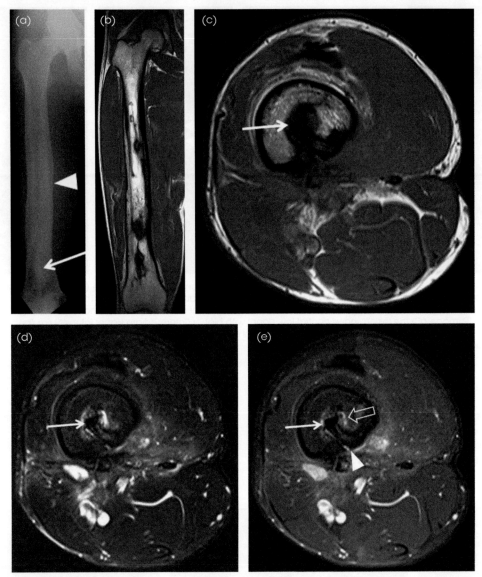

Figure 86.2. Chronic OM of the right femur in a 32-year-old man. (*A*) AP radiograph of the right femur shows cortical thickening, osseous expansion and bony remodeling, sclerotic changes, sequestrum (*arrow*), and involucrum (*arrowhead*). Coronal (*B*) and (*C*) axial T1W, (*D*) axial T2W FS, and (*E*) axial postcontrast T1W FS MR images show diffuse cortical thickening involving the right femur with medullary sequestrum (*arrow*), which is hypointense on all sequences, enhancing surrounding granulation tissue (*open arrow*) and cloaca (*arrowhead*), which is seen as a cortical defect.

Magnetic Resonance Imaging

- The earliest MRI finding is a focal area of decreased marrow signal on T1WI (Figure 86.5*A*) and an increased signal on fluid-sensitive sequences caused by BME and exudate (Figures 86.4*C* and 86.5*B*).
- BME and enhancement without associated low T1 signal comprises reactive changes/osteitis and is not diagnostic of OM.
- On postcontrast T1W FS images, the affected area shows significant marrow enhancement (Figures 86.4*D* and 86.5*C*).
- Imaging findings of acute OM are quite nonspecific. Other conditions such as noninfectious inflammation, healing fractures, bone contusion, and metastasis can also produce increased BME on T2W images similar to OM. Thus, MRI findings must be correlated with

secondary imaging abnormalities and the clinical background. The secondary findings include cortical bone destruction, cellulitis, soft tissue abscess, and sinus tract.
- On MRI, the normal cortical bone appears hypointense on T1W and T2W images. In case of OM with cortical erosion, there is loss of normal cortical hypointense signal.
- Soft tissue and intraosseous abscesses appear as hypointense, peripherally enhancing fluid collections on postcontrast T1W FS images (Figure 86.3*D*).
- Sinus tracts, if present, are seen as curvilinear or linear areas of increased signal on T2W images and may exhibit contrast enhancement.
- In chronic stages, sequestra and involucra demonstrate decreased signal on all the pulse sequences with no contrast enhancement (Figure 86.2*B–E*).

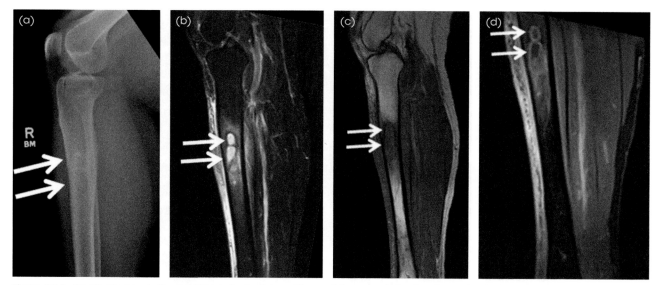

Figure 86.3. Brodie abscess in the right tibial diaphysis in a 48-year-old woman. Lateral radiograph (*A*) shows a bilobed lucent lesion with a thin sclerotic rim in the proximal tibial diaphysis consistent with Brodie abscess (*arrows*). (*B*) The lesion demonstrates high signal intensity on the sagittal STIR MR image with associated low signal rim of sclerosis (*arrows*) and adjacent high signal BME. On the sagittal T1W MR image (*C*) the lesion shows central low signal with higher/intermediate signal intensity rim (penumbra sign) and surrounding low signal sclerosis (*arrows*) and demonstrates rim enhancement (*arrows*) on the postcontrast T1W FS MR image (*D*) with enhancing adjacent BME.

- The granulation tissue surrounding the sequestrum, however, displays increased signal on fluid-sensitive sequences with contrast enhancement (Figure 86.2D,E).
- Brodie abscess is best seen on MRI and appears as a round, well-defined area with decreased signal on T1W images and increased signal on T2W FS/STIR images

with peripheral rim enhancement on postcontrast images. It is characteristically surrounded by a band of decreased signal on T2W images caused by bone sclerosis (Figure 86.3B-D).

- It may be challenging to distinguish subacute OM from tumor on MRI images. Rim of increased and/or

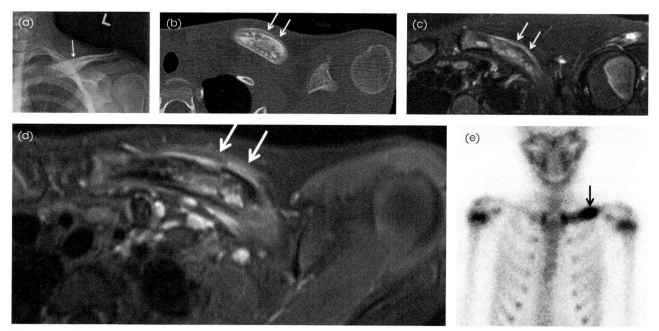

Figure 86.4. OM of the left clavicle in a 24-year-old man. (*A*) AP radiograph of the left shoulder shows osseous expansion of the proximal and mid clavicle with periosteal reaction (*arrow*). (*B*) Axial CT image of the left clavicle, taken in bone window, better demonstrates osteolytic and sclerotic changes with periosteal reaction (*arrows*). (*C*) Axial T2W FS MR image shows diffuse increased signal in the left clavicle with periosteal reaction (*arrows*) and surrounding reactive soft tissue edema. (*D*) Axial postcontrast T1W FS MR image shows diffuse periosteal (*arrows*), marrow and surrounding soft tissue enhancement in keeping with acute OM. (*E*) Corresponding ^{99m}Tc-MDP radionuclide bone scan shows intense increased uptake in the left clavicle (*arrow*), corresponding to the site affected by acute OM.

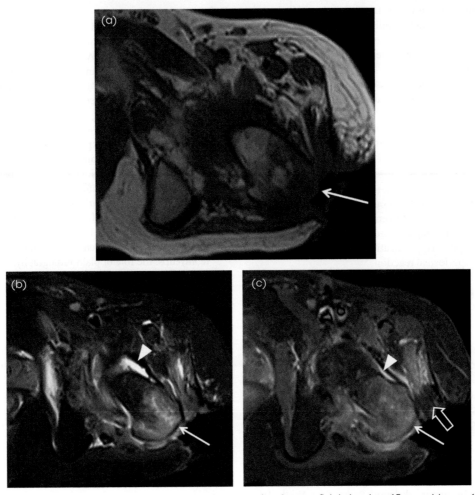

Figure 86.5. Contiguous focus OM in the left greater trochanter secondary to superficial ulcer in a 65-year-old man. (*A*) Axial T1W MR image shows large soft tissue defect/ulcer (*arrow*) by the greater trochanter with low signal in the adjacent soft tissues and in the greater trochanter. (*B*) Axial STIR MR image shows increased signal in the greater trochanter (*arrow*) and surrounding soft tissues with associated left hip joint effusion (*arrowhead*). (*C*) Corresponding axial postcontrast T1W FS MR image shows enhancement in the affected greater trochanter (*arrow*) and the soft tissues with enhancing synovitis (*arrowhead*) in the left hip. Note nonenhancing devitalized tissue (*block arrow*).

intermediate signal on T1W images (penumbra sign) (Figure 86.3*C*) favors OM over tumor.

- Distinguishing acute changes of Charcot arthropathy from OM in the diabetic foot may be challenging as they can share similar imaging features on MRI. Presence of adjacent sinus tracts and draining soft tissue abscess is considered helpful in diagnosis of OM. Additionally, correlation with contemporary radiographs is useful in differentiating foot fractures from OM, which may also display similar signal on MR images. It is easier to discern frequently complex anatomy of the partially amputated and deformed diabetic foot on radiographs when compared to MR images.

Nuclear Imaging

- The commonly used radionuclide, technetium-99m-labeled methylene diphosphonate (^{99m}Tc-MDP) demonstrates increased tracer uptake in acute OM (Figure 86.4*E*). Other agents used are gallium-67 citrate, and indium-111–labeled leukocytes.
- Radionuclide imaging is highly sensitive but has the disadvantage of low specificity and poor anatomical details. Consequently, it is at times difficult to differentiate

between OM and other entities such as fractures, neoplasia, or arthritis.

Differential Diagnosis

- Neoplasms such as osteosarcoma, Ewing sarcoma, lymphoma, and metastasis
- LCH
- Osteoid osteoma
- Charcot arthropathy in diabetic foot
- Fractures

Treatment Options

- OM treatment depends on the appropriate antibiotic therapy and often requires thorough surgical debridement removing infected and necrotic tissue, adequate drainage, postdebridement dead space obliteration, and proper wound care.
- If OM is secondary to host-related causes, such as diabetes mellitus, effort should be made to treat the underlying etiology and improve the host immune system.

- When possible, the antibiotic treatment should be based on the culture and susceptibility results. In cases of urgent surgical debridement, before the cultures can be obtained, empirical broad-spectrum antibiotics should be administered.
- Indications for surgical management include chronic OM, failed response to the antibiotic treatment, and infected surgical hardware.
- Surgical management helps remove dead necrotic tissues and decreases the bacterial load.

Key Points

- OM is caused by hematogenous spread, direct inoculation or contiguous spread from adjacent infection.
- Acute stage radiographic findings include soft tissue edema, osteoporosis, permeative bone erosion, cortical erosion, and periosteal reaction.
- Sequestra, involucra, and cloacae are markers of the chronic stage.
- Brodie abscess usually affects children and involves the metaphysis of the long bones.
- MRI is the modality of choice because of higher sensitivity and better soft tissue contrast.
- MRI protocol must include a T1W sequences together with fluid-sensitive sequences.
- Postcontrast T1W FS MR images improve delineation of nonenhancing fluid collections and necrotic tissue and rim-enhancing osseous and soft tissue abscesses.

Recommended Reading

Tehranzadeh J, Wong E, Wang F, Sadighpour M. Imaging of osteomyelitis in the mature skeleton. *Radiol Clin North Am.* 2001;39:223–50.

References

1. Calhoun JH, Manring MM, Shirtliff M. Osteomyelitis of the long bones. *Semin Plast Surg.* 2009;23:59–72.
2. Gilbertson-Dahdal D, Wright JE, Krupinski E, McCurdy WE, Taljanovic MS. Transphyseal involvement of pyogenic osteomyelitis is considerably more common than classically taught. *AJR Am J Roentgenol.* 2014;203(1):190–95.
3. Hatzenbuehler J, Pulling TJ. Diagnosis and management of osteomyelitis. *Am Fam Physician.* 2011;84:1027–33.
4. Ikpeme IA, Ngim NE, Ikpeme AA. Diagnosis and treatment of pyogenic bone infections. *Afr Health Sci.* 2010;10:82–88.
5. McGuinness B, Wilson N, Doyle AJ. The "penumbra sign" on T1-weighted MRI for differentiating musculoskeletal infection from tumour. *Skeletal Radiol.* 2007;36(5):417–21.
6. Oudjhane K, Azouz EM. Imaging of osteomyelitis in children. *Radiol Clin North Am.* 2001;39:251–66.
7. Pineda C, Espinosa R, Pena A. Radiographic imaging in osteomyelitis: the role of plain radiography, computed tomography, ultrasonography, magnetic resonance imaging, and scintigraphy. *Semin Plast Surg.* 2009;23:80–89.
8. Renton P. Periosteal reaction, bone and joint infections. In: Sutton D, ed. *Textbook of Radiology and Imaging.* 7th ed. Philadelphia, PA: Elsevier; 2003:1153–77.
9. Sanders J, Mauffrey C. Long bone osteomyelitis in adults: fundamental concepts and current techniques. *Orthopedics.* 2013;36:368–75.
10. Tehranzadeh J, Wong E, Wang F, Sadighpour M. Imaging of osteomyelitis in the mature skeleton. *Radiol Clin North Am.* 2001;39:223–50.

CHAPTER 87

Septic Arthritis

Sumer N. Shikhare and Wilfred C. G. Peh

Introduction

Septic arthritis is defined as purulent infection of a joint that leads to arthritis. It has a bimodal age distribution, occurring in very young children and elderly patients. It is slightly more prevalent in male patients. Larger joints are more often involved, with the knee most commonly affected in adults and the hip most at risk in children. The risk is higher when the joint has been traumatized. *Staphylococcus aureus (S. aureus)* is the most common causative organism in most cases in adults. Other common organisms are *Streptococcus* spp., *Neisseria gonorrhoeae*, and less commonly, aerobic gram-negative bacilli such as *Escherichia coli*. In children, *S. aureus* and non-group A and B streptococci are the most common causative agents. *Kingella kingae* is emerging as an important pathogen in children with septic arthritis. In neonates, *S. aureus* (40-50%) or group B *Streptococcus* (20-25%) are the most common causative organisms.

Individuals with open wounds are at a higher risk for septic arthritis. SI and sternoclavicular joints are particularly at risk in patients with human immunodeficiency virus infection, diabetes mellitus, and IV drug abusers. Other potential risk factors include prosthetic joints, alcoholism, recent intraarticular steroid injections, immune deficiency disorders, and cutaneous ulcers. Chronic inflammatory arthritis, such as juvenile idiopathic arthritis (JIA), may predispose to joint infection in children.

Pathophysiology

The 2 principal modes of joint infection are hematogenous and nonhematogenous spread. Hematogenous spread from a distant source such as pneumonia, endocarditis, or wound infection is most common. The less common nonhematogenous route includes infection by direct seeding through trauma or surgery or contiguous spread of infection from overlying soft tissues (eg, cellulitis, abscess) or bone (eg, osteomyelitis).

In the hips, shoulders, ankles, and elbows, the joint capsule overlies a portion of the metaphysis. Hence, if there is underlying metaphyseal osteomyelitis, it may break through and enter the joint, resulting in septic arthritis. The synovial membrane lining the vascularized synovium lacks a basement plate, allowing easy hematogenous entry of the bacteria. Once the organism enters the joint space, the low flow and replacement of joint fluid facilitates bacterial adherence and infection. Infection of the synovial membrane leads to edema and subsequent synovial hypertrophy. Exudative fluid produced by synovium releases proteolytic enzymes causing underlying cartilage destruction. This process eventually extends to the underlying bone, resulting in erosions and osteomyelitis.

Clinical Findings

The clinical symptoms of septic arthritis develop rapidly and mainly manifest with intense pain, joint swelling, and fever. Other symptoms may include chills, fatigue, generalized weakness, and inability to move the affected limb. The joint may appear swollen because of the accumulation of fluid within the joint and warm to touch because of increased blood flow. Intraarticular pathology leads to limitation of active and passive range of motion with the joint held in position to maximize intraarticular space. In contrast, pain from periarticular pathology is triggered when the joint is in active range of motion, and joint swelling is more localized. Laboratory parameters, such as leukocyte count, ESR, and CRP levels, are usually raised, which indicates the presence of infection or inflammatory response. They are also helpful in monitoring response to treatment. However, absence of fever or normal white cell count does not reliably exclude septic arthritis.

Imaging Strategy and Findings

The initial imaging modality should always be conventional radiography in suspected cases of septic arthritis. With suspected septic arthritis, joint aspiration/arthrocentesis should be performed.

MRI is the modality of choice in detecting septic arthritis because of its ability to detect infection at an early stage, as well as its superior contrast resolution and ability to provide multiplanar images. MRI may detect features of septic arthritis as early as 24 hours after the onset of infective process. Postcontrast MRI with fat saturation (FS) has high sensitivity (100%) and specificity (77%) to detect joint infection. CT, US, and radionuclide studies have a more limited role and are used as needed.

Radionuclide imaging is a highly sensitive modality for determining the site and distribution of joint infection. It can identify a septic focus at a very early stage of infection. However, radionuclide imaging has the disadvantage of low specificity. Consequently, it is at times difficult to differentiate between septic arthritis, inflammation, and other causes of synovitis (eg, JIA). Figures 87.1–87.4 show radiographic, MRI, US, and CT findings of septic arthritis.

Radiography

- Early radiographic findings in septic arthritis may include soft tissue edema, periarticular osteopenia, joint effusion, and loss of joint space (Figure 87.1*A*).
- In later or advanced stages of infection, radiographic findings include central or marginal erosions, periosteal

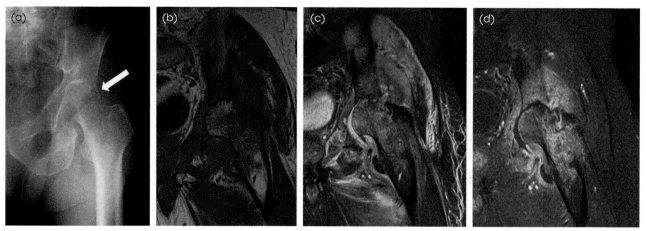

Figure 87.1. Pyogenic septic arthritis and concomitant osteomyelitis of the left hip joint in a 53-year-old man. (*A*) AP radiograph of the left hip joint shows periarticular osteoporosis, uniform narrowing of the joint space and articular erosions (*arrow*). (*B*) Coronal T1W MR image shows a low signal intensity synovial-fluid complex within the left hip joint with associated low bone marrow signal intensity in the acetabulum and patchy low signal in the proximal femur. Note ill-defined low signal in the periarticular soft tissues. (*C*) Coronal STIR MR image shows BME in the affected regions with marked periarticular soft tissue edema. Left hip joint effusion is also present. (*D*) Coronal postcontrast T1W FS MR image shows enhancement of the joint synovium, femoroacetabular bone marrow, and periarticular soft tissues. Bone marrow enhancement in the proximal femur and acetabulum is in keeping with concomitant osteomyelitis.

reaction, subchondral osteolysis, and joint subluxation or dislocation.

- In the chronic stage, there may be bony ankylosis.
- Air lucency may be seen in the joint space and surrounding soft tissues in any stage if there is infection by gas-producing organisms.
- In post arthroplasty patients, particularly hip or knee joints, infection may cause joint effusion, periprosthetic bone erosion, and loosening of the prosthesis (Figure 87.2*A,B*).

Ultrasound
- US is not the modality of choice to diagnose septic arthritis. However, in suspected cases, US is extremely sensitive for demonstrating joint effusion (Figure 87.3*A*).
- Color and/or power Doppler imaging may be helpful to detect periarticular hyperemia in the setting of acute synovitis.
- Nevertheless, joint effusion is not specific for septic arthritis and only indicates an underlying synovial disease.
- US cannot exclude underlying osteomyelitis or soft tissue infection.
- US may be used in needle-guided aspiration of the joint effusion (Figure 87.3*B*).

Computed Tomography
- CT is occasionally used, particularly when MRI cannot be performed.
- Early CT features of septic arthritis include synovial thickening on postcontrast imaging and minimal joint effusion, which are nonspecific findings.
- Other CT features that may be seen are narrowing of the joint space, surrounding soft tissue edema, subarticular erosions, lysis of subchondral bone, and synovial enhancement on postcontrast images.
- CT is very sensitive in detecting air within the joint space in infections caused by gas-forming organisms (Figure 87.2*C*).

- This modality is also effective in image-guided arthrocentesis.

Magnetic Resonance Imaging
- At an early stage of infection, joint effusion is seen as increased signal on fluid-sensitive sequences.
- It is believed that joint effusion and synovial enhancement have the highest association with the clinical diagnosis of septic arthritis (Figures 87.1*B-D*, 87.2*D-F*, and 87.4).
- Other MRI findings that may be seen in septic arthritis include narrowing of the joint space, cartilage destruction, subarticular bone erosion, subchondral bone destruction, and synovial enhancement on postcontrast T1W FS MR images (Figures 87.1*B-D* and 87.2*D-F*).
- Joint fluid may appear heterogeneous on fluid-sensitive (T2W FS or STIR) images because of debris and hemorrhagic components (Figures 87.2*E* and 87.4*A*). The surrounding soft tissues may demonstrate edema because of inflammation (Figures 87.2*E* and 87.4*A*).
- MRI may be useful in detecting coexistent osteomyelitis. In coexistent osteomyelitis, the adjacent bone marrow demonstrates decreased signal on T1W images and corresponding BME on fluid-sensitive images (Figure 87.1*B,C*). This finding may be easily confused with reactive BME/osteitis of septic arthritis. However, BME in bone infection is usually more extensive and multifocal than that seen in reactive BME.
- Lack of abnormal subchondral bone marrow signal intensity and presence of bone erosions favors a diagnosis of tuberculous arthritis rather than of pyogenic arthritis.
- Extraarticular abscesses in pyogenic arthritis show thick and irregularly enhancing rims, in contrast to smooth margins seen in tuberculous arthritis.

Nuclear Imaging
- The 3-phase technetium-99m-labeled methylene diphosphonate (^{99m}Tc-MDP) bone scan in the early stages of infection reflects hyperemia adjacent to the

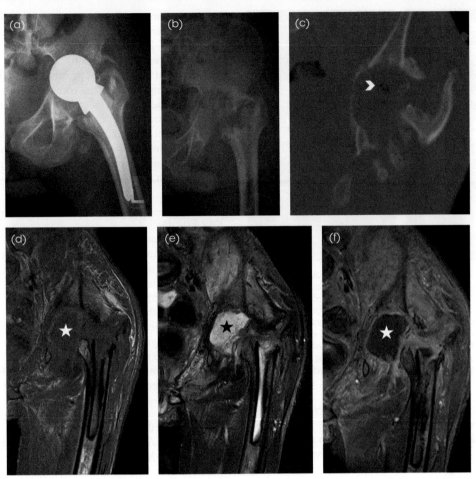

Figure 87.2. Periprosthetic left hip septic arthritis in a 61-year-old man. (*A*) AP radiograph of the left hip shows protrusion of prosthetic femoral head with erosive changes about the proximal femoral metaphysis. (*B*) Postremoval of prosthesis, AP radiograph of the left hip shows erosive changes involving proximal femoral metaphysis and acetabulum and superolateral displacement of the proximal femur. (*C*) Coronal reformatted CT image of the left hip shows erosive bone changes in the proximal femur and acetabulum, periosteal reaction, and a few small foci of gas within the joint space (*arrowhead*). Corresponding coronal MR images, (*D*) T1W, (*E*) T2W FS, and (*F*) T1W FS postcontrast, show a fluid collection in the acetabular fossa (*asterisk*), BME in the proximal femur and acetabulum, and periarticular soft tissue edema with low T1 signal (*D*), high T2 signal (*E*) and no enhancement of acetabular fossa fluid collection in (*F*). In (*F*) note synovial, bone marrow and diffuse high signal periarticular soft tissue enhancement.

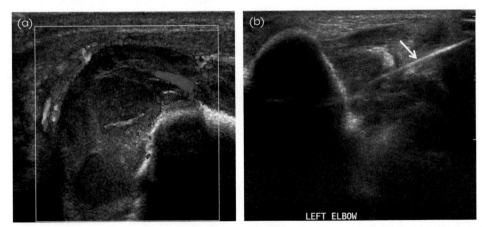

Figure 87.3. US of septic arthritis of the left elbow joint in a 40-year-old man. (*A*) Color Doppler US image of the posterior left elbow joint shows heterogeneous fluid collection with internal echoes and increased vascularity, predominantly peripherally (*colored areas*). (*B*) US-guided aspiration of the elbow joint fluid was performed. Note the echogenic needle within the complex effusion (*arrow*).

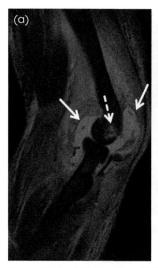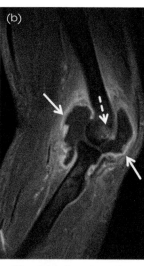

Figure 87.4. MRI of septic arthritis of the right elbow in a 46-year-old man. (*A*) Sagittal T2W FS MR image of the elbow shows a large joint effusion, synovial thickening (*arrows*), patchy BME in the posterior capitellum (*dashed arrow*), and extensive edema in the periarticular soft tissues. (*B*) Sagittal postcontrast T1W FS MR image of the elbow shows moderate synovial enhancement (*arrows*) and enhancement of the periarticular soft tissues, typical of septic arthritis. There is also patchy bone marrow enhancement in the posterior capitellum (*dashed arrow*).

joint and on blood pool images, shows increased activity on either side of the affected area.

- A delayed 24-hour phase bone scan can be helpful in equivocal cases where images usually reveal decreased activity, as opposed to osteomyelitis, which usually shows increased activity.
- Other radionuclides that may be used in the workup of septic arthritis include technetium-99m-hexamethylpropylene-amine-oxime (^{99m}Tc-HMPAO)–labeled leukocytes, indium-111–labeled leukocytes, and gallium-67 citrate scan.
- Gallium imaging may be used in conjunction with a technetium radionuclide study, improving the specificity of the latter technique.

Differential Diagnosis
- Inflammatory arthritis
- Crystal-induced arthritis
- OA
- Primary bone tumor or metastasis

Treatment Options
- Delayed or inadequate treatment of septic arthritis can lead to irreversible joint destruction and subsequent disability.
- Medical management focuses on administration of appropriate antibiotics and immobilization of the joint to control pain.
- Adequate and timely drainage (needle aspiration or open drainage) of the infected synovial fluid remains

the mainstay of treatment. Septic hip is a clinical emergency and warrants immediate aspiration. Radiologists should be proficient in performing imaging-guided arthrocentesis/aspiration.
- Surgical treatment for prosthetic joint infection involves removing the infected components and all cement, as any residual material can potentially serve as a nidus for progressive infection.
- Antibiotic-impregnated cement spacers are often placed at the defect for several weeks or months. The joint must be evaluated for the presence of any infection prior to revision arthroplasty.

Key Points
- Rapid and accurate diagnosis of septic arthritis is crucial, as any delay in diagnosis may irreversibly damage the affected joint.
- With suspected septic arthritis joint, aspiration/arthrocentesis should be performed.
- MRI is the modality of choice in suspected septic arthritis because of its ability to detect infection at an early stage, as well as its superior contrast resolution and ability to provide multiplanar imaging.
- Adequate and timely drainage of the infected synovial fluid remains the mainstay of treatment.

Recommended Reading
1. Greenspan A, Tehranzadeh J. Imaging of infectious arthritis. *Radiol Clin North Am.* 2001;39:267–76.
2. Karchevsky M, Schweitzer ME, Morrison WB, Parellada JA. MRI findings of septic arthritis and associated osteomyelitis in adults. *AJR Am J Roentgenol.* 2004;182:119–22.

References
1. Bodker T, Tottrup M, Petersen KK, Jurik AG. Diagnostics of septic arthritis in the sternoclavicular region: 10 consecutive patients and literature review. *Acta Radiol.* 2013;54:67–74.
2. Greenspan A, Tehranzadeh J. Imaging of infectious arthritis. *Radiol Clin North Am.* 2001;39:267–76.
3. Karchevsky M, Schweitzer ME, Morrison WB, Parellada JA. MRI findings of septic arthritis and associated osteomyelitis in adults. *AJR Am J Roentgenol.* 2004;182:119–22.
4. Lee SK, Suh KJ, Kim YW, et al. Septic arthritis versus transient synovitis at MR imaging: preliminary assessment with signal intensity alterations in bone marrow. *Radiology.* 1999;211:459–65.
5. Lin HM, Learch TJ, White EA, Gottsegen CJ. Emergency joint aspiration: a guide for radiologists on call. *Radiographics.* 2009;29:1139–58.
6. Mathews CJ, Kingsley G, Field M, et al. Management of septic arthritis: a systematic review. *Ann Rheum Dis.* 2007;66:440–45.
7. Margaretten ME, Kohlwes J, Moore D, Bent S. Does this adult patient have septic arthritis? *JAMA.* 2007;297:1478–88.
8. Morgan DS, Fisher D, Merianos A, Currie BJ. An 18 year clinical review of septic arthritis from tropical Australia. *Epidemiol Infect.* 1996;117:423–28.

9. Mue D, Salihu M, Awonusi F, et al. The epidemiology and outcome of acute septic arthritis: a hospital based study. *J West Afr Coll Surg.* 2013;3:40–52.

10. SH Hong, Kim SM, Ahn JM, Chung HW, Shin MJ, Kang HS. Tuberculous versus pyogenic arthritis: MR imaging evaluation. *Radiology.* 2001;218:848–53.

11. Shirtliff ME, Mader JT. Acute septic arthritis. *Clin Microbiol Rev.* 2002;15:527–44.

12. Zimmerli W. Infection and musculoskeletal conditions: prosthetic-joint-associated infections. *Best Pract Res Clin Rheumatol.* 2006;20:1045–63.

CHAPTER 88

Soft Tissue Infections

Sumer N. Shikhare and Wilfred C. G. Peh

Introduction

Soft tissue infection can affect any age group, although it is more common in the elderly population. Factors that may predispose to soft tissue infection are old age; IV drug abuse; immune-compromised status; surgery; trauma; systemic diseases, such as diabetes mellitus and peripheral vascular disease; and lower socioeconomic status. Some of the infections are more common in tropical climates than temperate ones.

Soft tissue infections commonly occur secondary to direct inoculation such as trauma, surgery, or foreign body injury. Other modes are hematogenous routes or contiguous spread of infection from nearby septic foci. Soft tissue infection can be mono- or polymicrobial, although the latter is more common. The organisms commonly cultured are *Streptococcus, Staphylococcus, Enterobacteriaceae, Enterococcus, Bacteroides* ssp., anaerobic gram-positive cocci, and *Clostridium* spp.

Pathophysiology and Clinical Findings

The soft tissues consist of skin, subcutaneous tissue, superficial and deep fascia, bursa, tendon sheath, and muscle. Soft tissue infections can be broadly classified into superficial and deep. Superficial soft tissue infections comprise cellulitis, superficial fasciitis, tenosynovitis, and infectious bursitis. Deep soft tissue infections include deep fasciitis, pyomyositis, and infected myonecrosis. Both superficial and deep soft tissue infections can evolve into abscesses. Soft tissue infection commonly occur after direct inoculation of the skin and subcutaneous tissues and extend into the deeper tissue. Apart from direct inoculation, the tendon sheath, bursa, and muscle can become infected via the hematogenous route as well as from a contiguous source such as joint infection.

Necrotizing fasciitis is a life-threatening infection of the superficial and deep fascia characterized by inflammation of the fascial planes, presence of air, and involvement of muscles in advanced cases. The commonly affected sites include the scrotum, perineum, lower extremity, and neck. Pyomyositis refers to pyogenic skeletal muscle infection characterized by muscle edema, which may lead to abscess formation. As skeletal muscle is quite resistant to infection, pyomyositis is relatively uncommon unless there is underlying injury, metabolic disorder, or systemic disease. Infectious bursitis commonly affects the prepatellar and olecranon bursae as they are more susceptible to direct trauma because of their superficial locations. Other locations commonly involved are the subacromial-subdeltoid, infrapatellar, gastrocnemius-semimembranosus, and iliopsoas bursae.

The clinical signs and symptoms are nonspecific and include fever, chills, malaise, pain, soft tissue edema, erythema, or crepitus caused by soft tissue gas. Useful laboratory investigations include complete blood count showing leucocytosis, with elevated inflammatory markers such as ESR and CRP.

Imaging Strategy

Imaging modalities useful in diagnosing soft tissue infections include radiography, US, CT, and MRI. The role of imaging is to define the extent of soft tissue infection, show coexisting complications, and identify areas where intervention may be useful. Figures 88.1 through 88.8 show imaging findings of various superficial and deep soft tissue infections.

Conventional radiographs are frequently not specific in diagnosing soft tissue infections and may show soft tissue edema (Figure 88.1A), displaced fat planes, radiolucent soft tissue gas in case of gas-forming organisms (Figure 88.2A), air-fluid level in the soft tissues, foreign body, or underlying reactive bone changes. MRI is the modality of choice in diagnosing soft tissue infections, but CT is better in detecting subtle foci of soft tissue air. US and CT examinations are useful for image-guided aspiration and drainage of loculated soft tissue collections.

Imaging Findings

Cellulitis

- The diagnosis of cellulitis is typically based on clinical history, and the role of imaging is to exclude any abscess formation or presence of other complications.
- Radiographs may show nonspecific soft tissue edema (Figure 88.1A).
- US characteristically shows diffuse skin thickening, subcutaneous edema, and linear anechoic fluid collections along the interlobular septa (Figure 88.1B). This finding is quite nonspecific and cannot be differentiated from other conditions causing soft tissue edema. Hyperemia is frequently present on power or color Doppler interrogation.
- CT examination usually is not recommended to diagnose cellulitis except where MRI cannot be performed. CT shows soft tissue edema, subcutaneous septations, and heterogeneous postcontrast enhancement.
- MRI shows subcutaneous tissue thickening and diffuse reticular increased signal in subcutaneous fat on

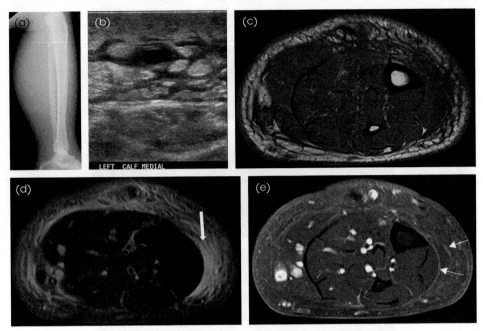

Figure 88.1. Cellulitis in a 50-year-old man. (*A*) Lateral radiograph of the left leg shows nonspecific soft tissue edema of the left calf. (*B*) Transverse US image shows soft tissue edema with anechoic linear fluid collections in the interlobular septa outlining hyperechoic fat lobules. (*C*) Axial T1W MR image shows decreased reticular signal intensity in the subcutaneous soft tissues and along superficial fascial planes of the left leg. (*D*) Axial STIR MR image shows corresponding increased signal intensity (*arrow*). (*E*) On the axial postcontrast T1W FS MR image, note mild enhancement in the affected tissues (*arrows*) consistent with cellulitis and superficial fasciitis.

fluid-sensitive sequences and decreased signal on T1W sequences, with variable degree of contrast enhancement (Figure 88.1*C-E*). Air within the subcutaneous tissue, if present is better demonstrated on GRE images as areas of signal voids (Figure 88.2*B*).

Superficial, Deep, and Necrotizing Fasciitis
- Superficial and/or deep fascial plane infection (infective fasciitis) shows fascial thickening and fluid tracking with variable contrast enhancement on both CT and MRI.

- MRI is the modality of choice in diagnosing necrotizing fasciitis.
  - On MRI, the most essential component to diagnose necrotizing fasciitis is increased signal on T2W images in the deep fascia (especially intermuscular fascia).
  - Extensive deep fascial involvement and deep fascial thickening of more than 3 mm are additional findings that may aid in the diagnosis (Figure 88.3*A*).
  - There is variable enhancement on postcontrast images along thickened deep fascial planes (Figure 88.3*B*).

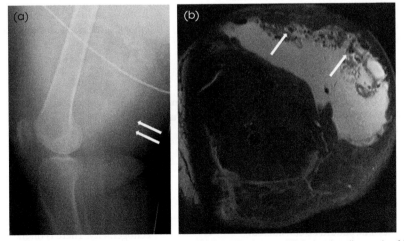

Figure 88.2. Necrotizing soft tissue infection in the right leg of a 58-year-old woman. (*A*) Lateral radiograph of the knee shows soft tissue edema with multiple foci of gas (*arrows*). (*B*) Axial T2W FS MR image shows mild scattered subcutaneous edema consistent with cellulitis and a large high signal subcutaneous fluid collection with multiple areas of signal void, typical of susceptibility artifacts caused by gas (*arrows*).

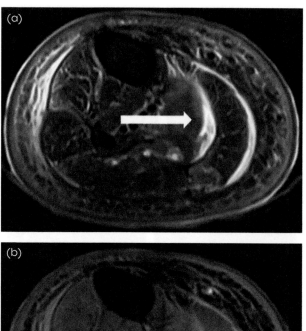

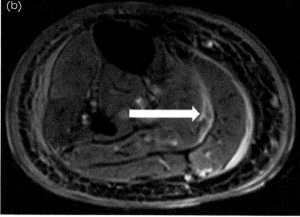

Figure 88.3. Necrotizing fasciitis in the right leg of a 62-year-old man. (*A*) Axial T2W FS MR image of the mid-calf shows thick hyperintense fluid signal in the intermuscular fascia abutting the calf muscles (*arrow*). Note additional subcutaneous, superficial fascial and patchy muscular edema. (*B*) Corresponding axial postcontrast T1W FS MR image shows heterogeneous enhancement of the affected tissues including the deep fascia (*arrow*), consistent with deep fasciitis associated with myositis, superficial fasciitis, and cellulitis.

- Lack of deep facial enhancement may be caused by tissue hypoperfusion and does not exclude necrotizing fasciitis.
- Diagnosis of necrotizing fasciitis can be excluded if the preceding findings are not present, but if seen, they are not specific and can be found in conditions such as lymphedema, venous congestion, muscle injury, neoplastic disease, and noninfectious fasciitis.
- Air in the deep fascia is a specific but inconsistent finding and is seen better on GRE images as areas of signal voids.
- The subcutaneous tissue demonstrates increased signal on T2W and STIR images, similar to cellulitis.
- Compartment syndrome is a complication that may be associated with fasciitis. In this condition, high pressure within a compartment reduces capillary blood supply with threatened tissue viability. Interstitial tissue pressure of 30 mm Hg has been suggested as a threshold at which the diagnosis of compartment syndrome should be considered.
- Although CT is not as sensitive as MRI, it is better in detecting subtle foci of soft tissue air and can additionally demonstrate fascial plane blurring, thickening of the fascial planes, and interfascial fluid.
- US is not an imaging modality of choice in evaluation of superficial and deep fasciitis.
  - It shows fluid in the affected fascial planes with variable degrees of associated color or power Doppler signal.
  - Air, if present, is seen as echogenic foci with posterior dirty shadowing.

Pyomyositis and Muscle Abscess
- US has a limited role and usually shows edematous, swollen muscle with increased or decreased muscle echogenicity and loss of the normal architectural striated pattern.
  - The inflamed muscle usually shows increased flow on power or color Doppler US.
  - In later stages, abscesses may be seen that are usually hypoechoic, anechoic (Figure 88.4*A*), or of mixed echogenicity. There is often peripheral hyperemia and occasionally internal septations, debris, or mobile hyperechoic air foci.

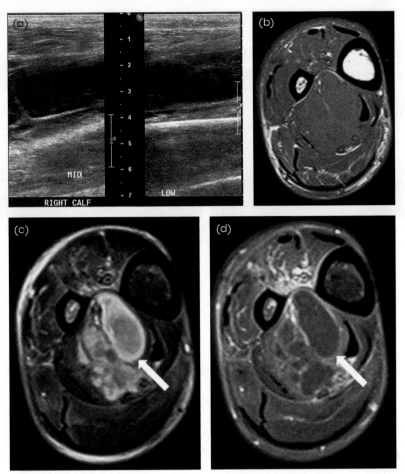

Figure 88.4. Pyomyositis and intramuscular abscess in a 63-year-old diabetic man with leg pain and swelling. (*A*) Long axis US images of the calf show an anechoic loculated intramuscular fluid collection with internal echoes. Corresponding axial MR images (*B-D*) show a large lobulated and multiloculated fluid collection (*arrows*) in the deep posterior muscle compartment of the calf with intermediate signal on the T1W MR image (*B*), heterogeneous increased signal on the T2W FS MR image (*C*), and with rim and septal enhancement on the postcontrast T1W FS MR image (*D*) consistent with an intramuscular abscess and pyomyositis. In (*C*), note additional patchy muscular and deep fascial edema in the anterior muscular compartments which show enhancement in (*D*).

- Surrounding soft tissue structures appear edematous and show increased vascularity on color Doppler US.
- Air, if present, is seen as echogenic foci with posterior dirty shadowing.
- CT shows thickened skin and fascial planes with asymmetric muscle thickness because of edema.
  - On postcontrast CT, the affected muscle usually shows less enhancement compared to the normal muscle.
  - In case of muscle necrosis or abscess, CT shows an ill-defined, low-attenuating region of the muscle with peripheral, thick-walled, rim enhancement on postcontrast images.
  - Air within the collection is easily seen on CT and shows low attenuation. These CT findings are useful in differentiating an abscess from a hematoma or tumor.
  - Another advantage of CT is in image-guided aspiration and drainage.
  - Concomitant deep vein thrombosis, if present, can be seen on contrast enhanced CT.
  - Concomitant osteomyelitis with associated destructive bone changes may also be seen if present.

- MRI is the preferred imaging modality to diagnose pyomyositis, which may show affected areas that are not evident on CT.
  - The affected muscles show heterogeneously increased signal on T2W images and minimally increased signal on T1W images with heterogeneous postcontrast enhancement on T1W FS images (Figure 88.5).
  - An abscess usually exhibits heterogeneously increased signal on T2W images, decreased signal on T1W images, with peripheral rim enhancement on postcontrast images (Figure 88.4*B-D*). Adjacent soft tissues demonstrate edema and reticulation on T2W images and enhancement following Gd-based contrast administration consistent with phlegmon.
  - Diffusion-weighted imaging may help in diagnosing abscess when Gd-based contrast cannot be given. Abscess will show restricted diffusion with high signal intensity on fractional anisotropy (FA) maps and low signal on apparent diffusion coefficient (ADC) maps.

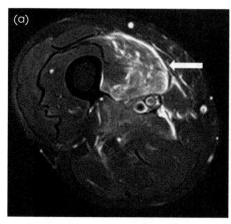
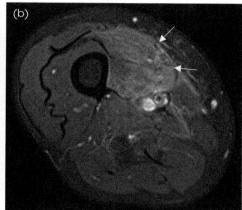

Figure 88.5. Pyomyositis in a 45-year-old woman. (*A*) Axial T2W FS MR image shows patchy areas of T2-hyperintense signal involving muscles of the anterior and medial compartments of the thigh (*arrow*). (*B*) Axial postcontrast T1W FS MR image shows heterogeneous enhancement in the affected muscles consistent with myositis (*arrows*).

Infectious Tenosynovitis

- On US, infectious tenosynovitis is characterized by a distended and thickened tendon sheath and may be associated with tendon thickening.
  - Color or power Doppler US shows a variable degree of hyperemia within the tendon sheath and tendon (Figure 88.6).
  - Tendon sheath fluid may show echogenic debris and/or septations.
- CT is rarely used and usually only indicated if MRI or US cannot be performed.
  - CT may only demonstrate a fluid-distended tendon sheath with variable synovial enhancement and a variable degree of tendon heterogeneity and thickening.
- MRI is the imaging modality of choice for evaluating tenosynovitis.
  - Normal tendon shows low signal on all pulse sequences.

- If infected, the tendon may appear thickened and indistinct and show increased signal on T2W sequences with variable postcontrast enhancement.
- Fluid within the tendon sheath demonstrates increased signal on T2W images with a variable degree of synovial enhancement on the postcontrast sequences (Figure 88.7).
- Tendon sheath fluid may appear heterogeneous if it contains debris, septations, blood, or gas.
- Adjacent soft tissues may show edema with high signal on fluid-sensitive sequences and variable degree of enhancement on the postcontrast sequences consistent with associated cellulitis.
- Differential diagnosis includes tenosynovitis associated with inflammatory arthritides such as RA.

Infectious Bursitis

- US shows fluid-filled distended bursae, thick bursal wall, and surrounding soft tissue edema.
  - In case of infection, bursal fluid is usually of mixed echogenicity showing internal debris and may have echogenic dirty shadowing in keeping with air.
  - Bursal wall and surrounding tissues reveal hyperemia on color or power Doppler imaging.
  - Another use of US is for image-guided fluid aspiration, which may be required for culture to identify a specific organism.
- CT usually demonstrates fluid-filled bursae and surrounding inflammatory changes with wall and peribursal soft tissue postcontrast enhancement which can mimic an abscess.
  - Bursal fluid may show air bubbles within, in case of gas-producing organism.
- MRI is very sensitive and is the modality of choice in evaluation of infectious bursitis.
  - On MRI, bursal fluid and adjacent inflamed soft tissues show heterogeneously increased signal on fluid-sensitive sequences (Figure 88.8A) with corresponding decreased signal on T1W images.
  - Foci of air may be seen as areas of signal voids.

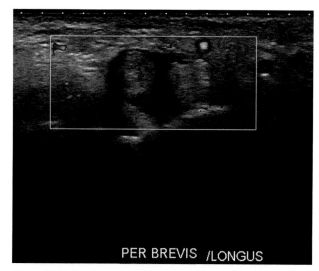

PER BREVIS /LONGUS

Figure 88.6. Septic peroneal tenosynovitis in a 52-year-old woman. Transverse power Doppler US image shows a fluid-distended peroneal tendon sheath with mild hyperemia.

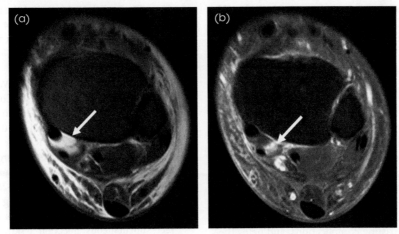

Figure 88.7. Septic tibialis posterior tibial tendon (PTT) tenosynovitis in a 29-year-old woman. (*A*) Axial T2W FS MR image of the ankle shows a distended PTT sheath with high signal intensity synovial-fluid complex (*arrow*). Note high signal intensity marked superficial soft tissue edema. (*B*) Corresponding axial postcontrast T1W FS MR image shows peripheral enhancement of the PTT sheath (*arrow*) with central nonenhancing fluid. Note heterogeneous enhancement of the superficial soft tissues consistent with cellulitis.

- On postcontrast images, the bursal wall and surrounding tissue typically show enhancement (Figure 88.8*B*).
- It may be difficult to differentiate inflammatory bursitis from pyogenic infectious bursitis, unless there are air foci or loose bodies within the bursal fluid. The latter is usually associated with RA, tuberculosis, PVNS, and synovial chondromatosis.

Treatment Options
- Uncomplicated cellulitis is treated with analgesics and antibiotics and correction of metabolic abnormalities. Elevation of the affected limb may be helpful.

- Necrotizing fasciitis requires urgent surgical debridement, decompression fasciotomy, and IV antibiotics. This may be supplemented by hyperbaric oxygen.
- Pyomyositis and muscle abscess are usually treated by IV antibiotics and surgical debridement. In some cases, image-guided drainage may be performed. Myoglobulinuria commonly associated with pyomyositis may cause renal tubular acidosis, thus the patient needs appropriate hydration and urine-alkalizing agents.
- Infective tenosynovitis is usually treated with IV antibiotics, limb elevation, and splinting and may need surgical intervention if there is no improvement after 24 hours.

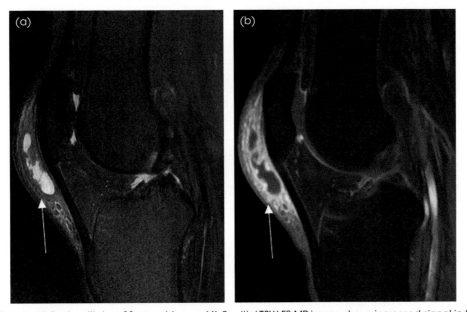

Figure 88.8. Septic prepatellar bursitis in a 38-year-old man. (*A*) Sagittal T2W FS MR image shows increased signal in the distended prepatellar bursa (*arrow*). (*B*) Sagittal postcontrast T1W FS MR image shows thick peripheral enhancement of the prepatellar bursa with areas of central nonenhancement representing fluid (*arrow*) in keeping with infectious bursitis.

■ Treatment options for septic bursitis include IV antibiotics, surgical drainage, or bursectomy, depending on complexity of the case.

Key Points

■ The most common route of soft tissue infection is direct inoculation.
■ Soft tissue infections broadly consist of cellulitis, superficial and deep fasciitis, tenosynovitis, infectious bursitis, and pyomyositis/muscle abscess.
■ Prompt imaging facilitates early diagnosis, thus facilitating early treatment and decreasing risk of complications.
■ Imaging accurately defines the extent of soft tissue infection, recognizes coexisting complications, and helps the clinicians in treatment management.
■ MRI is the imaging modality of choice in evaluation of soft tissue infections.
■ US and CT examinations are useful for image-guided drainage of loculated soft tissue collections.

Recommended Reading

Turecki MB, Taljanovic MS, Stubbs AY, et al. Imaging of musculoskeletal soft tissue infections. *Skeletal Radiol.* 2010;39:957–71.

References

1. Ali SZ, Srinivasan S, Peh WCG. MRI in necrotizing fasciitis of the extremities. *Br J Radiol.* 2014;87(1033):20130560.
2. Beauchamp NJ, Scott WW, Gottlieb LM, Fishman EK. CT evaluation of soft tissue and muscle infection and inflammation: a systematic compartmental approach. *Skeletal Radiol.* 1995;24:317–24.
3. Bureau NJ, Ali SS, Chhem RK, Cardinal E. Ultrasound of musculoskeletal infections. *Semin Musculoskelet Radiol.* 1998;2:299–306.
4. Chau CL, Griffith JF. Musculoskeletal infections: ultrasound appearances. *Clin Radiol.* 2005;60:149–59.
5. Chou H, Teo HE, Dubey N, Peh WCG. Tropical pyomyositis and necrotizing fasciitis. *Semin Musculoskelet Radiol.* 2011;15:489–505.
6. Chun CW, Jung JY, Baik JS, Jee WH, Kim SK, Shin SH. Detection of soft-tissue abscess: Comparison of diffusion-weighted imaging to contrast-enhanced MRI. *J Magn Reson Imaging.* 2018;47(1):60–68. doi:10.1002/jmri.25743.
7. Elliott D, Kufera JA, Myers RA. The microbiology of necrotizing soft tissue infections. *Am J Surg.* 2000;179:361–66.
8. Hadley AJ. Necrotizing soft tissue infections: a primary care review. *Am Fam Phys.* 2003;68:323–28.
9. Johnston C, Keogan MT. Imaging features of soft-tissue infections and other complications in drug users after direct subcutaneous injection ("skin popping"). *AJR Am J Roentgenol.* 2004;182:1195–202.
10. Kothari NA, Pelchovitz DJ, Meyer JS. Imaging of musculoskeletal infections. *Radiol Clin North Am.* 2001;39:653–71.
11. Pattamapaspong N, Sivasomboon C, Settakorn J, Pruksakorn D, Muttarak M. Pitfalls in imaging of musculoskeletal infections. *Semin Musculoskelet Radiol.* 2014;18:86–100.
12. Pretorius ES, Fishman EK. Helical CT of musculoskeletal infection. *Crit Rev Diagn Imaging.* 2001;42:259–305.
13. Schmid MR, Kossmann T, Duewell S. Differentiation of necrotizing fasciitis and cellulitis using MR imaging. *AJR Am J Roentgenol.* 1998;170:615–20.
14. Small LN, Ross JJ. Suppurative tenosynovitis and septic bursitis. *Infect Dis Clin North Am.* 2005;19:991–1005.
15. Struk DW, Munk PL, Lee MJ, Ho SG, Worsley DF. Imaging of soft tissue infections. *Radiol Clin North Am.* 2001;39:277–303.
16. Turecki MB, Taljanovic MS, Stubbs AY, et al. Imaging of musculoskeletal soft tissue infections. *Skeletal Radiol.* 2010;39:957–71.
17. Yoshida S, Shidoh M, Imai K, Imai A, Konishi Y, Kon S. Rice bodies in ischiogluteal bursitis. *Postgrad Med J.* 2003;930:220–21.

Atypical Infections

CHAPTER 89

Tuberculosis

Remide Arkun

Introduction

Tuberculosis (TB) is an infectious disease caused by *Mycobacterium tuberculosis*. Although TB is most common in areas with crowding, poor sanitation, and malnutrition, it is a worldwide disease nowadays because of the global emergence of acquired immunodeficiency syndrome (AIDS), increased number of immunocompromised patients, growing population suffering from chronic diseases, such as diabetes and chronic renal failure, and development of multidrug resistant strains. Extrapulmonary TB is seen in 20% of all TB cases. Musculoskeletal TB accounts for 1-3% of tuberculous infections.

Pathophysiology and Clinical Findings

Five different forms of musculoskeletal TB have been described. TB spondylitis (50%) is the most common presentation followed by peripheral TB arthritis (30%), TB osteomyelitis (19%), TB tenosynovitis, TB bursitis, and Poncet disease (1%). Poncet disease is characterized by polyarthritis occurring during active TB infection. Hematogenous dissemination of the organism from a visceral primary focus (lungs, kidneys, lymph nodes) to the musculoskeletal system is the most common pathway, but lymphatic spread or direct inoculation of the organism are also possible. After the causative organism has reached the site, it becomes ingested by the mononuclear cell followed by serial inflammatory reactions after which tubercle formation and central caseation of tubercle occur. The outcome depends on the characteristics and sensitivity of the organism, status of the host immune system, stage of disease at presentation, and treatment.

Approximately 50% of patients with osteoarticular TB will present with spinal involvement. The most common locations are the thoracic and thoracolumbar spine. However, any segment of the spine can be involved. Spinal TB is initially apparent in the anterior inferior portion of the vertebral body as spondylitis. Later on, it spreads into the central part of the vertebral body or intervertebral disc. Paradiscal, anterior, and central lesions are the common types of vertebral involvement. Because of subligamentous spread of infection, multiple contiguous vertebral involvement and cold abscess formation (abscesses with a paucity of intense inflammation usually seen with abscesses caused by bacteria) may occur. With central vertebral body involvement, the disc is not involved, and collapse of the vertebral body produces vertebra plana. Spinal canal narrowing by abscesses, granulation tissue, or direct dural invasion resulting in spinal cord compression and neurologic deficits are other pathologic changes in spinal TB.

In TB arthritis, tubercular bacilli disseminate to the synovium through the subsynovial vessels via hematogenous spread, but the joint can become involved from direct penetration of an epiphyseal focus in adults or metaphyseal focus in children. When the infection starts as synovitis, the synovial membrane becomes congested and thickened and joint effusion develops. Synovial granulation tissue proliferates at the joint periphery and leads to marginal erosions. Granulomatous synovial lesions expand further over the bone and may subsequently result in central and peripheral erosions and cartilage destruction. However, because the exudate in TB arthritis lacks proteolytic enzymes, cartilage loss occurs only late in the disease. If the disease process is not interrupted, it may lead to severe destruction of the joint and ankylosis. TB arthritis is usually seen as monoarthritis, and the knee and hip joints are the most common sites.

TB osteomyelitis comprises 19% of musculoskeletal TB cases. Infection spreads from an active focus by a hematogenous route. The femur, tibia, and small bones of the hands and feet are most commonly involved. Metaphyseal involvement is common. The disease process includes granuloma formation with caseating necrosis and fibrosis. Further progression may result in macroscopically visible bone destruction, transphyseal spread of disease, and joint involvement. Abscess formation may occur, and sinus tracts are common.

TB soft tissue involvement, such as tenosynovitis and bursitis, is rare and may result from hematogenous spread or because of periarticular extension of disease. Synovial hyperemia and inflammation may cause synovial ischemia and necrosis caused by hypoxia. The wall of the tendon sheath is replaced by TB granulation tissue. Rice bodies are formed by the necrotic particles in TB synovitis that detach from the synovium and adhere to fibrin in the joint space, tendon sheath, or inside the bursa.

Musculoskeletal TB can cause significant morbidity, and a high index of suspicion is needed for early diagnosis to avoid destruction and disability. Clinical findings are variable depending on the region involved. Generally, patients complain of low-grade fevers, night sweats, weight loss, anorexia, and malaise. Other complaints include swelling, stiffness, and pain (*night cries* may wake the patient from sleep). Osseous involvement is associated with localized warmth, swelling, and tenderness. Joint involvement is associated with tenderness, soft tissue swelling and/or effusion, and restriction of movement. Findings in patients with spinal disease include back pain/tenderness, neurologic deficit, and kyphotic deformity. Swelling and tenderness over a synovial bursa (especially the greater trochanter) or tendon sheath is seen less frequently. Lymphadenopathy is common, and sinus tracts are frequently seen. Laboratory investigations including complete blood count, ESR, CRP, and chest radiographs should be obtained, however, these tests may not be conclusive. Mantoux skin test has a limited role in adults in high prevalence areas but can be useful in children younger than 5 years. Tissue smear or culture are also not always positive.

Imaging Strategy

Several imaging modalities including radiography, CT, MRI, and US are available and helpful in the diagnosis of musculoskeletal TB. Radiography should be the first imaging modality. Imaging findings vary according to the location of TB infection. Spinal TB is the most common form in the musculoskeletal system, and early diagnosis of spinal TB is important to prevent advanced bone and/or joint destruction. However, radiography is often not effective in making an early diagnosis. MRI is the best imaging modality to evaluate TB spondylitis.

Imaging Findings

Spinal Tuberculosis
Figures 89.1 through 89.3 show imaging findings of the spinal TB.

Radiography
- Osteolytic destruction of the anterior part of the vertebral body
- Vertebral body collapse
- Increased paravertebral soft tissue density with or without calcification
- Disc space narrowing
- Irregular vertebral body endplate sclerosis
- Extensive vertebral body height loss with severe kyphotic angulation (gibbus deformity) in advanced cases

Computed Tomography
- Imaging findings are similar to radiographic findings but better seen on CT (Figure 89.1D).

Magnetic Resonance Imaging
- Decreased signal intensity on T1W MR images (Figures 89.1A, 89.2A, and 89.3A) and BME with high signal on fluid-sensitive sequences (Figures 89.2B, 89.3B, C) in the involved vertebral bodies with relative preservation of the disc space.
- Thin and smooth enhancement of associated paraspinal abscess walls and well-defined paraspinal abnormal signal are suggestive of TB spondylitis with subligamentous spread to 3 or more vertebral levels (Figures 89.1B, C, 89.2C, and 89.3D–F). Conversely, thick and irregular enhancement of abscess walls and an ill-defined paraspinal abnormal signal are suggestive of pyogenic spondylitis.
- With epidural involvement, cord compression can occur (Figures 89.1B, C and 89.2).

Tuberculosis Arthritis
This is commonly a monoarticular disease (Figures 89.4 and 89.5). The hip and knee are the most commonly involved joints.

Radiography
Refer to Figure 89.4

- Phemister triad-juxtaarticular osteoporosis, peripherally located osseous erosions, and gradual narrowing of the joint space are seen.
- Severe subchondral erosions, osseous destruction, and fibrous ankylosis are seen late in the disease.

Magnetic Resonance Imaging
Refer to 89.4B-D and 89.5.
- Synovitis and pannus formation are the early findings of TB arthritis. Active synovitis and pannus formation are

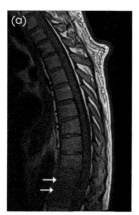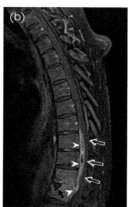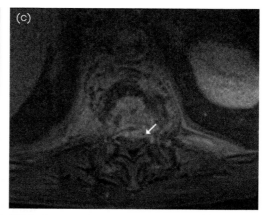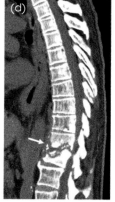

Figure 89.1. Tuberculous spondylitis at T11-T12. (*A*) Sagittal T1W MR image shows hypointense signal involving the T11 and T12 vertebral bodies (*arrows*) with indistinctness of vertebral endplates adjacent to the T11-T12 disc space. (*B*) Sagittal and (*C*) axial T1W FS postcontrast MR images show enhancement on the T11 and T12 vertebral bodies and posterior part of T11-T12 disc. Note rim-enhancing intraosseous (*black arrow*) and epidural abscesses with epidural subligamentous spread up to the T8-T9 level (*arrowheads*). Cord compression caused by epidural abscess is seen on sagittal (*open arrows*) and axial (*arrow*) postcontrast images. (*D*) Sagittal reformatted CT image demonstrates loss of the anterior part of T12 vertebral body height, irregular endplate sclerosis, and fragmentation on both the T11 and T12 vertebral bodies (*arrow*).

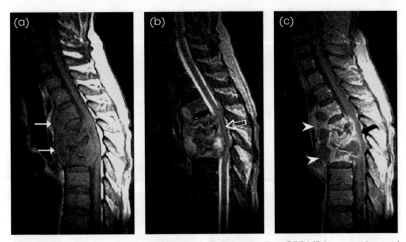

Figure 89.2. Tuberculous spondylitis at C7-T3. (*A*) Sagittal T1W and (*B*) fluid-sensitive GRE MR images show a large anterior paravertebral soft tissue mass (*arrows*) with collapse of the T1 and T2 vertebral bodies, collapse of the T1, T2, and T3 vertebral endplates and loss of the disc spaces at the T1-T2 and T2-T3 levels. Note epidural soft tissue mass/extension causing cord compression with myelopathy (*open arrow*). (*C*) Sagittal T1W FS postcontrast MR image shows avid heterogeneous enhancement of the affected vertebral bodies and thin and smooth enhancement of the anterior paravertebral abscess wall (*white arrowheads*). Note severe cord compression caused by an epidural abscess (*curved black arrow*).

seen as low-intermediate signal intensity on T1W, T2W, and PDW MR images. Whereas active pannus formation (inflamed synovium) shows early enhancement after IV Gd-based contrast administration, synovial fluid does not show enhancement.

- Cartilage and bone erosions—cartilage destruction can be seen as local or diffuse thinning that shows intermediate signal intensity on T1W, T2W, and PDW MR images and hyperintense signal on GRE images. Bone erosions may be central and/or peripheral and

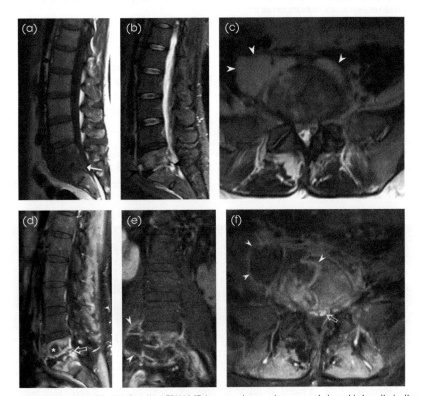

Figure 89.3. Tuberculous spondylitis at L5-S1. (*A*) Sagittal T1W MR image shows decreased signal intensity in the L5 and S1 vertebral bodies with a hypointense posterior epidural soft tissue mass (*arrow*). (*B*) Sagittal T2W FS MR image shows increased signal intensity in the L5 and S1 vertebral bodies and subligamentous spread (*black arrowheads*). (*C*) Axial T2W FS MR image shows a large anterior paravertebral abscess (*arrowheads*). (*D*) Sagittal T1W FS postcontrast MR image shows enhancement of the L5 and S1 vertebral bodies including the epidural mass (*open arrow*). There is also a rim-enhancing intraosseous abscess (*asterisk*). (*E*) Coronal and (*F*) axial T1W FS postcontrast MR images show thin and smooth rim enhancement of the paravertebral and intraosseous abscess walls (*arrowheads*) and epidural enhancement (*open arrow*).

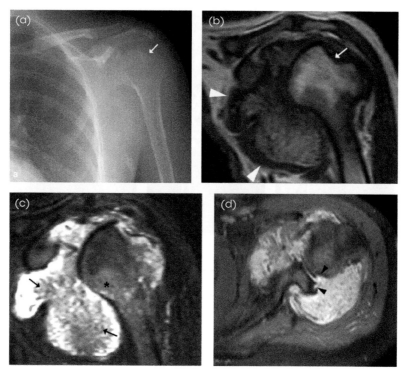

Figure 89.4. Tuberculous arthritis involving the glenohumeral joint. (*A*) AP radiograph of the left shoulder shows periarticular osteopenia and a large juxtaarticular erosion at the humeral head (*arrow*). (*B*) Coronal T1W MR image shows a bone erosion at the humeral head (*arrow*) and a large joint effusion with heterogeneous signal intensity (*arrowheads*). (*C*) Coronal T2W FS MR image shows hypointense pannus (*arrows*) and a joint effusion with BME (*asterisk*) in the medial part of humeral head. (*D*) Axial T1W FS postcontrast MR image shows juxtaarticular erosions at the posterior aspect of the glenohumeral joint (*arrowheads*) with associated joint-space narrowing and marked synovial enhancement.

appear hypointense on both T1W and fluid-sensitive sequences. There may be rim enhancement around bone erosions.

- BME and periarticular abscess formation also can be seen. These findings are more common in pyogenic than septic arthritis.
- Rice body formation may occur with a systemic inflammatory disease or in the localized form. Rice bodies are free particles that have a cartilage-like shiny appearance and can be numerous. These are

of synovial origin and can be seen in patients with RA and atypical mycobacterial tenosynovitis in addition to TB synovitis. On MRI, rice bodies are seen as numerous small hypointense nodules within the hyperintense synovial fluid on the fluid-sensitive sequences.

Tuberculosis Osteomyelitis

Femur, tibia, and small bones of the hands and feet are the most commonly involved bones (Figure 89.6).

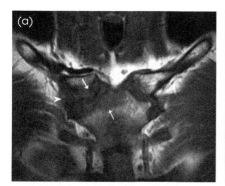
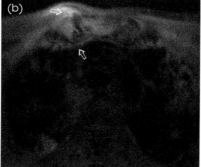
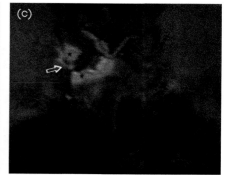

Figure 89.5. Tuberculous arthritis involving the sternoclavicular joint. (*A*) Coronal T1W MR image shows low bone marrow signal intensity in the clavicular head and adjacent sternal manubrium along the right sternoclavicular joint (*arrows*) with associated soft tissue mass (*arrowhead*). (*B*) Axial T2W FS MR image shows BME in the affected clavicle and sternum. Note an associated joint effusion (*open arrows*). There is also extensive pulmonary TB infection in the lung apices. (*C*) Coronal T1W FS postcontrast MR image shows heterogeneous enhancement of the affected clavicle and sternum (*asterisks*) together with associated synovial enhancement in the sternoclavicular joint (*open arrow*) consistent with TB arthritis and osteomyelitis.

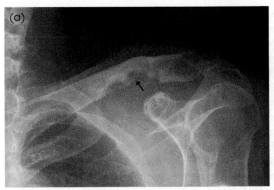
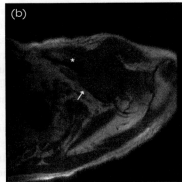
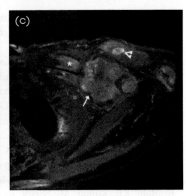

Figure 89.6. Tuberculous osteomyelitis. (*A*) AP radiograph of left clavicle shows cortical destruction and osteolysis at the inferior surface of the clavicle (*arrow*) with surrounding mild sclerosis. (*B*) Axial T1W MR image shows decreased signal intensity in the eroded middle third of the clavicle (*asterisk*) with destructive changes, expansion, low signal bone marrow replacement, and associated soft tissue mass involving the lateral third of the clavicle (*arrow*). (*C*) Axial T2W FS MR image shows BME in the middle third of the clavicle (*asterisk*) and heterogeneous signal in the destroyed lateral third of the clavicle (*arrow*). Note a small area of higher signal at the anterior aspect of the associated soft tissue component consistent with an abscess (*open arrowhead*). Courtesy of J. Monu MD.

Radiography

Refer to Figure 89.6*A*.

- Metaphyseal or diaphyseal lesions that may penetrate the physis or extend into an adjacent joint
- Osteopenia
- Osteolytic foci with poorly defined borders and varying degrees of sclerosis located eccentrically
- Three forms of TB osteomyelitis have been described:
  - TB dactylitis is also known as *spina ventosa* and characterized as an expansile osteolytic lesion with periosteal thickening and soft tissue swelling, which is more common in children in the metacarpal and metatarsal bones.
  - Cystic TB presents as multifocal well-defined, round or oval radiolucent lesions often accompanied by sequestra.
  - Honeycombing form is a diffuse uniform lesion associated with cavitation and relatively less-pronounced osteoporosis.

Magnetic Resonance Imaging Features of Tuberculosis Osteomyelitis

- Low intramedullary signal intensity on T1W (Figure 89.6*B*) and high signal on fluid-sensitive sequences (Figure 89.6*C*) similar to acute pyogenic osteomyelitis are seen.
- With TB granulomata, MRI may be suggestive of TB osteomyelitis. TB granulomata show low to intermediate signal on T2W MR images compared with the normal bone marrow and may be associated with soft tissue abscesses.

Treatment Options

- **TB spondylitis.** Treatment begins with TB-specific drug therapy with or without bed rest. Drug therapy duration is 9-18 months. In case of inadequate response, spinal orthosis and surgical debridement have been employed.
- **TB arthritis.** TB-specific drug therapy is recommended for all patients with active disease. The affected joint should be adequately immobilized/splinted to minimize joint destruction and preserve function. For patients presenting in the later stage of disease, joint arthroplasty is the method of choice for treatment.
- **TB osteomyelitis.** TB-specific drug therapy is recommended without weight-bearing.

Key Points

- Extrapulmonary TB is seen in 20% of all TB cases. Musculoskeletal TB accounts for 1-3% of TB infections.
- Five different forms of musculoskeletal TB have been described. TB spondylitis (50%) is the most common type followed by TB arthritis (30%), TB osteomyelitis (19%), TB tenosynovitis, TB bursitis, and Poncet disease (1%).
- Osseous involvement is associated with localized warmth, swelling, and tenderness. Joint involvement is associated with tenderness, soft tissue swelling/effusion, and restriction of movement. Findings in patients with spinal disease include back pain/tenderness, neurologic deficit, and kyphotic (gibbus) deformity.
- MRI is the best imaging modality to evaluate spinal infection including TB. Thin and smooth enhancement of the paraspinal abscess wall and a well-defined paraspinal abnormal signal are suggestive of TB spondylitis with subligamentous spread to 3 or more vertebral levels.
- MRI is also the modality of choice in evaluating all other forms of musculoskeletal TB because of higher sensitivity and superb soft tissue contrast resolution.

Recommended Reading

Burrill J, Williams CJ, Bain G, Conder G, Hine AL, Misra RR. Tuberculosis: a radiologic review. *Radiographics*. 2007;27(5):1255–73.

References

1. Amine B, Bahiri R, Hajjaj-Hassouni N. Multifocal tuberculous tenosynovitis. *Joint Bone Spine*. 2006;73:474–83.

2. Arathi N, Faiyaz A, Najmul H. Osteoarticular tuberculosis—a three years retrospective study. *J Clin Diagn Res.* 2013;7(10):2189–92.

3. Choi JA, Koh SE, Hong SH, Koh YH, Choi JY, Kang HS. Rheumatoid arthritis and tuberculous arthritis: differentiating MRI features. *AJR Am J Roentgenol.* 2009;193:1347–53.

4. Erdem H, Baylan O, Simsek I, Dinc A, Pay S, Kocaoglu M. Delayed diagnosis of tuberculous arthritis. *Jpn J Infect Dis.* 2005;58:373–75.

5. Jung NY, Jee WH, Ha KY, Park CK, Byun JY. Discrimination of tuberculous spondylitis from pyogenic spondylitis on MRI. *AJR Am J Roentgenol.* 2004;182:1405–10.

6. Raju KP, Kumar M, Shetty R. Tuberculous tenosynovitis of ankle with rice bodies. *Foot Ankle Online J.* 2013;6(10). doi:10.3827/faoj.2013.0610.001.

7. Rasuli MR, Mirkoohi M, Vaccaro AR, Yarandi KK, Rahimi-Movaghar V. Spinal tuberculosis: diagnosis and management. *Asian Spine J.* 2012;6:294–308.

8. Sawlani V, Chandra T, Mishra RN, Aggarwal A, Jain UK, Gujral RB. MRI features of tuberculosis of peripheral joints. *Clin Radiol.* 2003;58:758–62.

9. Sharma P. MR features of tuberculous osteomyelitis. *Skeletal Radiol.* 2003;32:279–85.

10. Spiegel DA, Singh GK, Banskota AK. Tuberculosis of musculoskeletal system. *Techniques Orthop.* 2005;20:167–78.

11. Sundaram VK, Doshi A. Infections of the spine: a review of clinical and imaging findings. *Appl Radiol.* 2016;10–20.

12. Vohra R, Kang HS, Dogra S, Saggar RR, Sharma R. Tuberculous osteomyelitis. *J Bone Joint Surg Br.* 1997;79(4):562–66.

CHAPTER 90

Atypical Mycobacterial Infections

Remide Arkun

Introduction

Atypical mycobacterial infections are caused by species of mycobacteria other than *Mycobacterium tuberculosis* (TB). They have different colonial characteristics and account for 0.5-30% of all mycobacterial infections. Atypical mycobacterial infection is typically acquired by contamination from penetrating injuries or surgical procedures and hematogenous spread. *Mycobacterium leprae*, the cause of leprosy, is described in Chapter 97, "Leprosy."

Because there is no evidence of human-to-human transmission, atypical mycobacterial infections do not pose public health hazards, but they are commonly drug resistant. Atypical mycobacteria typically colonize the host; however, the rate of clinical infection is low. Elderly and immunocompromised individuals are frequently affected. Involvement of the musculoskeletal system occurs in approximately 5-10% of patients. At least 15 species of nontuberculous atypical mycobacteria have been mentioned in the literature as the cause of musculoskeletal infection. In particular, atypical mycobacterial strains usually acquired by trauma are *Mycobacterium fortuitum*, *Mycobacterium chelonae*, and *Mycobacterium marinum*. These infections can present as nonhealing wounds or as skin lesions, tenosynovitis, osteomyelitis, or septic arthritis.

Pathophysiology and Clinical Findings

Atypical mycobacterial osteomyelitis resembles an acute pyogenic infection but is characterized by slower progression. Metaphyses or diaphyses of long bones are frequently involved. In the spine, abnormalities and pathogenesis of the disease are similar to TB spondylitis with involvement of one or several contiguous vertebral bodies that may result in kyphosis, destruction of intervertebral discs, absence of reactive sclerosis, and formation of soft tissue abscesses. Atypical mycobacterial arthritis can occur as a result of adjacent osteomyelitis or as a sequela of primary synovial inflammation. Typically, joint effusions and soft tissue edema without rapid progression of destructive arthritis are early findings. Subsequently, marginal and subchondral erosions and various degrees of cartilage destruction occur. In contrast to RA, joint-space loss is generally seen in advanced stages caused by lack of proteolytic enzymes.

Soft tissue manifestations of disease include cellulitis, superficial and deep fasciitis, abscess, pyomyositis, septic tenosynovitis, and CTS. If left untreated, infection progresses to cutaneous granulomata, ulcers, suppuration, deep necrotizing infection, and deep soft tissue abscesses. Pyomyositis caused by atypical mycobacteria has recently been recognized in association with human immunodeficiency virus (HIV) infection and IV drug abuse. Mycobacterial pyomyositis may also be observed in immunocompetent individuals after penetrating trauma or invasion from contiguous sites of infection. Atypical mycobacterial tenosynovitis is a rare condition. Most of the cases are located in the hand and wrist and occur with inoculation of the microorganism through minor penetrating injuries.

Clinically, musculoskeletal infections caused by atypical mycobacteria resemble those caused by TB, although the overall course of atypical mycobacterial disease is often milder than that of TB infection. In children, however, atypical mycobacterial disease can be more aggressive and can result in growth disturbance. Symptoms are nonspecific, and include local pain and swelling, joint stiffness, low-grade fever, sweats, chills, anorexia, malaise, and weight loss. Because of these nonspecific clinical findings, diagnosis is usually delayed and a high index of suspicion is needed for early diagnosis to avoid bone and/or joint destruction and disability. Living in endemic areas and certain occupations may increase the likelihood of developing atypical mycobacterial infections. Fluid aspiration and/or tissue sampling and culturing are needed for diagnosis. If the cultures are negative, DNA amplification and subsequent determination of the nucleic acid sequence have reportedly been helpful in identifying the causative pathogen. Increased awareness of the disease, familiarity with the imaging features, and identification of different *Mycobacterium* species by using polymerase chain reaction (PCR) lead to rapid detection of the causative agent and proper treatment of the disease.

Imaging Strategy

Imaging is widely used in the evaluation of musculoskeletal atypical mycobacterial infections. Imaging findings are nonspecific in early stages. In the late stages, imaging findings frequently resemble other granulomatous or mycobacterial infections. Evaluation usually begins with radiography. MRI and CT are more sensitive and are subsequently used to evaluate the extent of disease. Final diagnosis of osteomyelitis is made with bone biopsy and culture of the causative mycobacterial organism. Tissue sampling including biopsy and aspiration of joint effusions or soft tissue fluid collections is frequently performed under imaging guidance.

Imaging Findings

Radiography

- In acute osteomyelitis, an early finding is subtle soft tissue edema. Later on, osteoporosis and medullary and cortical bone resorption are seen in the metaphyses and diaphyses. Multiple osteolytic lesions surrounded with sclerosis are more common than in TB osteomyelitis (Figure 90.1).

- In subacute and chronic osteomyelitis, bone abscesses, sequestrum formation, osseous deformity, mature periosteal reaction, involucrum formation, and sinus tracts are characteristic radiographic findings.
- In the spine, involvement of one or several contiguous vertebral bodies that may result in kyphosis, destruction of the intervening discs, absence of reactive sclerosis, and formation of soft tissue abscesses are seen. The abscesses frequently contain calcifications, which may be paravertebral or extradural or may spread into adjacent structures, including the gluteal region, abdominal wall, and thigh. These diagnostic criteria for spinal atypical mycobacterial infections are similar to TB. Involvement of only a single endplate and of noncontiguous levels may be seen.
- Articular involvement occurs as a result of adjacent osteomyelitis or, less commonly, as a sequela of primary synovial inflammation and may result in destructive arthritis. Early in the disease, the joint space is normal and there is periarticular soft tissue edema associated with a joint effusion. Later on, regional osteoporosis and marginal or subchondral osseous erosions are seen. Because of the absence of proteolytic enzymes in the coexistent exudate in atypical mycobacterial arthritis, joint-space loss is a relatively late finding.

Computed Tomography

- CT shows early cortical bone erosions, periostitis, bone fragmentation, and accumulation of fluid and cloacae in osteomyelitis and helps to further characterize destructive bone changes in septic arthritis. It also helps in detection of soft tissue fluid collections and foreign bodies.
- In spondylitis, CT reveals supplemental diagnostic information regarding paraspinal and intraspinal extension of disease and may characterize the extent of bone and disc involvement. CT is the best imaging modality in detection of soft tissue calcifications, which are frequently associated with paraspinal abscesses.

Magnetic Resonance Imaging

- MRI is the most sensitive imaging modality for the early detection of osteomyelitis, infectious spondylitis, and septic arthritis.
- In osteomyelitis, there is decreased signal intensity on T1W and BME with high signal on fluid-sensitive sequences in the infected areas. Periosteal involvement is seen as high signal intensity on fluid-sensitive sequences and may enhance on Gd-enhanced postcontrast sequences. Contrast-enhanced sequences enable delineation of bone and soft tissue abscesses and differentiation between necrotic and living bone. Areas of cellulitis, superficial and deep fasciitis, and myositis show variable degrees of enhancement.
- In atypical mycobacterial spondylitis, MRI findings are similar to TB spondylitis. Contrast-enhanced MRI allows better delineation and extent of epidural and paraspinal soft tissue involvement. Furthermore, MRI is useful in differentiation between spondylitis and primary or metastatic spinal tumors and sarcoidosis.
- In joint infection, the presence and extent of inflammation can be accurately evaluated on MRI. Joint effusions and subarticular marrow signal abnormalities show low signal intensity on T1W and high signal intensity on fluid-sensitive sequences with variable degrees of synovial and bone marrow enhancement on postcontrast sequences.
- Exuberant tenosynovitis without tendon tear may be seen in atypical mycobacterial infection and is usually located in the hand and wrist. Imaging plays an important role in establishing the diagnosis of tenosynovitis (Figure 90.2). Tenosynovial fluid shows low signal on T1W and high signal on fluid-sensitive sequences. Active synovitis shows prominent enhancement on postcontrast sequences.

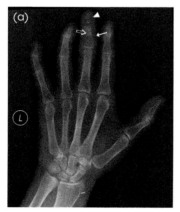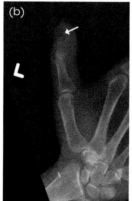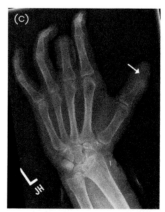

Figure 90.1. Atypical mycobacterial osteomyelitis in an immunocompetent patient. (*A*) PA radiograph of the left hand shows a permeative osteolytic lesion involving the proximal aspect of the middle phalanx of the middle finger with associated cortical destruction and increased mottled sclerosis of the distal aspect of the middle phalanx (*open arrow*). Note associated soft tissue edema (*arrow*). There is widening of the middle finger DIP joint with fragmentation and irregularity of the distal phalanx (*arrowhead*). (*B*) Five months later, PA radiograph of the same hand shows cortical destruction of the thumb distal phalangeal tuft with associated foci of soft tissue gas (*arrow*) and edema. (*C*) PA radiograph of the same hand obtained 3 months later shows complete resorption of the thumb distal phalanx with cortical irregularity of the proximal phalangeal head. Note adjacent soft tissue gas and edema (*arrow*). There was interval amputation of the middle finger at the level of PIP joint.

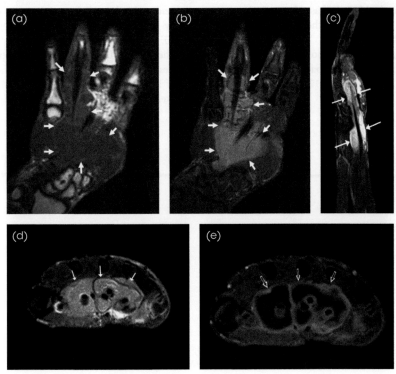

Figure 90.2. Tenosynovitis and ulnar bursitis caused by *Mycobacterium avium* complex. (*A*) Coronal T1W MR image of the left hand shows fusiform heterogeneous hypointense distension of the ring finger flexor tendon sheath in continuity with the distended ulnar bursa (*arrows*). (*B*) Coronal (*C*), sagittal, and (*D*) axial T2W FS MR images show heterogeneous intermediate to high signal intensity in the same regions consistent with tenosynovitis and bursitis (*arrows*). Note innumerable punctate areas of low signal intensity within the synovial fluid consistent with rice bodies. (*E*) Axial T1W FS postcontrast MR image shows thin enhancement of the synovial membrane in the ulnar bursa about the flexor tendons with associated nonenhancing fluid (*arrows*). Courtesy of A. Chhabra MD.

Ultrasound
- US reveals increased fluid in the tendon sheath with tendon thickening and possible rice bodies. Active synovitis shows hyperemia on color or power Doppler interrogation.
- Both US and MRI findings are nonspecific, and differential diagnosis includes pyogenic and fungal infections, GCT of the tendon sheath, RA, and PVNS.

Treatment Options
- There is no standard treatment for atypical musculoskeletal mycobacterial infections.
- Different antituberculous drugs and antibiotics to which the isolates are sensitive are recommended.
- In patients with insufficient response to medical treatment, surgical treatment and debridement are recommended.

Key Points
- Involvement of the musculoskeletal system occurs in approximately 5-10% of patients with atypical mycobacterial infections.
- Infection is typically acquired by contamination from penetrating injuries or surgical procedures and hematogenous spread.

- Because there is no evidence of human-to-human transmission, these infections do not pose public health hazards but are commonly drug resistant.
- Musculoskeletal atypical mycobacterial infections can present as nonhealing wounds or skin lesions, superficial and deep soft tissue infections, osteomyelitis, or septic arthritis.
- Imaging findings are nonspecific and differential diagnosis includes TB and various fungal and bacterial infections.
- Final diagnosis is made by tissue sampling and culturing. With negative cultures, identification of different *Mycobacterium* species can be made using PCR.

Recommended Reading
Theodorou JD, Theodorou SJ, Kakitsubata Y, Sartoris DJ, Resnick D. Imaging characteristics and epidemiologic features of atypical mycobacterial infections involving the musculoskeletal system. *AJR Am J Roentgenol.* 2001;176:341–49.

References
1. Piersimoni C, Scarparo C. Extrapulmonary infections associated with nontuberculous mycobacteria in immunocompetent persons. *Emerg Infect Dis.* 2009;15:1351–58.
2. Rohilla M, Khan K, Raza H. Musculoskeletal manifestations of atypical mycobacterium: case reports. *Surg Sci.* 2014;5:25–27.

3. Sanal HT, Zor F, Kacaoglu M, Bulakbasi N. Atypical mycobacterial tenosynovitis and bursitis of the wrist. *Diagn Interv Radiol*. 2009;15:266–68.

4. Saugat R, Chhabra M, Kumari S, Kapoor A. A case report pelvic abscess by non-tubercular mycobacterium: a very unusual presentation. *Int J Med*. 2015;1:10–12.

5. Seidl A, Lindeque B. Large joint osteoarticular infection caused by Mycobacterium arupense. *Orthopedics*. 2014;37(9):e848–50. doi:10.3928/01477447-20140825-93.

6. Theodorou JD, Theodorou SJ, Kakitsubata Y, Sartoris DJ, Resnick D. Imaging characteristics and epidemiologic features of atypical mycobacterial infections involving the musculoskeletal system. *AJR Am J Roentgenol*. 2001;176:341–49.

CHAPTER 91

Fungal and Higher Bacterial Infections

Remide Arkun

Introduction

In nature, there are numerous described species of fungi. Of those described, approximately 150 species are generally recognized as primary pathogens of humans and animals. They may cause a broad spectrum of diseases, which include simple superficial skin lesions to deep single or multiple organ involvement. Skeletal involvement is not frequent. However, there is an increasing number of cases with invasive fungal infection, including osteomyelitis or septic arthritis, particularly in immunocompetent patients. Incidence of fungal musculoskeletal infections may be endemic or sporadic and related to geographic distribution, ethnicity, nutrition, and occupation.

Pathophysiology and Clinical Findings

Fungal infections spread either by contiguity from an initial skin inoculation or hematogenously from a distant focus, usually the lungs. They almost all cause granuloma formation. Although there is a general concept for musculoskeletal involvement, each species can have special features.

Cryptococcosis is an infection caused by the encapsulated fungus *Cryptococcus neoformans*. It is a cosmopolite mycosis and can be seen throughout the world. This fungus can be found in the respiratory tract or skin in healthy individuals or can be recovered from the soil, pigeon droppings, fruit, and human intestinal tract and skin. It is initially inhaled into the lungs from where it can spread hematogenously, principally to the brain and meninges; however, other visceral organ, bone and joint involvement can also occur. Skeletal cryptococcosis is usually secondary to disseminated disease with a reported incidence of 5-10%. The pelvis, ribs, skull, tibia, and knees are other favorable sites. Spinal involvement is uncommon and can mimic tuberculosis (TB) with discitis. Extension from the vertebral body to the pedicle or contiguous rib can occur in vertebral cryptococcosis. Cryptococcal arthritis is quite uncommon and occurs with invasion of the contiguous joints from an osteomyelitic focus in the adjacent bone.

Candidiasis is the infection caused by the Candida species. The major etiologic agent of candidiasis is *Candida albicans*. Because this fungus is a part of the normal human flora, candidiasis is an opportunistic infection. It has no geographic predilection, and the disease mostly occurs in patients with central venous catheters, on broad-spectrum antibiotics and immunosuppressive medications, and in IV drug abusers. In disseminated disease, bone and joint involvement are relatively rare. Osteomyelitis can occur at any age group, involving the long bones or the flat bones such as the pelvis, sternum, scapula, and ribs. Spine involvement can occur either with direct extension of a contiguous infection or via hematogenous seeding from a distant focus of infection and cannot be differentiated from other bacterial or fungal osteomyelitis based on imaging findings. Septic arthritis can occur with hematogenous spread, by direct invasion from adjacent infected osseous or soft tissue structures or in association with joint replacement surgery. The knee joint is the most common site.

Aspergillosis is a fungal infection caused by the *Aspergillus* species. *Aspergillus fumigatus* is the most common causative organism. Humans are constantly exposed to these fungi which live in our environment. Aspergillosis is relatively uncommon and the severe, invasive form may affect both immunocompetent and immunocompromised hosts. Bone involvement is very rare and secondary to hematogenous dissemination from invasive pulmonary aspergillosis. The most common form is spinal infection; however, involvement of the ribs, sternum, wrist, pelvis, knee, and tibia has been reported. Osteomyelitis tends to be multifocal with osteolytic lesions. Septic polyarthritis has been described and can be multifocal.

Mucormycosis refers to several different diseases caused by infection with fungi in the order of *Mucorales* and is characterized by vascular invasion with hyphae, infarction, and tissue necrosis. The disease may have an acute or subacute course. Almost all patients have a serious underlying condition, such as diabetes mellitus, immunosuppression, starvation, burns, or other major trauma. The underlying disease influences the portal of entry and usually mucormycosis originates in the paranasal sinuses. Severe infectious sinusitis, which may extend into the brain, is the most common presentation. Pulmonary, cutaneous, and gastrointestinal infections are also recognized. Osteomyelitis without rhinocerebral disease in immunocompetent patients may occur.

Sporotrichosis is a chronic fungal infection usually limited to the cutaneous and subcutaneous tissues, although it may become disseminated. The causative organism is *Sporothrix schenckii*. The disease starts as an erythematous, ulcerated, or verrucous skin nodule. Subsequent nodular lymphangitic spread is common. This infection may also be hematogenously disseminated and involve the bones, joints, skin, eyes, central nervous system, or genitourinary tract. Sporotrichosis has a worldwide distribution and is found mainly in warm and tropical areas. With skeletal involvement, osteomyelitis or septic arthritis can occur. A frequent form of sporotrichosis presents as an indolent tenosynovitis, usually about the wrist or ankle. Nerve entrapment can occur. Although, radiological findings of sporotrichosis are similar to those of TB or other fungal disorders, involvement of the small joints of the hands and feet is more common in this fungal disease compared to others.

Coccidioidomycosis is a systemic fungal infection caused by the soil fungus *Coccidioides immitis* and *Coccidioides posadasii*, endemic to the southwestern United States, Mexico, and portions of South America. Infection occurs through inhalation of dust containing the organism. The primary site of infection is the lung, and the disease is commonly either asymptomatic or presents as a mild-to-moderate flulike illness that resolves spontaneously. A small proportion of patients (0.5-1%) can develop a potentially lethal progression of infection, involving the lungs or other organs through hematogenous dissemination. In disseminated disease, patients usually have primary pulmonary infection. With dissemination of disease, the skin and subcutaneous tissues, mediastinum, and skeletal system are sequentially involved. Bone and joint involvement is reported between 10% and 50% in previous studies. There are three factors for disseminated disease: (1) Filipino, African American, Native American, and Hispanic populations are at greater risk than those of European-descent ethnicities; (2) men are at greater risk than women; and (3) immunosuppressed patients are at greater risk than others. Skeletal involvement includes osteomyelitis and septic arthritis. In osseous involvement, lesions are often multicentric and the spine, ribs, sternum, pelvis, and skull are the most prevalent sites. Coccidioidomycosis frequently involves bony protuberances such as the iliac spine, femoral trochanters, or tibial tubercle with a tendency toward bilateral and symmetric distribution. Involvement of the patella, calcaneus, and olecranon have also been described.

The spine is the most frequently involved part of the skeletal system. Complete vertebral destruction and paravertebral soft tissue masses can be seen. Disc-space narrowing and gibbus deformity are not as common as in TB. In joint involvement, a self-limited migratory sterile polyarthritis (*desert rheumatism*) occurs as a hypersensitivity reaction in some cases of acute nondisseminated coccidioidomycosis. Coccidioidal arthritis is a granulomatous disease that develops by direct extension from an adjacent bone infection, although, rarely, direct hematogenous implantation of organisms to the synovium can occur. The most common sites are the knee and ankle joints. Coccidioidal soft tissue abscesses, tenosynovitis, and septic bursitis can also occur.

Maduromycosis (mycetoma) is a chronic granulomatous fungal infection caused by various *Actinomycetes* and true fungi (*Eumycetes*) species. It is mainly found in food and is prevalent in India, sub-Saharan Africa, the southern part of the Arabian Peninsula, and Central and South America. The disease commonly follows a thorn prick and involves the lower limbs in 70-75% of cases. After the initial skin lesion, granulomatous infection often extends from the subcutaneous facial planes to the first and second metatarsal bones, causing chronic osteomyelitis, either on the dorsal or plantar surface. Nodular skin and soft tissue thickening at the plantar aspect of the foot frequently suppurates and develops multiple skin sinuses draining yellow pus.

Blastomycosis, also called *North American blastomycosis*, is an infection caused by the fungus *Blastomyces dermatitidis*. The infection appears to begin in the lung and, in acute cases, may resolve without spread to other organs. Alternatively, it can progress from either the lungs or other sites via hematogenous spread. Skin, bone, and the genitourinary tract are the most common sites of hematogenous dissemination.

Blastomycosis has a very narrow geographic distribution and the disease is most prevalent in the southeastern United States, Ohio-Mississippi Valley area, and in the Mid-Atlantic region. Blastomycosis is now known to be endemic to wide geographic areas of Africa. Men and boys are affected slightly more frequently than women and girls. Osteomyelitis is found in 14-60% of all disseminated cases and can occur from hematogenous seeding or by direct extension from overlying soft tissues. The most common sites are the vertebrae, skull, ribs, and distal half of the extremities. In the long bones, the infection usually begins in the epiphysis or subarticular region. In the spine, blastomycosis invades the vertebral body, disc space, and paravertebral soft tissues, and the radiological findings cannot be differentiated from tuberculosis. Blastomycotic arthritis is also common and associated with lung involvement. The elbow, knee, and ankle are the most frequently affected sites.

Histoplasmosis is an infection caused by *Histoplasma capsulatum*, which is present in the United States, especially in the Mississippi River Valley, or *Histoplasma capsulatum var. duboisii*, which is present in Africa. Both can lead to the same disease. Histoplasmosis is a soil fungus and the disease starts in the lungs with inhalation of soil containing spores. The fungus proliferates in the reticuloendothelial system and can spread to the brain, lymph nodes, spleen, bones, mediastinum, and pericardium. With skeletal involvement, flat bones including the ribs and small tubular bones are affected. Radiological findings are similar to those of sarcoidosis and TB.

Chromoblastomycosis is a chronic mycosis of skin and subcutaneous tissue. Four or 5 different organisms, which include *Phialophora verrucosa*, *Fonsecaea pedrosoi*, *Fonsecaea compacta*, *Cladosporium carrionii*, and *Rhinocladiella aquaspersa*, cause the disease. Chromoblastomycosis has no geographic predilection. Infection results from inoculation through superficial injuries. Multifocal lesions may develop by lymphatic dissemination, and hematogenous spread from primary skin lesions is very rare. The brain and meninges are the most common sites of spread, and paranasal sinus involvement also commonly occurs. Skin lesions are similar to those in blastomycosis and sporotrichosis. Musculoskeletal involvement is very rare and as in other granulomatous disorders, osteomyelitis and septic arthritis may occur.

Similar to fungal infections, *actinomycosis* and *nocardiosis*, which are rare gram-positive filamentous bacterial infections can cause chronic, slowly progressive granulomatous disease.

Actinomycosis is a rare, chronic and slowly progressive granulomatous disease caused by filamentous gram-positive anaerobic bacteria from the Actinomycetaceae family (genus *Actinomyces*). Among several pathogenic *Actinomyces* species in humans, *Actinomyces israelii*, which is normally encountered in the mouth, gastrointestinal tract, and female genital tract flora, is the most common causative agent of actinomycosis. The organism is usually unable to cross the mucosal barrier. However, individuals with poor orodental hygiene, those with prolonged use of intrauterine devices, and those receiving bisphosphonate therapy are at high risk of actinomycosis infection. Disruption of the mucosal barrier because of trauma, surgery, or foreign bodies may allow bacterial entry into deep tissues. Typically, a densely fibrotic lesion is one of the features of actinomycosis, which tends to extensively spread beyond fascial and connective tissue planes. As the lesion progresses, it is accompanied by abscess formation centrally, which eventually leads to sinus tracts extending from the abscess to the skin or adjacent organ. Actinomycosis usually manifests with several features, such as abscess formation, dense fibrosis, and draining sinuses. From a diagnostic perspective, actinomycosis is further characterized by the histopathologic finding of *sulfur granules*. The presence of these sulfur granules, composed of bacterial elements and tissue debris, found in pus from an abscess, exudates from a sinus tract, or tissue specimen is the single most helpful histopathologic finding in the diagnosis of actinomycosis. The most common location is the cervicofacial region. Musculoskeletal involvement is rare. It can be caused by hematogenous spread of localized actinomycosis, contiguous spread of pulmonary actinomycosis to the spine, and polymicrobial bone and joint infection following bone exposure, especially in patients with paraplegia and osteomyelitis of the ischial tuberosity.

Nocardiosis is an uncommon gram-positive bacterial infection and is typically considered an opportunistic disease especially in immunocompetent patients. *Nocardia asteroides* is the most common species associated with human disease. Although the most common route of infection is inhalation, direct inoculation into the skin is the second most common pathway. Nocardiosis is a rare cause of osteomyelitis and is usually associated with localized and cutaneous infections. The spine is the most common location for infection, and the skull, sacrum, femur, and tibia are other rare locations.

Clinical Findings

Fungal and higher bacterial infections of the musculoskeletal system are uncommon and a challenging clinical problem. These infections are more common in patients taking immunosuppressant therapy, steroids, cytotoxic agents, and antibiotics. Individuals with diabetes, other neuropathies, sickle cell disease, human immunodeficiency virus (HIV), malnutrition, agricultural exposure, and thorn pricks, and travelers to endemic regions are prone to fungal infections. Clues to the clinical diagnosis of fungal infection are the presence of soft tissue nodules, discharging skin sinuses, multifocal chronic osteomyelitis, and chronic granulomatous joint involvement. Tendon and muscle involvement are uncommon and usually present as chronic nodular tenosynovitis or granulomatous myositis with abscess formation. Signs of infection can be mild, and chronic evolution and delayed diagnosis are common. Knowledge of predisposing factors, imaging findings, and a high index of clinical suspicion are necessary, but the final diagnosis requires aspiration or biopsy from the infected soft tissues, bones, or joints.

Imaging Strategy

Imaging findings are nonspecific in many fungal and higher bacterial infections and may mimic TB or malignancy. Evaluation usually begins with radiography. MRI and CT are more sensitive and are subsequently used to evaluate for the extent of disease. Radionuclide studies are frequently helpful in evaluation of multifocal and disseminated skeletal involvement. US is useful in the evaluation of soft tissue lesions and is frequently used to guide aspiration or biopsy.

Imaging Findings

- Imaging findings in *cryptococcosis* include the following:
  - Cryptococcal osteomyelitis is a rare entity, which is even rarer in children. Radiography shows osteolytic lesions. Most lesions are poorly marginated with variable periosteal reactions. Extensive periosteal reaction can be seen and may mimic malignant bone neoplasm.
  - Vertebral involvement is rare. Isolated vertebral body involvement may mimic metastatic disease.
  - In joint involvement, radiological changes may include synovial effusion, osteopenia, joint-space narrowing, bone destruction, and in some instances, ankylosis.
  - Technetium-99m and gallium-67 bone scans can detect early osseous and soft tissue lesions with higher sensitivity than radiographs.
- Imaging findings in *candidiasis* include the following:
  - Candida osteomyelitis is relatively rare. Periosteal reaction is usually absent. Other imaging findings are similar to bacterial or TB osteomyelitis.
  - Candida spondylitis (Figure 91.1) is the most common fungal spondylitis in the immunocompromised patients. Radiography and CT show erosive and destructive vertebral changes with limited disc-space narrowing (Figure 91.1).
  - MRI commonly reveals involvement of 2 adjacent vertebral bodies with small paraspinal abscesses or phlegmon that is typically smaller than those in pyogenic or TB infection, and relative sparing of the disc space (Figure 91.1A–C). The signal intensity of an abscess is typically lower on the fluid-sensitive sequences in contrast to the high signal intensity expected in inflammatory lesions caused by pyogenic or TB infection.
  - Candida arthritis is usually seen as a monoarticular disease. The knee joint is the most common location. Radiography reveals massive soft tissue swelling, joint-space narrowing, marginal erosions, and bone collapse and fragmentation. There is no osteopenia. After joint arthroplasty, the bone in contact with an infected prosthesis may eventually demonstrate osteolysis.
  - On MRI, synovial hypertrophy, joint effusion, periarticular soft tissue edema, and bone erosions are better delineated than on radiography.
- Imaging findings in *aspergillosis* include the following:
  - Aspergillus osteomyelitis is a debilitating and severe form of invasive aspergillosis and occurs at any age. The most common locations are the vertebral body, ribs, and sternum. Long bone involvement is uncommon, and the tibia is the most frequently involved bone.
  - Osteolysis, bone destruction, and bone erosions are the most common radiographic findings for *Aspergillus* osteomyelitis. Soft tissue extension, periosteal reaction, abscess, and sequestrum are less common findings.
  - Imaging findings include osteolytic destruction of the vertebral body endplates, paravertebral soft tissue

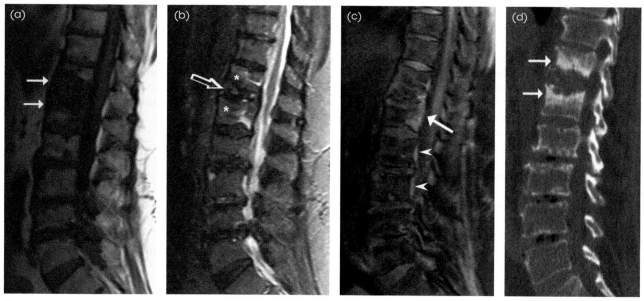

Figure 91.1. Fungal spondylitis caused by *Candida parapsilosis*. (*A*) Sagittal T1W MR image shows low signal intensity at the T12-L1 disc space with involvement of the T12 and L1 vertebral bodies (*arrows*). (*B*) Sagittal T2W FS MR image shows mild increased signal intensity in the T12 and L1 vertebral bodies (*asterisks*) with mild T12-L1 disc-space narrowing (*open arrow*). (*C*) Sagittal T1W FS postcontrast MR image shows mild enhancement of the posterior aspects of the T12 and L1 vertebral bodies (*arrow*) with associated linear epidural enhancement extending down to L3-L4 disc (*arrowheads*). (*D*) Sagittal reformatted CT image shows endplate erosions with sclerosis at the T12-L1 level (*arrows*) with disc-space widening.

edema, disc-space narrowing, and spinal cord compression caused by epidural or subdural abscess in spinal involvement. On MRI, there is decreased signal intensity on T1W and increased signal intensity on T2W images, with enhancement on postcontrast T1W FS images.

- Aspergillus-related septic arthritis is very rare without specific imaging findings.

- Imaging findings in *sporotrichosis* include the following:
  - Musculoskeletal involvement of sporotrichosis is unusual and is the result of local inoculation or hematogenous spread. The infection is typically chronic and indolent, which may result in delayed diagnosis.
  - The tibia is the most common location for sporotrichosis osteomyelitis. Hand and wrist bone lesions may result from trauma and subsequent spread from cutaneous lesions. On radiography, 2 different forms are reported. There may be solitary or multiple osteolytic lesions without periosteal reaction or proliferative and sclerotic bone changes.
  - Sporotrichosis septic arthritis is typically multifocal. Classical findings are osteoporosis of contiguous bone surfaces, periarticular soft tissue edema, and destruction of subchondral bone with discrete, *punched-out* bone lesions. Joint-space narrowing and cystlike changes are less common. Imaging findings are similar to other fungal arthritides, TB, and sarcoidosis.

- Imaging findings in *coccidioidomycosis* include the following:
  - In coccidioidomycosis osteomyelitis, the radiographic pattern is variable. Radiographs reveal either multiple lytic permeative lesions with periosteal

reaction, osteoporosis, and soft tissue edema or well demarcated, punched-out osteolytic lesions with variable degrees of surrounding sclerosis. Lesions involving the ribs can be associated with prominent extrapleural masses.

- Involvement of bony protuberances is common and may be symmetric.

- In coccidioidomycosis septic arthritis, osteoporosis, joint-space narrowing, and bone destruction may mimic other granulomatous infections (Figure 91.2A).

- Bone and joint lesions may be better delineated with multidetector CT. Fine cortical detail and sequestra are usually best visualized by CT. CT is particularly useful and probably now the most frequently used imaging modality for biopsy guidance.

- MRI is the preferred imaging modality to define extension of the infection not only in the bone and joint (Figure 91.2) but also in the soft tissues. Although MRI findings are nonspecific, contrast-enhanced images may help to estimate active infection.
  - Coccidioidal lesions typically reveal nonspecific intermediate-to-low signal intensity on T1W sequences and increased, frequently heterogeneous, signal on fluid-sensitive sequences.
  - In the spine, there is nonspecific involvement of several contiguous vertebral levels with or without skip lesions and paraspinal abscesses. Vertebral collapse and disc involvement are rare and late findings.
  - After IV contrast administration, rim enhancement of intraosseous and soft tissue abscesses and synovial proliferation in infected joints usually indicate active disease.

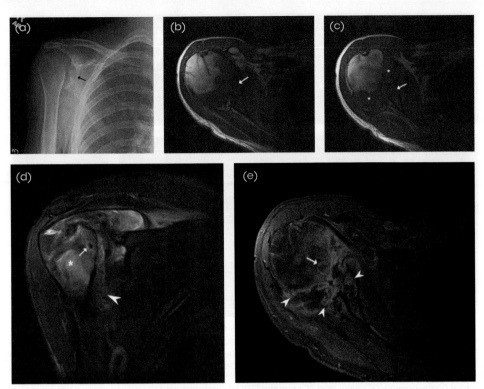

Figure 91.2. Coccidioidomycosis arthritis. (*A*) AP radiograph of the right shoulder shows periarticular osteoporosis, joint-space narrowing, and cortical destruction in both the glenoid (*arrow*) and humeral head. (*B, C*) Consecutive axial T1W MR images show a large heterogeneous low signal joint effusion (*asterisks*) with extensive erosive and destructive changes in the glenoid (*arrows*). Note the cortical destruction of the humeral head. (*D*) Coronal T2W FS MR image shows a large heterogeneous joint effusion with synovial thickening (*arrowhead*). Note BME in the proximal humerus (*asterisk*) with associated extensive erosive changes and a small low signal focus within the humeral head consistent with a sequestrum (*arrow*). There is edema in the supraspinatus muscle. (*E*) Axial T1W FS postcontrast MR image shows heterogeneous enhancement of the humeral head with a rim-enhancing intraosseous abscess (*arrow*) and enhancing thick synovial proliferation within the glenohumeral joint (*arrowheads*) with nonenhancing joint fluid invaginating into the eroded glenoid.

- Imaging findings in *maduromycosis* include the following:
  - *Madura foot* is a localized chronic suppurative infection characterized by exuberant granulation tissue formation. Radiological findings include loss of cortical definition, followed by periosteal reaction, coarse trabeculation, soft tissue edema, cortical erosions, rounded lucencies, joint destruction, a *moth-eaten* appearance, osteopenia, bone lysis, and in the terminal phase, a *melting snow* appearance of the bone. However, radiographically apparent changes occur late during the disease, and surgical treatment is usually required.
  - MRI can demonstrate pedal mycetoma and help early diagnosis. *Pedal mycetoma* is characterized by the formation of microabscesses consisting of aggregates of the organism (known as *grains* or *sulfur granules*) that are surrounded by abundant granulation tissue. These appear as small, round, hyperintense lesions surrounded by a low signal intensity hypointense rim on fluid-sensitive sequences, measuring 2-5 mm. The central low signal intensity dot is the result of susceptibility artifact caused by the presence of a conglomeration of fungal grains. This finding is known as the *dot-in-circle* sign.
- Imaging findings in *blastomycosis* include the following:

- On radiographs in blastomycosis osteomyelitis, there are well-defined eccentric osteolytic lesions with or without periosteal reaction associated with osteoporosis, and in some cases, diffuse moth-eaten bone destruction. These findings are often mistaken for bone tumors.
- Imaging findings in *actinomycosis* include the following:
  - Actinomycosis osteomyelitis is rare but most common in the facial bones, particularly the mandible and maxilla. The chronic and indolent course of actinomycosis resembles TB, fungal infections, and malignancy.
  - Because actinomycosis is often difficult to diagnose, it has been referred to as a forgotten or misdiagnosed disease.
  - On radiographs, there are multiple osteolytic lesions surrounded with sclerosis caused by intraosseous granulomas.
  - Rib involvement may be seen associated with pulmonary disease, and severe osseous eburnation, cutaneous sinus tracts, and pleuritis are suggestive radiographic findings.
  - In the spine, posterior element involvement is seen, and paravertebral abscesses do not calcify.
  - Penetrating plant thorn and human-bite injuries have been associated with actinomycosis, which produce a sinus tract that discharges sulfur granules in the hand.

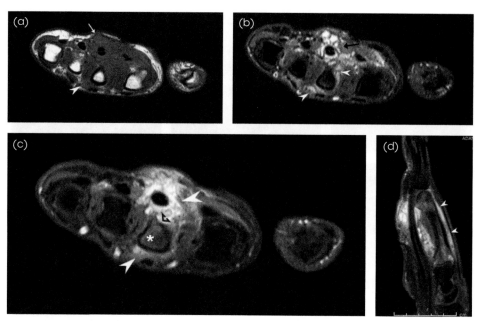

Figure 91.3. Actinomycosis in the hand soft tissues with invasion of the third metacarpal bone after thorn prick injury. (*A*) Axial T1W MR image shows a hypointense soft tissue lesion invading subcutaneous fat and skin along the palmar aspect of the hand (*arrow*) extending about the adjacent flexor tendons and along the radial aspect of the third metacarpal. Note decreased signal intensity soft tissue thickening at the dorsal aspect of third metacarpal bone (*arrowhead*). (*B*) On axial T2W FS MR image, note ill-defined heterogeneous increased signal intensity in the same regions, at the palmar aspect (*arrow*) and at the radial and dorsal aspects of the third metacarpal (*arrowheads*). (*C*) Axial and (*D*) sagittal T1W FS postcontrast MR images show prominent nodular and infiltrative soft tissue enhancement on both palmar and dorsal aspects of the hand about the third metacarpal (*white arrowheads*), cortical erosion at the palmar aspect of the third metacarpal (*open black arrow*), and enhancing BME in the third metacarpal bone (*asterisk*). Courtesy of A. Purbager MD.

This entity is known as *punch* actinomycosis. After trauma, microorganisms locate in the subcutaneous tissue and spread contiguously into deep soft tissue planes as well as subjacent tendon sheaths and bones (Figure 91.3).

- MRI reveals extensive soft tissue inflammatory and infiltrative changes in the affected soft tissues extending to the skin surface (Figure 91.3) and forming fistulae, which may be a diagnostic clue for actinomycosis.

Treatment Options
- Treatment options of fungal infections include the following:
    - After isolation of causative organism, long-term appropriate antifungal medication is indicated, frequently with surgical treatment including debridement.
- Treatment options of higher bacterial infections include the following:
    - In actinomycosis, penicillin D is the drug of choice. Treatment duration depends on the severity of infection. For more severe and complex cases, combined medical and surgical treatment may be required, with a high dosage of antibiotics for a prolonged period.
    - In nocardiosis, it is essential to perform surgical debridement to remove damaged necrotic tissue together with appropriate antibiotic treatment.

Key Points
- Fungal infections of the musculoskeletal system are uncommon.
- Fungal infections spread either by contiguity from an initial skin inoculation or hematogenously from a distant focus, usually the lungs. They almost all cause granuloma formation.
- Fungal infections are more common in immunosuppressed patients. Individuals with diabetes, other neuropathies, sickle cell disease, HIV, malnutrition, agricultural exposure, and thorn pricks, and travelers to endemic regions are also prone to fungal infections.
- Clues to the clinical diagnosis of fungal infection are the presence of soft tissue nodules, discharging skin sinuses, multifocal chronic osteomyelitis, and chronic granulomatous joint involvement.
- Imaging findings of fungal infections are nonspecific, and the differential diagnosis includes other fungal infections, TB, sarcoidosis, and malignancy.
- Actinomycosis and nocardiosis are rare higher bacterial infections characterized by slowly progressive granulomatous disease. Imaging findings are similar to fungal infections.

Recommended Reading
Corr PD. Musculoskeletal fungal infections. *Semin Musculoskelet Radiol.* 2011;15:506–10.
Arkun R. Parasitic and fungal disease of bones and joints. *Semin Musculoskelet Radiol.* 2004;8:231–42.

References

1. Arias F, Mata-Essayag S, Landaeta ME, et al. Candida albicans osteomyelitis: case report and literature review. *Int J Infect Dis.* 2004;8:307–14.

2. Arkun R. Parasitic and fungal disease of bones and joints. *Semin Musculoskelet Radiol.* 2004;8:231–42.

3. Çevik R, Tekin R, Gem M. Candida arthritis in patient diagnosed with spondylarthritis. *Rev Soc Bras Med Trop.* 2016;49:793–95.

4. Chaudhuri R, McKeown B, Harrington D, et al. Mucormycosis osteomyelitis causing avascular necrosis of the cuboid bone: MR imaging findings. *AJR Am J Roentgenol.* 1992;159:1035–37.

5. Corr PD. Musculoskeletal fungal infections. *Semin Musculoskelet Radiol.* 2011;15:506–10.

6. Cuéllar ML, Silveira LH, Espinoza LR. Fungal arthritis. *Ann Rheum Dis.* 1992;51:690–97.

7. Firth GB, Ntanjana T, Law T. Cryptococcal osteomyelitis in a clinically immune-competent child. *South Afr J Infect Dis.* 2015;30:138–40.

8. Gamaletsou MN, Rammaert B, Bueno MA, et al. Aspergillus osteomyelitis: epidemiology, clinical manifestations, management and outcome. *J Infect.* 2014;68:478–93.

9. Gamaletsou MN, Rammaert B, Bueno MA, et al. Candida arthritis: analysis of 112 pediatric and adult cases. *Open Forum Infect Dis.* 2015;3(1)ofv207. doi:10.1093/ofid/ofv/207.

10. Heo SH, Shin SS, Kim JW, et al. Imaging of actinomycosis in various organs: a comprehensive review. *Radiographics.* 2014;34:19–33.

11. Joo HS, Ha J, Hwang CJ, et al. Lumbar cryptococcal osteomyelitis mimicking metastatic tumor. *Asian Spine J.* 2015;9:798–802.

12. Khan MI, Goss G, Gotsman A, Asvat MS. Sporotrichosis arthritis. *S Afr Med J.* 1983;63:1099–101.

13. Lee SW, Lee SH, Chung HW, et al. Candida spondylitis: comparison of MRI findings with bacterial and tuberculous causes. AJR *Am J Roentgenol.* 2013;201:872–77.

14. Ledere HT, Sullivan E, Crum-Cianflone NF. Sporotrichosis as an unusual case of osteomyelitis: a case report and review of the literature. *Med Mycol Case Rep.* 2016;11:31–35.

15. Mert A, Bilir M, Bahar H, et al. Primary actinomycosis of hand: a case report and literature review. *Int J Infect Dis.* 2001;5:112–14.

16. Nayak AR, Kulkarnil SK, Khodnapur GP, Santhos V. Actinomycotic fungal infection of foot—a case report. *Int J Biomed Adv Res.* 2013;4:946–49.

17. Ramkillawan Y, Dawood H, Ferreira N. Isolated cryptococcal osteomyelitis in an immune-competent host: a case report. *Int J Infect Dis.* 2013;17:e1229–31.

18. Sethi S, Siraj F, Kalra KL, Chopra P. Aspergillus vertebral osteomyelitis in immunocompetent patients. *Indian J Orthop.* 2012;46:246–50.

19. Steinfeld S, Durez P, Hauzeur JP, Motte S, Appelboom T. Articular aspergillosis: two case reports and review of the literature. *Br J Rheumatol.* 1997;36:1331–34.

20. Taljanovic MS, Adam RD. Musculoskeletal coccidioidomycosis. *Semin Musculoskelet Radiol.* 2011;15:511–26.

21. Valour F, Senechal A, Celine D, et al. Actinomycosis: etiology, clinical features, diagnosis, treatment and management. *Infect Drug Resist.* 2014;7:183–97.

22. Venegas S, Franco-Cendejas R, Cicero A, et al. Nocardia brasiliensis-associated femorotibial osteomyelitis. *Int J Infect Dis.* 2014;20:63–65.

23. White EA, Patel DB, Forrester DM, et al. Madura foot: two case reports, review of the literature, and new developments with clinical correlation. *Skeletal Radiol.* 2014;43:547–33.

24. Williams RL, Fukui MB, Meltzer CC, et al. Fungal spinal osteomyelitis in the immunocompromised patient: MR findings in three cases. *AJNR Am J Neuroradiol.* 1999;20:381–85.

CHAPTER 92

Brucellosis

Remide Arkun

Introduction

Brucellosis is a zoonosis of worldwide distribution that is caused by small, gram-negative, nonencapsulated coccobacilli of the genus *Brucella*. It is particularly endemic in areas such as the Mediterranean region, Arabian Peninsula, Indian subcontinent, Mexico, and parts of Central and South America. Of the 4 species associated with human infection, *Brucella melitensis* is the most common, most virulent, and most invasive. Brucellosis occurs naturally in domestic animals. Human infection is contracted from infected animals and closely linked to poor animal handling, feeding habits, and hygiene standards. Human-to-human transmission is unusual; however, a few cases of suspected sexual transmission have been reported.

Pathophysiology and Clinical Findings

The first signs of *Brucella* infection usually appear 2–4 weeks after inoculation. The disease mainly affects organs rich in reticuloendothelial cells. Although any organ or system can be affected, the musculoskeletal system is the most frequent target site. The disease can present as infectious sacroiliitis, spondylitis/spondylodiscitis, arthritis, bursitis, tenosynovitis, and osteomyelitis with the incidence varying between 10% and 85%. Monoarthritis (usually of the knees and hips) and sacroiliitis are the most common types of musculoskeletal brucellosis in children and young adults, whereas the spine remains the most common site of involvement in elderly patients.

The lumbar spine, especially the L4 vertebra, is most commonly affected in cases of spinal involvement. Brucellar spondylitis may appear as either focal or diffuse. Focal spinal involvement is characterized by osteomyelitis, which is localized in the anterior superior endplate of a lumbar vertebra at the discovertebral junction. Localized osseous endplate erosions, defined as *brucellar epiphysitis*, bone sclerosis, anterior osteophyte formation (*parrot beak*), or a small amount of gas, probably representing localized tissue destruction, are the result of a slowly progressing infectious process. The intervertebral disc, paraspinal soft tissues, and spinal canal are typically not affected in early disease. Diffuse spinal involvement is characterized by osteomyelitis, which affects the entire vertebral endplate or the whole vertebral body. Spread of the infection occurs via the ligaments and vascular communications to involve the adjacent discs, vertebral bodies, paraspinal soft tissues, and epidural space. Spinal brucellosis usually starts in the superior endplate because of its rich blood supply, but occasionally the inferior endplate may also be involved. In the early stages, there is bone destruction of the superior vertebral endplate. When the bone starts to heal, the new bone formation, so-called parrot beak osteophytes, are seen in the focal form of disease. Most of the time, a single vertebra is involved, but multifocal and multilevel involvement may also be seen. Vertebral collapse, gibbus deformity, or spinal cord compression are very rare complications in *Brucella* spondylodiscitis.

The incidence of brucellar sacroiliitis is variable, ranging from 0 to 72% of musculoskeletal cases. Although unilateral sacroiliitis is more common, recent studies suggest bilateral sacroiliitis is more common than previously reported. SI joint involvement can be associated with spondylitis, which makes the differentiation between the infectious and reactive disease difficult.

Peripheral infectious arthritis, usually involving large joints, especially the hip, knee, and ankle, occurs more frequently in children and young adults and presents as monoarthritis. Peripheral joint disease manifests as an acute or subacute joint inflammation of variable severity, usually less intense than acute pyogenic infection. Periarticular inflammation including bursitis and tenosynovitis may occur, either isolated or associated with joint infection.

Extraspinal brucellar osteomyelitis is rare. Osteomyelitis can be associated with brucellar arthritis caused by concomitant involvement or caused by hematogenous spread. Muscles and soft tissue involvement with *Brucella* infection may also be seen. However, brucellar myositis and tumor-like soft tissue masses are extremely rare clinical manifestations.

Brucellosis with or without musculoskeletal involvement usually has nonspecific clinical manifestations such as fever, malaise, sweating, hepatomegaly, or splenomegaly. In clinical diagnosis, routine laboratory test results such as elevated ESR, white blood cell counts, and serum CRP level are not specific. Serologic tests, such as the enzyme-linked immunosorbent assay, counterimmunoelectrophoresis, and rose bengal plate test are useful to establish the disease and define its stage.

In countries where brucellosis is endemic, there should be a high index of suspicion in patients presenting with localized back pain or neurologic deficits, because these may be the only manifestations of the disease. However, the timely and accurate diagnosis of human brucellosis continues to be a challenge for clinicians because of its nonspecific clinical features, slow growth rate in blood cultures, and the complexity of its serologic diagnosis.

Imaging Strategy

In musculoskeletal brucellosis, evaluation usually begins with radiography. Radionuclide bone scan with technetium-99m-labeled methylene diphosphonate (^{99m}Tc-MDP) has been recommended when clinical suspicion is strong and the radiographic examination is normal. However, MRI and CT are more sensitive and are subsequently used to evaluate the extent of disease.

Imaging Findings

Spinal Involvement
Refer to Figures 92.1 and 92.2.

Radiography
- Can be normal in the early course of disease with abnormal findings seen later (Figure 92.1*A*, *B*).
- In the focal type, the earliest radiographic finding is epiphysitis of the anterosuperior corner of the vertebra followed by erosions, sclerosis, anterior osteophyte formation (parrot beak), and a small amount of gas. The disc and paraspinal soft tissues are normal.
- In the diffuse type, imaging findings can mimic degenerative disease because of the slow progression of disease.

Computed Tomography
- CT better delineates irregularity and destruction of the adjacent vertebral endplates with disc gas and invariable amount of bone sclerosis (Figure 92.2*F–G*) than radiography. CT is also useful in performing image-guided biopsies of the vertebral body or aspiration of paravertebral abscesses.

Magnetic Resonance Imaging
- MRI is the imaging modality of choice to show extension of the infection (Figures 92.1*C–F* and 92.2*A–E*).
- Imaging findings of spinal brucellosis are similar to other diseases that affect the spine, including but not limited to degenerative spondylosis; spondyloarthropathy infections, such as tuberculous (TB) spondylitis, actinomycosis, or pyogenic osteomyelitis; metastatic lesions; or plasmocytoma.
- In the acute phase of *Brucella* infection, the vertebral endplates and disc itself show low signal intensity on T1W images (Figure 92.1*C*) and high signal intensity on fluid-sensitive sequences. In subacute and chronic cases, T1W and fluid-sensitive sequences show heterogenous signal intensity in both affected vertebrae and the disc (Figure 92.2A, B).

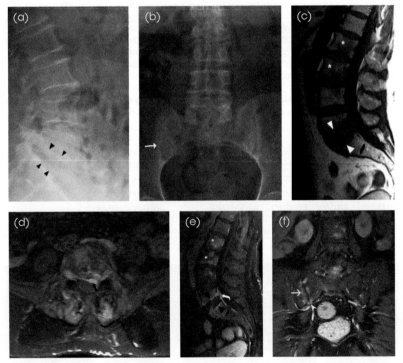

Figure 92.1. *Brucella* spondylodiscitis with multilevel osteitis and sacroiliitis. (*A*) Lateral radiograph of the lumbar spine shows indistinctness of the L5 inferior and S1 superior endplates about the L5-S1 disc space (*arrowheads*). (*B*) AP radiograph of the lumbosacral spine shows subchondral osseous blurring and indistinctness involving the right SI joint (*arrow*). (*C*) Sagittal T1W MR image shows decreased signal intensity involving the L5-S1 disc space and the opposing end plates (*arrowheads*). Patchy areas of hypointense signal are seen in the L2 and L3 vertebral bodies (*asterisks*). (*D*) Axial T1W FS postcontrast MR image at the L4-L5 level shows heterogeneous enhancement with epidural (*curved black arrow*) and anterior paravertebral phlegmon/abscesses (*black arrow*). (*E*) Sagittal T1W FS postcontrast MR image shows increased signal intensity with enhancement of the L5 and S1 endplates adjacent to a nonenhancing L5-S1 disc (*arrowheads*) and epidural enhancement (*curved arrow*). Patchy enhancement is seen in the L2 and L3 vertebral bodies (*asterisks*) suggestive of osteitis. (*F*) Coronal T1W FS postcontrast MR image shows enhancing subchondral bone marrow about the right SI joint (*arrow*) consistent with osteitis. Note enhancing synovium at the distal aspect of the right SI joint related to synovitis (*arrowhead*).

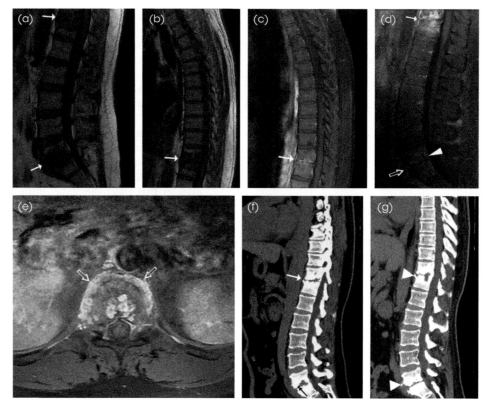

Figure 92.2. Noncontiguous multifocal *Brucella* spondylodiscitis. (*A*) and (*B*) Sagittal T1W MR images show decreased signal intensity in L5-S1 and T11-T12 vertebral bodies about the involved intervertebral disc spaces (*arrows*). (*C*) Sagittal T1W FS postcontrast MR image shows enhancement in T11 and T12 vertebral bodies and the intervening disc space with associated subligamentous enhancement (*arrow*). (*D*) Sagittal T1W FS postcontrast MR image shows irregularities and destructive changes of the vertebral endplates at the L5-S1 level with moderate disc space and vertebral body enhancement. Note anterior subligamentous enhancement (*open white arrow*) and enhancing epidural extension (*arrowhead*). There is intense enhancement in the T11-T12 vertebral bodies and intervening disc with subligamentous enhancement (*open arrows*). (*E*) Axial T1W FS postcontrast MR image shows an enhancing smooth anterior paravertebral mass (*open arrows*). (*F, G*) Consecutive sagittal reformatted CT images show endplate sclerosis and irregularities with disc-space narrowing at the T11-T12 (*white arrow*) and L5-S1 (*black arrow*) levels. There is gas formation in the L5-S1 disc (*black arrow*) and anterior osteophytes (parrot beak) at the T11-T12 and L5-S1 levels (*arrowheads*). Courtesy of BD Mete MD

- Contrast-enhanced sequences show enhancement with increased signal intensity of the affected vertebral endplates, intervertebral discs, and rim-enhancing paravertebral and/or epidural abscesses (Figures 92.1*D,E* and 92.2*C–E*). Paravertebral and/or epidural abscess formation is a rare finding compared to *Brucella* spondylodiscitis and spinal infections of other causes.

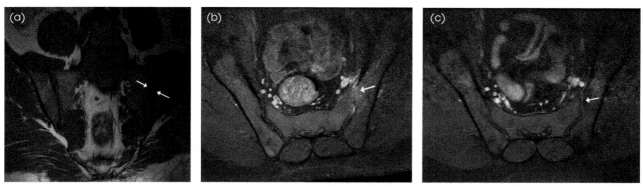

Figure 92.3. *Brucella* sacroiliitis. (*A*) Coronal oblique T1W MR image shows low signal intensity at the sacral and iliac sides of the left SI joint (*arrows*). (*B*) Axial T1W FS postcontrast MR image shows enhancement of the left SI joint and adjacent bone marrow (*arrow*). (*C*) Axial T1W FS postcontrast MR image shows no enhancement of the left SI joint region (*arrow*) 6 months after treatment. Courtesy of BD Mete MD.

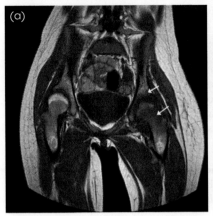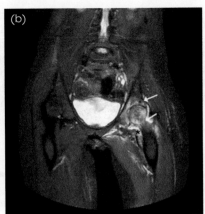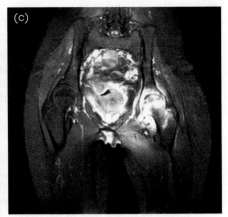

Figure 92.4. *Brucella* arthritis involving the left hip. (*A*) Coronal T1W MR image shows decreased signal intensity in the left proximal femur and acetabular roof (*arrows*) with femoroacetabular joint-space loss. (*B*) Coronal T2W FS MR image shows BME in the same affected regions (*arrows*). Note synovitis (*asterisk*) in the distended joint capsule and edema in the adjacent adductor musculature. (*C*) Coronal T1W FS postcontrast MR image shows intense osseous and synovial enhancement of the affected left hip consistent with infectious arthritis. Courtesy of BD Mete MD.

Brucella Sacroiliitis
Radiography
- Findings within the first 2 or 3 weeks include blurring and indistinctness of the subchondral bone and narrowing or widening of the joint space (Figure 92.1*B*). Erosions, subchondral sclerosis, and ankylosis may be seen in chronic cases.

Magnetic Resonance Imaging
Refer to Figure 92.3.

- BME and joint effusion are seen.
- SI joint involvement may be associated with spinal infection (Figure 92.1*F*).
- In chronic cases, subchondral sclerosis, erosions, and ankylosis of the joint may be seen.

Brucella Arthritis
Radiography
- Usually normal in the early course of disease

Magnetic Resonance Imaging
Refer to Figure 92.4.

- In early stages, MRI can reveal increased synovial-fluid complex, BME, and involvement of periarticular soft tissue.
- Joint-space narrowing and destruction, which are rarely reported, are usually observable only at the late phase of the disease (Figure 92.4).
- Imaging findings are indistinguishable from pyogenic or TB arthritis.
- Periarticular bursitis and tenosynovitis can occur alone or may accompany brucellar arthritis.

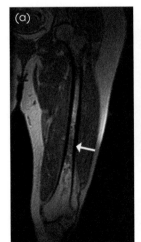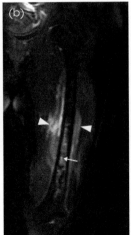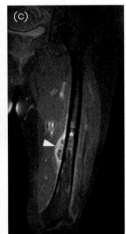

Figure 92.5. *Brucella* osteomyelitis. (*A*) Coronal T1W MR image shows patchy decreased intramedullary signal intensity in the distal diaphysis of the left femur (*arrow*). (*B*) Coronal T2W FS MR image shows BME in the affected medullary bone (*arrow*) with adjacent soft tissue edema (*arrowheads*). (*C*) Coronal T1W FS postcontrast MR image shows heterogeneous bone marrow enhancement (*asterisk*) with a rim-enhancing subperiosteal abscess (*arrowhead*). Courtesy of A. Purbager MD.

Brucella Osteomyelitis

- *Brucella* osteomyelitis is very rare and can be associated with concomitant involvement of the neighboring joints.
- Radiographs show ill-defined osteolytic lesions, typically in the metaphysis. However, well-defined osteolytic lesions, which can mimic GCTs or multiple myeloma, located at the proximal metaphysis of the tibia have been reported.
- MRI findings for *Brucella* osteomyelitis are nonspecific (Figure 92.5).

Soft Tissue Infection

- Bursitis and tenosynovitis are rare in brucellosis patients. Tenosynovitis is usually seen in the hand and wrist. MRI reveals increased fluid in the tendon sheath and thickening of the tendon itself. Synovial enhancement can be seen. However, imaging findings are nonspecific.
- Myositis and soft tissue abscesses are also other rare manifestations of *Brucella* infection. The psoas and paraspinal muscles are most commonly involved.

Treatment Options

- The treatment goal is to avoid relapses. Combined double or triple antibiotic therapy has been recommended for a minimum of 3 months depending on the clinical signs and complications.
- In muscle abscess and tenosynovitis, the combination of percutaneous drainage and antibiotic therapy is effective for treatment.

Key Points

- Brucellosis is a zoonosis of worldwide distribution that is caused by a small, gram-negative, nonencapsulated coccobacilli of the genus *Brucella*. Among the 4 species associated with human infection, *B. melitensis* is the most common, most virulent, and most invasive.
- Human infection is contracted from infected animals and closely linked to poor animal handling, feeding habits, and hygiene standards especially in endemic areas.
- Musculoskeletal infection may manifest as sacroiliitis, spondylitis/spondylodiscitis, arthritis, bursitis, tenosynovitis, and osteomyelitis.
- Brucellosis should be included in the differential diagnosis of any patients with arthralgia or symptoms of osteomyelitis or spondylodiscitis in endemic regions.

Recommended Reading

Arkun R, Mete BD. Musculoskeletal brucellosis. *Semin Musculoskelet Radiol*. 2011;15:470–79.

References

1. Al-Shahed MS, Sharif HS, Haddad MC, Aabed MY, Sammak BM, Mutairi MA. Imaging features of musculoskeletal brucellosis. *Radiographics*. 1994;14:333–48.
2. Arkun R, Mete BD. Musculoskeletal brucellosis. *Semin Musculoskelet Radiol*. 2011;15:470–79.
3. Bozgeyik Z, Aglamis S, Bozdag PG, Denk A. Magnetic resonance imaging findings of musculoskeletal brucellosis. *Clin Imaging*. 2014;719–23.
4. Fowler TP, Keener J, Bucwalter JA. Brucella osteomyelitis of the proximal tibia: case report. *Iowa Orthop J*. 2004;24:30–32.
5. Geyik MF, Gür A, Nas K, et al. Musculoskeletal involvement in brucellosis in different age groups: a study of 195 cases. *Swiss Med Wkly*. 2002;132:98–105.
6. Pourbagher A, Pourbagher MA, Savas L, et al. Epidemiologic, clinical, and imaging findings in brucellosis patients with osteoarticular involvement. *AJR Am J Roentgenol*. 2006;187:873–80.
7. Tekin R, Cevik FC, Tekin RC, Cevik R. Brucellosis as a primary cause of tenosynovitis of the extensor muscle of the arm. *Infez Med*. 2015;3:257–60.

CHAPTER 93

Syphilis

Remide Arkun

Introduction

Syphilis is an infection caused by the bacterium *Treponema pallidum* and is acquired by sexual intercourse or vertical transmission from mother to baby. It is transmitted by intimate contact with moist infectious lesions of the skin and mucous membranes. The primary lesion is vasculitis.

Pathophysiology and Clinical Findings

In congenital syphilis, the fetus is infected by transmission of the organism through the placenta. The causative organism spreads directly into the fetal circulation resulting in spirochetemia with subsequent widespread dissemination to all organs. Because of inflammatory response, infection can be apparent in the fetus, the newborn, or if the infant is not treated later, in childhood. The microorganism invades perichondrium, periosteum, cartilage, bone marrow, and enchondral ossification sites in the fetus. The spirochetes inhibit osteogenesis and lead to degeneration of osteoblasts. In the fetus, neonate, and young infant, bone abnormalities include osteochondritis, diaphyseal osteomyelitis, and periostitis.

Acquired syphilis, which is seen in adults, is divided into primary, secondary, latent, and tertiary stages.

Early acquired syphilis is characterized by proliferative periostitis, which is prominent in the tibia, skull, ribs, and sternum. Bilateral tibial and clavicular periostitis in adults is suggestive of syphilis. Destructive bone lesions with a permeative or moth-eaten pattern in the skull, periostitis, cortical sequestration, and epiphyseal separation in the long bones also occur.

In late acquired syphilis, bone changes can be related to gummatous or nongummatous inflammation. Large destructive gummatous lesions may be seen in any organ of the body, particularly the skin and the bones in the tertiary stage. In acquired syphilis, bone and joint manifestations are seen in the latent and/or tertiary stages of the disease.

Gummatous bone lesions are characterized by severe bone resorption, lytic and sclerotic bone lesions, and periostitis. Nongummatous bone lesions, including periostitis, osteitis, and osteomyelitis, can occur independently or in conjunction with gummas in the bone marrow. Both types of lesions are located in the cranial vault, nasal bones, maxilla, mandible, long tubular bones, spine, and pelvis. Extreme periosteal reaction resembles the late stage of congenital syphilis, including saber shin deformity. Joint involvement is less frequent than osteomyelitis and mostly seen in the tertiary stage of the disease. Neuropathic changes also occur.

There are early and late presentations of congenital syphilis. In neonates, clinical findings include a bullous rash, anemia, jaundice and hepatosplenomegaly, rhinitis, and cutaneous lesions. Late congenital syphilis in a child or an adolescent corresponds to tertiary syphilis in an adult. Manifestations that may appear include Hutchinsonian triad, consisting of Hutchinson teeth, interstitial keratitis, and nerve deafness. Additional manifestations include fissuring about the mouth and anus, anterior bowing of the lower leg, saddle nose, and perforation of the palate.

In acquired syphilis, clinical manifestations depend on the stage of the disease. The primary lesion, called a *chancre*, represents an anogenital ulcer that appears 9–90 days after exposure. After that, secondary (latent) syphilis manifests with a generalized rash affecting the palms and soles, generalized lymphadenopathy, and orogenital mucosal lesions. Patients can also present with patchy alopecia, anterior uveitis, retinitis, cranial nerve involvement, meningitis, laryngitis, gastritis, hepatosplenomegaly (including hepatitis), glomerulonephritis, and periostitis. Tertiary (gummatous) syphilis can involve any organ, including the bones and joints, and can result in infiltrative or destructive lesions.

Imaging Strategy

Radiography is the first imaging technique for evaluation of syphilis bone lesions. MRI is more sensitive in detection of early bone, joint, and soft tissue involvement. In the prenatal period, high-frequency US may give additional information about syphilis-related fetal abnormalities.

Imaging Findings

In *early congenital syphilis*, periostitis, metaphysitis (osteochodritic changes), and diaphyseal osteomyelitis are seen, which is usually symmetric (Figure 93.1).

- **Periostitis**. Periosteal reaction can be seen as single layer or lamellar form in long bones.
- **Metaphysitis**. In tubular bones, the epiphyseal–metaphyseal junction is affected. This is also seen at the costochondral regions and flat bones.
  - In the growing metaphysis of the long bones, widening of the provisional calcification zone, serrations, and adjacent osseous irregularity are seen.
  - Erosive lesions develop along the contour of the bone at the metaphyseal–growth plate junction.
  - Broad horizontal radiolucent bands are also seen.

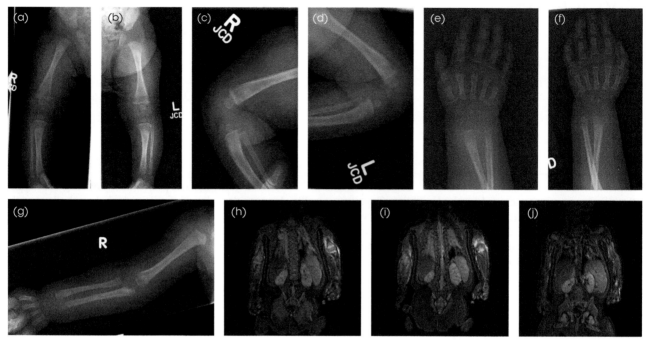

Figure 93.1. Congenital syphilis in an 8-week-old fussy infant with history of maternal syphilis who was not moving arms spontaneously. (*A-G*) Radiographs of the lower limbs, right upper extremity, and both hands and wrists show generalized demineralization of the long bone metaphyses, diametaphyseal periostitis, small bony fragments at the metaphyseal corners and cupping, fraying, and loss of the zone of provisional ossification in the distal radial and ulnar metaphyses. (*H-J*) Coronal T1W FS postcontrast MR images of upper extremities show inflammatory changes involving the bone marrow, musculature, and periarticular soft tissues with enhancement of the upper extremities from the distal humeral metaphyses through the wrist joints, left greater than right, consistent with congenital syphilis.

- In advanced disease, metaphyseal irregularities are more prominent, especially at the medial surface of the proximal tibial shaft, which is known as *Wimberger sign*. This finding, however, is also seen in rickets, scurvy, neuroblastoma, and battered baby syndrome.
- **Diaphyseal osteomyelitis.** In long bone diaphysis, moth-eaten osteolytic lesions with surrounding bony eburnation and overlying periostitis are seen.
  - Osteomyelitis usually occurs in infants who have not received therapy or in whom treatment is inadequate or inappropriate.
- Syphilitic dactylitis and skull lesions are uncommon radiographic features.
- Skull lesions may be purely sclerotic or may appear as a combination of osteosclerosis and osteolysis.
- Clinical manifestations of *late congenital syphilis* occur in children older than 2 years. Imaging findings resemble the changes that are seen in acquired syphilis and include the following:
  - Osteomyelitis and periostitis are seen in long tubular and flat bones and even the cranium.
  - In the tibia, a typical saber shin with anterior bending of the bone is seen.
- Imaging findings of *early acquired syphilis* include the following:
  - Proliferative periostitis is prominent in the skull, ribs, and sternum.

- There may be solitary or lamellated periosteal reaction, which may result in cortical thickening.
- Exaggerated periosteal reaction may mimic osteosarcoma.
- Destructive bone lesions are less common and mostly seen in the skull. CT reveals osteolytic lesions with ill-defined contours in the skull. On MRI, these lesions are hyperintense on fluid-sensitive sequences and show enhancement on postcontrast sequences including enhancement of associated soft tissue components.
- Imaging findings of *late acquired syphilis* include the following:
  - Gummatous or nongummatous osteomyelitis in the skull, radius, tibia, and ulna. These lesions have osteolytic and osteosclerotic components with associated periosteal reaction.
  - Excessive periosteal reaction causes saber shin deformity in the tibia similar to late stage congenital syphilis.

Treatment Options
- According to the treatment guidelines for syphilis from WHO, intramuscular benzathine penicillin is the mainstay of treatment in developing countries.
- In pregnant women, benzathine penicillin has been recommended.
- In infants, crystalline penicillin is the treatment of choice.

Key Points

- Syphilis is an infection caused by the bacterium *Treponema pallidum* and is acquired by sexual intercourse or vertical transmission from mother to baby. It is transmitted by intimate contact with moist infectious lesions of the skin and mucous membranes.
- In congenital syphilis, radiographic changes are related to periostitis, metaphysitis, and diaphyseal osteomyelitis.
- In acquired syphilis, bone and joint involvement is seen in the latent and/or tertiary stages of the disease.

Recommended Reading

Naraghi AM, Salonen DC, Bloom JA, Becker EJ. Magnetic resonance imaging features of osseous manifestations of early acquired syphilis. *Skeletal Radiol.* 2010;39:305–309.

Rasool MN, Govender S. The skeletal manifestation of congenital syphilis: a review of 197 cases. *J Bone Joint Surg Br.* 1989;71(5):752–55.

References

1. Goh BT. Syphilis in adults. *Sex Transm Infect.* 2005;81:448–52.
2. Huang I, Leach JL, Fictenbaum CJ, Narayan NK. Osteomyelitis of the skull in early- acquired syphilis: evaluation by MR imaging and CT. *AJNR Am J Neuroradiol.* 2007;28:307–308.
3. Murali MV, Nirmala MC, Rao JV. Symptomatic early congenital syphilis: a common but forgotten disease. *Case Rep Pediatr.* 2012;2012:934634. doi:10.1155/2012/934634.
4. Naraghi AM, Salonen DC, Bloom JA, Becker EJ. Magnetic resonance imaging features of osseous manifestations of early acquired syphilis. *Skeletal Radiol.* 2010;39:305–309.
5. Rasool MN, Govender S. The skeletal manifestation of congenital syphilis: a review of 197 cases. *J Bone Joint Surg Br.* 1989;71(5):752–55.
6. Sharma M, Solanki RN, Gupta A, Shah AK. Different radiological presentation of congenital syphilis—four cases. *Indian J Radiol Imag.* 2005;15:53–57.
7. Taljanovic MS. Atypical infections. In: Pope T, Bloem HL, Beltran J, Morrison WB, and Wilson DJ, ed. *Musculoskeletal Imaging.* 2nd ed. Philadelphia, PA: Elsevier; 2015:858–62.

CHAPTER 94

Cat Scratch Disease

Remide Arkun

Introduction

Cat scratch disease is an infection caused by *Bartonella henselae,* a gram-negative intracellular *Bacillus,* which causes granulomatous inflammation in the tissues. This disease is one of the most common causes of chronic lymphadenopathy in children and adolescents. Typically, there is a history of exposure to cats and cat scratch, bite, or licking. Enlarged lymph nodes are located proximal to the site of inoculation. In immunocompromised patients, severe systemic disease or other atypical manifestations may develop. These may include oculoglandular syndrome, encephalitis, neuroretinitis, pneumonia, osteomyelitis, spondylodiscitis, erythema nodosum, arthralgia, arthritis, and thrombocytopenic purpura.

Pathophysiology and Clinical Findings

There is a granulomatous and suppurative response with neovascularization in systemic involvement. Clinical presentation may mimic malignancy. Osteomyelitis is very rare and usually associated with ipsilateral lymphadenopathy. However, with hematogenous spread, infection may be seen in the contralateral side or axial skeleton. Cat scratch disease is more common in children. Although any bone can be involved, the most common location is the spine.

Clinical Findings

Clinical findings depend on site of involvement. Most of the patients present with fever and regional lymphadenopathy. The upper extremity is the most commonly involved site. After hand injury, 2 weeks following the inoculation, the epitrochlear lymph nodes at the elbow are first involved with secondary involvement of axillary lymph nodes. With musculoskeletal involvement, patients have prolonged fever, enlarged lymph nodes, and localized pain. Bone infection can be associated with multiple organ involvement caused by hematogenous spread. In patients with lymph node involvement, clinical presentation may mimic a soft tissue tumor. A history of cat exposure, polymerase chain reaction (PCR), and other serologic tests are helpful in diagnosis and supported by imaging findings. Histological examination of lymph nodes or bone tissue will show granulomatous infection with central necrosis, surrounded by palisading epithelioid cells and lymphocytes. *Bartonella henselae* must be added to the list of organisms that can produce cryptogenetic granulomatous bone lesions. The cat scratch skin test is not recommended because of possible seeding of infection.

Imaging Strategy

Because cat scratch disease may have different clinical presentations, imaging should be tailored according to clinical findings. Radiographs are usually the first imaging modality employed in the evaluation of cat scratch disease. Cross-sectional imaging is used to evaluate the extent of disease. MRI is the most sensitive imaging technique for detection of bone and soft tissue changes. With lymph node involvement, US and MRI are used to detect soft tissue lesions and make the differential diagnosis. Radiography and CT are additional imaging modalities in evaluation of bone involvement.

Imaging Findings

Radiography

- Nonspecific permeative osteolytic lesions surrounded by a soft tissue mass are revealed. Additional sclerosis and periosteal reaction may be seen.
- Soft tissue masses reveal subcutaneous fat irregularity and blurring of the adjacent soft tissue planes at the elbow. Elbow joint effusions, periosteal reaction, and adjacent bone erosions can also be detected.

Computed Tomography

- Similar imaging findings to radiography with bone involvement are revealed. Soft tissue extension of osseous lesions shows peripheral contrast enhancement with central necrosis.
- Enlarged lymph nodes show similar attenuation to adjacent skeletal muscle on CT studies. Irregular margins and adjacent inflammatory fat stranding and skin thickening without mineralization are additional findings.

Magnetic Resonance Imaging

- In bone lesions, there is low signal intensity on T1W and high signal intensity on fluid-sensitive sequences in the infected part of the bone. There is no specific MRI finding regarding *B. henselae* osteomyelitis.
- Enlarged lymph nodes demonstrate surrounding inflammatory changes in the adjacent fat and along the skin and fascial planes.
- Most enlarged lymph nodes are round (Figure 94.1). Usually central enhancement is seen; however, central necrosis of lymph nodes has also been reported. These findings are nonspecific but suggestive of an inflammatory process such as any bacterial, fungal, granulomatous, or parasitic infection. The differential diagnosis

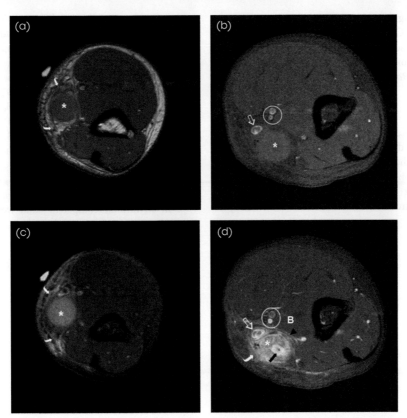

Figure 94.1. Cat scratch disease in a 13-year-old boy who presented with epitrochlear lymphadenopathy. Patient was treated with azithromycin. (*A*) T1W, (*B*) T1W FS, (*C*) T2W FS, and (*D*) T1W FS postcontrast axial MR images of the elbow show a round epitrochlear soft tissue mass consistent with an enlarged lymph node (*asterisk*). The lesion is hypointense but mildly hyperintense to muscle in (*A*) and (*B*) and hyperintense in (*C*) with surrounding inflammation (*curved white arrows*). In (*D*), note moderate peripheral enhancement and intense central enhancement (*solid black arrow*) with enhancing surrounding inflammatory soft tissue stranding (*curved white arrow*). The epitrochlear lymph node is located posterior to the basilic vein (*open white arrow*), medial and superficial to the brachialis muscle (*B*) and brachial fascia (*black arrowhead*), and posterior to the median neurovascular bundle (*dotted circle*). Courtesy of KB Hoover MD, PhD.

includes lymphoma, metastatic disease, and soft tissue sarcoma. However, malignant lymph nodes are relatively well defined, and there is no surrounding edema in the adjacent soft tissues.

- Enlarged epitrochlear lymph nodes have 3 characteristic features about their anatomic location (Figure 94.1):
  1. They reside posterior to the basilic vein.
  2. They are superficial to the brachialis muscle separated by fascia from the brachial artery and median nerve neurovascular bundle.
  3. They are superficial to the brachial fascia and medial intermuscular septum covering the medial head of the triceps and ulnar nerve.

Ultrasound

- US is useful in evaluating cat scratch-related lymphadenopathy and soft tissue lesions.
- Enlarged lymph nodes appear as mildly hypoechoic and lobular or oval soft tissue masses with preserved central hilar vascularity and increased surrounding echogenicity in the adjacent soft tissues.
- There is markedly increased Doppler signal within the involved lymph nodes.

Treatment Options

- In systemic disease, antibiotic treatment is necessary. However, it is still not clear which antibiotic is the most useful and whether antibiotics are even useful in treatment.

Key Points

- Cat scratch disease is an infection caused by *Bartonella henselae*, a gram-negative intracellular *Bacillus*, which causes granulomatous inflammation of the tissues.
- There is usually a history of exposure to cats and cat scratch, bite, or licking.
- The upper extremity is the most commonly involved site.
- After hand injury, 2 weeks following the inoculation, the epitrochlear lymph nodes at the elbow are first involved with secondary involvement of axillary lymph nodes.
- Osteomyelitis is very rare and usually associated with ipsilateral lymphadenopathy.
- Bone involvement is more common in children.
- Clinical findings are related to the site of involvement.
- A history of cat exposure, PCR, and other serologic tests are helpful in diagnosis and are supported by imaging findings.
- Tissue diagnosis reveals granulomatous infection.

Recommended Reading

Bernard SA, Walker EA, Carroll JF, Klassen-Fischer M, Murphey MD. Epitrochlear cat scratch disease: unique imaging features allowing differentiation from other soft tissue masses of the medial arm. *Skeletal Radiol.* 2016;45:1227–34.

References

1. Atici S, Kadayifci EK, Karaaslan A, et al. Atypical presentation of cat-scratch disease in an immunocompetent child with serological pathological evidence. *Case Rep Pediatr.* 2014;2014:397437. doi:10.1155/2014/397437.
2. Bernard SA, Walker EA, Carroll JF, Klassen-Fischer M, Murphey MD. Epitrochlear cat scratch disease: unique imaging features allowing differentiation from other soft tissue masses of the medial arm. *Skeletal Radiol.* 2016;45:1227–34.
3. Heye S, Matthisj P, Wallon J, van Campenhoudt M. Cat-scratch disease osteomyelitis. *Skeletal Radiol.* 2003;32:49–51.
4. Holt PD, de Lange EE. Cat scratch disease: magnetic resonance imaging findings. *Skeletal Radiol.* 1995;24:437–40.
5. Melville DM, Jacobson JA, Downie B, et al. Sonography of cat scratch disease. *J Ultrasound Med.* 2015;34:387–94.
6. Verdon R, Geffray L, Collet T, et al. Vertebral osteomyelitis due to *Bartonella henselae* in adults: a report of two cases. *Clin Infect Dis.* 2002;35:e141–44.
7. Woestyn S, Moreau M, Munting E, Bigaignon G, Delme'e M. Osteomyelitis caused by *Bartonella henselae* genotype I in an immunocompetent adult woman. *J Clin Microbiol.* 2003;41:3430–32.

CHAPTER 95

Melioidosis

Remide Arkun

Introduction

Melioidosis is a frequently fatal infection caused by the gram-negative bacillus *Burkholderia pseudomallei* (former name *Pseudomonas pseudomallei*). The causative organism is commonly found in soil and fresh water. Melioidosis is seen in tropical regions, mainly between the latitudes 20 degrees north and 20 degrees south. The main endemic areas are in Southeast Asia, particularly northeastern Thailand, Singapore, parts of Malaysia, and northern Australia. This disease is also seen in South America, Central America, various Pacific and Indian Ocean islands, and some countries in Africa. It has a wide range of clinical manifestations and can involve any organ including the musculoskeletal system.

Pathophysiology and Clinical Findings

A common route of transmission is percutaneous inoculation by contaminated soil or water, but the disease can be acquired by inhalation of aerosols, aspiration (including near drowning), and ingestion of contaminated water. Melioidosis is more common in immunocompromised patients compared to those who are immunocompetent and in those with diabetes mellitus, chronic renal failure, or chronic lung disease.

Musculoskeletal involvement accounts for 5-27% of melioidosis. The most common form is septic arthritis, followed by osteomyelitis, pyomyositis, and soft tissue abscess. Musculoskeletal disease is usually associated with additional organ involvement. The infection is usually chronic and relapsing. In disseminated form, mortality rate is up to 80%.

Clinical Findings

Clinical manifestations of melioidosis range from asymptomatic and subclinical to acute localized forms, acute septicemia, and chronic forms. Chronic disease (symptoms >2 months) can mimic other diseases such as tuberculosis (TB) or cancer. A diagnosis of melioidosis is not possible by clinical features alone. The definitive diagnosis is made by positive culture of the organism from the blood or infected organs. Sometimes, biopsy of an infected organ or culture of material obtained from a drained abscess may be required for diagnosis.

Imaging Strategy

Imaging findings in musculoskeletal melioidosis are nonspecific and may mimic other infections. Evaluation usually begins with radiography. MRI and CT are more sensitive and are subsequently used to evaluate for the extent of disease.

Imaging Findings

- Osteomyelitis occurs in both the axial and appendicular skeleton. Long bones and vertebrae are the most common locations.
  - Radiographic findings of melioidotic osteomyelitis include profound osteoporosis, osteosclerosis, cortical and medullary osteolysis, and sequestrum. Periosteal reaction is uncommon. A sinus tract is present in chronic relapsing disease.
  - In the spine, both the vertebral bodies and posterior elements can be involved. The disease may be limited to a single vertebra or associated with disc involvement and multilevel disease. MRI is used in the evaluation of paravertebral and epidural abscesses and the extent of infection to the spinal cord.
- In septic arthritis, large weight-bearing joints, such as the knee, ankle, and hip, are the most common locations.
  - Radiographic findings include soft tissue edema, periarticular osteoporosis, and joint effusion. Concomitant osteomyelitis also can be seen.
  - US can identify joint effusion and periarticular abscess and can guide aspiration.
  - CT shows similar findings to radiography, although bone erosions are better seen with CT.
  - MRI demonstrates synovitis, associated BME, and intraosseous and soft tissue abscesses.
- Muscle and soft tissue infection occur as a result of direct spread from the infected adjacent skin or bone or from hematogenous spread (Figure 95.1). Patients present with pain and soft tissue edema and subsequently develop abscesses in the affected tissue.
  - MRI may show muscle enlargement, muscle edema, and focal abscesses (Figure 95.1A–C).
  - Sinus tracts and soft tissue calcification can be present.

Treatment Options

- Melioidosis may relapse even in apparently cured disease. Combined IV antibiotic treatment of at least 2 weeks followed by oral antibiotic therapy for 12-20 weeks is necessary to prevent relapse.
- In addition to appropriate IV and oral antibiotic treatment, musculoskeletal melioidosis frequently requires surgical intervention. Drainage of soft tissue

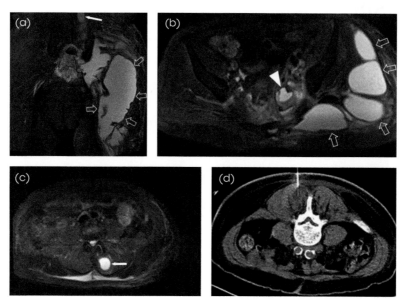

Figure 95.1. Soft tissue melioidosis of the left gluteal region in a 51-year-old man with history of end-stage renal disease and hemodialysis, and previously treated melioidosis of the lungs. (A) Coronal and (B) axial T2W FS MR images show a high signal intensity multiloculated, large left gluteal intramuscular -abscess with adjacent edema predominantly involving the gluteus maximus (*open arrows*). In (B), note pelvic extension with involvement of the piriformis muscle (*arrowhead*). In (A) and (C) axial T2W FS MR image, note left paraspinal extension with intramuscular abscess formation (*arrow*). (D) Axial CT image obtained during aspiration shows a needle within the paraspinal abscess. Culture of the aspirate grew *Burkholderia pseudomallei.* Courtesy of S. Srinivasan MD.

abscesses and debridement of infected tissue and necrotic bone are the most important processes to eradicate musculoskeletal infection.

Key Points

- Melioidosis is a frequently fatal infection caused by the gram-negative bacillus *Burkholderia pseudomallei.*
- The disease has a wide range of clinical manifestations and can involve any organ including the musculoskeletal system.
- The most common form of musculoskeletal disease is septic arthritis, followed by osteomyelitis and soft tissue infection.
- Imaging findings in musculoskeletal melioidosis are nonspecific and may mimic other infections.
- Definite diagnosis is made by positive culture of the organism from the blood or infected organs.

Recommended Reading

Pattamapaspong N, Muttarak M. Musculoskeletal melioidosis. *Semin Musculoskelet Radiol.* 2011;15:480–88.

References

1. Hoffmaster AR, AuCoin D, Baccam P, et al. Melioidosis diagnostic workshop, 2013. *Emerg Infect Dis.* 2015;21:1–9.
2. Inglis TJJ, Rolim DB, Rodriguez JLN. Clinical guideline for diagnosis and management of melioidosis. *Rev Inst Med Trop.* 2006;48:1–4.
3. Muttarak M, Peh WCG, Euathrongchit J, et al. Spectrum of imaging findings in melioidosis. *Br J Radiol.* 2009;82:514–21.
4. Pattamapaspong N, Muttarak M. Musculoskeletal melioidosis. *Semin Musculoskelet Radiol.* 2011;15:480–88.
5. Pui MH, Tan APA. Musculoskeletal melioidosis: clinical and imaging features. *Skeletal Radiol.* 1995;24:499–503.

CHAPTER 96

Musculoskeletal Echinococcosis (Hydatid Disease)

Remide Arkun

Introduction

Human echinococcosis is a parasitic disease caused by tapeworms of the genus *Echinococcus*. The 2 most important forms of the disease in humans are cystic echinococcosis (hydatidosis) and, less frequently, alveolar echinococcosis. Human echinococcosis, generally called *hydatid disease*, is a zoonotic infection with widespread infestation in the Mediterranean region, Central Asia, South America, southern Europe and Australia. Musculoskeletal involvement is rare and reported in 1-4% of cases.

Pathophysiology and Clinical Findings

Dogs and other carnivores are definitive hosts, whereas sheep and other ruminants are intermediate hosts. Humans are infected secondarily by ingestion of food or water contaminated by dog feces containing parasite eggs. Most of the embryos, which are released from eggs, lodge in the hepatic capillaries, while some pass through capillaries and lodge in the lungs and other organs. The wall of the parasitic cyst consists of the endocyst (germinal layer), ectocyst (laminated membrane), and pericyst. The germinal layer produces the laminated membrane and the scolices that represent the larval stage. Scolices are also produced by brood capsules, which are small spheres of disrupted germinal membrane. These may remain attached to the germinal membrane, but free-floating brood capsules and scolices form white sediment known as *hydatid sand*.

Muscular hydatid cysts are rare, with the prevalence at primary presentation being only 0.5-4%. This is because muscle is an unfavorable site for infestation due to its high levels of lactic acid. The most frequent locations are the paravertebral, pelvic/gluteal and lower extremity muscles. Cystic lesions can also be found in other soft tissues, such as the subcutaneous tissues. A multivesicular cystic lesion represents a characteristic appearance of hydatid disease. However, unilocular cyst formation or atypical complex or solid lesions may be seen. The presence of abundant intracystic debris and inflammatory changes may alter typical cystic morphology, transforming it into complex or solid lesions mimicking soft tissue tumors.

Bone involvement is also rare (0.5-2% cases) and occurs mostly in heavily vascularized areas such as vertebrae and long bones. The spine is the most common location followed by the pelvis, hip, femur, tibia, ribs, and scapula. In early stages of disease, microvesicular infiltration of medullary bone with embryos results in osteolytic and inflammatory changes without bone expansion, which can mimic pyogenic or atypical osteomyelitis (eg, tuberculosis or actinomycosis). Later, cystic lesions without pericyst formation develop and extend into the bone with resultant bone marrow infiltration and replacement. The cysts progressively enlarge, filling the medullary cavity to a variable extent and destroy the cortex. They then spread from bone to surrounding tissues such as muscle and spinal cord. The radiologic appearance may be confused with ABC, GCT, multiple myeloma, atypical osteomyelitis, cystic metastases, or FD. Periosteal reaction and sclerosis are uncommon. Bony extension into the adjacent joints can occur. Extraosseous hydatid cysts may have peripheral calcifications, whereas intraosseous hydatid cysts rarely show calcification.

Clinically, osseous lesions may present with pain, pathologic fracture, secondary infection, deformity, or neurovascular symptoms caused by compression. With extremity involvement, the most common finding is a palpable soft tissue mass.

Immunodiagnosis is useful in primary diagnosis and follow-up of patients after surgical or pharmacological treatment. Detection of circulating *Echinococcus granulosus* antigens in serum is less sensitive than antibody detection, which remains the method of choice. The enzyme-linked immunosorbent assay (ELISA), indirect hemagglutination antibody assay, latex agglutination test, and immunoblot test are the most commonly used immunological methods. However, serological tests may aid in the diagnosis but are not always positive in all histopathologically proven cases. Hence, a negative test does not exclude the diagnosis of echinococcosis. Imaging remains more sensitive than serodiagnostic techniques, and characteristic imaging findings in the presence of negative serologic results still suggest the diagnosis. Fine needle aspiration (FNA) still has a limited value in diagnosing musculoskeletal hydatid disease.

Imaging Strategy

Evaluation usually begins with radiography. CT and MRI examinations are useful to show extension of disease. The CT appearances of bone lesions are nearly identical to those demonstrated on radiographs. However, CT enables better evaluation of bony lesions. MRI provides excellent definition of lesion size and extension. US is useful in characterization of soft tissue lesions and may be used to guide biopsy.

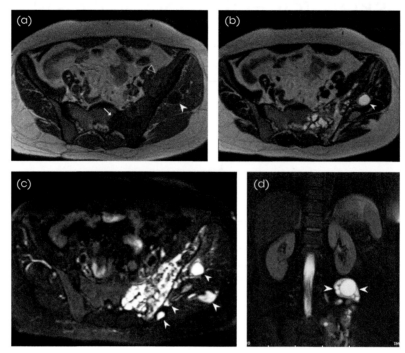

Figure 96.1. Pelvic echinococcosis in a 50-year-old woman. (*A*) Axial T1W MR image shows an expansile left iliac bone lesion with heterogeneous decreased signal intensity and pelvic soft tissue extension (*open arrowhead*). The lesion crosses the left SI joint and extends into the sacrum (*arrow*). There is also a round hypointense soft tissue mass in the adjacent gluteal muscle (*arrowhead*). (*B*) Axial T2W FS and (*C*) STIR MR images show multiple small heterogeneous predominantly hyperintense cystic lesions in the left iliac bone and sacrum. There are multiple, round, hyperintense left gluteal soft tissue masses adjacent to bone (*arrowheads*). (*D*) Coronal STIR MR image shows a multiloculated cystic mass adjacent to the left iliac crest (*arrowheads*). Daughter cysts are smaller compared to the mother cyst. There are also multiple heterogeneous cystic lesions in the left iliac bone. Courtesy of A. Purbager MD.

Imaging Findings of Skeletal Echinococcosis
Refer to Figures 96.1.

- Radiographic findings are different according to the stage of disease (Figure 96.3C).

- Initially, there are ill-defined, multilocular lucent areas without periosteal reaction located at the meta-epiphyseal regions. Later, because of development of larger cystic lesions, bone expansion with trabecular distortion and thickening occurs. Pathologic fractures may occur. This pattern of bone involvement may mimic

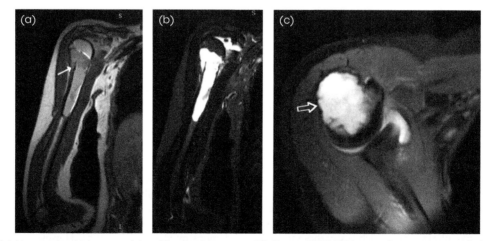

Figure 96.2. Right humeral echinococcosis in a 50-year-old woman. (*A*) Coronal T1W MR image shows an expansile lesion with increased signal intensity compared with muscle involving the proximal humeral metadiaphysis. The lesion is well demarcated with normal signal in the adjacent bone marrow. Note a pathologic fracture at the proximal humeral metaphysis (*arrow*). (*B*) The lesion demonstrates hyperintense signal on the coronal STIR image without associated periosteal reaction. (*C*) On the axial T2W FS MR image, note endosteal scalloping (*open arrow*) about the hyperintense expansile lesion in the humeral head. There is an associated glenohumeral joint effusion. Imaging findings mimic cystic FD.

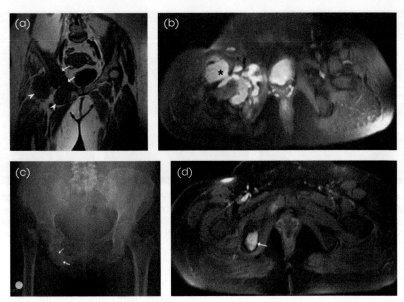

Figure 96.3. Recurrent pelvic echinococcosis in a 39-year-old woman. (*A*) Coronal T1W MR image shows an expansile low signal intensity lesion in the right acetabulum with extension into the superior pubic ramus, cortical discontinuity at the iliopectineal line (*arrows*), and associated soft tissue masses (*arrowheads*). (*B*) On axial T2W FS MR image, note hyperintense cystic lesions about the right hip (*asterisk*) and associated joint effusion. (*C*) AP radiograph of the pelvis obtained 8 years after surgery shows a new osteolytic lesion with a sclerotic margin in the right ischium (*arrows*). Note postoperative changes of the right hip joint. (*D*) Axial T2W FS MR image reveals slightly heterogeneous increased signal intensity in the right ischium (*arrow*) suggestive of disease recurrence..

bone tumors such as ABC, GCT, multiple myeloma, or metastasis.

- In chronic cases, there is trabecular thickening, sclerosis, and osteolytic areas resembling osteomyelitis. In advanced cases, cortical penetration caused by cyst enlargement and increased soft tissue density can be seen.
- CT appearances of bone lesions are similar to those demonstrated on radiographs. A well-defined typically multiloculated osteolytic lesion, sometimes with coarse trabeculae, is usually seen, which gives it a honeycomb appearance, and is accompanied by bone expansion and cortical thinning.
- MRI reveals unilocular or multilocular expansile bone lesions with irregular boundaries, with intermediate to low signal intensity on T1W images and high signal intensity on fluid-sensitive sequences. Multiple daughter cysts embedded in a large cystic lesion can also be detected. Soft tissue extension and bone marrow changes is best evaluated with MRI (Figures 96.1, 96.2, and 96.3*A*,*B*,*D*).

- In spinal involvement, vertebral expansion, extension into the spinal canal, and spinal cord and/or nerve root compression may occur. The differential diagnosis primarily includes tuberculous (TB) spondylitis. Lack of sclerosis in the host bone and absence of disc space involvement, extension into the contiguous ribs, and paraspinal extension are typical for vertebral hydatid disease and may narrow the diagnosis.

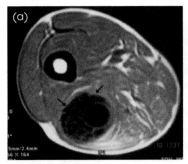 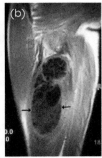 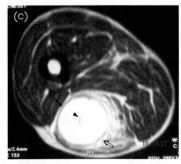

Figure 96.4. Intramuscular echinococcosis. (*A*) Axial and (*B*) coronal T1W MR images show a well-defined heterogeneous soft tissue mass at the posterior aspect of the right thigh containing multiple round hypointense nodules (*black arrows*). (*C*) Axial T2W MR image shows a well-defined hyperintense lesion surrounded with a hypointense peripheral rim (*black arrow*). There is also a round hyperintense lesion surrounded by a hypointense rim inside the large lesion corresponding to a daughter cyst (*arrowhead*) and perilesional soft tissue edema (*open arrow*). Courtesy of S. Orguc MD.

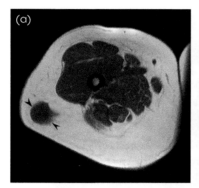
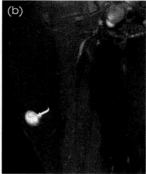
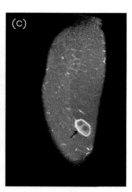

Figure 96.5. Soft tissue echinococcosis in a 45-year-old woman. (*A*) Axial T1W MR image shows an intermediate signal (isointense to skeletal muscle) soft tissue mass with multiple internal round hypointense nodules situated in the subcutaneous fat at the lateral aspect of the right thigh (*arrowheads*). (*B*) On coronal STIR image, note a corresponding hyperintense multicystic soft tissue mass (*curved arrow*) in the subcutaneous fat. (*C*) Sagittal T1W FS postcontrast MR image shows peripheral enhancement of the same lesion (*arrow*). Courtesy of B. D. Mete MD.

Imaging Findings of Soft Tissue Echinococcosis
Refer to Figures 96.4 and 96.5.

- US examination reveals well-defined multiseptated cystic soft tissue lesions including daughter cysts, floating membranes, calcifications, and hydatid sand. However, unilocular cyst formation or atypical complex or solid lesions may also be seen. The presence of abundant intracystic debris and inflammatory changes may alter typical cystic morphology, transforming it into a complex or solid lesion mimicking a tumor.
- On MRI, soft tissue echinococcosis generally appears as a cyst typically containing multiple vesicles in the mother cyst also named as *cyst* or *cysts within a cyst*. These internal cysts (daughter cysts) have low signal intensity on T1W images, and low or high signal intensity on fluid-sensitive sequences, when compared to the mother cyst (Figure 96.4).
- A *rim sign* is described on T2W MR images and consists of 2 layers with a hypointense inner rim representing an acellular laminating membrane ectocyst and outer hyperintense layer representing vascularized pericyst. The vascularized pericysts show enhancement after Gd-based IV contrast administration (Figure 96.5).
- The *water-lily sign, hydatid sand sign,* and *fluid-fluid level* are additional findings that may be seen with MRI. Separation of the laminated membrane from the pericyst produces a split wall or floating membrane appearance.

Treatment Options
- Curative treatment of osseous echinococcosis requires surgery. Ideally, the lesions should be removed using the same technique as for a malignant tumor. The combination of target-specific drug treatment, including benzimidazoles, mebendazole, or albendazole; wide resection; and if necessary, filling the defect with polymethylmethacrylate (PMMA) has been recommended for good outcome and to prevent recurrence.

- It is necessary to combine wide surgical excision with target-specific drug treatment including benzimidazoles, mebendazole, or albendazole for soft tissue echinococcosis.

Key Points
- Musculoskeletal echinococcosis caused by tapeworms of the genus *Echinococcus* is a zoonotic disease, which can be seen even in nonendemic areas.
- Echinococcal involvement of bones and soft tissues is rare.
- Differential diagnosis includes but is not limited to bone and soft tissue tumors, tumor-like lesions, and osteomyelitis.
- Radiological, laboratory, and clinical findings combined with a strong element of suspicion are the key in diagnosis.

Recommended Reading
Arkun R, Dirim Mete B. Musculoskeletal hydatid disease. *Semin Musculoskelet Radiol.* 2011;15:527–40.

References
1. Arkun R, Dirim Mete B. Musculoskeletal hydatid disease. *Semin Musculoskelet Radiol.* 2011;15:527–40.
2. Hui M, Tandon A, Prayaga AK, Patnaik S. Isolated musculoskeletal hydatid disease: diagnosis on fine needle aspiration and cell block. *J Parasit Dis.* 2015;39:332–35.
3. Memis A, Arkun R, Bilgen I, et al. Primary soft tissue hydatid disease: report of two cases with MRI characteristics. *Eur Radiol.* 1999;9:1101–103.
4. Polat P, Kantarci M, Alper F, et al. Hydatid disease from head to toe. *Radiographics.* 2003;23:475–94.
5. Ratnaparkhi CR, Mitra KR, Kulkarni A, et al. Primary musculoskeletal hydatid mimicking a neoplasm. *J Case Rep.* 2014;4:424–27.
6. Song XH, Ding LW, Wen H. Bone hydatid disease. *Postgrad Med J.* 2007;83:536–42.

CHAPTER 97

Leprosy

Remide Arkun

Introduction

Leprosy (Hansen disease) is a chronic granulomatous infection caused by the obligate intracellular bacillus, *Mycobacterium leprae (M. leprae)*. Skin and peripheral nerves are primarily affected. The disease is prevalent in Southeast Asia with 70% of cases seen in India, Myanmar, and Nepal. The disease is also prevalent in Brazil.

Pathophysiology and Clinical Findings

Mycobacterium leprae is an acid-alcohol-fast, gram-positive obligate intracellular bacillus that shows tropism for cells of the reticuloendothelial system and peripheral nervous system (notably Schwann cells). Contamination is possible either via nasal mucosa or skin puncture especially in immunocompromised patients.

The disease can present in different forms, depending on the host response to the organism. The tuberculoid form of the disease usually involves the skin and peripheral nerves. Nerve involvement is usually asymmetric and skin lesions are of limited number in association with hypoesthesia. The lepromatous form of disease is characterized by extensive skin involvement. Skin lesions are often described as infiltrated nodules and plaques, and nerve involvement tends to be symmetric in distribution.

Nerve involvement results in loss of sensory and motor function, which may lead to frequent trauma and amputation. Nerve abscesses may occur in various forms of leprosy because of caseation of nerve fasciculi leading to cold abscess formation. The ulnar nerve is most commonly involved.

Osseous involvement is seen in 15-29% of patients and most commonly involves the feet. Plantar ulcers, osteomyelitis, periostitis, and other neuropathic changes in the tarsal bones are the result of prolonged anesthetic changes in the feet experienced by leprosy patients. Similar changes also occur in the hands. Osseous involvement can also occur because of direct invasion by *M. leprae*.

The clinical presentation and histopathologic changes depend on the immune status of the patient at the time of infection and over the course of the disease. Diagnosis is currently based on 3 cardinal signs specified by the World Health Organization (WHO): hypopigmented or erythematous macules with sensory loss, thickened peripheral nerves, and positive acid-alcohol-fast smear or skin biopsy. The musculoskeletal system is affected in 95% of cases. The most common skeletal signs are nonspecific, as sensory loss secondary to nerve damage leads to ulcers, deformities, and fractures in hands and feet. Osteoporosis

is the second most common skeletal finding in patients with leprosy.

Imaging Strategy

Radiography is the initial imaging technique in the evaluation of leprosy bone lesions. High-frequency US and MRI have increasingly been used for noninvasive assessment of peripheral nerve disease.

Imaging Findings

Radiography

- Bone invasion by the microorganism, whether with direct inoculation or hematogenous spread, results in significant bone destruction and cystic degeneration.
- Radiographic findings include formation of bone cysts, honeycombing, enlarged nutrient foramina, subarticular erosions, concentric cortical erosions, acroosteolysis, and periostitis. Healing is characterized by sclerosis. In advanced disease, findings of neuropathic arthropathy may be seen.

Ultrasound

- Nerve hypertrophy is considered a main feature of leprosy. The sites of nerve swelling are similar to those of entrapment neuropathies.
- US appearance of nerve involvement is variable.
  - In group 1, nerves appear normal.
  - In group 2, nerves are enlarged/markedly swollen with fascicular abnormalities (Figure 97.1A). Swollen nerves appear hypoechoic on US imaging with associated hyperemia on color or power Doppler interrogation.
  - In group 3, nerve fascicular pattern is absent without significant change in size.
    - On US, these nerves appear either hypoechoic or hyperechoic. There is no hyperemia on color or power Doppler imaging.

Magnetic Resonance Imaging

- Imaging typically shows enlargement/swelling, and enhancement of the nerve (Figure 97.1B). This is nonspecific and can be seen in hypertrophic neuropathy, amyloid infiltration, and chronic relapsing polyneuropathy.
- Additional nodule or granuloma and abscess formation in the nerve or nerve sheath is suggestive of leprosy. Nodules or granulomata are isointense on T1W

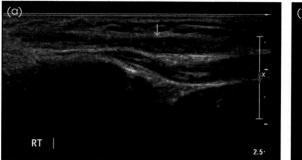
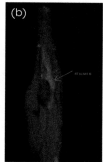

Figure 97.1. Leprosy of a peripheral nerve in a 28-year-old man with right elbow pain. (*A*) Long-axis grayscale US image depicts abnormal enlarged ulnar nerve (group 2) with decreased echogenicity (*arrow*). (*B*) Sagittal T1W FS postcontrast MR image of the right elbow shows diffuse ulnar nerve enlargement with avid contrast enhancement (*arrow*). Courtesy of A. Chhabra MD.

images and hyperintense on fluid-sensitive sequences surrounded with perineural soft tissue edema. Associated abscesses show rim enhancement on postcontrast T1W FS MR images.

Treatment Options

- Combined antibiotic treatment is necessary for a prolonged period.
- Multidrug therapy has led to a rapid decline of the contagious disease and decreased rates of recurrence and reactions.
- Steroid treatment has been used for nerve involvement. If steroid therapy has failed, surgical intervention in the form of epineurotomy by multiple longitudinal incisions and external decompression to relieve the internal pressure throughout the involved segment is the treatment of choice. Nerve abscesses should be drained.

Key Points

- Leprosy (Hansen disease) is a chronic granulomatous infection caused by the obligate intracellular bacillus, *M. leprae*. Skin and peripheral nerves are primarily affected.
- Leprosy can present in different forms, depending on the host response to the organism.
- Nerve involvement results in loss of sensory and motor function, which may lead to frequent trauma and amputation. The ulnar nerve is the most commonly involved peripheral nerve.
- Skin ulcers, osteomyelitis, periostitis, and other neuropathic changes in the hands and feet bones are the result of prolonged anesthetic changes.

Recommended Reading

Martinolli C, Derchi LE, Bertolotto M, et al. US and MR images of peripheral nerves in leprosy. *Skeletal Radiol*. 2000;29:142–50.

Taljanovic MS. Atypical infections. In: T Pope, HL Bloem, J Beltran, WB Morrison, and DJ Wilson, ed., *Musculoskeletal Imaging*. 2nd ed. Philadelphia, PA: Elsevier; 2015: 851–54.

References

1. Ankad BS, Halawar RS. Bone involvement in leprosy: early changes. *Radiol Infect Dis*. 2015;1:88–89.
2. Ankad BS, Hombal A, Rao S, Naidu VM. Radiological changes in the hands and feet of leprosy patients with deformities. *J Clin Diagn Res*. 2011;5:703–707.
3. Eichelmann K, Gonzalez SEG, Salas-Alanis JC, Ocampo-Candia J. Leprosy. An update: definition, pathogenesis, classification, diagnosis, and treatment. *Actas Dermosifiliogr*. 2013;104:554–63.
4. Hari S, Subramanian S, Sharma R. Magnetic resonance imaging of ulnar nerve abscess in leprosy: a case report. *Lepr Rev*. 2007;78:155–59.
5. Kulkarni M, Chauhan V, Bharucha M, Desmukh M, Chhabra A. MRI imaging of ulnar leprosy abscess. *J Assoc Physicians India*. 2009;57:175–76.
6. Martinolli C, Derchi LE, Bertolotto M, et al. US and MR images of peripheral nerves in leprosy. *Skeletal Radiol*. 2000;29:142–50.

Section Six

Arthrography

Edited by Mihra S. Taljanovic and Tyson S. Chadaz

CHAPTER 98

Shoulder Arthrography

Matthew DelGiudice

Indications

- Indications include evaluation of glenoid labrum in shoulder instability and trauma (ie, dislocation), evaluation of pre- and postoperative rotator cuff, fluoroscopic guidance for therapeutic injections (most commonly steroid), or therapy for adhesive capsulitis.
- In the author's institution, diagnostic injections of the glenohumeral joint are performed in patients younger than 40 years and in the postoperative setting regardless of patient age. Most patients undergo subsequent MRA imaging with a small number having computed tomography arthrography (CTA).
- CTA may also be performed for evaluation of total shoulder arthroplasty (TSA) loosening and conversion from anatomic to reverse TSA.

Technique

- The patient is in the supine position with the affected shoulder in external rotation (palm up). A weight, such as sandbag can be used to hold the hand in external rotation.
- Use a modified anterior technique with needle in the anteroposterior position through the rotator interval to avoid ligaments, rotator cuff tendons, and labrum (Figure 98.1).
- Use a 22- to 20-gauge, 3.5-inch needle (or 1.5-inch needle for low body mass index [BMI] patients) using sterile technique.
- For MRA, combine 10 mL of normal saline and 10 mL of iodinated radiopaque contrast (such as iohexol [Omnipaque 300]) at a ratio of 1:1 with 0.1 mL of Gd-based contrast and inject 10-12 mL (depending on the joint size) into the glenohumeral joint. For CTA, 10-12 mL of iodinated contrast is injected into the glenohumeral joint.
- Some operators prefer injection of Gd and saline mixture and only minimal injection of iodinated contrast at the beginning of the procedure for confirmation of intraarticular needle position. This amount of iodinated

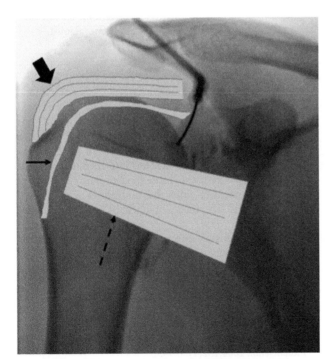

Figure 98.1. Fluoroscopic image with cartoon display of relevant anatomy during right shoulder arthrogram for MRA. Contrast can partly be seen in the glenohumeral joint arising from the needle within the rotator cuff interval. Thick arrow—supraspinatus tendon; small arrow—long head of biceps tendon; dashed arrow—subscapularis tendon.

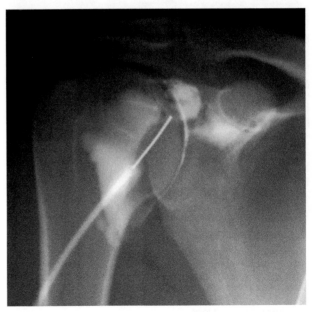

Figure 98.2. Right shoulder arthrogram for MRA with anterior rotator interval approach shows contrast in the glenohumeral joint indicating successful needle positioning.

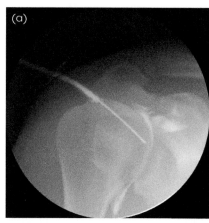 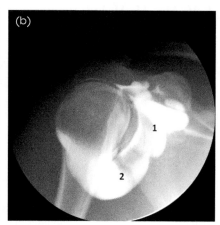 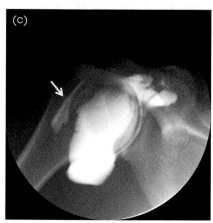

Figure 98.3. Normal shoulder arthrogram. (*A*) AP fluoroscopic image of the shoulder shows needle positioning for trans-subscapularis contrast injection. (*B*) Internal rotation AP view demonstrates normal distribution of intraarticular contrast including the subscapularis recess (*1*) and axillary pouch (*2*). (*C*) On external rotation AP view, note normal extension of the contrast into the long head of biceps tendon sheath (*arrow*).

contrast does not provide diagnostic arthrographic images or conversion of the procedure to CTA, which is occasionally needed if the patient cannot tolerate MRI.

- Contrast should be easy to inject and disperse throughout the joint (Figure 98.2); if contrast stays in one spot then the needle in not in the joint.
- There are alternate techniques for contrast injection including the subscapularis or posterior approaches. In some institutions, injections are performed under US guidance.

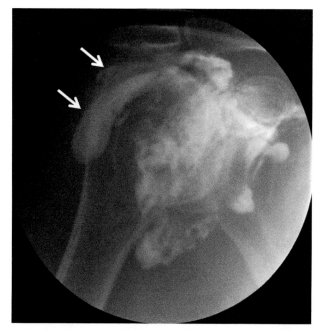

Figure 98.4. Full-thickness rotator cuff tear on right shoulder arthrogram. AP radiograph shows multiple contrast filling defects in the glenohumeral joint capsule consistent with synovitis and joint bodies and abnormal communication with the subacromial-subdeltoid bursa (*arrows*) in keeping with a full-thickness rotator cuff tear.

- Complications are rare but include infection and bleeding.

Normal Findings

- Contrast opacifies the glenohumeral joint without extension into the tendon substance, glenoid labrum, or subacromial-subdeltoid bursa (Figure 98.3).
- The joint capsule attaches to the anatomic neck of the humerus and forms 2 normal anterior recesses: the axillary pouch/recess at the inferior aspect and the subscapular recess at the superomedial aspect of the glenohumeral joint. The long head of the biceps tendon sheath normally communicates with the glenohumeral joint.

Abnormal Findings

- Abnormal communication between the glenohumeral joint and subacromial-subdeltoid and subcoracoid bursae is diagnostic of a full-thickness rotator cuff tear unless the contrast is accidentally injected into the bursa (Figure 98.4). However, in the setting of prior rotator cuff repair, contrast may extend into the bursa even in the absence of re-tear because the cuff is not watertight.
- Contrast extension into the undersurface of the rotator cuff is diagnostic of partial-thickness articular surface tear.
- Contrast extension into the glenoid labral substance is diagnostic of labral tear.

Recommended Reading

Dépelteau H, Bureau NJ, Cardinal E, Aubin B, Brassard P. Arthrography of the shoulder: a simple fluoroscopically guided approach for targeting the rotator cuff interval. *AJR Am J Roentgenol.* 2004;182(2):329–32.

Lungu E, Moser TP. A practical guide for performing arthrography under fluoroscopic or ultrasound guidance. *Insights Imaging.* 2015;6(6):601–10.

CHAPTER 99

Elbow Arthrography

Matthew DelGiudice

Indications

- Indications include injury to ulnar or radial collateral ligaments, evaluation of osteochondral lesions or joint bodies, or therapeutic injections (most commonly steroid).
- The patient should be positioned prone with a pillow under the body for comfort, with the affected arm above the head with the elbow flexed 90 degrees with the wrist in a neutral position (thumb up).
- The elbow can be injected via the lateral approach, aiming for the radiocapitellar joint (Figure 99.1).
- Some operators prefer the posterior transtriceps approach (Figure 99.2), which they consider easier to perform than the radiocapitellar approach. The posterior transtriceps approach still allows adequate evaluation of medial and lateral structures should there be extravasation. The entry point for the posterior transtriceps technique is at the level of the olecranon fossa, midpoint between the humeral epicondyles, with the needle endpoint being the olecranon fossa. This approach is preferred when the clinical concern is for radial collateral ligament injury.

Technique

- Use a 22-gauge, 1.5-inch spinal needle using sterile technique.
- For MRA, combine 10 mL of normal saline and 10 mL of iodinated radiopaque contrast (such as iohexol [Omnipaque 300]) at a ratio of 1:1 with 0.1 mL of Gd-based contrast and inject 6-8 mL or less of contrast. Greater than 8 mL has an increased rate of extravasation. Iodinated contrast allows conversion of the procedure to CTA if needed. Alternatively, for CTA, 6-8 mL of iodinated contrast is injected.
- Contrast should easily inject and disperse throughout the joint with contrast in the anterior joint easy to identify.
- Complications are rare but include infection and bleeding.

Normal Findings

- Contrast opacifies the anterior (coronoid), posterior (olecranon), and periradial (annular) recesses, which are easily depicted on the lateral radiograph (Figure 99.3A).
- In the frontal projection, there are 2 normal contrast outpouchings overlying the distal humerus, which have an appearance of rabbit ears (Figure 99.3B).

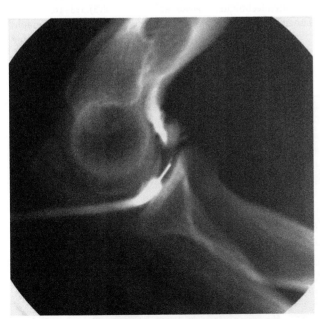

Figure 99.1. Elbow arthrogram using the radiocapitellar approach. Contrast is seen dispersing into the anterior recess of the elbow joint.

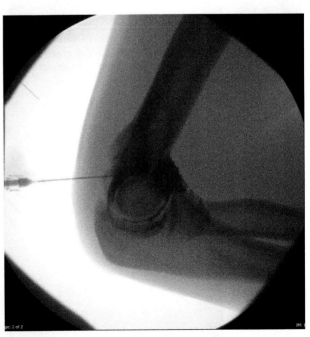

Figure 99.2. Elbow arthrogram using the posterior transtriceps approach. Note needle position for posterior transtriceps approach with intraarticular contrast extending into anterior elbow.

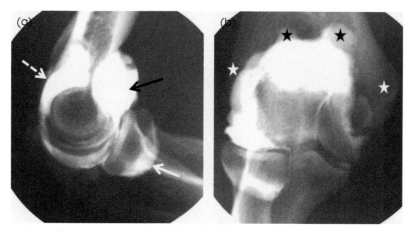

Figure 99.3. Normal contrast opacified recesses on lateral (*A*) and AP (*B*) elbow arthrogram images. In (*A*), note anterior (coronoid) recess (*black arrow*), posterior (olecranon) recess (*dashed white arrow*), and periradial (annular) recess (*white arrow*). In (*B*), note normal *rabbit ear-like* contrast outpouchings (*black asterisks*) and medial and lateral humeral epicondyles outside the joint capsule (*white asterisks*).

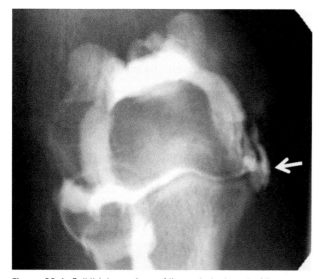

Figure 99.4. Full-thickness tear of the anterior band of the UCL. On the AP arthrogram image, note contrast extravasation through the torn UCL (*arrow*).

- Please note that the medial and lateral humeral epicondyles are extraarticular and not opacified by intraarticular contrast (Figure 99.3*B*).

Abnormal Findings

- Leaking of the intraarticular contrast through the torn elbow ligaments, usually the anterior band of the ulnar collateral ligament (UCL) (Figure 99.4)
- Contrast undermining an unstable osteochondral defect (Figure 99.5)
- Filling defects within the intraarticular contrast related to joint bodies or synovitis

Recommended Reading

Lohman M, Borrero C, Casagranda B, Rafiee B, Towers J. The posterior transtriceps approach for elbow arthrography: a forgotten technique? *Skeletal Radiol.* 2009;38(5):513–16.

Lungu E, Moser TP. A practical guide for performing arthrography under fluoroscopic or ultrasound guidance. *Insights Imaging.* 2015;6(6):601–10.

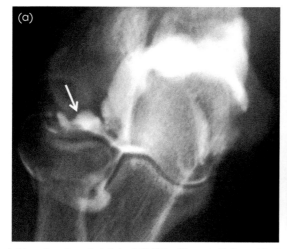
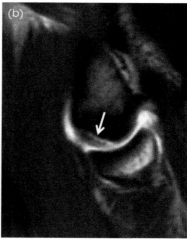

Figure 99.5. Unstable osteochondral defect (OCD) of the capitellum. (*A*) On the AP elbow arthrogram image, note contrast undermining an unstable capitellar OCD (*arrow*), which is easier to see on the subsequent (*B*) sagittal T1W FS MRA image (*arrow*).

CHAPTER 100

Wrist Arthrography

Matthew DelGiudice

Indications

- Indications include evaluation of intrinsic wrist ligaments (scapholunate and lunotriquetral) and TFCC injuries.

Technique

- The patient should be positioned prone with a pillow under the body for comfort and the affected wrist above the head with the palm down and wrist slightly flexed. A rolled-up cloth can be used under the wrist to keep mild flexion.
- A radiocarpal joint injection can be performed aiming for the proximal most aspect of the scaphoid (Figure 100.1) or alternatively, the radioscaphoid joint (Figure 100.2), with a 5/8-inch 25-gauge needle using sterile technique. Some authors perform arthrography in all 3 wrist compartments including the midcarpal and distal radioulnar joints if there is no contrast extravasation into the other 2 compartments with radiocarpal joint injection (Figure 100.3).
- For MRA, combine 10 mL of normal saline and 10 mL of iodinated radiopaque contrast (such as iohexol [Omnipaque 300]) at a ratio of 1:1 with 0.1 mL of Gd-based contrast and inject 3-5 mL of solution. Iodinated contrast allows conversion of the procedure to CTA if needed. Alternatively, for CTA, 3-5 mL of iodinated contrast is injected.
- Inject approximately 2 mL of contrast into the midcarpal joint and 1 mL of contrast into the distal radioulnar joint.
- Complications are rare and include infection and bleeding.

Normal Findings

- Contrast should easily inject and disperse throughout the radiocarpal joint space (Figure 100.4).
- With midcarpal joint injection, there is normal communication with the common (second through fifth) carpometacarpal (CMC) joint (Figure 100.3A).

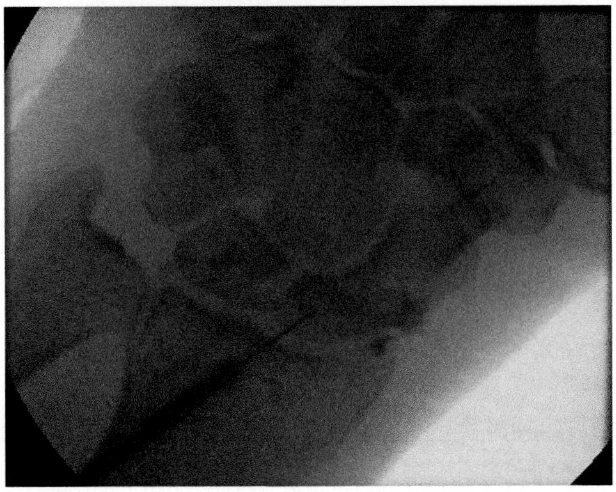

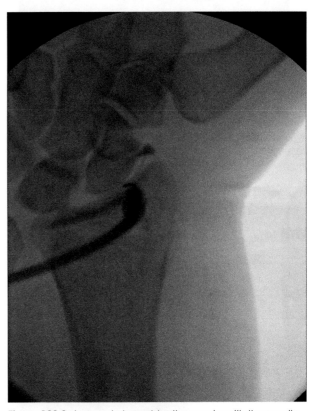

Figure 100.1. Wrist arthrogram demonstrates technique aiming for the proximal most aspect of the scaphoid. Contrast can be seen extending into the radial aspect of the radiocarpal joint.

Figure 100.2. Image during wrist arthrography with the needle in the more traditional radioscaphoid joint. Contrast can be seen extending into the radial aspect of the radiocarpal joint.

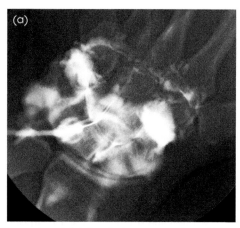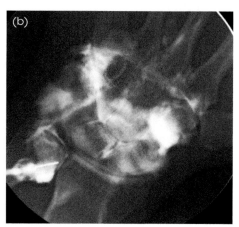

Figure 100.3. Midcarpal and distal radioulnar compartment injections following normal radiocarpal joint injection. (*A*) PA wrist arthrogram image shows needle positioning between the lunate, triquetrum, capitate, and hamate for midcarpal joint injection. Note normal contrast extension into the common (second through fifth) CMC joint. (*B*) PA wrist arthrogram image shows needle positioning for injection of the distal radioulnar joint.

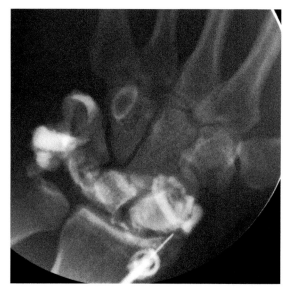

Figure 100.4. Normal radiocarpal joint arthrogram. Note needle in the radioscaphoid joint with normal contrast dispersion throughout the radiocarpal joint space.

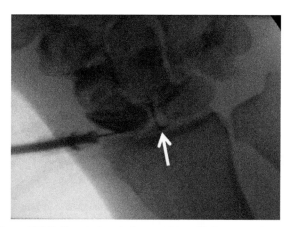

Figure 100.5. Scapholunate ligament tear. PA fluoroscopic image of the wrist during radiocarpal joint injection shows abnormal communication with the midcarpal joint through the torn scapholunate ligament (*arrow*).

Abnormal Findings

- Full-thickness tearing of any of the 3 components of the scapholunate and/or lunotriquetral ligament allows abnormal communication with the midcarpal joint (Figure 100.5).
- Central tearing of the TFC disc allows abnormal communication with the distal radioulnar joint (Figure 100.6).

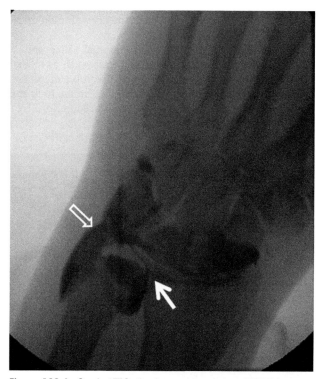

Figure 100.6. Central TFC disc tear and peripheral TFCC tear. PA wrist arthrogram image after radiocarpal joint injection shows abnormal communication with the distal radioulnar joint through the central tear of the TFC disc (*arrow*) and contrast extravasation through the ulnar joint capsule (UCL) related to the peripheral TFCC tear (*open arrow*).

- Peripheral tearing of the TFCC allows extravasation of the radiocarpal joint contrast through the ulnar joint capsule (Figure 100.6).
- Communication of the midcarpal joint with the first CMC joint.

Recommended Reading

Lungu E, Moser TP. A practical guide for performing arthrography under fluoroscopic or ultrasound guidance. *Insights Imaging.* 2015;6(6):601–10.

Moser T, Dosch JC, Moussaoui A, Buy X, Gangi A, Dietemann JL. Multidetector CT arthrography of the wrist joint: how to do it. *Radiographics.* 2008;28(3):787–800; quiz 911.

CHAPTER 101

Hip Arthrography

Matthew DelGiudice

Indications

- Indications include hip pain thought to be caused by acetabular labral injury, femoroacetabular impingement syndromes, as well as therapeutic steroid injections. The technique can also be used for arthrocentesis with suspected infection, but contrast should not be injected.

Technique

- Patients should be positioned supine with the affected hip in mild internal rotation. A sandbag can be used to hold the leg in internal rotation (10-15 degrees). The femoral artery should be marked on the patient's skin to avoid puncture.
- Various anterior approaches for hip injection are preferred by different operators, including femoral neck and head recesses, to avoid the tight capsular ligamentous structures (zona orbicularis [ZO]).

- An anterior oblique approach is used with the skin entry site at the base of the greater trochanter (at the C) and the target being the lateral aspect of the femoral head/neck junction (Figure 101.1). Aiming toward the umbilicus can serve as a guide to needle trajectory. Anecdotally, with this technique, the author of this chapter found lower first puncture failure rates than with straight AP approach.
- Alternative approaches include a straight AP needle position at the lateral femoral head/neck junction (Figure 101.2), or medial femoral head/neck junction and medial femoral neck recess (Figure 101.3).
- Use a 20- to 22-gauge, 3.5-inch spinal needle (or 5- to 7-inch spinal needle for larger patients) using sterile technique.
- For MRA, combine 10 mL of normal saline and 10 mL of iodinated radiopaque contrast (such as iohexol [Omnipaque 300]) at a ratio of 1:1 with 0.1 mL of Gd-based contrast. Inject 10-15 mL of contrast into the hip joint. Iodinated contrast allows conversion of the

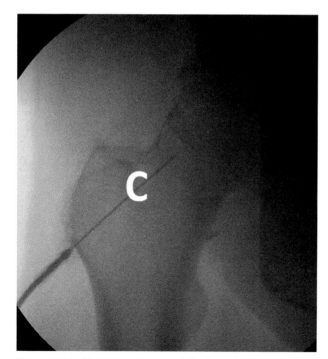

Figure 101.1. Right hip arthrogram injection using an anterior oblique approach. The C outlines the greater trochanter skin entry site. Intraarticular contrast can be seen about the femoral neck and head.

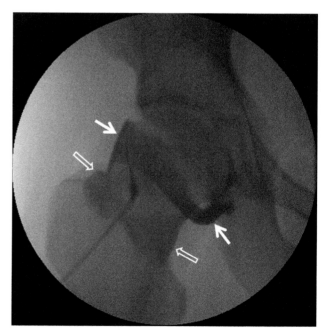

Figure 101.2. Right hip arthrogram injection using an anterolateral approach. Note normal contrast distribution through the femoral neck (*open arrows*) and femoral head recesses (*arrows*).

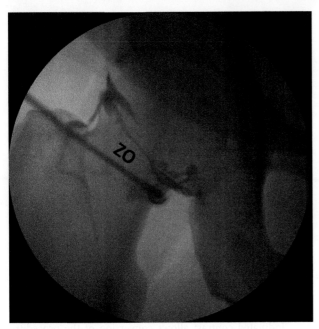

Figure 101.3. Right hip arthrogram injection using an anteromedial approach. Intraarticular contrast is seen in the femoral neck and head recesses outlining the ZO.

procedure to CTA if needed. Alternatively, for CTA, 10-15 mL of iodinated contrast is injected.

- Complications include infection, bleeding (especially if arterial puncture), and femoral nerve injury.

Normal Findings

- Contrast should easily inject and disperse throughout the joint away from the needle, opacifying the femoral head and neck recesses and outlining the ZO (Figures 101.2 and 101.3).
- There is no extension of the contrast into the acetabular labral substance.

Abnormal Findings

- Extension of the joint contrast into the acetabular labral substance may be occasionally depicted on standard arthrography images. However, it is nowadays evaluated by MRA or sometimes CTA.
- Contrast extension through the torn/incompetent joint capsule especially post total hip arthroplasty (THA), as well as through the torn gluteal tendons can occur.

Recommended Reading

Duc SR, Hodler J, Schmid MR, et al. Prospective evaluation of two different injection techniques for MR arthrography of the hip. *Eur Radiol.* 2006;16(2):473–78.

Lungu E, Moser TP. A practical guide for performing arthrography under fluoroscopic or ultrasound guidance. *Insights Imaging.* 2015;6(6):601–10.

CHAPTER 102

Knee Arthrography

Matthew DelGiudice

Indications

- Indications include evaluation for meniscal re-tear after prior repair, osteochondral injuries, and therapeutic injections (most commonly steroid).

Technique

- The patient should be positioned supine with knee in slight flexion.
- Different approaches for knee injection are favored by different operators. These include the lateral (Figure 102.1) or medial (Figure 102.2) patellofemoral joint approaches or aiming for the lateral femoral condyle (Figure 102.3).
- The author of this chapter prefers an anterior approach lateral to the patellar tendon, staying sufficiently superior to the tibial plateau to avoid the lateral meniscus, aiming slightly medial with the endpoint being the lateral femoral condyle (Figure 102.3).

- Use a 20- to 22-gauge, 3.5-inch spinal needle using sterile technique. Frequently a 1.5-inch needle would be sufficient.
- For MRA, combine 20 mL of normal saline and 20 mL of iodinated radiopaque contrast (such as iohexol [Omnipaque 300]) at a ratio of 1:1 with 0.2 mL of Gd-based contrast and inject 20-40 mL (depending on the joint size) into the knee joint, making sure contrast is dispersing away from needle into the rest of the joint. Iodinated contrast allows conversion of the procedure to CTA if needed. Alternatively, for CTA, 20-40 mL of iodinated contrast is injected.
- For MRA or CTA, a compression band may be applied to the suprapatellar recess to direct the larger amount of contrast about the articular surfaces for better outlining of the menisci and cruciate ligaments.
- Complications are rare but include infection and bleeding.

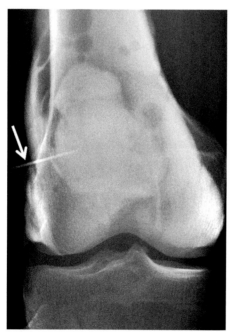

Figure 102.1. Lateral patellofemoral approach for knee arthrogram. Note needle projecting over the lateral aspect of the patellofemoral joint (*arrow*).

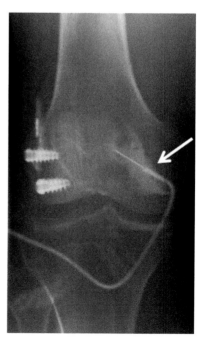

Figure 102.2. Medial patellofemoral approach for knee arthrogram. Note needle projecting over the medial aspect of the patellofemoral joint (*arrow*).

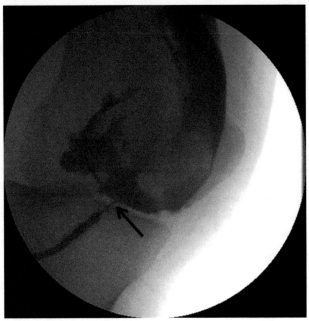

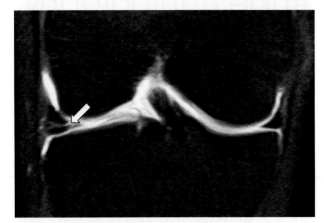

Figure 102.4. New horizontal cleavage tear of the lateral meniscus in a 21-year-old patient with history of ACL reconstruction and inner partial lateral meniscectomy who presented with new lateral knee pain. Coronal T1W FS MRA image of the knee shows horizontal contrast extension into the meniscal substance consistent with a new horizontal cleavage tear (*arrow*).

Figure 102.3. Anterolateral approach for knee arthrogram. Fluoroscopic image during knee arthrogram for CTA in a patient unable to get an MRI showing successful intraarticular knee injection using an anterolateral approach (*arrow*) with the knee internally rotated.

Normal Findings
- There is no contrast extension into the meniscal substance or into the pathway of the cruciate ligaments.

Abnormal Findings
- Extension of intraarticular contrast into the meniscal substance indicating a tear or re-tear (Figure 102.4)
- Abnormal course of the cruciate ligament fibers indicating a tear
- Contrast undermining an unstable osteochondral defect/lesion
- Extension of the contrast into the hyaline cartilage defects (Figure 102.5)

Recommended Reading
Lungu E, Moser TP. A practical guide for performing arthrography under fluoroscopic or ultrasound guidance. *Insights Imaging*. 2015;6(6):601–10.

Reference
Moser, T. Moussaoui A, Dupuis M, Douzal V, Dosch JC. Anterior approach for knee arthrography: tolerance evaluation and comparison of two routes. *Radiology*. 2008;246(1):193–97.

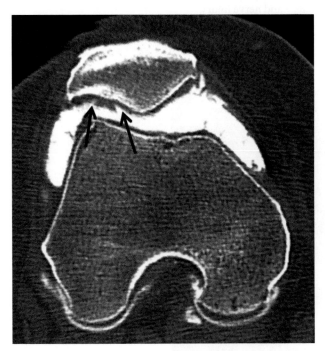

Figure 102.5. Chondromalacia patellae. Axial CT arthrogram image shows thinning and irregularity of the patellar hyaline articular cartilage with contrast extension into the cartilage defects (*arrows*).

CHAPTER 103

Ankle Arthrography

Matthew DelGiudice

Indications

- Ankle arthrography is performed predominantly for the evaluation of the talar dome for stability of osteochondral lesions/defects.

Technique

- Place the patient in the supine position with the anterior aspect of the ankle facing the examiner.
- The main approach is anterior, lateral to the tibialis anterior tendon. It is important to localize the neurovascular bundle by marking the anterior tibial artery/dorsalis pedis artery. However, moving the ankle into the lateral position during the procedure is sometimes needed for confirmation of adequate needle positioning.
- Position the needle between the tibialis anterior and extensor hallucis longus tendons, medial to the neurovascular bundle, with the endpoint being the talar dome.
- Insert a 22-gauge needle (usually a 1.5-inch long needle is sufficient) under sterile conditions into the tibiotalar joint with slight superior needle angulation to avoid the anterior lip of distal tibia (Figure 103.1).
- For MRA, combine 10 mL of normal saline and 10 mL of iodinated radiopaque contrast (such as iohexol [Omnipaque 300]) at a ratio of 1:1 with 0.1 mL of Gd-based contrast and inject approximately 10 mL or less of contrast, making sure the contrast disperses away from the needle tip throughout the joint space. Iodinated contrast allows conversion of the procedure to CTA if needed. Alternatively, for CTA, 10 mL or less of iodinated contrast is injected.
- Complications are rare but include infection, bleeding, and nerve injury.

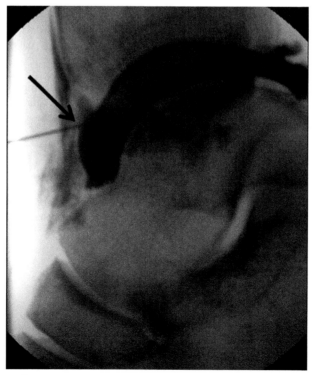

Figure 103.1. Left ankle arthrogram with needle positioned between the tibialis anterior tendon and extensor hallucis longus tendons (*arrow*). Contrast is seen dispersing throughout the tibiotalar joint.

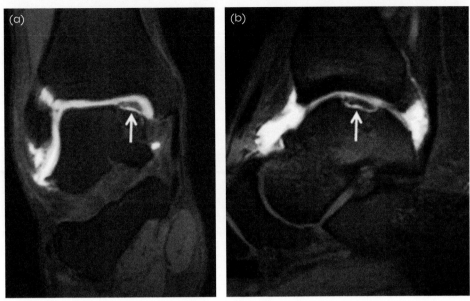

Figure 103.2. Unstable osteochondral defect/lesion of the talar dome. (*A*) Coronal and (*B*) sagittal T1W FS MRA images of the ankle show contrast undermining an unstable osteochondral defect (*arrows*).

Normal Findings

- Contrast opacifies the tibiotalar joint without subchondral/osseous extension.

Abnormal Findings

- Contrast undermining an unstable osteochondral defect (Figure 103.2)
- Extravasation of the contrast through the lateral or medial joint capsule consistent with a ligamentous tear

- Filling defects within the intraarticular contrast related to joint bodies or synovitis

Recommended Reading

Cerezal L, Abascal F, García-Valtuille R, Canga A. Ankle MR arthrography: how, why, when. *Radiol Clin North Am.* 2005;43(4):693–707, viii. Review.

Lungu E, Moser TP. A practical guide for performing arthrography under fluoroscopic or ultrasound guidance. *Insights Imaging.* 2015;6(6):601–10.

Internal Derangements of the Joints

Edited by Mihra S. Taljanovic, Imran M. Omar, Kevin B. Hoover, and Tyson S. Chadaz

CHAPTER 104

Internal Derangement of the Shoulder

David Brandel and Girish Gandikota

Introduction

As is common in musculoskeletal imaging, evaluation of the shoulder begins with radiography, which provides an accessible and accurate assessment of the osseous structures and their alignment. However, when injury to the soft tissues is suspected, MRI and MR arthrography (MRA) offer numerous advantages. The spectrum of indications for MRI examination of the shoulder includes pathology related to the rotator cuff tendons, biceps tendon, articular cartilage, glenoid labrum, and the glenohumeral joint capsule, including the glenohumeral ligaments. As part of the preimaging assessment, many institutions ask the patients to fill out a questionnaire (Box 104.1). This clinical information can facilitate focused and relevant reporting and assists the interpreting radiologist in relating the observed findings to the appropriate clinical context.

Indications for Imaging and Protocols for Magnetic Resonance Imaging and Magnetic Resonance Arthrography

Indications for Magnetic Resonance Imaging

Acute shoulder injury

- Radiographically occult fractures and osseous contusions
- Traumatic tendon and muscle tears/strains
- Acute ligamentous injury to the AC and coracoclavicular ligaments
- Assessment of traumatic joint effusion/hemarthrosis

Overuse injuries

- Tendinosis and tendon tears, with assessment of rotator cuff muscle bulk
- Glenoid labral tears
- Shoulder impingement syndromes
- Long head of biceps tenosynovitis, tendon tear, and subluxation/dislocation
- OA, including assessment of cartilage integrity and presence of intraarticular bodies
- Subacromial-subdeltoid bursitis

Miscellaneous conditions

- Nerve entrapment, including denervation changes in muscle
- Inflammatory arthritis, including assessment of synovitis and effusion
- Septic arthritis and osteomyelitis
- ON

- Diagnosis, staging, and follow-up of soft tissue or osseous tumors

Imaging Technique and Protocol

- Arm imaged at patient's side, palm up
- Shoulder-specific coil allows for higher image signal-to-noise ratio (SNR) and resolution.
- A saturation band may be placed along the medial boundary of the imaging volume to decrease effects of motion from the thoracic cavity.
- Image planes
  - *Axial:* Prescribe axial images off coronal plane, parallel to the glenohumeral joint and perpendicular to humeral shaft; cover from AC joint through proximal humeral shaft
  - *Coronal oblique:* Prescribe coronal images off axial images, parallel to the supraspinatus muscle/tendon; cover all rotator cuff muscles and tendons.
  - *Sagittal oblique:* Prescribe sagittal imaging plane off axial images parallel to bony glenoid (perpendicular to coronal plane); cover from mid supraspinatus muscle through deltoid muscle.
- Fluid-sensitive (T2W and PDW with fat suppression [FS]) sequences to highlight pathology (often acquired in all 3 planes)
- T1W images to delineate anatomic structures and assess for fatty atrophy of the rotator cuff muscle bellies (oblique sagittal plane usually most helpful)

Best Imaging Plane by Anatomic Structure

- Supraspinatus = coronal oblique, sagittal oblique
- Infraspinatus = coronal oblique, sagittal oblique
- Subscapularis = axial, sagittal oblique
- Long head of the biceps tendon (LHBT) = axial, sagittal oblique
- Acromion/AC joint = coronal oblique, sagittal oblique
- Os acromiale = axial
- Glenoid labrum = coronal oblique (superior), axial and abduction and external rotation (ABER) (anterior and inferior)

Indications for Magnetic Resonance Arthrography

Refer to Box 104.2.

Assessment and characterization of labral tears

- Assessment of hyaline articular cartilage

Box 104.1 Preimaging Questionnaire

- Current symptoms
- Prior diagnoses
- Traumatic events
- Prior surgical procedures
- Pacemaker or other implant

- Evaluation of glenohumeral joint instability, including assessment of the joint capsule and intrinsic capsular ligaments
- Postoperative rotator cuff for reinjury

Imaging Technique and Protocol

The glenohumeral joint injection technique is described in detail in Chapter 98, "Shoulder Arthrography."

Imaging Protocol

- T1W sequences with FS performed in at least 2 orthogonal planes
- Include at least 1 fluid-sensitive sequence with FS to assess for bursal side tendon tears, tendinosis, bursitis, paralabral cyst, BME, and soft tissue injury.
- Include at least one T1W sequence without FS to assess the bone marrow and for degree of fatty atrophy.
- GRE sequence can be helpful to optimize cartilage assessment.
- ABER view assists in visualization of the anteroinferior labrum and inferior glenohumeral ligament (IGHL).

Rotator Cuff—Normal Anatomy

The rotator cuff, responsible for much of the dynamic motion and stability of the shoulder joint, consists of 4 muscles: the supraspinatus, infraspinatus, teres minor, and subscapularis (Figures 104.1 through 104.3)). Distally, the tendons of the supraspinatus, infraspinatus, and teres minor muscles fuse to form a supportive cuff around the superior and posterior aspects of the glenohumeral joint (Figure 104.4), hence the name *rotator cuff*.

The subacromial-subdeltoid bursa is a potential space and can become one of the largest bursae of the entire body when distended with fluid. As the name suggests, it is located deep to the acromion process and deltoid muscle and superficial to the underlying rotator cuff tendons and musculature. The glenohumeral joint capsule lies immediately caudal to the articular surface of the tendon.

Box 104.2 Indications for MRA

- Articular surface rotator cuff injury
- Full-thickness rotator cuff injury
- Labral pathology in a young patient (eg, younger than 40 years)
- Cartilage evaluation
- Rotator interval pathology

The subscapularis tendon does not fuse with the rest of the rotator cuff tendons; instead it courses along the anterior aspect of the shoulder joint, attaching to the lesser tuberosity of the humerus (Figure 104.4A). The space between the subscapularis and the supraspinatus tendons is called the *anterior rotator interval* and contains the LHBT, coracohumeral (CHL), and superior glenohumeral (SGHL) ligament complex.

The supraspinatus muscle, as the name indicates, originates superior to the dorsal spine of the scapula, and its fibers course laterally and horizontally, primarily toward the superior (horizontal) facet of the greater tuberosity of the humeral head. The superior (horizontal), middle (oblique), and posterior (vertical) facets of the greater tuberosity are best appreciated in the sagittal oblique plane and can be identified in most shoulders. The myotendinous junction of the supraspinatus is typically centered along the course of a vertical line drawn through the medial humeral head and acromial center, passing directly inferior to the AC joint. The supraspinatus tendon inserts on the superior facet of the greater tuberosity of the humerus, immediately lateral to the lateral boundary of the joint capsule (Figure 104.4A). Some anterior supraspinatus tendon fibers extend to the bicipital groove.

The infraspinatus muscle, as its name suggests, originates inferior to the dorsal spine of the scapula. Its fibers course laterally to insert primarily on the middle facet of the greater tuberosity (Figure 104.4A). The anterior-superior fibers of the infraspinatus tendon converge with the posterior inferior supraspinatus tendon fibers, called *junctional fibers*. At this overlap, infraspinatus tenon fibers are superficial to the supraspinatus fibers and closely adherent. Anatomic studies describe the surface area of the supraspinatus and infraspinatus tendon insertion, known as the *rotator cuff footprint*. The anteroposterior dimension of the footprint measures approximately 25 mm and the medial-lateral dimension measures approximately 14 mm.

The teres minor muscle arises from the inferior aspect of the posterior scapula, immediately caudal to the infraspinatus muscle and courses laterally to insert onto the posterior facet of the greater tuberosity of the humerus (Figure 104.4A). The teres minor tendon is very short, often not discretely identified, and almost never involved in rotator cuff tears. The teres minor muscle is notable for forming the cephalic boundary of the quadrilateral space (the space between the teres minor, teres major, long head of triceps, and medial border of humerus), through which the axillary nerve and superior circumflex humeral vessels pass.

The subscapularis muscle originates from the anterior aspect of the scapula in the subscapular fossa and courses laterally to insert onto the lesser tuberosity. Some of the superficial subscapularis tendon fibers extend over the bicipital groove along the anteromedial aspect of the proximal humeral shaft, forming the *transverse humeral ligament*, and serve as one of the anterior stabilizers for the LHBT as it passes through the bicipital groove. The deep fibers of the subscapularis tendon blend with the middle glenohumeral ligament (MGHL) and anterior joint capsule. Normal rotator cuff muscles and tendons are shown in Figures 104.1 through 104.4.

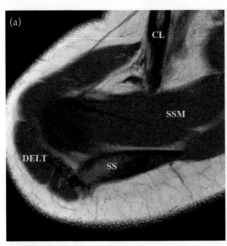
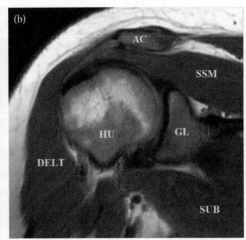

Figure 104.1. Normal supraspinatus. Normal supraspinatus muscle and tendon depicted on T1W images in the axial (*A*) and coronal oblique planes (*B*). SSM = supraspinatus muscle; CL = clavicle; DELT = deltoid; SS = scapular spine; AC = acromion; HU = humerus; GL = glenoid; SUB = subscapularis muscle.

Coracoacromial Arch

The coracoacromial arch is a protective osteo-ligamentous structure, which overlies the head of the humerus, preventing its upward displacement from the glenoid fossa. It is formed by the smooth inferior aspect of the acromion and the coracoid process of the scapula with the coracoacromial ligament spanning between them. The subacromial-subdeltoid bursa, supraspinatus tendon, and the LHBT are located within the coracoacromial arch. Several anatomic variations in acromial morphology and configuration have been implicated as factors that may predispose to impingement and, over time, rotator cuff injury. Many of these morphological considerations are

developmental, such as an os acromiale or lateral downsloping of the acromion, and some are acquired, such as subacromial spurs or degenerative disease of the AC joint.

- Three acromial morphologic types (best identified on sagittal oblique plane) (see Table 104.1 for the Bigliani classification) (Figure 104.5)
  - Type 1: Flat undersurface
  - Type 2: Curved undersurface, paralleling the contour of the humeral head
  - Type 3: Curved undersurface with prominent anterior hook
  - An additional subsequently described type 4 acromial morphology is noted when there is a convex undersurface near its distal end.

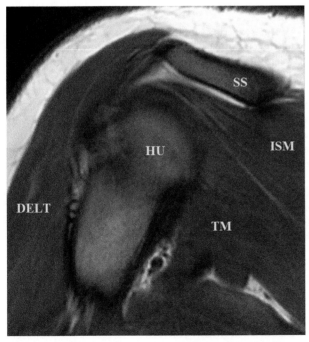

Figure 104.2. Normal infraspinatus and teres minor muscles and tendons depicted on a coronal oblique T1W image. DELT= deltoid; HU = humerus; ISM = infraspinatus muscle; SS = scapular spine; TM = teres minor muscle.

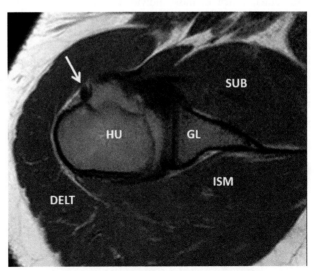

Figure 104.3. Normal subscapularis muscle depicted on an axial T1W image. Normal LHBT is seen within its groove (*arrow*) just lateral to the subscapularis tendon insertion. DELT= deltoid; GL = glenoid; HU = humerus; ISM = infraspinatus muscle; SUB = subscapularis muscle.

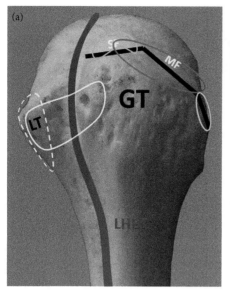 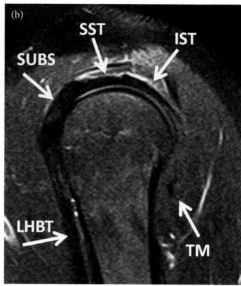

Figure 104.4. Rotator cuff tendon attachment sites from anterolateral perspective. (*A*) Drawing shows attachment sites of the supraspinatus tendon at the greater tuberosity superior facet (*blue crescent*), infraspinatus tendon (*red oval*) at the superior (SF) and middle (MF) facets, teres minor tendon at the posterior facet (*green oval*), and subscapularis tendon, which attaches primarily at the medial aspect of the lesser tuberosity (*dashed yellow outline*). LHBT course through the intertubercular groove is depicted by a *purple line*. Superficial subscapularis tendon fibers extend over the bicipital groove and attach onto the greater tuberosity (*yellow outline*). (*B*) Sagittal oblique T2W FS MR image shows normal low signal intensity rotator cuff tendons about the humeral head. SST = supraspinatus tendon; IST = infraspinatus tendon; TM = teres minor; SUBS = subscapularis tendon; and LHBT = long head of the biceps tendon.

- Acromial position (best identified on coronal oblique plane) (Figure 104.6)
  - Variable angulation of the lateral portion, which may be relatively flat, or may demonstrate a degree of lateral downsloping (>15 degrees is considered significant)
  - Variable relationship to the clavicle, with possible caudal offset

Development of the acromion occurs through an ossification center, which in most individuals, fuses with the remainder of the scapula. Although there is a wide age range over which this fusion can occur, it is unlikely to occur after age 25 years. Therefore, an unfused acromial apophysis in an individual older than 25 years is diagnostic of an *os acromiale*, a nonfused developmental variant. The lack of a true osseous connection between this ossicle and the scapula predisposes to hypermobility at this junction, which can be symptomatic and promotes degenerative change (as evidenced by sclerosis

at the junction) that may narrow the outlet space occupied by the supraspinatus tendon (Figure 104.7).

Rotator Cuff Impingement

Rotator cuff impingement is typically categorized into 2 main varieties: extrinsic, (subacromial and subcoracoid) and intrinsic.

Primary extrinsic impingement has been the most studied and is the best understood. It refers to narrowing of the space between the bursal surface of the supraspinatus muscle and the overlying coracoacromial arch.

Secondary extrinsic impingement is characterized by narrowing of the space between the humeral head and acromion during motion, caused by an underlying instability of the glenohumeral joint. This phenomenon is most commonly seen in patients who participate in sports that demand repetitive overhand throwing.

Intrinsic impingement is characterized by increased friction between the glenoid-labrum complex and undersurface of the rotator cuff tendons. Overhand athletes are predisposed to this type of impingement pathology, the concept of which has gained more attention in recent years.

Regardless of etiology, MRI is able to identify the anatomic features frequently associated with rotator cuff impingement with high reliability.

Subacromial Impingement

- Developmental factors
  - Anterior acromial "hook" (Bigliani type 3)

Table 104.1. Bigliani Classification of Acromial Morphology		
TYPE	DEFINING MORPHOLOGY	CONTRIBUTES TO IMPINGEMENT?
1	Flat undersurface	No
2	Concave undersurface	No
3	Anterior hook	Yes

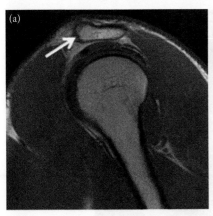
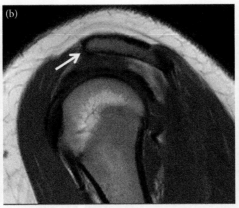
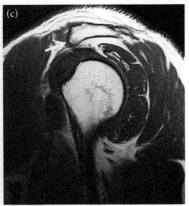

Figure 104.5. Bigliani classification of acromial morphology. Sagittal oblique T1W MR images demonstrate a flat type 1 (*arrow*) acromion (*A*), a curved type 2 (*arrow*) acromion (*B*), and an anteriorly hooked type 3 (*arrow*) acromion (*C*).

- Lateral acromial downsloping (>15 degrees) (Figure 104.6*B, C*)
- Caudal offset of the acromion relative to the clavicle
- Acquired factors
  - AC joint degenerative changes with inferior articular surface osteophytosis
  - Degenerative changes at synchondrosis of os acromiale (if present)
- Can result in injury (tendinosis or eventual tear) of the supraspinatus tendon (Figure 104.8)
- Best imaging planes = coronal oblique, sagittal oblique

Subcoracoid Impingement
- Narrowing of the space between the lateral margin of the coracoid process relative to the lesser tuberosity/medial humeral head
  - Normal coracohumeral distance is 10 mm or greater.

- Narrow interval (<10 mm) may predispose to injury of the subscapularis tendon (tendinosis or tear).
- Best imaging plane = axial

Internal shoulder impingements are divided into 2 major types: posterosuperior and anterosuperior.

Posterosuperior Internal Impingement
- Frequent in throwing athletes
- May cause tear of the posterosuperior labrum and associated undersurface rotator cuff tendon tear with typical involvement of the posterior distal supraspinatus and anterior distal infraspinatus tendon fibers

Anterosuperior Internal Impingement
- Repetitive forceful shoulder adduction and internal rotation above the horizontal plane lead to friction damage

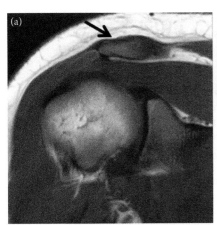
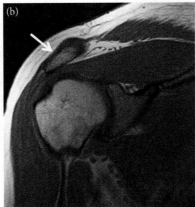
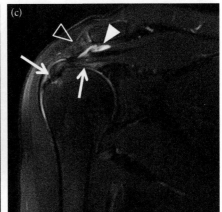

Figure 104.6. Acromial downsloping. (*A*) Coronal oblique T1W MR image demonstrates an acromion without lateral downsloping (*arrow*). (*B*) Coronal oblique T2W FS MR image shows an acromion with significant (>15 degrees) lateral downsloping (*arrow*). (*C*) Coronal oblique T2W FS MR image shows downsloping of the acromion (*open arrowhead*) causing subacromial impingement. Note heterogeneously increased signal and mild thickening of the supraspinatus tendon (*arrows*) consistent with severe tendinosis. There is predominantly bursal surface low-grade partial-thickness tearing of the supraspinatus tendon with associated thickening of the subacromial-subdeltoid bursa consistent with bursitis (*white arrowhead*).

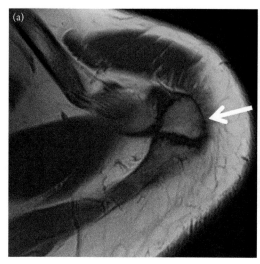
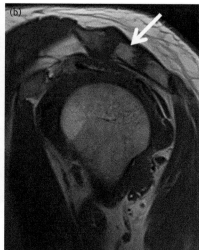

Figure 104.7. Os acromiale. Axial (*A*) and sagittal oblique (*B*) T1W MR images demonstrate an unfused acromial ossification center in a 50-year-old patient consistent with an os acromiale (*arrows*).

as the undersurface of the biceps pulley system impinges against the anterior-superior glenoid rim.
- Manifests clinically in overhead-throwing athletes, as a weakness with horizontal adduction and internal rotation of the shoulder, as well as anterior shoulder pain during the follow-through phase of throwing
- Associated with biceps pulley lesion and instability of the LHBT, medial subluxation of the LHBT and biceps tendinopathy, and articular surface supraspinatus and subscapularis tears

Rotator Cuff Pathology

Rotator cuff pathology includes tendinosis/tendinopathy (Figure 104.9) and tears (partial and full thickness). Rotator

cuff tears are most commonly degenerative in etiology, related to impingement and overuse injuries, and are rarely associated with acute traumatic events.

The most commonly affected tendon is the supraspinatus. The tear usually starts anteriorly involving the anterior most fibers of the supraspinatus, within 1 cm of its greater tuberosity insertion site, and can extend posteriorly to involve the infraspinatus tendon.

Rotator Cuff Tendinosis

Rotator cuff tendinosis is characterized as mechanical degeneration of tendon fibers. Because no inflammation is generally noted, the term *tendinitis* is usually erroneous and avoided. It can also result from attrition, which represents gradual degeneration with wear and tear of the tendon.

- On MRI, tendinosis appears as tendon thickening with increased signal on fluid-sensitive sequences (Figure 104.9).
- Attritional tendinosis is manifested as tendon thinning.
- Treatment is conservative, often involving physical therapy.
- Can progress to tendon tearing

Rotator Cuff Tears

Rotator cuff tear represents disruption of tendon fibers following progressive mechanical degeneration or trauma. Figure 104.10 shows the common types of rotator cuff tears that are described in this chapter.

- On MRI, tears appear as fluid-signal cleft within the tendon substance.
- Partial-thickness tears are classified arthroscopically based on the thickness of the tendon measured from the bursal to the articular surface of the involved tendon (Table 104.2).

Articular Surface Tears

Refer to Figures 104.11.

Figure 104.8. Advanced AC joint degenerative change. Coronal oblique T2W FS MR image reveals high signal within the adjacent articular clavicle (*arrow*) and acromion (*dashed arrow*) consistent with BME. Inferior osteophytes have likely contributed to supraspinatus tendinosis (*arrowhead*).

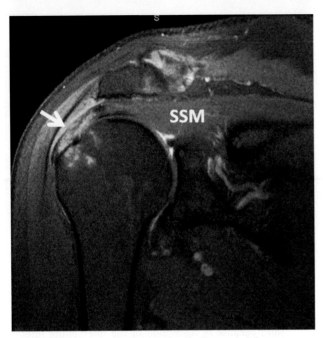

Figure 104.9. Supraspinatus tendinosis. Coronal oblique T2W FS MR image demonstrates high signal within the distal supraspinatus tendon consistent with tendinosis (*arrow*). BME is seen within the adjacent portion of the humeral head. SSM = supraspinatus muscle.

- Commonly originate at the tendon footprint (distal attachment site)
- Rim rent tear (a.k.a. partial articular surface tendon avulsion [PASTA]): a type of partial-thickness rotator cuff tear that involves the articular surface of the

supraspinatus footprint at the greater tuberosity attachment site; relatively common and also may involve the infraspinatus tendon

- Delamination partial-thickness rotator cuff tears are recognized as fluid-signal defects that parallel the long axis of the tendon and typically occur between the superficial and deep layers of the tendon. They may remain entirely within the tendon substance or communicate with 1 of the cuff surfaces. Delamination tears frequently originate from the distal articular surface. They may extend over great distances and be associated with intramuscular (myotendinous) cysts.
- Overall sensitivity of diagnosing subtle articular surface partial-thickness tears is suboptimal in routine MRI (Box 104.3). However, these are often considered nonsurgical.
- MRA can better characterize these tears.

Bursal Surface Tears
Refer to Figure 104.14.

- Commonly thought to be caused by subacromial impingement and AC joint degenerative change
- Some patients are more prone because of genetically determined body mechanics, hence these can be bilateral.
- Associated with distention/thickening of the subacromial-subdeltoid bursa
- Detection not improved with MRA

Intrasubstance Tears
Tears within the substance of the supraspinatus and/ or infraspinatus tendons that do not extend to either the

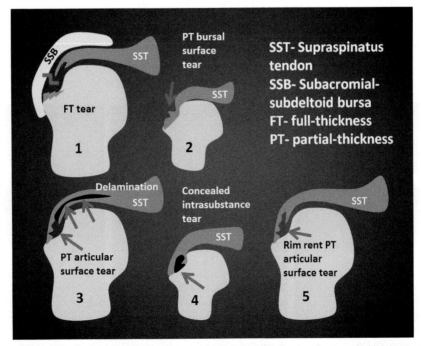

Figure 104.10. Drawings of common types of rotor cuff tears. 1, full-thickness; 2, bursal surface partial-thickness; 3, articular surface partial-thickness (note longitudinal intratendinous extension consistent with delamination); 4, intrasubstance concealed tear without extension to articular or bursal surface; 5, rim rent partial-thickness articular surface tear with extension into the footprint.

Table 104.2. Grading of Partial-Thickness Supraspinatus Tears		
GRADE	PERCENTAGE OF TENDON HEIGHT INVOLVED	THICKNESS (MM)
1	<25	<3
2	25-50	3-6
3	>50	>6

Box 104.3 Sample Routine MRI and MRA sequences

- Routine MRI
  - Axial PDW FS
  - Oblique coronal T2W FS
  - Oblique sagittal T2W FS
  - Oblique sagittal T1W NFS
- MRA
  - Axial T1W FS
  - Oblique coronal T1W FS
  - Oblique sagittal T1W FS
  - ABER T1W FS
  - Oblique coronal T2W FS
  - Axial water-sensitive sequence (WATS)—3D GRE
  - Sagittal T1W NFS

articular or bursal surface are referred to as *intrasubstance (concealed) tears*.

- Characterized by high T2 fluid signal within the fibers that do not communicate with the glenohumeral joint or subacromial-subdeltoid bursa
- Can be subtle on imaging and are also difficult to visualize at arthroscopy
- MRA typically does not improve visualization of intrasubstance tears because of lack of continuity with the joint space.

Full-Thickness Tears
Refer to Figures 104.15 and 104.16.

- Can be of any size, shape, and magnitude causing a direct communication between the glenohumeral joint and the subacromial-subdeltoid bursa
- Full-thickness tears can be quantified based on the width of the involved tendon, as measured on the sagittal oblique image (Table 104.3), which is essentially the degree of propagation in the direction perpendicular to the tendon fiber trajectory.
- Larger tears may be associated with retraction of the torn fibers and can lead to rotator muscle atrophy and/or fatty infiltration over time.

- *High-riding humerus* (acromiohumeral interval <7 mm) and *geyser sign* (cyst extending superiorly from the AC joint, from fluid communicating with glenohumeral joint because of disruption of the intervening inferior AC joint capsule and longstanding full-thickness rotator cuff tear or rotator interval injury) are associated signs.
- Size of the tear and degree of fatty atrophy are important predictors of surgical outcome (Figures 104.17 and 104.18) (Table 104.4)
- Massive rotator cuff tear: greater than 5-cm tear dimension
  - Full-thickness involvement of multiple tendons or 2 or more tendons in the European classification

Glenoid Labrum—Normal Anatomy and Pathology

Normal Anatomy
The glenoid labrum is a rim of tough fibrocartilaginous tissue that lines the peripheral aspect of the glenoid

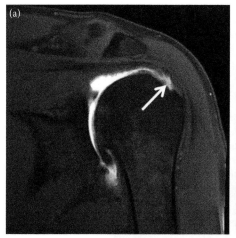
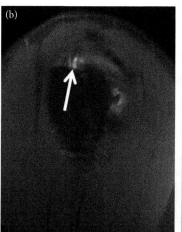
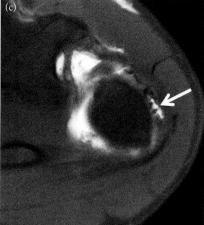

Figure 104.11. Rim rent tear. (*A*) Coronal oblique, (*B*) sagittal oblique, and (*C*) axial T1W MRA images of the shoulder in a patient with OA show a small partial-thickness tear involving the articular surface of the distal supraspinatus tendon insinuating into the footprint, often called a rim rent tear (*arrows*).

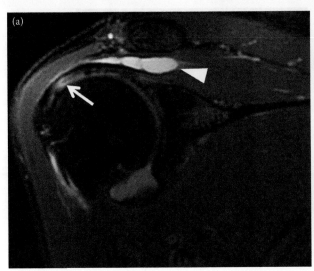
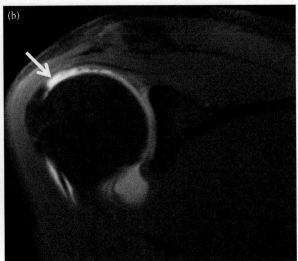

Figure 104.12. Articular surface partial-thickness supraspinatus tendon tear. (*A*) Coronal oblique T2W FS MR image and (*B*) coronal oblique T1W FS MRA image demonstrate the difference in conspicuity of a low-grade articular surface supraspinatus tendon tear (*arrow*) without and with intraarticular contrast in the same patient. In (*A*), note also the lobulated hyperintense intramuscular cyst, likely related to chronic tendon pathology and a delaminating tear (*arrowhead*).

surface, effectively deepening the glenoid fossa and leading to increased glenohumeral joint stability. The inner margin of the labrum is continuous centrally with the glenoid hyaline cartilage, which forms the articular surface for the humeral head. The labral outer margin joins with the fibrous joint capsule, which attaches to the labrum via redundant synovial folds.

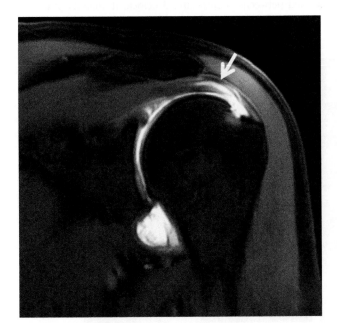

Figure 104.13. Partial-thickness articular surface supraspinatus delamination tear. T1W FS coronal oblique MRA image shows an articular surface partial-thickness tear of the supraspinatus tendon with intrasubstance contrast extending longitudinally along the tendon fibers consistent with a delamination component (*arrow*).

- On MRI, the normal glenoid labrum appears mostly as a hypointense triangular structure on all pulse sequences, with a characteristic *black* appearance (Figure 104.19).
- Slight variations in labral signal intensity are possible, particularly at the junction of the labrum with the hyaline cartilage.
- Additionally, given that the posterosuperior aspect of the labrum is near a 55-degree angle relative to the main magnetic field on the sagittal oblique images, magic angle artifact is common.
- Labral shape, although often described as triangular on axial and oblique coronal images, may normally demonstrate a more rounded contour.
- Further adding to the complexity of interpretation, there are several common normal variants of labral morphology that occur at the labral-chondral junction that can mimic a tear. Fortunately, these normal variants occur at specific locations along the glenoid rim, mostly involving the superior and anterior-superior glenoid.
- MRA improves visualization of the glenoid labrum and can greatly increase the conspicuity of both normal variants and labral tears, as contrast can freely enter these gaps within the labral tissue.

Glenoid Labral Variants

When viewed in the oblique sagittal plane, the glenoid labrum demonstrates an ellipsoid appearance and can be roughly approximated as a clock face (Figure 104.20). By convention, the most cephalad point of the labrum is labeled as 12 o'clock, and the most anterior point is labeled 3 o'clock regardless of side. Labral attachment to the underlying glenoid is not always watertight in all people, and the gaps can represent tears or normal variants. There may be a recess between the superior labrum and glenoid termed the *superior labral/sublabral recess* and a foramen between anterior-superior labrum and glenoid termed the *sublabral foramen*. These anatomic variants should

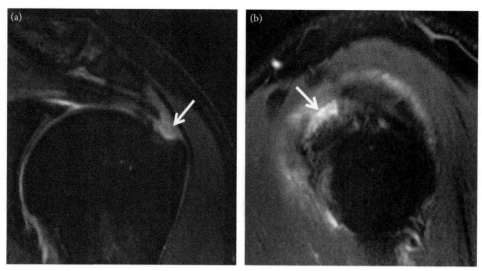

Figure 104.14. Bursal-sided partial-thickness supraspinatus tendon tear. T2W FS coronal oblique (*A*) and sagittal oblique (*B*) MR images show a fluid-signal intensity cleft (*arrows*) deep to the deltoid muscle extending into the bursal aspect of the distal supraspinatus tendon, consistent with a high-grade partial-thickness tear.

not to be confused with labral tears. The normal glenoid labrum, anatomic variants, and normal CHL and glenohumeral ligaments are shown in Figures 104.19 through 104.25.

Superior Labral/Sublabral Recess

The superior labral recess is a normal synovial recess between the labrum and glenoid between the 11 o'clock and 1 o'clock positions (Figure 104.23).

- Seen as a curvilinear focus of fluid-signal intensity on T2W imaging and routinely fills with intraarticular contrast on MRA images (Figure 104.23)

- There are a few key features that allow one to accurately distinguish a superior recess from a tear:
  - A recess follows the natural curvature of the underlying superior glenoid and does not cut into the labral substance.
  - Demonstrates smooth, regular margins and uniform width

Sublabral Foramen

An important variant, the sublabral foramen (incidence 10-20% of the population) occurs in the anterior-superior labrum, located between 1 o'clock and 3 o'clock. It consists of an intact anterosuperior labrum that does not firmly adhere to the

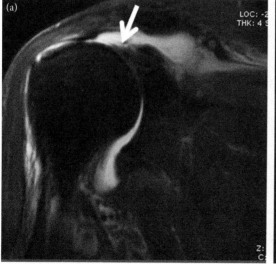
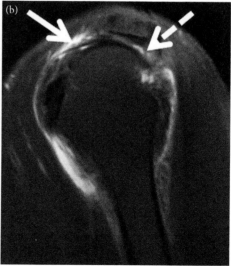

Figure 104.15. Massive full-thickness supraspinatus tendon tear. (*A*) T2W FS coronal oblique MR image shows a massive supraspinatus tendon tear with tendon retraction to the glenoid (*arrow*), allowing wide communication between the glenohumeral joint and the subacromial-subdeltoid bursa. Note proximal subluxation of the humeral head. (*B*) T2W FS sagittal oblique MR image shows a proximally migrated humeral head, pseudoarticulating with the overlying acromion. The humeral head lacks any tendon attachment (naked tuberosity sign) related to a massive rotator cuff tear with completely torn supraspinatus (*arrow*) and infraspinatus (*dashed arrow*) tendons.

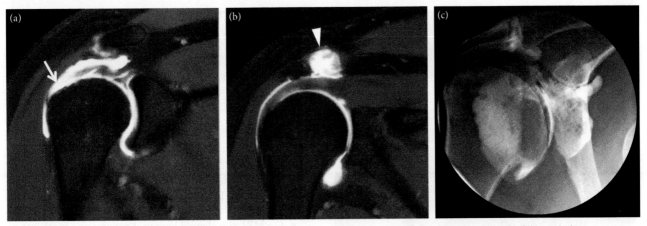

Figure 104.16. Geyser sign. Coronal oblique T1W FS MRA images reveal a chronic full-thickness tear (*arrow*) of the anterior supraspinatus tendon (*A*), and extension of glenohumeral joint contrast into the AC joint (*arrowhead*), consistent with AC joint capsular disruption (*B*). A fluoroscopic spot image obtained during contrast injection demonstrates the same finding (*C*).

Table 104.3.	Grading of Full-Thickness Rotator Cuff Tears
GRADE	**AP WIDTH OF TENDON INVOLVED (CM)**
Small	<1
Medium	1-3
Large	3-5
Massive	>5 (In the European classification, a massive tear is defined as involving 2 or more tendons.)

glenoid, leaving a foramen adjacent to the labrum. Anatomically speaking, this normal *detachment* may extend from the origin of the MGHL superiorly, to the origin of the anterior band of the IGHL inferiorly. The presence of a sublabral foramen often predicts a coexistent superior recess, as the former is more prevalent in patients possessing the latter.

- The sublabral foramen is commonly best assessed on axial images, although the contrast cleft can often be visualized on sagittal oblique images as well (Figure 104.24).

Buford Complex

In some cases, the anterosuperior labrum is not merely unattached, but entirely absent or diminutive. In these patients, there is characteristic *cordlike* thickening of the MGHL. This configuration is known as a *Buford complex*, and although less common than the sublabral foramen, may exist in up to 7% of patients.

- A Buford complex is best diagnosed on axial and sagittal oblique images, where the absence of the anterosuperior labrum and thickening of the MGHL are well visualized.

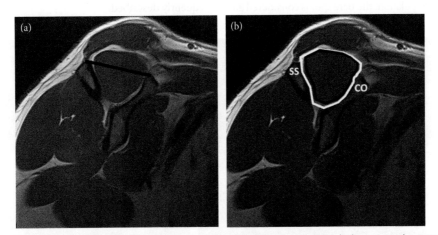

Figure 104.17. Normal supraspinatus muscle bulk. Sagittal oblique T1W MR images demonstrate a normal supraspinatus muscle as determined by a tangential line drawn from the scapular spine to the coracoid (*A*) and occupancy ratio of the supraspinatus fossa (*B*). Note also the normal muscle signal without fatty infiltration. CO = coracoid; SS = scapular spine. It is important to select the appropriate image medial to the region of the retracted tendon/myotendinous junction to avoid overcalling the degree of muscular atrophy.

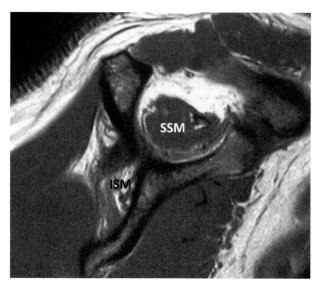

Figure 104.18. Muscular atrophy—sequela of chronic rotator cuff tear. Sagittal oblique T1W MR image in a patient with a longstanding massive rotator cuff tear involving both the supraspinatus and infraspinatus tendons reveals volume loss of these muscle bellies, with severe fatty infiltration of the infraspinatus. ISM = infraspinatus muscle; SSM = supraspinatus muscle.

MRA improves visualization of this anatomic variant (Figure 104.25).

Interestingly, although the sublabral foramen and Buford complex are considered normal variants, they may contribute to altered biomechanics and are associated with a higher incidence of superior labral tears.

Glenoid Bare Spot
A final variant, known as the *glenoid bare spot*, although not truly labral, is worth mentioning because of its frequency. The bare spot represents an area of focal cartilage thinning and is usually located near the center of the glenoid. In fact, orthopedic surgeons historically used the bare spot as a landmark for the center point of the glenoid, although this has now been shown to be less accurate than originally believed. Although common in the adult population, the bare spot is considered an

Table 104.4. Quantitative Cross-Sectional Assessment of Supraspinatus Muscle Bulk

DEGREE OF MUSCLE ATROPHY	OCCUPANCY RATIO
Normal/Mild	1.0-0.6
Moderate	0.6-0.4
Severe	<0.4

acquired finding because it is essentially absent in all children younger than age 10 years and rare in the second decade of life.

- On MRI, the glenoid bare spot appears as a focal area of cartilage thinning in the central glenoid, ranging from 2 to 9 mm in diameter, without evidence of underlying osseous irregularity or BME.

Coracohumeral Ligament
Refer to Figure 104.22.
The CHL forms a bridge between the supraspinatus and infraspinatus tendons and is anchored to the coracoid process.

- Arises from the lateral aspect of the coracoid process and divides into 2 discrete bands as it courses laterally through the anterior rotator interval
- The CHL medial band passes directly above the biceps tendon, and most fibers blend with the superior subscapularis.
- The CHL larger band continues more laterally to merge with the most superficial bursal and deep articular fibers of supraspinatus tendon.

Glenohumeral Ligaments
Refer to Figure 104.21.
The glenohumeral ligaments represent infoldings of the joint capsule and provide capsular reinforcement. Their presence is variable. Also, there are significant variations noted involving their attachments. The most common ones are subsequently described.

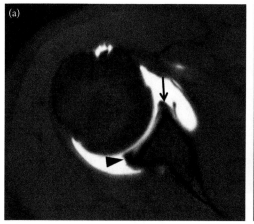
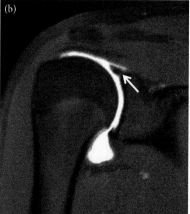

Figure 104.19. Normal glenoid labrum. (*A*) Axial T1W FS MRA image demonstrates a normal anterior labrum (*arrow*) and posterior labrum (*arrowhead*). (*B*) Coronal oblique T1W FS MRA image shows subtle intermediate signal intensity at the labral-cartilaginous junction (*arrow*), which is a normal variant.

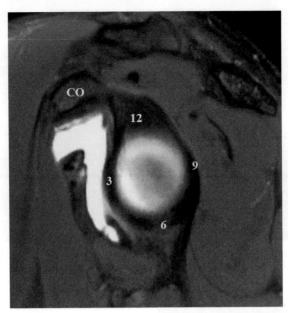

Figure 104.20. Clock face labrum. Sagittal oblique T1W FS MRA image demonstrates normal appearance of the glenoid labrum in this plane, which is analogous to a clock. 3, 6, 9, and 12 o'clock as indicated. CO = coracoid. When interpreting MRI, the 3 o'clock position is conventionally anterior, although many orthopedic surgeons use a conventional clock face in which the 3 o'clock position may be anterior or posterior depending on which side is involved. The clock face notations should be discussed with the referring orthopedic surgeons to avoid confusion on MRI reports.

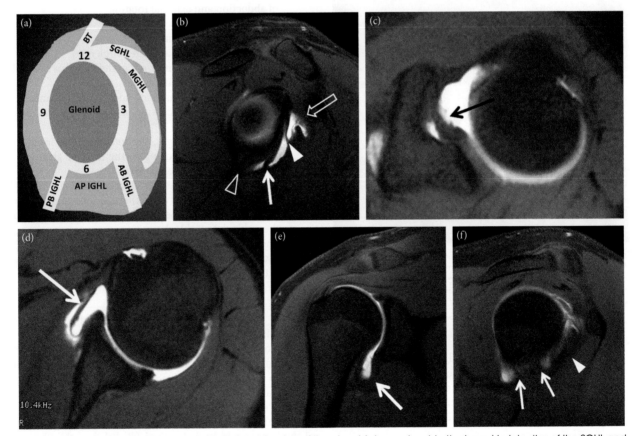

Figure 104.21. Glenohumeral ligaments. (*A*) En face drawing of the glenoid shows glenoid attachment/origin sites of the SGHL and MGHL ligaments and anterior (AB IGHL) and posterior (PB IGHL) bands of the inferior glenohumeral ligament with intervening axillary pouch (AP IGHL). Note glenolabral origin of the long head of biceps tendon (BT). 12 o'clock, midline superior; 6 o'clock, midline inferior; 3 o'clock, midline anterior; 9 o'clock, midline posterior. On T1W FS sagittal oblique MRA image (*B*), note SGHL (*open arrow*), MGHL (*arrowhead*), AB IGHL (*arrow*), and part of the PB IGHL (*open arrowhead*). Axial T1W FS MRA images show normal SGHL (*arrow*) in (*C*) and MGHL (*arrow*) in (*D*). (*E*) Coronal oblique T1W FS MRA image shows a normal AB IGHL (*arrow*) with a normal U-shaped axillary recess. (*F*) Sagittal oblique T1W FS MRA image shows portion of the normal humeral attachment of the IGHL (*arrows*). Note multipennate subscapularis tendon at the anterior aspect of the humeral head (*arrowhead*).

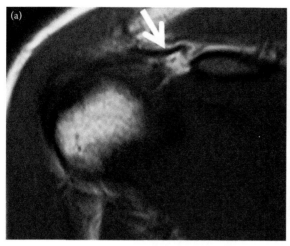 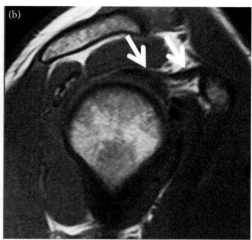

Figure 104.22. Coracohumeral ligament. (*A*) Coronal oblique and (*B*) sagittal oblique T1W MR images show a normal low signal coracohumeral ligament (*arrows*) originating from the coracoid process and extending toward the humeral head.

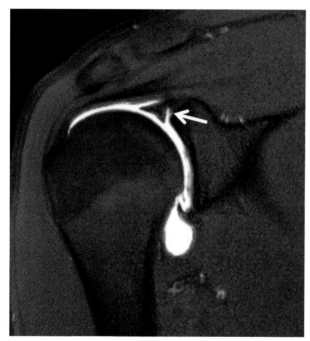

Figure 104.23. Superior labral recess. Coronal oblique T1W FS MRA image shows a thin, fluid signal, smoothly marginated cleft (*arrow*) insinuating into the superior labrum and tracking along the superior surface of the osseous glenoid, consistent with a normal variant.

Superior Glenohumeral Ligament

- The most consistently identified glenohumeral ligament arises directly anterior to the LHBT origin/biceps anchor and adjacent glenoid, passes anterior to and then beneath the proximal biceps tendon, and then courses laterally to attach onto the lesser tuberosity of the humerus.
- SGHL provides static restraint with arm at the side.
- The SGHL and CHL limit inferior translation of the adducted shoulder and posterior translation of the flexed, adducted, and internally rotated shoulder.

Middle Glenohumeral Ligament

- Originates beneath the superior glenoid tubercle and inserts on the anterior aspect of the anatomic neck of the humerus
- Can be absent in up to 27% of individuals
- MGHL provides static restraint with arm in 45 degrees of abduction and external rotation.

Inferior Glenohumeral Ligament

- Originates at the mid and inferior glenoid
- Attaches to the anatomic neck of the humerus in a collar or V-shaped configuration
- Consists of defined anterior and posterior bands, and along with the joint capsule, makes up the interposed axillary pouch
- On coronal MR images, the intact IGHL forms a U-shaped structure attaching to the inferior glenoid rim and the humeral anatomic neck.
- When viewed en face, the anterior band of the IGHL usually originates between the 2 o'clock and 4 o'clock positions, whereas the posterior band originates from the 7 o'clock to 9 o'clock positions.
- The IGHL is the primary static anterior stabilizer of the shoulder when the arm is at 90 degrees of abduction and external rotation.

Labral Tears and Glenohumeral Joint Instability

In spite of its resiliency, the glenoid labrum can be injured in the setting of chronic overuse or substantial acute trauma. Subtle changes within the labral contour with associated degenerative fraying and blunting are relatively common with advancing age and are often asymptomatic, which is why labral pathology is not commonly investigated in patients older than age 40 years. Labral tears are identified as fluid-filled clefts within the labral substance, not consistent with normal variation.

Discrete tears are best characterized on MRA. Superior labral anterior-posterior (SLAP) tears are common, often seen in throwing athletes (Figure 104.26). Anterior labral tears are

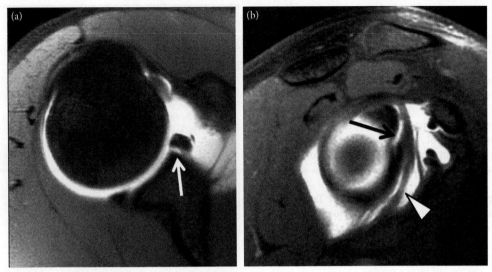

Figure 104.24. Sublabral foramen. (*A*) Axial T1W FS MRA image demonstrates a fluid-signal cleft (*arrow*) separating the glenoid from the anterosuperior labrum, which can be difficult to visualize as separate from the MGHL. (*B*) Sagittal oblique T1W FS MRA image also shows the fluid cleft (*arrow*) invaginating into the expected position of the normal anterosuperior labrum. The MGHL is now more easily visualized as a discrete structure (*arrowhead*).

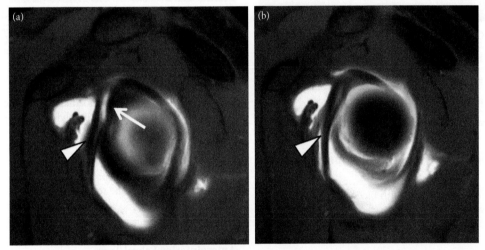

Figure 104.25. Buford complex. Two adjacent sagittal oblique T1W FS MRA images (*A,B*) reveal an absent or diminutive anterior labrum (*arrow*) and a thickened MGHL (*arrowhead*) consistent with a normal anatomic variant.

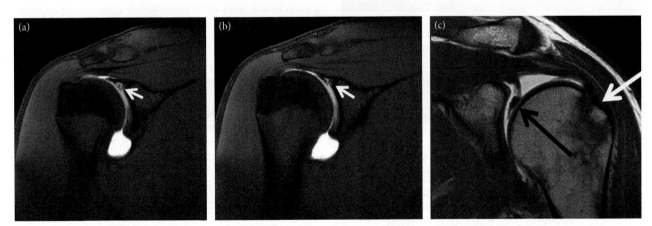

Figure 104.26. SLAP tears. Sequential coronal oblique T1W FS MRA images (*A, B*) of an 18-year-old male baseball player demonstrate contrast extending into the superior labral substance and undercutting the biceps anchor consistent with SLAP type II tear (*arrow*).
(*C*) Coronal oblique T1W MRA image in a different patient with acute trauma shows detached and laterally flipped/displaced superior labrum consistent with a SLAP type III tear (*black arrow*). Note mildly impacted nondisplaced fracture of the greater tuberosity (*white arrow*).

associated with anterior glenohumeral joint instability (Figures 104.27 through 104.33), whereas posterior labral tears are associated with posterior glenohumeral joint instability, particularly in throwing athletes (Figures 104.34 through 104.37).

Superior Labral Anterior-Posterior Tears

SLAP tears occur in overhead-throwing athletes. Snyder et al initially described 4 types, although currently, 10 types of SLAP tear have been described (Tables 104.5A and 104.5B). The most common is the SLAP type II tear (Figure 104.26*A*, *B*). SLAP tears may contribute to glenohumeral joint instability and a *catching sensation*.

Features of Superior Labral Anterior-Posterior Tears That Help Distinguish Them from Normal Superior Recesses on Magnetic Resonance Imaging and Magnetic Resonance Arthrography

- Tears have irregular margins.
- Lateral course toward biceps tendon

Table 104.5A. SLAP Tear Classification Scheme (Snyder and Morgan)

TYPE	MORPHOLOGY
I	Undersurface fraying
II A	Tear of anterosuperior labrum
II B	Tear of posterosuperior labrum
II C	Tear of both anterosuperior and posterosuperior labrum
III	Bucket handle tear without biceps anchor involvement
IV	Bucket handle tear with biceps anchor involvement

Table 104.5B. Expanded SLAP Tear Classification Scheme

TYPE	MORPHOLOGY
V	Bankart lesion (anteroinferior tear) with extension superiorly
VI	*Flap tear* with separation of the biceps tendon superiorly
VII	Extension of tear into the middle glenohumeral ligament
VIII	Tear of biceps labral complex with pronounced posterior extension (more so than type II B)
IX	Superior tear with extensive anterior and posterior extension, resulting in global abnormality and near total detachment
X	Superior labral tear with extension into the rotator interval

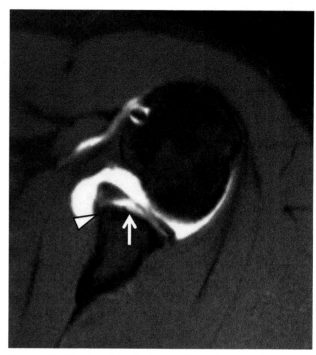

Figure 104.27. Glenolabral articular disruption (GLAD). Axial T1W FS MRA image shows contrast entering the space between the anteroinferior labrum and glenoid cartilage (*arrow*). Note that the anterior scapular periosteum (*arrowhead*) is not avulsed from the glenoid.

- Extension beyond the normal confines of the recess (11 to 1 o'clock positions), involving the posterior third of the superior labrum
- "Double Oreo cookie sign"—2 high signal intensity lines within the superior labrum at the biceps anchor. The more medial line represents a superior recess, whereas the more lateral line represents the labral tear.

Best imaging plane = coronal oblique

Anteroinferior Labral Tears

Refer to Figures 104.27 through 104.30.

Anteroinferior labral tears often occur because of anterior glenohumeral joint dislocation, which accounts for approximately 95% of all shoulder dislocations. Several variants/types have been described:

- Glenolabral articular disruption (GLAD) is defined as a superficial labral tear with injury of the adjacent articular cartilage.
  - It can be associated with pain and accelerated degenerative changes, but not instability (Figure 104.27).
- A Perthes lesion is defined as an anteroinferior labral tear with partial avulsion, but intact anterior glenoid periosteum (Figure 104.28).
  - The torn labrum could relocate to assume its normal place, but is not adherent and therefore does not provide functional stability.
  - Best imaging planes = axial, ABER
  - Because of its potential to appear normal, it is a difficult diagnosis on arthroscopy.

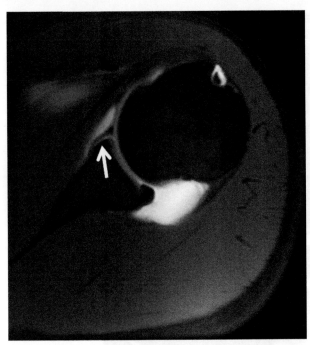

Figure 104.28. Perthes lesion. Axial T1W FS MRA image shows abnormal appearance of contrast insinuating between the anteroinferior labrum and glenoid cartilage and continuing under the anterior scapular periosteum to *lift* it away from the glenoid (*arrow*).

- Anterior labroligamentous periosteal sleeve avulsion (ALPSA) is a variant of the Perthes lesion in which the periosteum is medially displaced and *balled up*; in chronic cases, the displaced anteroinferior labrum is medialized relative to the glenoid rim (Figure 104.29).
- A Bankart lesion is defined as an anterior inferior labral tear with complete disruption of the anterior scapular periosteum, resulting in formation of a loose labroligamentous fragment (Figure 104.30).
  - Can be associated with an anterior inferior glenoid fracture (osseous/*bony* Bankart) (Figure 104.30*C, D*). With significant bone loss, the normal pear-shaped glenoid seen en face acquires an inverted pear-shaped configuration.

- Substantial glenoid bone loss (involving >25% of the glenoid surface) may require osseous augmentation such as the Bristow-Latarjet procedure to prevent chronic instability and recurrent dislocation.
- A glenoid labrum ovoid mass (GLOM) lesion comprises the detached anteroinferior labrum and associated scarring/fibrosis at the level of the inferior glenoid.

Additional Injuries Related to Anterior Glenohumeral Joint Dislocation

When the humeral head translates anteriorly and inferiorly relative to the glenoid, an impaction injury to the posterior superolateral humeral head against the anterior inferior glenoid during reduction may result in a Hill-Sachs fracture of the humeral head (Figure 104.31) and Bankart fracture of the anterior inferior glenoid.

Imaging Pearls for Hill-Sachs Fracture
- Measure depth and width on axial series; more than 15% bone loss may warrant bone augmentation such as remplissage procedure.
- On the axial series, the defect must be seen in the posterior superior humeral head at or above the level of the coracoid process.
- Seen at the 3 most superior axial slices where the humeral head is visible (when progressing in a caudal direction)
- Posterior aspect of the humeral head becomes relatively flat at and below the coracoid (a pitfall, not to be diagnosed as Hill-Sachs lesion).
- In acute injuries, Hill-Sachs lesions usually demonstrate BME on fluid-sensitive sequences. However, this may resolve in chronic injuries.

Engaging Dislocation and Glenoid Track
In addition to the amount of glenoid bone loss, the size of Hill-Sachs lesions when determining the treatment of recurrent anterior shoulder dislocation has more recently received attention. In the ABER position, as the humeral head glides over the glenoid, it contacts 83% of the anterior glenoid surface, referred to as the *glenoid track*. The glenoid track can be measured in the anteroposterior dimension on the sagittal MR

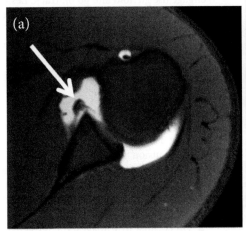
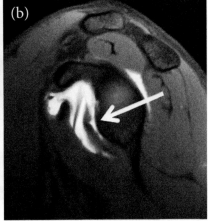

Figure 104.29. ALPSA lesion. Axial (*A*) and sagittal oblique (*B*) T1W FS MRA images reveal an anteriorly and medially displaced anteroinferior labrum (*arrows*). In (*A*), the anterior scapular periosteum is lifted away from the glenoid but not discontinuous.

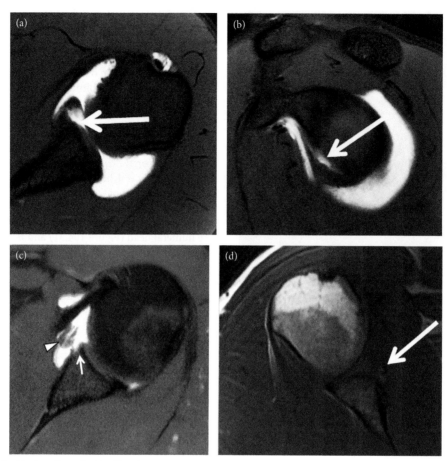

Figure 104.30. Bankart lesions in patients with prior anterior shoulder dislocation. (*A*) Axial and (*B*) sagittal oblique T1W FS MRA images show complete detachment of the anteroinferior labrum consistent with a cartilaginous Bankart lesion (*arrows*). (*C*) Axial T1W FS MRA image in a different patient shows complete disruption of the anteroinferior labrum and anterior scapular periosteum, as well as frank fracture of the underlying glenoid (*arrow*) consistent with a bony Bankart. An irregularly shaped intermediate signal intensity structure just deep to the subscapularis muscle is consistent with displaced labral tissue (*arrowhead*). (*D*) Axial T1W MR image in another patient shows a displaced, high T1 signal bone fragment (bony Bankart lesion) arising from the anterior inferior glenoid (*arrow*).

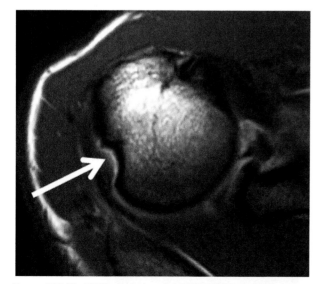

Figure 104.31. Hill-Sachs lesion. Axial T1W MRA image in a patient with history of anterior shoulder dislocation shows an impaction fracture at the posterosuperolateral aspect of the humeral head consistent with a Hill-Sachs lesion (*arrow*).

images. In the presence of bony Bankart lesions with glenoid bone loss, the glenoid track becomes smaller and the likelihood of engaging *off-track* dislocation of the humeral head increases. Similarly, if the Hill-Sachs lesion is very large or far medial, it also makes it more likely for the Hill-Sachs lesion to engage the glenoid and go off track. Lesions are considered engaging, or off-track (Figure 104.32), if the Hill-Sachs index (measured from the most medial aspect of the Hill-Sachs lesion to the supraspinatus/infraspinatus footprint) exceeds the glenoid track. They are considered nonengaging, or on-track, if the Hill-Sachs index measures smaller than the glenoid track.

Injuries of the Inferior Glenohumeral Ligament

Stretching forces during anterior dislocation can result in humeral avulsion of the anterior band of the IGHL called an *HAGL* (which stands for humeral avulsion of the inferior glenohumeral ligament) lesion (Figure 104.33). More extensive injuries may involve the axillary pouch and the posterior band.

- On coronal MR images, the retracted IGHL is seen as a displaced, thickened, and wavy structure. This appearance is analogous to the letter J.

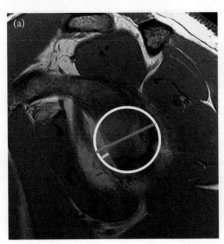
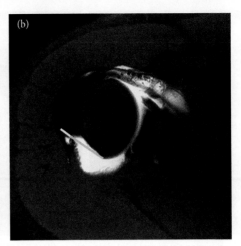

Figure 104.32. Off-track glenoid lesion in a patient with recurrent anterior glenohumeral joint dislocations. (*A*) On a sagittal oblique MRA image, draw a circle over the distal two-thirds of the glenoid (*white circle*) and measure the diameter (*red line*), 83% of which represents the estimated glenoid track. From the estimated glenoid track, subtract the amount of anterior glenoid bone loss (*green line*) to calculate the actual glenoid track [AGT: (glenoid diameter × 0.83) – anterior bone loss]. (*B*) On the axial MRA image, measure the length of the Hill-Sachs lesion (*blue line*) and add the length of the bone bridge between the lateral aspect of the Hill-Sachs lesion and the rotator cuff footprint (*yellow line*) to calculate the Hill-Sachs index (HIS). If the HIS > AGT, the Hill-Sachs lesion is characterized as an off-track lesion at risk of engagement. If the HIS < AGT, it is characterized as on-track lesion with low risk of engagement.

- MRA substantially improves detection of the HAGL lesion by demonstrating leakage of contrast material through the disrupted inferior joint capsule (Figure 104.33).
- Pitfall: Sometimes contrast may leak through the inferior joint capsule because of overdistension of the

joint capsule, which should not be mistaken for a HAGL lesion.
- Can avulse osseous fragment from its humeral attachment site (*bony* HAGL or BHAGL)
- Anterior band of the IGHL may also be avulsed at the glenoid side (called a GAGL or *glenoid avulsion of the inferior glenohumeral ligament*).
- IGHL avulsion from both the humeral and glenoid sides results in floating IGHL.
- Best imaging planes = axial, coronal oblique

Posterior Glenohumeral Joint Dislocation
Posterior translation of the humerus relative to the glenoid accounts for less than 5% of glenohumeral joint dislocations and is usually the result of convulsion, electrocution, or high-energy trauma.

- More difficult to detect clinically and can be subtle on AP radiographs
- Persistent internal rotation of humeral head even in attempted external rotation view is a clue on radiographs.
- May be associated with a reverse Hill-Sachs lesion at the anteromedial aspect of the humeral head and reverse cartilaginous (labral) or bony Bankart lesion (fracture of the posterior inferior glenoid) (Figure 104.34).

Figure 104.33. HAGL lesion. Coronal oblique T1W FS MRA image of an 18-year-old female gymnast with a history of recurrent right shoulder injuries shows a large anterior HAGL lesion with humeral avulsion of the anterior band (*arrow*) and axillary pouch (*arrowhead*) of the IGHL. Note J-shaped anterior band of the IGHL and leak of the joint contrast through the inferior joint capsule.

Posterior Labroligamentous Injuries
The posterior glenohumeral capsular complex provides posterior stability to the joint. Anatomic structures that contribute to posterior stability include the posterior capsule, posterior labrum, osseous glenoid, posterior band of the IGHL, infraspinatus, and teres minor. Tears of the posterior labrum and capsule (Figure 104.35) are less common than anterior ones and are associated with posterior and multidirectional instability. Several variants/

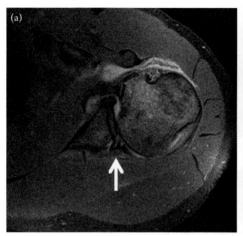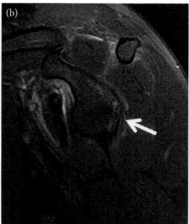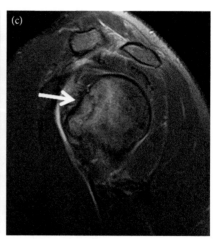

Figure 104.34. Posterior glenohumeral joint dislocation. (*A*) Axial PDW and (*B*) sagittal oblique T2W FS MR images of the shoulder show posterior subluxation of the humeral head with fractured posterior inferior glenoid consistent with a reverse bony Bankart lesion (*arrows*). In (*A*), note BME at the anterior aspect of the humeral head. (*C*) On T2W FS sagittal oblique MR image, note an impaction fracture with BME at the anteromedial aspect of the humeral head consistent with a reverse Hill-Sachs lesion (*arrow*).

types of the posterior glenoid labral tear have been described:

- Posterior labroligamentous periosteal sleeve avulsion (POLPSA) lesion is similar to ALPSA, but involves the posterior inferior labrum and is associated with posterior instability (Figure 104.36).
- Bennett lesion represents ossification (frequently linear and paralleling posterior glenoid) of the posterior band of the IGHL or the posterior joint capsule, often as a result of the posterior avulsion of the IGHL (posterior HAGL lesion). As with any calcified lesion, it is better seen on CT studies and radiographs and may represent a chronic form of POLPSA lesion.
- Axial MRA imaging in flexion, adduction, and internal rotation performed in the short axis of the proximal humerus (FADIR [flexion, adduction and internal rotation] position) may improve visualization of posterior labral tears (Figure 104.35).

Posterior Glenohumeral Joint Instability

Overhead-throwing athletes may experience alteration of normal mechanics, with tightening of posterior or posteroinferior joint capsule, which leads to posterosuperior shifting of the humeral head and decreased internal rotation, termed *glenohumeral internal rotation deficit* (GIRD) (Figure 104.37). This is often seen in baseball pitchers and occurs in the late cocking and early acceleration phases.

- GIRD is defined by the altered glenohumeral joint kinematics with posterior superior shift of the humeral head and decrease in internal rotation usually with a greater than 25-degree difference as compared to the nonthrowing shoulder.
- Posterosuperior translation of the humeral head during late cocking of the throwing arm forces the LHBT superiorly and rotates it posteriorly causing a SLAP type II posterior superior labral tear also known as *peel-back lesion*.

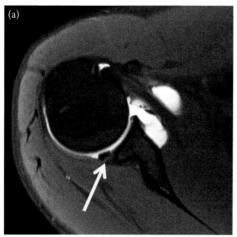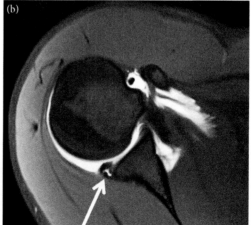

Figure 104.35. Posterior superior labral tear better depicted in FADIR projection. (*A*) Axial and (*B*) FADIR, T1W FS MRA images show posterior superior labral tear (*arrows*). This tear is better seen in (*B*) with contrast extension into the torn labrum.

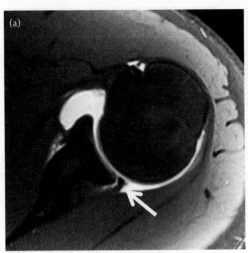
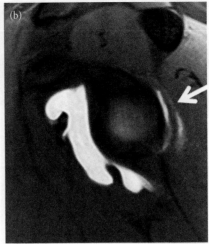

Figure 104.36. POLPSA lesion. (*A*) Axial and (*B*) sagittal oblique T1W FS MRA images in a 15-year-old boy with posterior instability reveal a torn posteriorly displaced posteroinferior labrum (*arrows*). In (*A*), the posterior scapular periosteum is lifted away from the glenoid but not frankly disrupted.

Multidirectional Instability

Mutidirectional glenohumeral joint instability is characterized by symptomatic involuntary subluxation or dislocation of the glenohumeral joint in more than 1 direction.

The etiology is multifactorial and includes:
- Congenital laxity
- Acute trauma
- Repetitive microtrauma

Anterior Rotator Cuff Interval

Normal Anatomy

The anterior rotator cuff interval is defined as the anatomic space between the anterior margin of the supraspinatus tendon and the cranial margin of the subscapularis tendon, with no overlying cuff musculature.
- Roughly encompasses the 1 o'clock to 2 o'clock positions of the glenoid labrum

- The rotator interval joint capsule is reinforced by several fibrous ligaments, including the SGHL and CHL.
- The LHBT arises from the superior glenolabral junction, and courses anterolaterally through the rotator interval to enter the bicipital groove of the humerus.
- The SGHL and CHL form a sleeve-like investment around the long head of biceps tendon, known as the *biceps pulley* (Figure 104.38).

Rotator Cable

The rotator cable is a variably present fibrous band coursing along the articular surface of supraspinatus and infraspinatus tendons, perpendicular to their fibers and continuous with the CHL anteriorly. It acts to stabilize the glenohumeral joint, especially in younger patients, and to shield the more lateral rotator cuff fibers (the crescent) from stress, especially in older patients (Figure 104.39). Its function has been likened to the cable of a suspension bridge. Rotator cuff tears

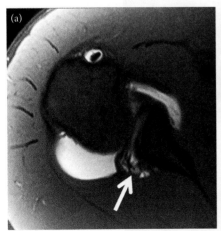
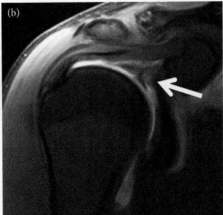
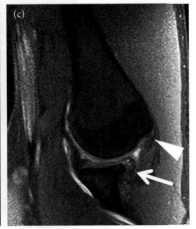

Figure 104.37. Posterior glenohumeral joint instability. (*A*) Axial, (*B*) coronal oblique, and (*C*) ABER T1W FS MRA images of the shoulder in a 20-year-old male diver with chronic right shoulder pain and posterior instability show posterior superior and superior labral tear with associated paralabral cyst (*arrows*). In (*C*), note posterior subluxation of the humeral head (*arrowhead*).

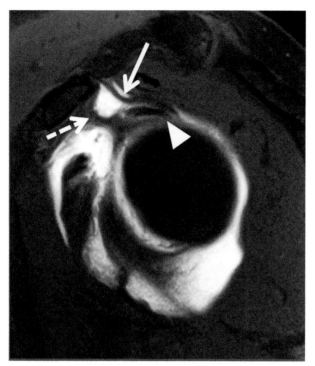

Figure 104.38. Anterior rotator interval and normal biceps pulley. Sagittal oblique T1W FS MRA image in the region of the anterior rotator interval shows the CHL (*arrow*) and SGHL (*dashed arrow*) forming a pulley about the biceps tendon (*arrowhead*).

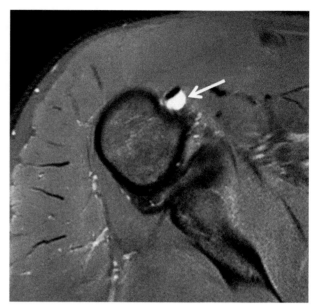

Figure 104.40. Long head of biceps tenosynovitis. PDW FS axial MR image shows an intact LHBT surrounded by fluid within the tendon sheath (*arrow*), suggestive of tenosynovitis in this patient with anterior shoulder pain and focal tenderness. This is especially true in the absence of significant associated glenohumeral joint effusion, which could also give similar appearance.

that involve the anterior or posterior cable insertion increase tension on the crescent and may increase tear size.

- Visibility of the rotator cuff cable in the non-ABER projections is suggestive of a partial-thickness articular surface supraspinatus and/or infraspinatus tendon tear.

Biceps Pulley Lesions
Acutely, the CHL and SGHL may be torn during a direct blow to the shoulder or fall onto an outstretched hand.

- Acute tears will appear as fibers disruption.
- Fibers may be displaced or balled up in the setting of a full-thickness tear.

In the chronic setting, frequent overhead movements can predispose to progressive biceps pulley injury.

- Chronic injury can be seen as either thickening or thinning of ligament fibers.
- In conjunction with subscapularis tendon tears, injuries of the pulley can predispose to LHBT subluxation/dislocation.

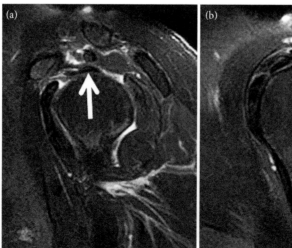
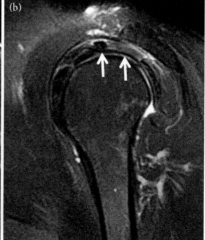

Figure 104.39. Rotator cable. Sagittal oblique T2W FS MR images (*A, B*) show a low signal band extending along the undersurface of the supraspinatus tendon consistent with rotator cable (*arrows*).

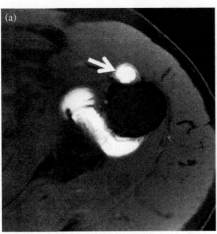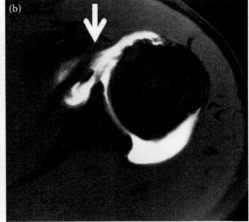

Figure 104.41. LHBT rupture and subscapularis tendon tear. (*A*) Axial T1WFS MRA image at the level of the proximal bicipital groove reveals complete LHBT tear with empty bicipital groove (*arrow*). (*B*) Additional axial T1WFS MRA image in the same patient reveals a full-thickness tear of the subscapularis tendon with retraction (*arrow*).

- Best imaging planes = axial, sagittal oblique

Intrinsic Biceps Tendon Injury
- Tendinosis—mechanical degeneration of the tendon substance, which is characterized by thickening and/or increased signal intensity on fluid-sensitive sequences
- A large amount of fluid within the biceps tendon sheath on routine MRI in the absence of a significant joint effusion raises the possibility of biceps tenosynovitis (Figure 104.40), but this can also be seen with adhesive capsulitis.
- Tear—can occur acutely but more likely as chronic progression of tendinosis
    - Partial-thickness tears tend to propagate in the longitudinal direction and appear as a fluid-filled cleft or *split* within the tendon substance.
    - Full-thickness tears result in tendon retraction and an *empty* bicipital groove on MRI (Figure 104.41).
- Best imaging planes = axial, sagittal oblique

Miscellaneous Conditions

Adhesive Capsulitis
Adhesive capsulitis is a clinical condition characterized by the gradual onset of increased shoulder pain and significantly decreased range of motion from unknown cause. This entity is associated with reactive fibrosis of the joint capsule, including the glenohumeral ligaments (IGHL involvement most notable) and rotator interval (Figure 104.42).

- On routine MRI, no abnormality may be appreciated. The most specific findings, when present, are thickening of the CHL and replacement of the normal subcoracoid fat with heterogeneous intermediate signal intensity in the rotator interval.
- Additional MRI findings associated with adhesive capsulitis include thickening/stranding and edema of the anterior rotator cuff interval and thickening of the axillary pouch joint capsule with pericapsular edema.

Calcific Tendinosis
Calcium hydroxyapatite crystal deposition is a common entity that can occur in various tendons and peritendinous locations (see Chapter 37, "Calcific Hydroxyapatite Deposition Disease"). This includes tissue deposition of basic calcium phosphate crystals, predominantly hydroxyapatite. The disease course is usually self-limiting. Intratendinous calcifications may extrude into the subacromial-subdeltoid bursa and cause calcific bursitis. They may also erode into bone and appear aggressive on MRI.

- Diagnosis of calcific tendinosis is typically made on radiographs and can be missed on MRI because both the calcium and tendon are low signal.
- MRI shows foci of low signal intensity on all sequences in the affected tendon (Figure 104.43). There may be associated variable degree of adjacent increased signal.
- GRE sequence may be helpful to detect susceptibility artifact (*blooming*) associated with calcifications.

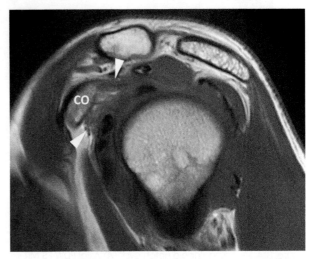

Figure 104.42. Adhesive capsulitis. Sagittal oblique T1W MR image in a patient with reduced range of motion demonstrates replacement of the normal subcoracoid fat with abnormal soft tissue stranding (*arrowheads*). CO = coracoid.

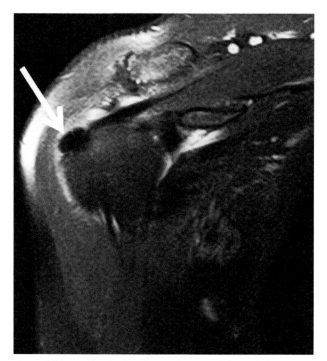

Figure 104.43. Calcific tendinosis. Coronal oblique T2W FS MR image shows a low signal intensity focus in the distal supraspinatus tendon consistent with calcific tendinosis (*arrow*). Note mild thickening of the adjacent subacromial-subdeltoid bursa in keeping with bursitis.

- With intrabursal extrusion of calcifications, MRI shows bursal calcifications, bursal thickening, and peribursal edema.
- With intraosseous extension, MRI shows erosive changes and BME, which can mimic an infectious process or tumors.

Denervation Injuries

The nerves supplying the rotator cuff arise from the brachial plexus and proceed through distinct anatomic planes. Impingement of or injury to these nerves results in specific and predictable patterns of muscle denervation seen on MRI (Table 104.6).

Normal Nerve Supply
- Suprascapular nerve
  - Derived from C5 and C6 nerve roots
  - Branches to supply the supraspinatus muscle just distal to the suprascapular notch
  - More distally, this nerve passes through the spinoglenoid notch to supply the infraspinatus muscle.
- Axillary nerve
  - Also supplied by C5 and C6 nerve roots
  - Motor supply to teres minor and deltoid and sensory cutaneous supply over the inferior deltoid.
  - Passes through the quadrilateral space (defined by the teres minor, teres major, long head of triceps, and medial cortex of the proximal humerus shaft)

Table 104.6. Muscle Denervation Patterns

NERVE(S) IMPLICATED	MUSCLE(S) INVOLVED
Suprascapular (at or proximal to suprascapular notch)	Supraspinatus, infraspinatus
Suprascapular (at spinoglenoid notch)	Infraspinatus
Axillary	Deltoid, teres minor
C5, C6	Multiple

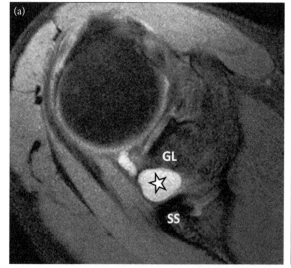
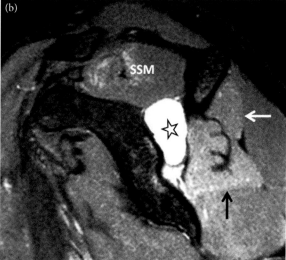

Figure 104.44. Spinoglenoid notch cyst. (*A*) Axial PDW FS MR image shows a lobulated hyperintense cystic structure (*asterisk*) in the spinoglenoid notch arising from the posterior labrum consistent with a paralabral cyst. (*B*) Sagittal oblique T2W FS MR image demonstrates increased signal within the infraspinatus muscle (*arrows*) consistent with neurogenic edema related to compressed suprascapular nerve by the ganglion cyst (*asterisk*) at the spinoglenoid notch. GL = glenoid; SS = scapular spine; SSM = supraspinatus muscle.

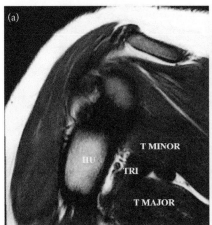 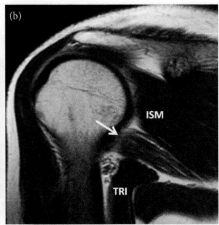 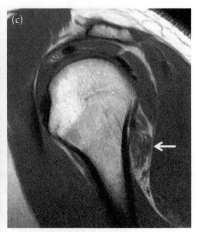

Figure 104.45. Isolated teres minor atrophy. (*A*) Coronal oblique T1W MR image demonstrates normal appearance and boundaries of the quadrilateral space. (*B*) Coronal oblique and (*C*) sagittal oblique T1W MR images in a patient with axillary neuropathy reveal isolated fatty infiltration of the teres minor muscle (*arrows*). No mass is present within the quadrilateral space. TRI = long head triceps muscle; T MINOR = teres minor muscle; T MAJOR = teres major muscle; ISM = infraspinatus muscle; HU = humerus.

Patterns of denervation (muscle edema, fatty infiltration, muscle atrophy) are based on location of nerve impingement/injury:

- Suprascapular nerve
  - Suprascapular notch → affects supraspinatus and infraspinatus
  - Spinoglenoid notch → isolated infraspinatus involvement (Figure 104.44)
- Axillary nerve
  - Quadrilateral space → isolated involvement of teres minor and posterior deltoid (Figure 104.45)
- Parsonage-Turner syndrome
  - Idiopathic denervation of rotator cuff and shoulder girdle muscles in multiple peripheral nerve distributions
  - Associated with recent viral infection, implicating inflammation of brachial plexus or autoimmune response as potential causes
  - Should exclude a more proximal brachial plexus lesion
  - Recovery is usually complete.
- MRI appearance
  - Increased muscular signal intensity on fluid-sensitive sequences compatible with edema (Figure 104.46)
  - Pattern of muscle edema does not correspond to a single peripheral nerve distribution.
  - In the chronic setting, volume loss and fatty infiltration may be present.
- Best imaging plane = sagittal oblique

Distal Clavicular Osteolysis
Distal clavicular osteolysis is considered to be sequela of repetitive microtrauma. It results in subchondral cystlike changes, BME, and resorption of the distal clavicle.

- MRI appearance

- BME (Figure 104.47) and cystlike changes in the distal clavicle often demonstrating a low signal intensity *fracture line* in acute stages
- Fluid distention of the AC joint
- Relative sparing of the acromion articular surface (in contradistinction to primary joint-related pathology)
- Over time, the distal clavicle may undergo healing, resulting in the chronic appearance of a truncated distal clavicle that has regained its distal sclerotic cortex.

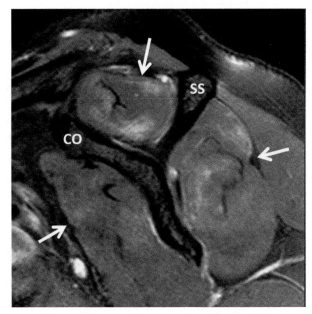

Figure 104.46. Parsonage-Turner syndrome. Sagittal oblique T2W FS MR image demonstrates patchy high signal intensity consistent with edema (*arrows*) in all of the rotator cuff muscles, consistent with a polyneuropathy. CO = coracoid; SS = scapular spine.

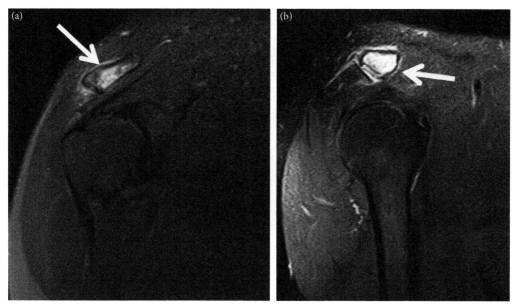

Figure 104.47. Distal clavicular osteolysis. (*A*) Coronal oblique and (*B*) sagittal oblique T2W FS MR images demonstrate marked BME in the distal clavicle (*arrows*) with sparing of the acromion.

Key Points

- *Rotator cuff tears* are common, especially in patients older than 40 years, and usually degenerative in etiology; partial-thickness tears may involve the articular or bursal surfaces or be intrasubstance. Full-thickness tears involve the entire tendon thickness, establishing a communication between the glenohumeral joint and the subacromial-subdeltoid bursa.

- It is important to describe the size of the rotator cuff tear, the amount of tendon retraction, and the degree of associated muscle atrophy, because these factors may influence surgical treatment and predict outcome.

- *Rotator cuff impingement* is typically categorized into 2 main varieties: extrinsic (subacromial and subcoracoid) and intrinsic.

- Primary extrinsic impingement refers to narrowing of the space between the supraspinatus muscle and the overlying coracoacromial arch.

- Intrinsic impingement is characterized by increased friction between the glenoid-labrum complex and undersurface of the rotator cuff tendons, which is commonly seen in overhand-throwing athletes.

- The *glenoid labrum* is a rim of tough fibrocartilaginous tissue that lines the rim of the glenoid surface, effectively deepening the glenoid fossa and leading to increased glenohumeral joint stability.

- Superior labral tears/lesions (SLAP = superior labrum anterior-posterior) are most common among overhead-throwing athletes with 10 different types recognized. SLAP type II is the most common.

- Anterior glenohumeral joint dislocation comprises 95% of all shoulder dislocations and is associated with various types of anterior labroligamentous injuries (Bankart lesion variants). There may be an associated impaction fracture at the posterior superolateral aspect of the humeral head (Hill-Sachs lesion) and a fracture of the anterior inferior glenoid (bony Bankart lesion).

- *HAGL* (humeral avulsion of the inferior glenohumeral ligament) lesion is associated with glenohumeral joint instability.

- *Posterior glenohumeral joint dislocation* accounts for less than 5% of all glenohumeral joint dislocations (often associated with a typical history of convulsions, electrocution) and is associated with various types of posterior labroligamentous injuries (reverse Bankart lesion variants). There may be an associated impaction fracture at the anteromedial aspect of the humeral head (reverse Hill-Sachs lesion) and fracture of the posterior inferior glenoid (reverse bony Bankart lesion).

- The *anterior rotator cuff interval* is located under the coracoid process, between the leading edge of the subscapularis tendon and anterior to the supraspinatus tendon and covered by the joint capsule. It contains the LHBT and the CHL and SGHL, which form the sling about the biceps tendon that is termed the *biceps pulley*. Disruption of the pulley allows abnormal movement of the biceps tendon in the anteromedial direction, which may become perched on the lesser tuberosity and indicates subluxation.

- *MRA* is the study of choice for diagnosing glenoid labral tears and also improves diagnostic accuracy in the diagnosis of partial-thickness undersurface rotator cuff tears.

- The nerves supplying the rotator cuff arise from the brachial plexus and proceed through distinct anatomic planes. Impingement of or injury to these nerves results in specific and predictable patterns of muscle denervation seen on MRI with muscular edema in the acute phase and atrophy in the chronic phase.

- *Distal clavicular osteolysis* occurs in the distal clavicle as a result of chronic stress. MRI shows BME in the distal clavicle, with possible visualization of a sclerotic fracture line. As the injury progresses, there is often progressive loss of the normal cortical margin of the distal clavicle and development of subchondral cystlike changes.

Recommended Reading

Morag Y, Jacobson JA, Miller B, De Maeseneer M, Girish G, Jamadar D. MR imaging of rotator cuff injury: what the clinician needs to know. *Radiographics*. 2006;26(4):1045–65. Review.

Jarraya M, Roemer FW, Gale HI, Landreau P, D'Hooghe P, Guermazi A. MR-arthrography and CT-arthrography in sports-related glenolabral injuries: a matched descriptive illustration. *Insights Imaging*. 2016;7(2):167–77. doi:10.1007/s13244-015-0462-5. Review.

References

1. Antonio GE, Griffith JF, Yu AB, Yung PSH, Chan KM, Ahuja AT. First-time shoulder dislocation: high prevalence of labral injury and age-related differences revealed by MR arthrography. *J Magn Reson Imaging*. 2007; 26:983–91.

2. Cothran Jr., RL, Helms C. Quadrilateral space syndrome: incidence of imaging findings in a population referred for MRI of the shoulder. *AJR Am J Roentgenol*. 2005;184(3):989–92.

3. Gustas CN, Tuite MJ. Imaging update on the glenoid labrum: variants versus tears. *Semin Musculoskelet Radiol*. 2014;18:365–73.

4. Gyftopoulos S, Yemin A, Beltran L, Babb J, Bencardino J. Engaging Hill-Sachs lesion: is there an association between this lesion and findings on MRI? *AJR Am J Roentgenol*. 2013;201(4):W633–38. doi:10.2214/AJR.12.10206.

5. Ilahi OA, Cosculluela P, Ho D. Classification of anterosuperior glenoid labrum variants and their association with shoulder pathology. *Orthopedics*. 2008;31:1–4.

6. Kassarjian A, Bencardino JT, Palmer WE. MR imaging of the rotator cuff. *Radiol Clin North Am*. 2006;44:503–23.

7. Larribe M, Laurent PE, Acid S, Aswad R, Champsaur P, Le Corroller T. Anterior shoulder instability: the role of advanced shoulder imaging in preoperative planning. *Semin Musculoskelet Radiol*. 2014;18:398–403.

8. Lin E. Magnetic resonance arthrography of superior labrum anterior-posterior lesions: a practical approach to interpretation. *Curr Probl Diagn Radiol*. 2009;38:91–97.

9. Llopis E, Montesinos P, Guedez MT, Aguilella L, Cerezal L. Normal shoulder MRI and MR arthrography: anatomy and technique. *Semin Musculoskelet Radiol*. 2015;19:212–30.

10. Modarresi S, Motamedi D, Jude CM. Superior labral anteroposterior lesions of the shoulder: part 1, anatomy and anatomic variants. *AJR Am J Roentgenol*. 2011;197:596–603.

11. Modarresi S, Motamedi D, Jude CM. Superior labral anteroposterior lesions of the shoulder: part 2, mechanisms and classification. *AJR Am J Roentgenol*. 2011;197:604–11.

12. Mellado JM, Salvadó E, Camins A, et al. Fluid collections and juxta-articular cystic lesions of the shoulder: spectrum of MRI findings. *Eur Radiol*. 2002;12:650–59.

13. Morag Y, Jacobson JA, Shields G, et al. MR arthrography of rotator interval, long head of the biceps brachii, and biceps pulley of the shoulder. *Radiology*. 2005;235:21–30.

14. Opsha O, Malik A, Baltazar R, et al. MRI of the rotator cuff and internal derangement. *Eur J Radiol*. 2008; 68:36–56.

15. Pandey T, Slaughter AJ, Reynolds KA, David RM, Hasan SA. Clinical orthopedic examination findings in the upper extremity: correlation with imaging studies and diagnostic efficacy. *Radiographics*. 2014;34:E24–40.

16. Petchprapa CN, Beltran LS, Jazrawi LM, Kwon YW, Babb JS, Recht MP. The rotator interval: a review of anatomy, function, and normal and abnormal MRI appearance. *AJR Am J Roentgenol*. 2010;195:567–76.

17. Rao AG, Kim TK, Chonopoulos E, McFarland EG. Anatomical variants in the anterosuperior aspect of the glenoid labrum: a statistical analysis of seventy-three cases. *J Bone Joint Surg Am*. 2003;85:653–59.

18. Scalf R, Wenger DE, Frick MA, Mandrekar JN, Adkins MC. MRI findings of Parsonage-Turner syndrome. *AJR Am J Roentgenol*. 2007;189:W39–44.

19. Walz DM, Burge AJ, Steinbach L. Imaging of shoulder instability. *Semin Musculoskelet Radiol*. 2015;19:254–68.

20. Woertler K. Rotator interval. *Semin Musculoskelet Radiol*. 2015;19:243–53.

21. Yablon CM, Jacobson JA. Rotator cuff and subacromial pathology. *Semin Musculoskelet Radiol*. 2015;19:231–42.

CHAPTER 105

Internal Derangements of the Elbow

Kathryn J. Stevens

Introduction

Indications for Imaging and Protocols for Magnetic Resonance Imaging and Magnetic Resonance Arthrography
Acute Elbow Injury
- Radiographically occult fractures and osseous contusions
- Apophyseal injuries or avulsions
- Acute ligamentous injuries to the medial and LCL complexes
- Tendon and muscle tears or strains

Overuse Injuries
- Osseous stress reaction and stress fractures
- Osteochondral pathology, including osteochondritis dissecans and Panner disease
- OA including the presence of joint bodies
- Tendinopathy and tendon tears
- Cubital or olecranon bursitis

Miscellaneous Conditions
- Nerve entrapments and neuropathies, including denervation changes in muscle
- Inflammatory arthritis
- Septic arthritis and osteomyelitis
- Osseous infarction
- Diagnosis, staging and follow-up of soft tissue or osseous tumors

General Magnetic Resonance Imaging Technique

Position

Prone Position
- Affected arm extended over head in so-called superman position with elbow near center of magnetic bore enabling uniform fat suppression
- Position uncomfortable and images therefore prone to motion artifact
- Pronating forearm can alleviate some of discomfort, but may distort anatomy of collateral ligaments and tendons in coronal plane.

Supine Position
- Affected arm placed at patient's side, which is more comfortable for most patients
- Elbow off-center in the magnet resulting in nonuniform fat suppression and poor SNR, thereby degrading image quality
- May be insufficient room in magnetic bore to place limb at side in obese patients

Flexed, Abducted, and Supinated Position
- Affected arm placed in the FABS (flexed, abducted, supinated) position: overhead with elbow flexed and forearm supinated to show entire distal biceps tendon under tension on 1 longitudinal image
- Occasionally useful to differentiate high-grade and complete tears of biceps tendon

Coil Choice
- Dedicated high-resolution surface coil essential to maximize SNR and obtain high-quality images
- Circumferential and cylindrical coils constructed in saddle, birdcage, or phased array configuration provide best receptive field homogeneity.
- Multichannel coils composed of 8 or more elements are required if parallel imaging techniques are used to decrease acquisition times of pulse sequences.

Protocols
- T1W and PDW images with short TE good to delineate anatomic structures
- Fluid-sensitive T2W FS or PDW FS images highlight pathology.
- Combination of T1, PDW, and T2W FS or PDW images acquired in axial, coronal oblique, and sagittal oblique imaging planes
- Imaging in the FABS position (*f*lexed elbow, *ab*ducted shoulder, and *s*upinated forearm), with the hand placed behind the patient's head can provide a more detailed view of the distal biceps tendon
- Axial images should extend from distal humeral diaphysis through the level of bicipital tuberosity of the radius.
- Coronal and sagittal images are prescribed parallel and perpendicular to transepicondylar axis of the humerus respectively.
- GRE sequences can demonstrate calcification, hemosiderin, or micrometallic artifact from prior surgical intervention.
- STIR sequences can be used if fat suppression is poor, caused by patient's arm position being off isocenter.
- IV Gd and FS T1W imaging may be used with strong clinical concern for underlying neoplastic or inflammatory

process, or to distinguish between solid and cystic lesions if imaging findings are equivocal.

Magnetic Resonance Arthrography: Indications, Technique, and Protocol
Indications
- Evaluation of articular cartilage—chondromalacia, thinning, chondral defects, or delamination
- Stability of osteochondral lesion (OCL)
- Increased visibility of joint bodies
- Improve diagnostic accuracy in detecting ligamentous tears, particularly subtle undersurface ligament tears

Technique
- T1W FS sequences in 3 orthogonal planes
- Include at least one T1W sequence without FS to evaluate bone marrow, detect muscle atrophy or fatty infiltration, and characterize soft tissue lesions.
- Include at least 1 fluid-sensitive sequence to detect soft tissue edema, BME, and fluid collections.

Normal Magnetic Resonance Imaging Anatomy

Bones
The elbow is a complex joint comprising of 3 separate bony articulations contained within a single joint cavity: The humeroulnar articulation between the trochlea of the distal humerus and deep trochlear notch of the ulna forms a hinge joint, which allows flexion and extension of the elbow; the radiocapitellar articulation between the radial head and capitellum allows a hinge and pivoting motion; and the proximal radioulnar articulation also permits a pivoting motion facilitating pronation and supination of the forearm.

Ligaments
The supporting ligamentous structures are formed by thickenings of the joint capsule both medially and laterally and are well seen on MRI. The UCL is divided into 3 main bundles or bands: anterior, posterior, and transverse (Figure 105.1). The anterior bundle is the largest and most important of the 3 components and provides the primary constraint to valgus stress. The anterior bundle is best identified on coronal MR images as a low signal intensity structure extending from the anteroinferior aspect of the medial epicondyle to the sublime tubercle of the ulna at the edge of the coronoid process, just distal to the proximal ulnar cartilage (Figure 105.2). The ligament also has a more distal insertion into a small bony ridge, called the *medial ulnar collateral ridge*, along the medial aspect of the proximal ulna. The anterior band is often mildly flared at its medial epicondylar attachment, with linear areas of higher signal caused by interspersed fat, particularly on T1W or PDW sequences with a short TE. Mildly increased signal may also be seen along the deep fibers proximally because of normal invagination of the synovium. The anterior bundle itself can be subdivided into anterior and posterior components: The anterior band is most taut in extension, whereas the posterior band is lax in extension, but becomes taut as the elbow is flexed. The posterior bundle of the UCL is a fan-shaped capsular

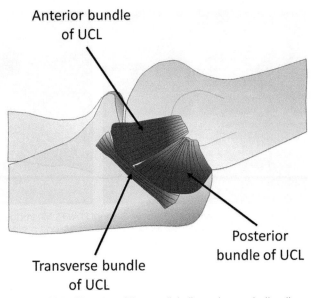

Figure 105.1. Diagram of the medial elbow demonstrating the 3 components of the UCL complex. The anterior bundle extends from the anteroinferior aspect of the medial epicondyle to the sublime tubercle of the ulna at the edge of the coronoid process, just distal to the proximal ulnar cartilage. The posterior bundle is a fan-shaped capsular thickening, arising from the inferior aspect of the medial epicondyle and inserting into the posteromedial margin of the trochlear notch, forming the floor of the cubital tunnel.

thickening, arising from the inferior aspect of the medial epicondyle and inserting into the posteromedial margin of the trochlear notch, forming the floor of the cubital tunnel. The posterior bundle acts as a secondary stabilizer of the elbow when the joint is flexed beyond 90 degrees. The thin transverse bundle bridges the ulnar attachment of the anterior and posterior bundles and does not play a significant role in elbow stability.

The LCL complex has 3 main components: the radial collateral ligament (RCL), annular ligament, and lateral ulnar collateral ligament (LUCL) (Figure 105.3). The annular ligament encircles the radial head, attaching into the margins of the sigmoid notch of the ulna and can be visualized on both coronal and axial images (Figure 105.2). The RCL arises from the lateral epicondyle and has a broad insertion into the annular ligament. The LUCL arises from the lateral epicondyle, passes behind the radial head, blends with fibers of the annular ligament, and inserts into the supinator crest of the ulna (Figure 105.2). The LUCL acts as a sling to support the radial head and provides the primary restraint to varus stress at the elbow. There may also be an accessory collateral ligament, but this is variably present.

Muscles and Tendons
Muscles and tendons around the elbow provide dynamic stability to the elbow and can be divided into anterior, posterior, medial, and lateral compartments. The anterior compartment contains the biceps brachii and brachialis muscles, which are the 2 main flexors of the elbow. Proximally, the long head of biceps brachii arises from the supraglenoid tubercle of the scapula and the short head arises from the coracoid process. The 2 heads unite to form a common tendon, which courses

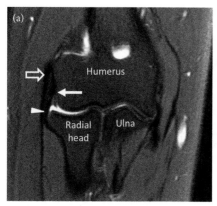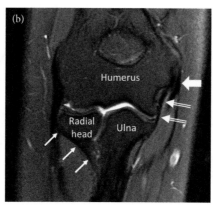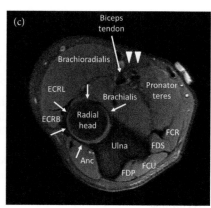

Figure 105.2. Ligaments of the elbow. Coronal PDW FS MR images of the elbow. (*A*) The RCL (*arrow*) arises from the lateral epicondyle deep to the common extensor tendon (*open arrow*), and merges with the annular ligament surrounding the radial head (*arrowhead*). (*B*) On the lateral side, the LUCL (*small arrows*) arises from lateral epicondyle, passes behind the radial head, merging with fibers of the annular ligament to insert into the supinator crest of the ulna. The anterior bundle of the UCL (*double line arrows*), courses from the medial epicondyle to the sublime tubercle of the ulna just deep to the common flexor tendon (*block arrow*). (*C*) Axial PDW FS MR image of the elbow demonstrates the annular ligament encircling the radial head (*arrows*) and attaching to the margins of the sigmoid notch of the ulna. The biceps tendon can be seen anteriorly, with a thin filamentous structure, the lacertus fibrosus (*arrowheads*) passing between the biceps tendon and pronator teres. ECRL = extensor carpi radialis longus; ECRB = extensor carpi radialis brevis; Anc = anconeus; FCR = flexor carpi radialis; FDS = flexor digitorum superficialis; FCU = flexor carpi ulnaris; FDP = flexor digitorum profundus.

through the antecubital fossa to insert onto the radial tuberosity of the proximal radius (Figures 105.4 and 105.5). The biceps tendon is best visualized on sagittal MR images (Figure 105.6). Superficial tendon fibers sweep across the antecubital fossa to blend with the fascia of the flexor-pronator mass, forming the lacertus fibrosus or bicipital aponeurosis, which is best identified on axial images (Figure 105.2). The lacertus fibrosus is usually torn in conjunction with avulsion injuries of the distal biceps tendon, but if the lacertus fibrosus remains

Radial collateral ligament

Annular ligament

Lateral ulnar collateral ligament

Figure 105.3. Diagram of the lateral elbow showing the 3 components of the LCL complex. The annular ligament encircles the radial head, attaching into the anterior and posterior margins of the sigmoid notch of the ulna. The RCL arises from the lateral epicondyle and has a broad insertion into the annular ligament. The LUCL arises from the lateral epicondyle, passes behind the radial head, blends with the fibers of the annular ligament, and inserts into the supinator crest of the ulna.

intact, it can prevent retraction of the tendon stump into the upper arm, making the diagnosis more challenging on clinical examination. Two bursae are associated with the distal biceps tendon: The bicipitoradial bursa is interposed between the distal biceps tendon and radial tuberosity, and the interosseous bursa lies between the proximal radius and ulna and may communicate with the bicipitoradial bursa (Figure 105.5). The brachialis muscle arises from the distal half of the humerus and inserts onto the ulnar tuberosity of the ulna and anterior surface of the coronoid process (Figure 105.6).

The medial flexor-pronator muscle group is formed by the pronator teres, flexor carpi radialis, palmaris longus (present in 90% of the population), flexor digitorum superficialis, flexor carpi ulnaris, and flexor digitorum profundus, arising from a common flexor tendon superficial and proximal to the UCL (Figure 105.2). Pathology within the individual muscle groups is best seen on axial imaging.

On the lateral elbow, the common extensor tendon originates from the lateral epicondyle of the humerus, superficial to the RCL, receiving contributions from the brachioradialis, extensor carpi radialis longus and brevis, extensor digitorum, extensor carpi ulnaris, and supinator (Figure 105.2).

The posterior compartmental muscles include the triceps brachii and anconeus. The triceps muscle has 3 heads arising from the infraglenoid tubercle of the scapula and proximal humerus. The long and lateral heads unite to form the triceps tendon proper, inserting into the tip of the olecranon (Figure 105.6). The contribution from the medial head lies deep to this and has a more muscular insertion into the olecranon. The medial head tendon may appear to have a separate insertion from the superficial triceps tendon on MRI, but histologically, the tendinous components are seen merging just above the distal insertion. The superficial olecranon bursa is a thin bursal space lying between the olecranon and overlying subcutaneous tissues and commonly becomes inflamed with distal triceps tendon pathology. The anconeus muscle arises

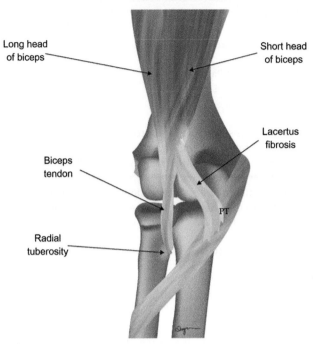

Figure 105.4. Diagram of the distal biceps tendon, which is formed by contributions from the long and short heads. The biceps tendon rotates approximately 90 degrees as it traverses the antecubital fossa to insert onto the radial tuberosity. The long head inserts proximally and the short head distally on the tuberosity, which enables supination of the forearm as well as flexion of the elbow. PT= pronator teres.

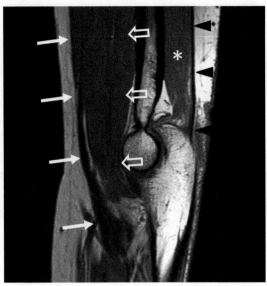

Figure 105.6. Sagittal T1W MR image of the elbow—normal anatomy. The biceps muscle forms the biceps tendon (*arrows*), which inserts onto the radial tuberosity of the proximal radius. The brachialis muscle lies deep to the biceps muscle (*open arrows*) and the muscle and tendon insert onto the ulnar tuberosity of the proximal ulna and anterior aspect of the coronoid process. Posteriorly, the triceps tendon proper is formed by the long and lateral heads of the triceps (*black arrowheads*) and inserts onto the olecranon. The medial head lies deep to the triceps tendon (*asterisk*) and has a more muscular insertion onto the olecranon.

from the posterior aspect of the lateral humeral epicondyle and passes medially to insert onto the lateral margin of the olecranon (Figure 105.2), acting to tighten the joint capsule. The anconeus also plays a minor role in extension of the elbow.

Nerves

Three major nerves are found around the elbow: the ulnar, radial, and median nerves (Figure 105.7). The ulnar nerve takes a

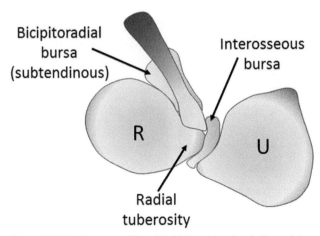

Figure 105.5. Diagram of the distal biceps tendon in the axial plane, demonstrating the tendon insertion onto the radial tuberosity. The bicipitoradial bursa lies between the distal biceps tendon and radial cortex and wraps itself around the biceps tendon in supination. Note also the interosseous bursa between the proximal radius and ulna.

superficial course along the posteromedial aspect of the distal humerus and enters the cubital tunnel, a tight fibroosseous tunnel on the posterior aspect of the medial epicondyle and medial aspect of the olecranon. The floor of the cubital tunnel is formed by the joint capsule and posterior bundle of the UCL. The roof is formed by the cubital tunnel retinaculum (Osborne ligament) proximally and the aponeurosis of the flexor carpi ulnaris (arcuate ligament) distally. There are a number of anatomic variants that can predispose to ulnar nerve compression. These include absence of the cubital tunnel retinaculum in 10% of the population, allowing anterior subluxation of the ulnar nerve when the elbow is flexed and predisposing to friction neuritis. A small accessory muscle, the anconeus epitrochlearis, may be present in some individuals, forming the roof of the cubital tunnel. Occasionally this may result in compression of the underlying ulnar nerve. Distally the ulnar nerve passes between the 2 heads of the flexor carpi ulnaris to enter the forearm and innervates the muscles of the posteromedial forearm.

The median nerve courses between the pronator teres and brachialis muscles and lies adjacent to the brachial artery and vein, just deep to the bicipital aponeurosis. The nerve passes between the humeral and ulnar heads of the pronator teres under a fibrous arch formed by the 2 heads of flexor digitorum superficialis into the forearm. The major branch of the median nerve in the forearm is the anterior interosseous nerve, which provides the motor supply to the deep forearm flexors.

The radial nerve lies between the brachioradialis and brachialis muscles in the antecubital fossa and runs through an anatomic space known as the *radial tunnel*, which starts at

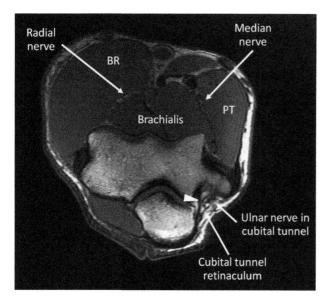

Figure 105.7. Axial T1W MR image shows the location of the major neurovascular bundles of the elbow. The radial nerve lies between the brachioradialis (BR) and brachialis, and the median nerve lies between the brachialis and pronator teres (PT). The ulnar nerve is in the cubital tunnel posterior to the medial epicondyle, with the floor formed by the posterior band of the UCL (*arrowhead*), and the roof is formed by the cubital tunnel retinaculum.

the level of the capitellum and terminates at the lower border of the supinator. At the proximal border of the supinator muscle, the radial nerve divides into a superficial sensory branch and a deep motor branch, the posterior interosseous nerve. The posterior interosseous nerve passes between the deep and superficial heads of the supinator muscle to enter the posterior compartment of the forearm. A fibrous band called the *arcade of Frohse* may be found along the superior border of the superficial supinator muscle. The superficial branch of the radial nerve passes between the supinator and brachioradialis muscles.

Imaging Findings of Elbow Pathology

Osseous and Chondral Pathology

Osteochondral Pathology
Refer to Box 105.1.

Trauma
- MRI sensitive to bone marrow changes
- Ideal to detect occult fracture (Figure 105.8)
- Best imaging modality to show osseous contusions or stress injuries (Figure 105.9)
- Location of osseous contusions helps determine mechanism of injury and predict associated soft tissue injury (Figure 105.10).

Panner Disease (Osteochondrosis of the Capitellum)
- In patients ages 5-10 years
- Affects blood supply to capitellar epiphysis
- Presents with intermittent pain and stiffness of elbow
- Radiographs may show demineralization in early disease
- Irregularity and fragmentation of articular surface in more advanced disease
- Geographic or diffuse low T1 and high T2 signal intensity within the capitellar epiphysis on MRI (Figure 105.11) with or without fragmentation of the articular surface
- Spontaneous healing 1-2 years
- Rarely results in joint bodies

Osteochondritis Dissecans
- In patients ages 10-16 years
- Repetitive valgus overload of elbow in sports such as baseball and gymnastics
- Fragmentation of capitellum and overlying cartilage may lead to joint bodies.

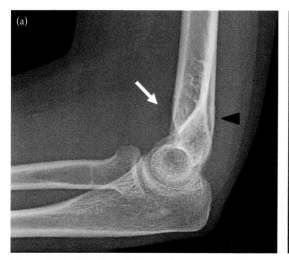
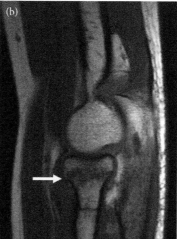
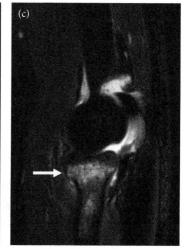

Figure 105.8. Occult radial head fracture. Lateral radiograph (*A*) shows a moderate joint effusion, with elevation of the anterior (*arrow*) and posterior (*arrowhead*) fat pads, but no visible fracture. Sagittal T1W MR image (*B*) demonstrates a linear low signal intensity fracture line across the radial neck (*arrow*), with corresponding BME (*arrow*) on the sagittal T2W FS MR image (*C*).

Box 105.1. Osteochondral Pathology

Panner Disease

- In patients aged 5-10 years
- Demineralization and resorption of entire capitellum
- Irregularity and fragmentation of articular surface
- Spontaneous healing 1-2 years
- Rarely results in joint bodies

Osteochondritis Dissecans

- In patients aged 10-16 years
- Repetitive valgus forces
- Fragmentation of capitellum and overlying cartilage
- May be unstable and lead to joint bodies

Pitfall

Pseudodefect of capitellum—contour change on posterolateral margin of capitellum simulating an osteochondral defect on coronal images

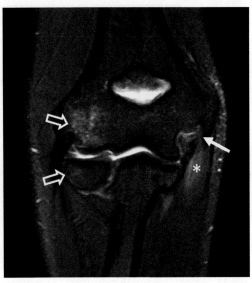

Figure 105.10. Complete UCL tear. A 20-year-old male water polo player with acute elbow pain. Coronal T2W FS MR image demonstrates a complete tear of the proximal UCL (*arrow*), with edema in the adjacent flexor-pronator mass (*asterisk*) and kissing contusions in the capitellum and radial head (*open arrows*). The UCL appears thickened from chronic repetitive valgus extension overload.

- Unstable lesions characterized by fluid tracking around OCL or underlying cystlike change on MRA (Figure 105.12); may need surgical intervention
- Stable lesions usually treated conservatively

Pitfall
- Pseudodefect of capitellum—contour change or cystlike change along the nonarticular posterolateral margin of capitellum simulating an osteochondral defect on coronal images (Figure 105.13).

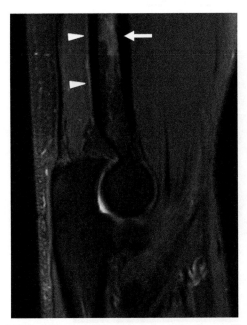

Figure 105.9. A 21-year-old female water polo player with medial elbow pain and stress reaction. Sagittal T2W FS MR image shows BME in the distal humeral diaphysis (*arrow*) with overlying periosteal edema (*arrowheads*) but no visible fracture.

Ligamentous Injury
Ulnar Collateral Ligament
Refer to Box 105.2.

Pathophysiology and Clinical Presentation
- Injuries of UCL common in sports requiring overhead throwing motion, for example, baseball, javelin, tennis, and volleyball
- Chronic repetitive microtrauma to UCL from valgus stresses during the late cocking and acceleration stages of throwing → microtears and reparative changes leading to weakening and eventual rupture
- Acute rupture of the UCL can also occur from acute valgus stress injury or elbow dislocation.

Imaging Findings
- Best imaging plane = coronal or coronal oblique
  - Low-grade sprain = intact ligament with surrounding high T2 signal (Figure 105.14)
  - Grade 2 sprain = irregular, thickened or attenuated ligament (Figure 105.15); look for partial-thickness undersurface tear of distal fibers forming T-sign (Figure 105.16), best seen on MRA
  - Grade 3 sprain = focal discontinuity—mid > distal > proximal fibers (Figure 105.10)
- Look for associated bone contusions in capitellum and radial head, or common flexor tendon tear/strain
- Injuries usually treated conservatively with NSAIDs, splinting, and physical therapy
- Surgical repair or reconstruction of UCL using semitendinosus or palmaris longus tendon graft

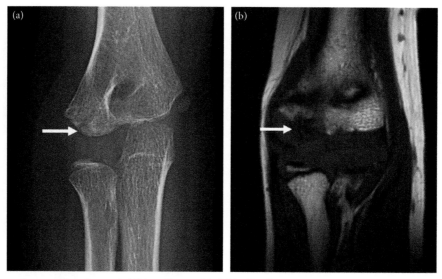

Figure 105.11. Panner disease. AP radiograph (*A*) in a 7-year-old child with elbow pain demonstrates irregularity and flattening of the capitellum with early fragmentation and adjacent sclerosis (*arrow*). Coronal T1W MR image (*B*) demonstrates diffuse low signal intensity within the capitellar epiphysis (*arrow*).

Valgus Extension Overload
Pathophysiology and Clinical Presentation
- Repetitive overhead throwing action results in valgus extension overload (VEO) → pain, stiffness, occasional locking of the elbow, and decrease in throwing velocity
- Valgus extension overload in skeletally immature individuals → medial epicondylar apophysitis, osteochondritis dissecans of the capitellum, and olecranon apophysitis
- *Medial epicondylar apophysitis* (Little League elbow)
  - Baseball pitchers younger than age 10 years

Imaging Findings
- Distractive valgus forces on UCL → thickened UCL (Figure 105.10) with or without heterotopic ossification or hypertrophic spurring at ulnar insertion
- Compressive forces in radiocapitellar joint → osteochondral injury
- Shearing forces along posteromedial olecranon → posteromedial OA, joint bodies, and olecranon stress injuries (Figure 105.17 and Figure 105.18)
- *Medial epicondylar apophysitis*
  - Widening and increased T2 signal along the physis with adjacent BME

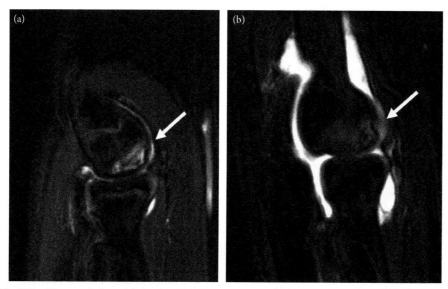

Figure 105.12. Stable OCL of the capitellum. (*A*) Sagittal T2W FS MR image of the elbow in an 11-year-old female gymnast demonstrates an OCL of the capitellum (*arrow*), with flattening of the subchondral bone plate and prominent BME, but no fluid undermining the osteochondral fragment to suggest instability. The patient was treated with synovectomy and osteochondral drilling. (*B*) Follow-up T1W FS MR image from an MRA demonstrates persistent irregularity and flattening of the articular surface (*arrow*), but intact overlying cartilage.

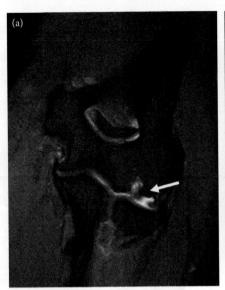
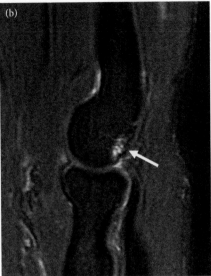

Figure 105.13. Pseudodefect of the capitellum. Coronal T2W FS MR image (*A*) shows an apparent OCL along the capitellum (*arrow*). However, on the corresponding sagittal T2W FS MR image (*B*), the cystlike change is located along the nonarticular sloping posterior margin of the capitellum (*arrow*).

■ Progresses to displacement or fragmentation of the apophysis (Figure 105.19)

Treatment Options

In most cases, treatment is conservative (rest and physical therapy):

■ Surgery occasionally required if significant displacement, instability, or loose bodies

Lateral Collateral Ligament Complex

Refer to Box 105.3.

Pathophysiology and Clinical Presentation

■ Acute varus stress on elbow or elbow dislocation → tears of RCL or LUCL—proximal more common than distal (Figure 105.20)

■ May result in posterolateral rotatory instability (PLRI) → radial head subluxates posterolaterally relative to the capitellum when the elbow is extended and the forearm is supinated

■ PLRI may present with lateral elbow pain, locking, and a catching sensation on moving the elbow → surgical intervention often needed to repair or reconstruct the torn or deficient LUCL

Box 105.2. Ulnar Collateral Ligament Injuries

■ Acute vs. chronic repetitive valgus stress to anterior or posterior bundles
■ Occur during late cocking and acceleration phases of throwing
■ Best imaging plane = coronal
■ Low-grade sprain = intact ligament with surrounding high T2 signal
■ Grade 2 sprain = irregular, thickened, or attenuated ligament (look for undersurface tear of distal fibers)
■ Grade 3 sprain = focal discontinuity: mid > distal > proximal fibers

Ancillary findings = bone contusions in capitellum and radial head, common flexor tendon tear/strain

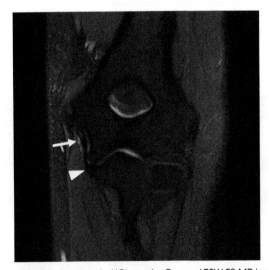

Figure 105.14. Low-grade UCL sprain. Coronal T2W FS MR image in a 32-year-old man after golfing injury demonstrates minimal increased signal in the proximal fibers of the anterior band of the UCL with periligamentous edema (*arrow*) compatible with a low-grade sprain. Note the distal insertion is 4 mm distal to the ulnar articular surface, a normal variant (*arrowhead*).

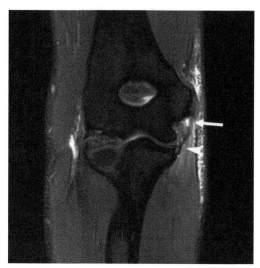

Figure 105.15. High-grade partial UCL tear. A 20-year-old male gymnast with acute right elbow injury. Coronal T2W FS MR image demonstrates a high-grade partial-thickness tear of the proximal fibers of the posterior band of the UCL (*arrow*), with interstitial tearing distally (*arrowhead*) and edema in the overlying flexor-pronator muscles. The injury was treated nonoperatively.

Imaging Findings

- RCL and LUCL tears best seen on coronal MR images as irregularity or focal discontinuity of ligament, with surrounding periligamentous edema.
- Sagittal images helpful to assess posterior subluxation of the radial head and incongruity of the radiocapitellar joint.
- RCL or LUCL pathology also seen in patients with moderate to severe lateral epicondylosis caused by degeneration/tearing in the adjacent common extensor tendon (Figure 105.21)
- Annular ligament injuries are less common but can occur with elbow dislocations.

Treatment Options

- Surgical intervention often needed to repair or reconstruct the torn or deficient LUCL.

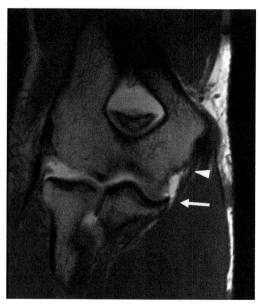

Figure 105.16. Partial-thickness undersurface tear of the distal UCL—T-sign. A 20-year-old male javelin thrower with chronic medial elbow pain. Coronal T1W MRA image demonstrates a partial-thickness undersurface tear of the distal UCL, with a cleft of fluid or T-sign between the distal attachment and sublime tubercle (*arrow*). Note the slightly flared appearance of the proximal fibers with interspersed high signal (*arrowhead*), which is a normal finding.

Tendon Pathology
Lateral Compartment
Refer to Box 105.4.

Pathophysiology and Clinical Presentation

- *Lateral epicondylosis* (tennis elbow) is a degenerative overuse-type injury of the common extensor tendon in individuals aged 40-60 years.
- Repetitive microtrauma to the extensor tendon → microtears→ fill in with granulation tissue, fibrosis, and neovascularity (Figure 105.21)

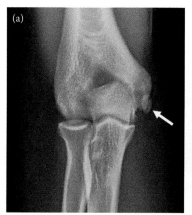 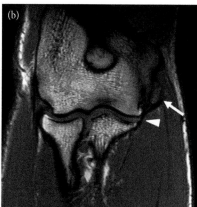 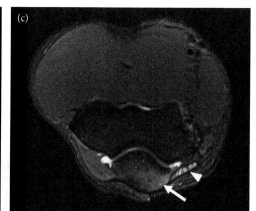

Figure 105.17. Pitcher's elbow. A 21-year-old baseball pitcher with medial elbow pain. AP radiograph (*A*) shows ossification distal to the medial epicondyle (*arrow*). (*B*) Corresponding coronal T1W MR image shows ossification in the thickened UCL (*arrow*) and early osteophytes of the humeroulnar joint medially (*arrowhead*). Axial T2W FS MR image (*C*) shows BME in the olecranon compatible with a stress reaction (*arrow*) and thickened hyperintense fascicles of the ulnar nerve (*arrowhead*), compatible with ulnar neuritis.

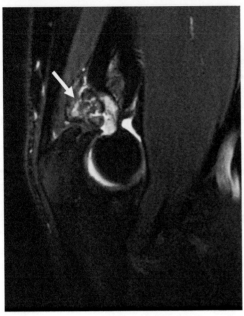

Figure 105.18. Pitcher's elbow. Sagittal T2W FS MR image in a 19-year-old baseball pitcher with intermittent locking of the elbow demonstrates chondral thinning in the posterior humeroulnar joint, with multiple joint bodies and synovitis in the olecranon fossa (*arrow*).

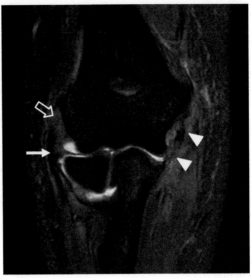

Figure 105.20. Common extensor tendon and LUCL avulsion and high-grade UCL tear. Coronal T2W FS MR image in a 37-year-old male patient who sustained a posterior elbow dislocation demonstrates avulsion of the common extensor tendon (*open arrow*) and proximal LUCL (*arrow*). The anterior band of the UCL is diffusely thickened and irregular with interspersed high signal (*arrowheads*), compatible with a high-grade tear.

- *Complete tears of the common extensor tendon* can occur after elbow dislocation or acute varus injury (Figure 105.20) → focal defect in the tendon often outlined with fluid

Imaging Findings
- Manifests as increased T1 and T2 signal within a thickened, attenuated or irregular tendon, (Figure 105.21) with or without adjacent soft tissue edema and reactive BME in the lateral epicondyle
- Focal fluid within the common extensor tendon seen with macroscopic tears, usually involving the extensor carpi radialis brevis (Figure 105.21)

- Diagnosis of lateral epicondylosis usually made clinically, but MRI is helpful in refractory cases to evaluate the extent of disease and detect any associated pathology, for example, lateral ligaments.

Treatment Options
- Initial treatment is conservative with NSAIDs, activity modification, physical therapy, splinting, peritendinous injection of steroid, or needle fenestration with injection of platelet-rich plasma or autologous blood.
- Surgery may be necessary in patients who fail to respond to conservative therapy → debridement of the diseased portion of tendon and surgical reattachment to the lateral humeral epicondyle.

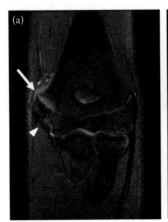
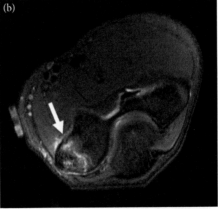

Figure 105.19. Little league elbow in a 15-year-old baseball pitcher. Coronal (*A*) and axial (*B*) T2W FS MR images demonstrate mild widening of the medial epicondylar physis (*arrow*) with adjacent osseous and soft tissue edema. Of note, the UCL is also thickened (*arrowhead*).

Box 105.3. Lateral Collateral Ligament Injuries

- Acute varus stress, elbow dislocation, or chronic repetitive microtrauma
- Tear of LUCL leads to posterolateral rotatory instability
- Best imaging planes = coronal (RCL, LUCL) and axial (LUCL, annular ligament)
- Low-grade sprain = intact ligament with surrounding high T2 signal
- Grade 2 sprain = irregular, thickened, or attenuated ligament (look for undersurface tear of distal fibers)
- Grade 3 sprain = focal discontinuity

Ancillary findings = lateral epicondylosis, common extensor tendon tear/strain, posterior subluxation of radial head

Medial Compartment
Refer to Box 105.5.

Pathophysiology and Clinical Presentation
- *Medial epicondylosis* (golfer's elbow) is less common than lateral, usually in high-level athletes participating in sports requiring repetitive valgus and flexion forces at the elbow, for example, golf, tennis, squash, baseball pitching, javelin, football, archery, and swimming (Figure 105.22)
- Repetitive valgus overload → degeneration and microtearing of the flexor-pronator muscle group → immature fibrovascular repair
- *Avulsion of the flexor-pronator muscle group* may occur with elbow dislocations in conjunction with tears of the UCL.

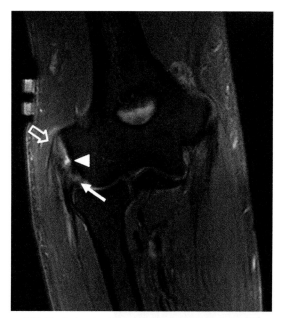

Figure 105.21. Lateral epicondylosis. Coronal T2W FS MR image in a 56-year-old man with lateral elbow pain for 3 months demonstrates thickening and increased signal within the common extensor tendon (*open arrow*), with a small focal tear in the extensor carpi radialis brevis (*arrowhead*). There is also a high-grade tear of the proximal LUCL (*arrow*).

Box 105.4. Lateral Epicondylosis (Tennis Elbow)

- Repetitive varus stress on elbow
- In patients aged 40-60 years
- Best imaging plane = coronal and axial
- Increased T1 and T2 signal in a thickened/attenuated tendon with adjacent edema
- Tear usually involves extensor carpi radialis brevis component

Ancillary findings = tears of lateral collateral ligament complex, BME in lateral epicondyle

Imaging Findings
- Presents with chronic medial elbow pain, and MRI is very helpful as the diagnosis is more challenging clinically because of overlap of symptoms from UCL injuries, ulnar neuritis, or intraarticular pathology.
- Medial epicondylosis manifests as increased T1 and T2 signal in the common flexor tendon (Figure 105.22 online), which may be thickened with areas of interstitial tearing with or without reactive BME in the medial epicondyle.

Treatment Options
- Treatment usually conservative, but surgical debridement of the diseased portion of tendon is occasionally necessary, with reattachment of the tendon to the medial epicondyle

Anterior Compartment
Refer to Box 105.6.

Pathophysiology and Clinical Presentation
- *Tears of distal biceps tendon* are predominantly seen in the dominant arm of men aged 40-60 years, particularly if smokers or on anabolic steroids:
  - Result from sudden extensor force applied to arm with elbow in 90 degrees of flexion or forceful hyperextension against resistance, for example, weightlifting
  - Pathology usually seen at distal insertion into the radial tuberosity, where the tendon is less well vascularized → degenerative tendinopathy, partial tears, or complete tears (Figure 105.23)
  - Bony hypertrophy of the radial tuberosity from repetitive traction forces and inflammatory changes

Box 105.5. Medial Epicondylosis (Golfer's Elbow)

- Repetitive valgus and flexion forces on elbow
- Less common than lateral epicondylosis
- High-performance athletes
- Best imaging plane = coronal and axial
- Increased T1 and T2 signal in a thickened/attenuated tendon with adjacent edema

Ancillary findings = BME in medial epicondyle, strain of overlying flexor-pronator muscle group

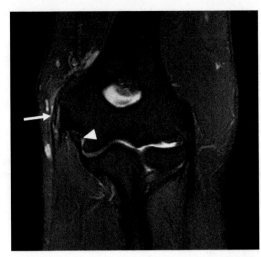

Figure 105.22. Medial epicondylosis. Coronal T2W FS MR image in an active 41-year-old mechanic with chronic medial elbow pain demonstrates focal increased signal within the common flexor tendon (*arrow*) and mild adjacent soft tissue edema. The underlying UCL also appears mildly thickened with intermediate signal proximally (*arrowhead*) suggesting remote injury.

in the bicipitoradial or interosseous bursae can increase mechanical impingement on the distal biceps tendon (Figure 105.24), particularly if the forearm is pronated.

■ Avulsed tendon stump will retract into the upper arm if lacertus fibrosus is torn producing a palpable defect and making clinical diagnosis easy.

■ If the lacertus fibrosus remains intact, there is no significant retraction of the tendon and diagnosis on clinical examination is more challenging.

■ *Brachialis muscle injuries* are also uncommon but may result from eccentric muscle contraction against resistance or posterior elbow dislocations.

Imaging Findings

■ Biceps pathology best seen on axial and sagittal images → thickened, irregular or attenuated distal tendon or focal

tendon gap with or without bursal distension or hypertrophied radial tuberosity with BME.

■ Integrity of lacertus fibrosus assessed on axial images

■ Imaging in FABS position places the distal biceps tendon under tension and can be useful for grading the degree of distal tendon involvement.

■ Bifid biceps tendon may occur as a normal variant, with separate tendinous components for the short and long heads, and isolated rupture of a single head may occur.

Treatment Options

■ Complete tears usually require immediate surgical reattachment to radial tuberosity, as delayed reconstruction can be challenging and lead to a poorer functional outcome.

■ Partial tears usually treated conservatively with immobilization, ice, NSAIDs, and physical therapy.

■ Tears of the biceps muscle belly or myotendinous strains are less common, but occur in military parachutists where the static line is accidentally wrapped around the upper arm or in watersports using a towline, such as water skiing or wakeboarding, where a handle is hooked around the upper arm.

Posterior Compartment
Refer to Box 105.7.

Pathophysiology and Clinical Presentation

■ *Triceps tendon rupture* is rare, and rupture of the triceps muscle belly or myotendinous strains are even less common.

■ Result from a direct blow or a fall on an outstretched hand → sudden flexion of an extended forearm and decelerating counterforce on contracted triceps muscle

■ Predisposing factors include anabolic steroids, oral or injected corticosteroids, olecranon bursitis, inflammatory arthropathies, or renal insufficiency with hyperparathyroidism.

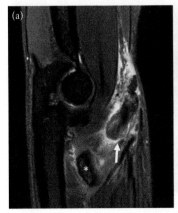
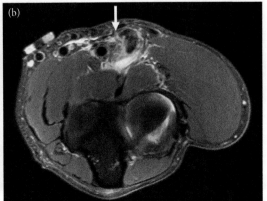

Figure 105.23. Distal biceps tendon avulsion in a 55-year-old man with acute lifting injury. Sagittal T2W FS MR image (*A*) demonstrates avulsion of the distal biceps tendon (*arrow*) from the radial tuberosity (*asterisk*) with surrounding hemorrhage and edema. On the axial T2W FS MR image (*B*), the lacertus fibrosus is also avulsed (*arrow*) from the retracted biceps tendon.

Box 105.6. Distal Biceps Tendon Injury

- Forceful overload of elbow in mid flexion
- Common in men aged 40-60 years
- Complete tears more common than partial tears
- Best imaging plane = sagittal and axial
- Intrasubstance degeneration with increased T1 and T2 signal intensity
- Partial tear or focal discontinuity of distal tendon

Ancillary findings = tear of lacertus fibrosus, bicipitoradial bursitis, bony hypertrophy of bicipital tuberosity

Imaging Findings
- Triceps tendon best evaluated on axial and sagittal images with tendinopathy manifesting as increased T1 and T2 signal in a thickened or partially torn tendon with or without BME (Figure 105.25)
- Entire tendon can avulse from olecranon process with retraction of the tendon stump with or without small accompanying fracture (Figure 105.26), or superficial or deep components may avulse in isolation.

Often the superficial tendinous component is torn, whereas the deeper, muscular component is still attached.

Treatment Options
- Partial tears usually treated conservatively with rest, NSAIDs, ice, and splinting unless tear progresses
- Complete tears require surgical reattachment to the olecranon process, or surgical reconstruction if the tear is chronic.

Nerve Pathology
- Nerve pathology around the elbow is common as the main nerves are relatively superficial and adjacent to underlying bones, making them vulnerable to acute injury from a direct blow or underlying fracture.
- Nerves pass through narrow fibromuscular/fibroosseous tunnels around the elbow where they can be compressed and result in entrapment neuropathy.
- Nerves pass through muscles activated during the throwing motion, making throwing athletes prone to dynamic compression injuries.
- MRI demonstrates changes in caliber or signal intensity of affected nerve, mass lesions or anatomic variant compressing the nerve, and denervation changes in muscles supplied by the nerve.

Ulnar Nerve
Refer to Box 105.8.

Pathophysiology and Clinical Presentation
- Ulnar nerve compression is most common peripheral neuropathy around the elbow → local pain, paresthesia, and sensory loss in the fourth and fifth digits and hand weakness.
- Most common site of entrapment is the cubital tunnel, particularly in elbow flexion when the aponeurosis of the flexor carpi ulnaris becomes taut, increasing pressure in the cubital tunnel.
- Anatomic variants predisposing to ulnar neuritis include
  - Thickening or absence of the cubital tunnel retinaculum
  - Replacement of retinaculum with an accessory anconeus epitrochlearis muscle (Figure 105.27)
  - Low-lying medial head of the triceps muscle
- Ulnar nerve pathology also seen following fractures, UCL injury, or in overhead athletes with valgus extension overload syndrome
- Other sites of potential entrapment include
  - Arcade of Struthers
  - Fascial bands where nerve passes into the forearm between the 2 heads of the flexor carpi ulnaris muscle
  - Deep flexor-pronator aponeurosis

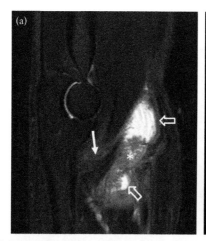
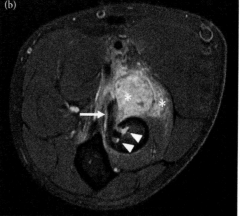

Figure 105.24. Bicipitoradial bursitis in a 65-year-old man with a palpable mass in the antecubital fossa. Sagittal (*A*) and axial (*B*) T2W FS MR images show thickening, irregularity, and increased signal within the distal biceps tendon (*arrow*), compatible with tendinopathy and partial tear. There is marked distension of the bicipitoradial bursa with fluid (*open arrows*) and severe synovitis (*asterisks*), resulting in the palpable mass. Reactive cystlike changes or erosions (*arrowheads*) are seen in the radial tuberosity.

Box 105.7. Triceps Tendon Injury

- Fall on outstretched hand vs. repetitive overuse
- Best imaging plane = sagittal and axial
- Intrasubstance degeneration, partial tear, or avulsion of distal tendon

Ancillary findings = Avulsion fractures of olecranon process, olecranon bursitis, ulnar neuritis

Imaging Findings

- Ulnar nerve best seen on axial MR images and may appear flattened at the site of compression (Figure 105.17) with obliteration of the fat plane surrounding the nerve, focal or diffuse swelling of the ulnar nerve proximal or distal to the point of compression, and increased T2 signal intensity (Figure 105.28), likened to a cobra head or spring onion
- Must correlate imaging findings with clinical findings as high T2 signal in ulnar nerve is common in asymptomatic patients
- MRI may show denervation changes in muscles supplied by the ulnar nerve → edema, fatty infiltration, or atrophy in the flexor digitorum profundus, flexor carpi ulnaris, or intrinsic muscles of hand.

Treatment Options

- Treatment of ulnar nerve compression is conservative, with rest, modification of activity, and occasionally local injection of corticosteroid.
- Surgical decompression may be indicated if patients fail to respond to conservative treatment, often in

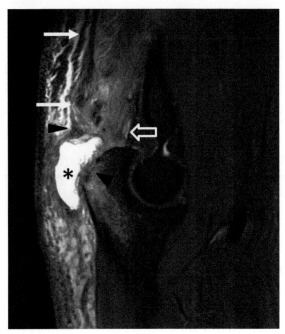

Figure 105.26. Near complete avulsion of the distal triceps tendon. Sagittal T2W FS MR image in a 41-year-old man shows avulsion of the distal triceps tendon from the olecranon process (*arrows*) with an associated avulsion fracture (*black arrowhead*). A few of the muscular fibers of the medial head remain intact (*open arrow*). There is prominent surrounding edema and overlying olecranon bursitis (*asterisk*).

conjunction with transposition of the ulnar nerve or medial epicondylectomy.

Median Nerve
Refer to Box 105.9.

Pathophysiology and Clinical Presentation

- Median nerve entrapment occurs at 1 of 4 main sites around the elbow:
  - Supracondylar process and ligament of Struthers (Figure 105.29)
  - Thickened lacertus fibrosus in antecubital fossa
  - Fibrous band between superficial and deep heads of the pronator teres muscle (most common)

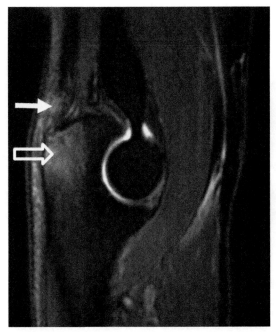

Figure 105.25. Partial tear of the triceps tendon. Sagittal T2W FS MR image in a 45-year-old man with posterior elbow pain demonstrates partial tearing of the distal triceps tendon (*arrow*) and reactive BME in the olecranon (*open arrow*).

Box 105.8. Ulnar Nerve Injury

- Presents with pain, paresthesia, and sensory loss in the fourth and fifth digits and hand weakness
- Commonest site of compression is cubital tunnel
- Best imaging plane = axial and sagittal
- Imaging findings include focal or diffuse thickening of ulnar nerve with high T2 signal intensity

Ancillary findings = thickening or absence of cubital tunnel retinaculum, anconeus epitrochlearis, low-lying medial head of triceps muscle, UCL injury, malunited or ununited medial condylar fracture

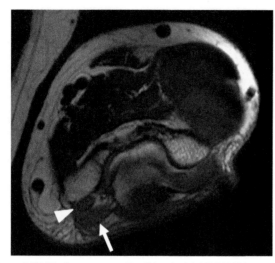

Figure 105.27. Anconeus epitrochlearis. Axial T1W MR image in a 60-year-old man with ulnar neuritis demonstrates an accessory anconeus epitrochlearis muscle (*arrow*) overlying a mildly thickened ulnar nerve (*arrowhead*).

- Fibrous arch formed between 2 heads of the flexor digitorum superficialis muscle in the proximal forearm
- Other causes of compression include humeral fracture; anomalous muscles, such as an accessory head of the flexor pollicis longus (Gantzer muscle); anomalous vessels; vascular pathology; or a distended bicipitoradial bursa.
- Clinically median nerve compression can present in 2 ways:
  1. *Pronator syndrome* (most common) → gradual onset of pain over volar aspect of the forearm with numbness and paresthesia in the radial most three and a half digits

2. *Anterior interosseous syndrome* (Kiloh-Nevin syndrome) caused by selective compression of anterior interosseous branch of the median nerve (motor) → weakness of flexor pollicis longus, flexor digitorum profundus tendons to the second and third digits, and pronator quadratus muscle

Imaging Findings
- MRI may demonstrate space-occupying lesions or accessory muscles and denervation changes of muscles supplied by the median nerve:
  - Pronator syndrome → edema or fatty infiltration in pronator teres (Figure 105.30), flexor carpi radialis, palmaris longus, and flexor digitorum superficialis
  - Anterior interosseous syndrome → edema or fatty infiltration in pronator quadratus, flexor pollicis longus, and portion of flexor digitorum profundus

Treatment Options
- Treatment of median nerve compression usually conservative including rest, modification of activity, physical therapy, and perineural steroid injection
- Surgical decompression reserved for those who fail to respond to conservative measures and compression by ligament of Struthers

Radial Nerve
Refer to Box 105.10.

Pathophysiology and Clinical Presentation
- Causes of radial nerve entrapment include:
  - Fibrous band along the proximal margin of supinator (arcade of Frohse)
  - Fibrous bands in distal supinator muscle
  - Fibrous bands around the radiocapitellar joint
  - Tendinous edge of the extensor carpi radialis brevis
  - Vascular arcades of recurrent radial artery (leash of Henry)

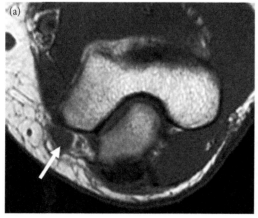
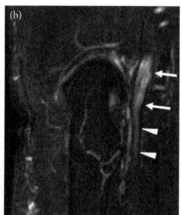

Figure 105.28. Cubital tunnel syndrome. A 38-year-old woman with pain and numbness in her ulnar forearm and hand, most marked in elbow flexion. Axial T1W MR image (*A*) demonstrates focal enlargement of the ulnar nerve just proximal to the cubital tunnel (*arrow*). On the coronal T2W FS MR image (*B*), the nerve is enlarged with high T2 signal above the cubital tunnel (*arrows*) and of normal caliber and more normal signal intensity within and distal to the cubital tunnel (*arrowheads*).

Box 105.9. Median Nerve Injury

- Pronator syndrome—presents with pain, numbness, and paresthesia in the radial most three and a half digits
- Anterior interosseous syndrome (Kiloh-Nevin syndrome)—presents with weakness of flexor pollicis longus, flexor digitorum profundus tendons to the second and third digits, and pronator quadratus
- Commonest site of compression is fibrous band between deep and superficial heads of pronator teres
- Best imaging plane = axial
- Imaging findings include denervation changes of innervated muscles, with high T2 signal in acute denervation and fatty infiltration or atrophy in chronic denervation

Ancillary findings = supracondylar process, humeral fracture, accessory muscles, distended bicipitoradial bursa, other space-occupying lesions

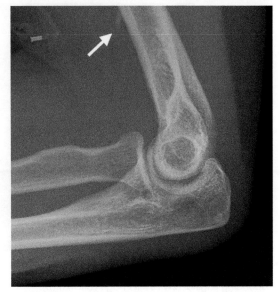

Figure 105.29. Supracondylar process. Lateral radiograph of the elbow demonstrates a small bony spur arising from the anterior aspect of the distal humerus (*arrow*), compatible with a supracondylar process, which can be associated with median nerve entrapment.

- Fractures
- Space-occupying lesions or inflamed bursae
- Radial nerve divides into superficial radial nerve (sensory) and deep posterior interosseous nerve (motor) at the proximal border of supinator.
- Compression of superficial radial nerve → pain in distal forearm and paresthesia in hand (*Wartenberg syndrome*)
- Compression of the posterior interosseous nerve proximally → vague pain over the lateral elbow and forearm (*radial tunnel syndrome*), usually with no sensory or motor defect, closely mimicking symptoms of lateral epicondylosis
- Distal compression of the posterior interosseous nerve → gradual onset of weakness in supinator and proximal forearm extensor muscles (*supinator syndrome*)

Imaging Findings

- On MRI, radial tunnel syndrome and posterior interosseous nerve syndrome → edema or fatty infiltration in supinator and extensor muscles (Figure 105.31), depending on whether compression is acute or chronic.
- MRI may show neural compressive lesion, for example, inflamed bicipitoradial bursa, ganglion, thickening of leading edge of extensor carpi radialis brevis, or humeral fracture.

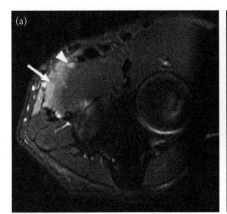
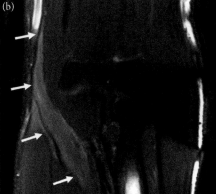

Figure 105.30. A 46-year-old man with pronator syndrome. Axial T2W FS MR image (*A*) shows edema within the pronator teres muscle (*arrow*) and high T2 signal in the median nerve (*arrowhead*). Coronal T2W FS MR image (*B*) shows diffuse edema in the pronator teres (*arrows*).

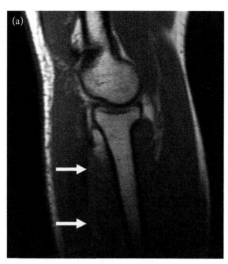
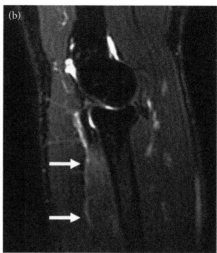

Figure 105.31. Posterior interosseous nerve syndrome. A 27-year-old man with painless motor loss in the posterior interosseous nerve distribution. Sagittal T1W MR image (*A*) demonstrates early fatty infiltration in the supinator muscle (*arrows*) with edema on the corresponding sagittal T2W FS MR image (*arrows*) (*B*).

Box 105.10. Radial Nerve Injury

- Wartenberg syndrome (superficial radial nerve) presents with pain in the distal forearm and paresthesia in the hand
- Radial tunnel syndrome (proximal posterior interosseous nerve) presents with vague pain over the lateral elbow and forearm
- Supinator syndrome (distal posterior interosseous nerve) presents with gradual onset of weakness of the supinator and proximal forearm extensor muscles
- Commonest sites of compression are fibrous bands along proximal margin of supinator (arcade of Frohse) or distal supinator muscle
- Best imaging plane = axial
- Imaging findings include denervation changes of supinator and extensor muscles supplied by posterior interosseous nerve, with high T2 signal in acute denervation and fatty infiltration or atrophy in chronic denervation

Ancillary findings = humeral fracture, inflamed bicipitoradial bursa, ganglion, thickening of the leading edge of the extensor carpi radialis brevis

---

Treatment Options

- Initial treatment usually conservative, consisting of splinting, activity modification, and perineural steroid injection
- Surgical decompression only recommended once conservative management has failed

---

Key Points
- MRI is an invaluable diagnostic tool for the evaluation of patients with elbow pain, particularly when pain is poorly localized.

- Many elbow injuries can be diagnosed on clinical history and physical examination alone. However, MRI is helpful to confirm the diagnosis, determine the extent of disease, and detect any associated bony or soft tissue pathology.
- The multiplanar imaging capabilities of MRI are ideal to evaluate the complex anatomy around the elbow and detect acute or chronic injury of the ligaments, tendon, muscles, and nerves.
- STIR and T2W FS images are exquisitely sensitive for BME and therefore ideal for detecting osseous stress injuries, occult fractures, and osteochondral pathology.
- MRA with injection of dilute Gd into the joint is helpful to detect subtle chondral defects or undersurface ligament tears.
- MRI plays a pivotal role in guiding clinical management and is helpful for planning operative intervention.

Recommended Reading
Hauptfleisch J, English C, Murphy D. Elbow magnetic resonance imaging: imaging anatomy and evaluation. *Top Magn Reson Imaging.* 2015;24(2):93–107.

References
1. Andreisek G, Crook DW, Burg D, Marincek B, Weishaupt D. Peripheral neuropathies of the median, radial, and ulnar nerves: MR imaging features. *Radiographics.* 2006;26(5):1267–87.
2. Bach BR Jr., Warren RF, Wickiewicz TL. Triceps rupture. A case report and literature review. *Am J Sports Med.* 1987;15(3):285–89.
3. Belentani C, Pastore D, Wangwinyuvirat M, et al. Triceps brachii tendon: anatomic-MR imaging study in cadavers with histologic correlation. *Skeletal Radiol.* 2009;38(2):171–75.

4. Bredella MA, Tirman PF, Fritz RC, Feller JF, Wischer TK, Genant HK. MR imaging findings of lateral ulnar collateral ligament abnormalities in patients with lateral epicondylitis. *AJR Am J Roentgenol.* 1999;173(5):1379–82.

5. Farrow LD, Mahoney AJ, Stefancin JJ, Taljanovic MS, Sheppard JE, Schickendantz MS. Quantitative analysis of the medial ulnar collateral ligament ulnar footprint and its relationship to the ulnar sublime tubercle. *Am J Sports Med.* 2011;39(9):1936–41.

6. Hackl M, Wegmann K, Ries C, Leschinger T, Burkhart KJ, Muller LP. Reliability of magnetic resonance imaging signs of posterolateral rotatory instability of the elbow. *J Hand Surg Am.* 2015;40(7):1428–33.

7. Hauptfleisch J, English C, Murphy D. Elbow magnetic resonance imaging: imaging anatomy and evaluation. *Top Magn Reson Imaging.* 2015;24(2):93–107.

8. Husarik DB, Saupe N, Pfirrmann CW, Jost B, Hodler J, Zanetti M. Elbow nerves: MR findings in 60 asymptomatic subjects—normal anatomy, variants, and pitfalls. *Radiology.* 2009;252(1):148–56.

9. Kijowski R, De Smet AA. Magnetic resonance imaging findings in patients with medial epicondylitis. *Skeletal Radiol.* 2005;34(4):196–202.

10. Kobayashi K, Burton KJ, Rodner C, Smith B, Caputo AE. Lateral compression injuries in the pediatric elbow: Panner's disease and osteochondritis dissecans of the capitellum. *J Am Acad Orthop Surg.* 2004;12(4):246–54.

11. Magee T. Accuracy of 3-T MR arthrography versus conventional 3-T MRI of elbow tendons and ligaments compared with surgery. *AJR Am J Roentgenol.* 2015;204(1):W70–75.

12. Patel RM, Lynch TS, Amin NH, Calabrese G, Gryzlo SM, Schickendantz MS. The thrower's elbow. *Orthop Clin North Am.* 2014;45(3):355–76.

13. Stevens K, Kwak A, Poplawski S. The biceps muscle from shoulder to elbow. *Semin Musculoskelet Radiol.* 2012;16(4):296–315.

CHAPTER 106

Internal Derangement of the Wrist and Hand

Apostolos H. Karantanas

Introduction

The wrist is perhaps the most complex joint in the body. A wide spectrum of disorders affects the wrist and hand. Evolving surgical techniques, including arthroscopy, and improving treatments for inflammatory disorders have increased the demand for accurate diagnostic imaging.

Internal derangement is a general and nonspecific term describing internal damage to the intraarticular structures following previous trauma, asymmetric loading with repetitive microinjuries, and long-standing inflammation. This term is often used by clinicians in cases that the clinical tests are nonspecific and the examiners are not able to suggest a specific cause of pain and functional limitation. Thus, not only isolated intraarticular structures are involved in this clinical entity. The spectrum of abnormal findings in the wrist and hand area include occult fractures, fracture nonunion, ON, TFCC injury, torn ligaments with associated instability, tendon disorders, and inflammatory disorders that can lead to advanced OA.

Magnetic Resonance Imaging Protocols

MRI and MRA play an important role in depicting the source of wrist and hand pain and limited function.

- Ideally, the imaging is performed in the prone position with the wrist/hand above the head (superman position) in the isocenter of the magnet using the dedicated wrist/hand coils.
- However, the imaging is commonly performed in the more comfortable, but less optimal supine position with the hand on the side of the patient's body.
- For MRI, T1W sequences without fat saturation and fluid-sensitive sequences with fat saturation are typically performed in 3 planes (axial, coronal, and sagittal). With suspected scaphoid or lunate ON, additional sequences after IV Gd-based contrast administration are frequently helpful.
- For MRA, in addition to T1W sequences with fat saturation in 3 planes, at least one T1W sequence without fat saturation and 1 fluid-sensitive sequence with fat saturation are added for the evaluation of bone marrow and adjacent soft tissues.
- Frequently, a thin submillimeter cut GRE sequence with near isotropic resolution in the coronal plane is added for both MRI and MRA.

- Additional axial oblique sequences of the wrist ligaments or sagittal oblique sequence of the scaphoid bone may improve evaluation of these structures. MRA improves the assessment of the TFCC and intrinsic and extrinsic wrist ligaments.

Occult Fractures and Osteonecrosis of the Scaphoid and Lunate

Pathophysiology and Clinical Findings

With its superb contrast resolution, MRI is the imaging modality of choice for evaluation of occult wrist fractures, bone contusions, and fracture complications.

The scaphoid bone is important in carpal stability and acts as a supporting rod bridging the 2 carpal rows (Figure 106.1). Scaphoid fractures account for 60-90% of all wrist fractures. The unique blood supply through the proximal pole predisposes scaphoid fractures to delayed union, nonunion, and ON. Approximately 12% of scaphoid fractures fail to heal and require surgical treatment. Scaphoid fracture nonunions may remain asymptomatic and undiagnosed. If left untreated for more than 2 years, particularly in cases with associated ligamentous injuries, nonunions have an increased risk for instability and OA. Scaphoid fractures are complicated with ON in approximately 30% of cases when located in the waist and in 80-100% when located in the proximal pole. Anatomic snuffbox tenderness is a highly sensitive test for scaphoid fracture, but compression pain and tenderness of the scaphoid tubercle tend to be more specific. Clinical examination alone cannot depict complications related to scaphoid fractures because of lack of specific clinical signs. SNAC wrist refers to the development of OA that usually occurs within 5-10 years after injury and can result in significant functional impairment. The *humpback* deformity results from malunion of the scaphoid waist fracture with volar angulation (flexion) of the proximal and distal poles. The dorsal aspect of the scaphoid forms the palpable humpback deformity. This leads to DISI because of dorsal rotation of the lunate, which may also lead to wrist OA.

Preiser disease represents an idiopathic form of ON of the scaphoid bone. In most of the cases, however, a history of repetitive microinjuries or overloading exists.

Kienböck disease is defined as ON of a part of or the entire lunate. ON of the lunate may result from repetitive microtrauma; interruption of blood supply including acute

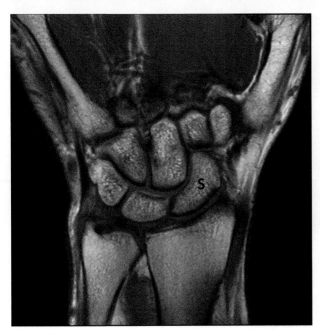

Figure 106.1. Anatomic position of the scaphoid bone. Coronal T1W MR image of the wrist shows normal anatomic position of the scaphoid bone (S) with high signal intensity of the bone marrow fat.

fracture, steroid use, hypercoagulability, and altered biomechanics, such as in the context of negative ulnar variance, decreased radial inclination, and type I lunate morphology. Type II lunate, which shows and extraarticulation to the hamate, may resist against fractures. Isolated fracture of the lunate bone is very rare, accounting for approximately 1-2% of all wrist fractures. The proximal pole of the lunate is vulnerable to ischemia because it does not have soft tissue attachments. In addition, in up to 20% of the population, there is a single arterial supply for the entire lunate bone, which can be interrupted with palmar pole fractures. Delayed diagnosis may lead to ON and instability. Kienböck disease typically affects manual workers who present with intermittent or constant dorsal pain, often related to activity, limited motion, swelling,

and weakness of the hand. On physical examination, there is tenderness between the extensor digitorum and extensor carpi radialis tendons with provoked pain during forceful extension. Typically, flexion and extension are limited, and there is reduced grip strength.

Imaging Strategy
- Radiographs, including PA, lateral, semipronated oblique, and PA with ulnar deviation views are the first-line imaging studies for detecting complications related to scaphoid fractures.
- CT is superior to radiographs to depict trabecular bridging, but also to assess the postoperative status despite the presence of metallic hardware/screws.
- A helpful tool for the assessment of movement at the site of the scaphoid fracture is real-time US. However, US cannot fully assess proximal pole nonunion.
- MRI without and with IV contrast is the preferred approach in chronic wrist pain as nonunion, ON, or other arthropathies, including inflammation may be the cause of symptoms. Contrast-enhanced MRI improves assessment of scaphoid nonunion with proximal pole ON in majority of cases.
- PA, oblique, and lateral radiographs should be obtained in cases of clinically suspected Kienböck disease, both for diagnosis and staging.
- Contrast-enhanced MRI is the preferred approach for assessing the viability of lunate bone marrow.

Imaging Findings
- Scaphoid nonunion is suggested if no bony trabeculae crossing the fracture line are detected 6 months following the initial injury (Figure 106.2).
- CT is more sensitive in evaluation of healing, showing the bony trabeculae crossing the fracture site, and can assess the percentage of solid bony union. Solid bony bridging of more than 25% of the cross-sectional area allows for safe mobilization and will proceed to full union.
- A fracture line associated with cystlike changes on either side suggests nonunion, which is better seen on CT and MRI studies compared to radiographs. The presence

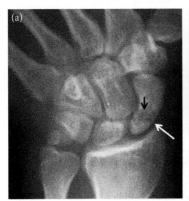
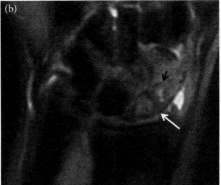

Figure 106.2. Scaphoid fracture nonunion with pseudoarthrosis 6 months after injury. (*A*) PA radiograph of the wrist shows scaphoid fracture nonunion (*white arrow*) with adjacent cystlike formation (*black arrow*). The sclerotic appearance of the proximal pole suggests ON development. (*B*) Coronal STIR MR image shows the nonunited low signal intensity fracture line (*white arrow*), improved visualization of the cystlike formation (*black arrow*), and BME on both sides of the fracture. Punctate bleeding, in keeping with viable marrow, was detected before surgical fixation indicating viable marrow.

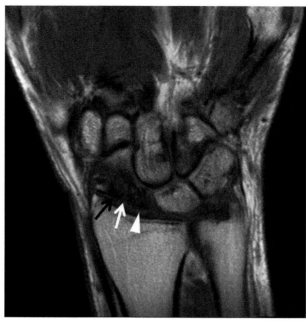

Figure 106.3. Scaphoid facture nonunion with proximal pole ON. Coronal T1W MR image shows a nonunited scaphoid waist fracture (*white arrow*) with cystlike formation (*black arrow*) and diminutive, irregular low signal at the proximal pole consistent with ON (*arrowhead*). The patient was treated with a vascularized bone graft.

of pseudarthrosis, with or without a sclerotic proximal pole, is not pathognomonic for nonviable bone marrow (Figure 106.2*A*).

- The preservation of normal fatty signal in the proximal fragment on T1W MR images suggests viable bone marrow. However, mummified fat in early ON may display *normal* high signal intensity with false-negative findings on the T1W sequences without fat saturation. Otherwise, early ON shows lower signal of the necrotic bone with respect to the surrounding normal bones on T1W sequences and variable signal on fluid-sensitive sequences (Figure 106.3).
- Vascularity within the bone marrow is suggested by the presence of enhancement. Homogeneous enhancement suggests viable bone marrow; inhomogeneous enhancement suggests coexistence of ON and viable tissue to variable degree and the absence of enhancement suggests ON. False-negative cases may still exist, possibly because of fibrous tissue ingrowth.
- The value of dynamic contrast-enhanced MRI is debatable. Nondynamic contrast-enhanced MRI is a valuable tool for assessing postoperative bone grafting in both the scaphoid and lunate bones.
- Lichtman staging of Kienböck disease with imaging is important for patient management (Table 106.1; Figures 106.4 and 106.5).

Treatment Options

Scaphoid Fracture Complications

- Nonoperative treatment of scaphoid nonunions with casting for 4-6 months is only indicated for patients who are not suitable for surgery, for any reason.

- In scaphoid nonunions with preserved vascularity, a nonvascularized bone graft fixated with screws is able to achieve a successful union.
- In cases of poor blood supply as shown on MRI and/or in absence of punctate bleeding at surgery, a vascularized bone graft is preferred (Figure 106.6).
- Scaphoid nonunions with OA require salvage procedures such as limited carpal or total wrist arthrodesis, proximal row carpectomy, scaphoid excision, or arthroplasty.

Kienböck Disease

- Treatment options for Kienböck disease include conservative and operative measures and vary depending on the stage, associated findings, and the surgeon's expertise.
- Depending on the severity, in stage I, casting and immobilization is suggested. Others suggest core decompression.
- In stages II and IIIA, unloading of the lunate bone by means of ulnar lengthening or radial shortening, with or without core decompression, may be applied. Vascularized bone grafting may also be used.
- In stages IIIb and higher, more aggressive salvage procedures such as proximal row carpectomy or arthrodesis with or without lunate excision aim to prevent further destruction of the wrist.

Triangular Fibrocartilage Complex

Pathophysiology and Clinical Findings

The TFCC acts as a primary stabilizer of the distal radioulnar joint and lies on the ulnar side of the wrist (Figure 106.7). It consists of the triangular disc (TFC), the dorsal and volar radioulnar ligaments, the UCL (between the ulnar styloid

Table 106.1. Lichtman Staging of Kienböck Disease

STAGE	RADIOGRAPHIC/CT FINDINGS	MRI FINDINGS
I	Normal morphology	Normal morphology, BME
II	Normal morphology, bone marrow sclerosis	Normal morphology, low signal on T1W, and variable on fluid-sensitive sequences
IIIa	Collapse of lunate bone, radioscaphoid angle <60 degrees	Collapse of lunate bone, low signal on T1W, and variable on fluid-sensitive sequences
IIIb	Collapse of lunate bone, radioscaphoid angle >60 degrees	Collapse of lunate bone, low signal on T1W, and variable on fluid-sensitive sequences
IIIc	Collapse of lunate bone, coronal lunate fracture (chronic)	Collapse of lunate bone, low signal on T1W, and variable on fluid-sensitive sequences coronal lunate fracture
IV	Radiocarpal and midcarpal osteoarthritis	Radiocarpal and midcarpal osteoarthritis, low signal on T1W, and variable on fluid-sensitive sequences

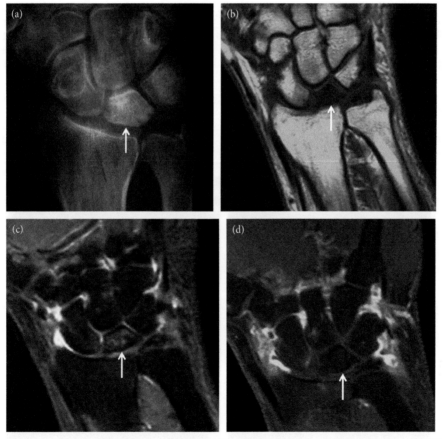

Figure 106.4. Lichtman stage II Kienböck disease. (*A*) PA radiograph of the wrist shows osteosclerosis of the lunate bone (*arrow*). (*B*) Coronal T1W MR image of the wrist shows low signal intensity throughout the lunate bone marrow (*arrow*). (*C*) Coronal STIR MR image shows patchy BME, which is false positive for viable bone marrow in the lunate in this patient (*arrow*). (*D*) Contrast-enhanced coronal T1W FS MR image shows lower signal intensity with nonenhancement of the lunate bone marrow as compared with the other carpal bones consistent with ON (*arrow*). Extensive enhancing synovitis is also seen in the carpal joints.

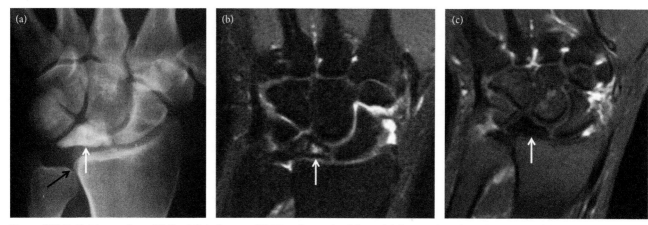

Figure 106.5. Lichtman stage IIIB Kienböck disease. (*A*) PA radiograph of the wrist shows sclerosis and collapse of the lunate bone (*white arrow*). Note associated negative ulnar variance (*black arrow*). (*B*) Coronal STIR MR image of the wrist shows patchy BME, which is false positive for viable bone marrow in the lunate (*arrow*). (*C*) Contrast-enhanced coronal T1W FS MR image shows lower signal intensity of the lunate bone marrow with nonenhancement as compared with the other carpal bones consistent with ON (*arrow*).

process and triquetrum), the meniscus homologue, and the tendon sheath of the extensor carpi ulnaris (ECU) tendon. The TFC (Figure 106.8) is thicker peripherally than centrally and attaches at the articular cartilage of the distal margin of the sigmoid notch at the ulnar aspect of the distal radius. The peripheral attachment of the TFC is named the *triangular ligament* and has 2 proximal and distal attachments (proximal and distal laminae). Peripherally, the TFC courses toward the ulnar head, and at its proximal lamina, it attaches in the fovea at the base of the ulnar styloid process. The attachment of the distal lamina is variable and extends to and beyond the ulnar styloid process and blends with the fibrous connective tissue of the ECU tendon sheath. The space between the proximal and distal laminae of the triangular ligament is termed the *ligamentum subcruentum*, which represents vascular tissue. The meniscus homologue (ulnomeniscal homologue) is a fibrous tissue on the ulnar aspect of the TFC, which merges

from the tip of the ulnar styloid process and inserts to the ulnar aspect of the triquetrum and lunate.

TFCC injury most commonly results from axial loading on the extended wrist in pronation. Racket sports athletes may present with TFCC injury caused by repetitive distraction loading on the volar aspect of the wrist. The presence of positive ulnar variance predisposes to TFC injury, either acute or chronic. TFC tears are classified according to the Palmer scheme as traumatic (class 1) and degenerative (class 2) (Table 106.2; Figures 106.9, 106.10, and 106.11). The class 2 tears are often the result of ulnocarpal impaction from a positive ulnar variance (abutment on the lunate bone) or rarely from an elongated ulnar styloid process (abutment on the triquetral bone) and secondary ulnar lengthening following malunion of distal radius fracture.

Patients with TFCC pathology usually present with ulnar-sided wrist pain, variable instability, and often with a

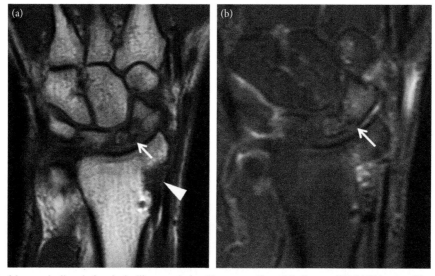

Figure 106.6. Scaphoid pseudarthrosis, treated with vascularized bone grafting. (*A*) Coronal T1W MR image 11 weeks following surgery, shows the vascularized bone graft placed between the proximal pole and distal scaphoid bone (*arrow*). The distal radial bone graft donor site is also seen (*arrowhead*). (*B*) T1W FS coronal MR image after IV contrast shows enhancement throughout the scaphoid bone suggesting normal incorporation of the bone graft (*arrow*).

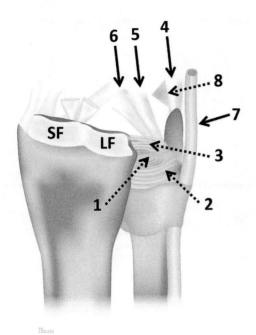

Figure 106.7. Artist drawing of the triangular fibrocartilage (TFCC) complex. 1 = triangular fibrocartilage (TFC); 2 = dorsal radioulnar ligament; 3 = volar radioulnar ligament; 4 = ulnar collateral ligament of the wrist; 5 = palmar ulnotriquetral ligament (extrinsic); 6 = palmar ulnolunate ligament (extrinsic); 7 = extensor carpi ulnaris tendon sheath; 8 = meniscus homologue. Also note distal radial articulating fossae for the scaphoid (SF) and lunate (LF).

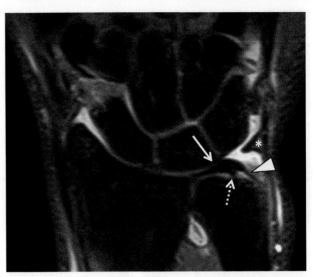

Figure 106.8. Normal TFC in a patient with joint effusions/synovitis. Coronal PDW FS MR image of the wrist shows normal low signal of the TFC (*arrow*) with normal appearance of its ulnar foveal/proximal lamina (*dashed arrow*) and ulnar styloid/distal lamina (*arrowhead*) attachment sites. Note the meniscus homologue (*asterisk*) at the ulnar aspect of the ulnocarpal joint. Also note mildly heterogeneous increased synovial-fluid complexes in all 3 compartments of the wrist including the distal radioulnar, radiocarpal, and midcarpal joints.

clicking or snapping sensation with rotation. Communicating tears represent full-thickness defects, whereas noncommunicating tears comprise partial-thickness defects of the TFC. Noncommunicating defects of the ulnar attachment of the disc, usually on its proximal side, are often symptomatic and result from trauma rather than from degeneration. Degenerative tears and perforations are age-related and usually occur in the central disc. Radial/central communicating tears are often bilateral and may be asymptomatic.

The dorsal and volar radioulnar ligaments are striated bands, arising from the dorsal and volar sigmoid notch cortex of the radius and inserting to the ulnar styloid process, blending with the TFC. Disruption of these ligaments may cause instability of the distal radioulnar joint (DRUJ), which is otherwise rare and characterized by dorsal subluxation of the ulna.

Imaging Strategy
- The complex anatomy of the TFCC, requires high-resolution MRI with high SNR and high-contrast resolution. This can be achieved with 1.5 or 3 T scanners, dedicated coils, and proper selection of various parameters such as FOV, slice thickness, and matrix size in order to maximize spatial resolution.
- Both 2D and 3D MR images are effective in detecting pathology. Coronal, sagittal, and axial PDW FS and coronal T2W* MRI sequences are routinely used.
- Direct MRA achieves the highest accuracy in detecting TFCC tears. A single radiocarpal injection is routinely adequate in assessing the contrast leak into the DRUJ or through the ulnar joint capsule suggesting capsular or UCL tear. In cases of no findings, a second injection of the DRUJ might be beneficial. High-resolution T1W FS images in 3 planes are acquired.

Table 106.2. Palmer Classification of TFCC Injuries

CLASS 1: TRAUMATIC INJURIES		CLASS 2: DEGENERATIVE INJURIES	
1A	Central perforation or tear	2A	TFC wear and thinning
1B	Ulnar avulsion	2B	Lunate and/or ulnar chondromalacia + 2A
1C	Distal avulsion (origin of ulnolunate and ulnotriquetral ligaments)	2C	TFC perforation + 2B
1D	Radial avulsion	2D	Ligament disruption + 2C
		2E	Ulnocarpal and DRUJ arthritis + 2D

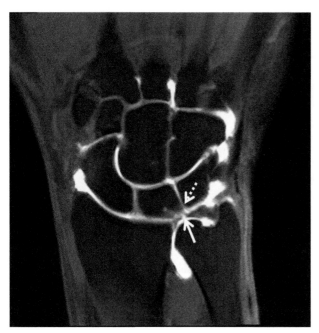

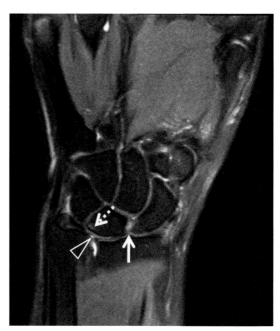

Figure 106.9. Central TFC tear and a small perforation of the central/proximal LTL band in a 59-year-old man with persistent pain status post fall 3 months prior to presentation. Coronal T1W FS MRA image of the wrist after radiocarpal joint injection shows extension of the radiocarpal joint contrast into the DRUJ through a central perforation of the TFC (*arrow*). A small amount of contrast extended into the midcarpal joint through a small perforation/tear of the central/proximal band of the LTL (*dashed arrow*).

Figure 106.10. Ulnar abutment syndrome and SLL tear in a 37-year-old woman with radial-sided wrist pain. Coronal PDW FS MR image of the wrist shows positive ulnar variance with small subchondral cystlike changes in the proximal ulnar aspect of the lunate (*dashed arrow*) with a degenerative central TFC tear (*arrowhead*). Note mild widening of the scapholunate interval with associated increased signal intensity consistent with a SLL tear (*arrow*).

- Indirect MRA following IV injection of 0.1 mmol/kg of Gd-based contrast was reported to be inferior to direct MRA and not superior to plain MRI.
- CTA is reserved for patients who are unable to undergo MRI.
- Direct MRA shows the highest accuracy for central and radial-sided disc tears (Palmer IA, ID, II). Moderate accuracy is achieved for peripheral tears of the ulnar attachment (Palmer IB, IC).
- DRUJ instability is best assessed with CT in pronation and supination with comparison of both wrists. Supination better shows the dorsal subluxation of the ulna.

Imaging Findings
- Normal TFC has a biconcave morphology, shows low signal intensity on all pulse sequences and is best seen on coronal (Figure 106.8), followed by sagittal images. It is important to be familiar with various pitfalls when reporting MRI of the TFCC.
- The hyaline cartilaginous extension of the radius on the sigmoid notch may simulate a tear at the central part of the TFC.
- The dorsal and volar radioulnar ligaments (best seen on the axial images) run parallel to the disc and may give an appearance of a split tear.
- Increased signal on fluid-sensitive MR sequences may be normally detected within the ligamentum subcruentum located between the 2 ulnar attachments of the disc

(proximal lamina/foveal attachment and distal lamina/styloid attachment).
- A focal abnormal signal intensity not extending to the surface of TFC probably represents mucoid degeneration.
- Abnormal MRI findings include partial- or full-thickness noncommunicating or communicating TFC tears with intraarticular contrast extending into the proximal or distal surface or through the whole substance of the TFC respectively (Figure 106.9).
- Pinhole disruptions located in the horizontal part of the disc are considered degenerative and have an increased prevalence in older patients.
- No specific imaging features can discriminate traumatic from degenerative tears. MRI findings in addition, may be similar in symptomatic and asymptomatic patients.
- The ulnar attachment is better delineated with MRA as opposed to PDW/T2W FS MR images because of the presence of fibrovascular tissue.
- With communicating TFC tears, MRA shows extension of the contrast from the radiocarpal to the DRUJ or the other way around, if single injection is performed (Figure 106.9).
- Two-compartment injection is required for depiction of noncommunicating tears of either the distal or proximal parts of the TFC.
- Ulnocarpal impaction or abutment is characterized by BME at the radial aspect of ulnar head and the proximal ulnar aspect of the lunate, and sometimes the triquetrum with later cystlike formation, associated with cartilage

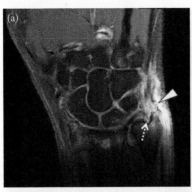
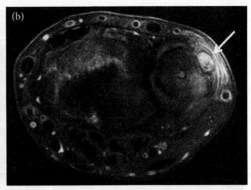

Figure 106.11. Peripheral TFCC tear and ECU tendon rupture in a 50-year-old man with history of a distal right radius fracture 3 months ago and persistent ulnar-sided wrist pain. (*A*) Coronal PDW FS MR image of the wrist shows marked increased signal at the TFC peripheral attachment site consistent with a tear (*dashed arrow*). There is high signal in the torn ulnar collateral ligament/ulnar joint capsule (*arrowhead*). Note mild increased signal related to BME about the healing distal radial metaphyseal and ulnar styloid process fractures. (*B*) Axial T2W FS MR image shows high signal synovial-fluid complex within the ECU tendon sheath in the ulnar groove at the dorsal aspect of the ulnar head. The ECU tendon is not visualized in keeping with rupture (*arrow*). Note adjacent high signal subcutaneous edema.

degeneration and central disc tear (Figure 106.10). Ulnar positive variance may, but does not have to, be present.

- Leak of the radiocarpal joint contrast through the ulnar joint capsule and/or into the ECU tendon sheath is indicative of peripheral TFCC injury (Figure 106.11).

Treatment Options

- Surgery is reserved for those patients who show no improvement after conservative treatment.
- Surgery aims at debridement or repair either with arthroscopy or open access.
- As a rule, elite athletes with acute tears are treated with surgical repair in order to quickly return to previous level of performance.
- Peripheral tears respond better to repair because of rich blood supply, whereas central disc tears show better outcome with debridement.
- Arthroscopic debridement is the preferred treatment approach for central Palmer class II tears.
- Ulnar shortening is a surgical option in patients with ulnocarpal impaction syndrome.

Ligaments of Wrist and Hand

Pathophysiology and Clinical Findings

Intrinsic (Interosseous) and Extrinsic (Capsular) Ligaments of the Wrist

Apart from the ligaments supporting the TFCC, the wrist consists of many ligaments, classified as *intrinsic* (interosseous) (Figures 106.12 and 106.13) and *extrinsic* (capsular) (Figure 106.14). The former connect the carpal bones and are important for maintaining the integrity of the proximal carpal row. The extrinsic ligaments connect the carpal bones either to the radius and ulna or to the metacarpal bones. Injuries may result in partial-thickness, full-thickness incomplete, and full-thickness complete tears. Depiction of the kind and extent of ligamentous injury contributes to patient management. The

most commonly injured ligaments and the most important ones for supporting the proximal carpal row are the intrinsic scapholunate (SLL) and lunotriquetral (LTL) (Figure 106.15). Common mechanism of injury to these ligaments is extension, ulnar deviation, and carpal supination, and their disruption leads to altered biomechanics. Repetitive stress-induced by crutch walking for SLL and ulnar impingement for LTL may also be the cause of injury.

The SLL is C-shaped and consists of dorsal, central, or membranous and volar or palmar bands (Figures 106.12 and 106.13). The dorsal band of the SLL is the most important for the stability of the wrist. Ligamentous tears of the dorsal SLL

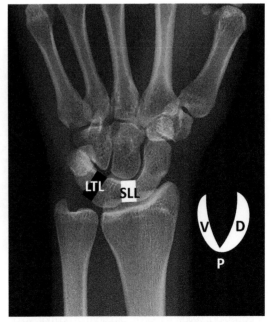

Figure 106.12. Diagram of the intrinsic scapholunate (SLL) and lunotriquetral (LTL) intrinsic (interosseous) wrist ligaments superimposed on a wrist radiograph. The inset illustrates the C-shaped SLL consisting of dorsal (D), central (proximal) or membranous (P), and volar/palmar (V) bands.

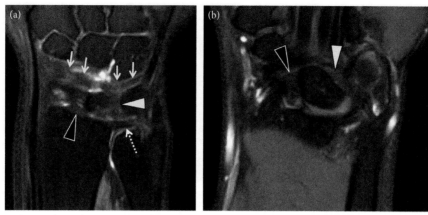

Figure 106.13. Normal MRI appearance of the dorsal and volar bands of the SLL and LTL. (*A*) Coronal PDW FS MR image of the wrist shows hypointense somewhat striated appearance of the normal dorsal band of the SLL (*black arrowhead*) and hypointense normal dorsal band of the LTL (*white arrowhead*). Note hypointense striated appearance of the normal dorsal intercarpal ligament (*white arrows*) and low signal of the normal TFC (*dashed white arrow*). (*B*) Coronal PDW FS MR image of the wrist shows a normal hypointense striated appearance of the volar bands of the SLL (*black arrowhead*) and LTL (*white arrowhead*).

band and at the lunate attachment are usually symptomatic and result from trauma rather than from degeneration. SLL disruption results in rotatory subluxation of the scaphoid and DISI (Figure 106.16), leading to SLAC wrist with proximal migration of the capitate with dorsal tilting of the lunate and OA changes of the radiocarpal and intercarpal joints. Scapholunate instability is associated with pain, tenderness, and swelling located at the dorsal and radial aspect of the wrist.

The LTL is V-shaped and consists of dorsal, central or membranous, and volar or palmar bands (Figures 106.12 and 106.13). This ligament is smaller than the SLL. The volar component blends with the TFCC and is the strongest. LTL disruption results in volar intercalated segmental instability (VISI)

with volar tilting of the lunate, which clinically presents with atypical pain and *clunking* during ulnar deviation. VISI may be a normal variant in patients with lax joints.

The extrinsic wrist ligaments are divided into palmar/volar and dorsal (Figure 106.14). The volar extrinsic wrist ligaments are stronger than dorsal and more important than dorsal for proper wrist function, but show variation in anatomy. The most important ones are the volar radioscaphocapitate, which prevents rotatory subluxation of the scaphoid and the volar radiolunotriquetral (a.k.a. long radiolunate), which connects the distal radius with the proximal carpal row. Tears of volar/palmar extrinsic wrist ligaments may contribute to the presence of DISI.

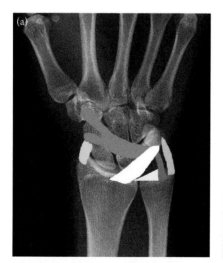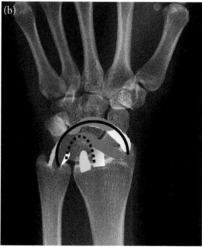

Figure 106.14. Diagram of extrinsic capsular and collateral ligaments of the wrist. (*A*) Diagram of dorsal extrinsic capsular wrist ligaments and collateral ligaments, superimposed on a wrist radiograph. *white* = dorsal radiocarpal ligament; *blue* = dorsal intercarpal ligament; *red* = dorsal ulnotriquetral ligament region; *green* = radial collateral ligament; *orange* = ulnar collateral ligament (ulnar capsular); *yellow* = TFC. (*B*) Diagram of palmar/volar extrinsic capsular wrist ligaments superimposed on wrist radiograph. *yellow* = radioscaphocapitate; *red* = long radiolunate; *gray* = radioscapholunate; *green* = short radiolunate; *white* = palmar ulnolunate; *blue* = palmar ulnotriquetral; *purple* = ulnocapitate; *pink* = palmar scaphotriquetral. The radioscaphocapitate and ulnocapitate ligaments interdigitate with the palmar scaphotriquetral ligament and form an arclike ligamentous structure termed the *arcuate ligament* (*black line*), which is the zone of perilunate fractures-dislocations. The *black dashed line* represents the lesser arc that outlines the radial, distal, and ulnar aspect of the lunate, which is the zone of perilunate and lunate dislocations.

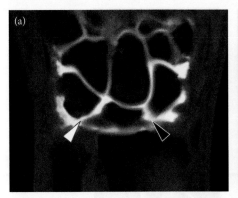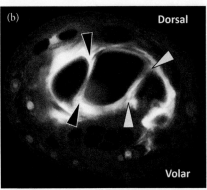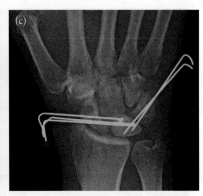

Figure 106.15. Complete acute posttraumatic tears of the SLL and LTL, which were treated surgically. (*A*) Coronal T1W FS MRA image of the wrist after radiocarpal joint injection shows contrast extension into the midcarpal joint through the complete tears of the central/proximal bands of the SLL (*black arrowhead*) and LTL (*white arrowhead*). (*B*) Axial T1W FS MRA image of the wrist shows complete tears of the dorsal and volar bands of the SLL (*black arrowheads*) and LTL (*white arrowheads*). (*C*) Postoperative PA radiograph of the wrist shows percutaneous K-wire fixation of the scapholunate and lunotriquetral intervals.

Two ulnar-sided volar extrinsic wrist ligaments are the palmar ulnolunate and palmar ulnotriquetral, which share the common proximal origin side from the volar radioulnar ligament. These ligaments contribute to stability of the TFCC.

The most important dorsal extrinsic ligament is the dorsal radiocarpal or radiolunotriquetral. An additional dorsal capsular wrist ligament is dorsal intercarpal, which extends from the scaphoid to the triquetrum and variably to the second metacarpal base.

A torn dorsal radiocarpal ligament may contribute to the presence of VISI, whereas a torn dorsal intercarpal ligament may contribute to DISI (Figure 106.16).

The RCL of the wrist is located at the radial aspect between the radial styloid and scaphoid bones and does not play a significant role in wrist stability (Figure 106.14*A*).

Overall, carpal instability is characterized by symptomatic malalignment and is classified as dissociative resulting from scaphoid fracture and intrinsic ligamentous disruption and nondissociative where interosseous ligaments are intact. Another classification is based on radiographs. In static instability, there is carpal malalignment on radiographs, whereas dynamic malalignment is depicted only with specific maneuvers during fluoroscopy or with specific views (ie, clenched fist).

Ligamentous/Supporting Structures of the Metacarpophalangeal and Interphalangeal Joints of the Hand

Radial and ulnar collateral ligaments support the radial and ulnar aspect of the MCP and interphalangeal (IP) joints of the hand, whereas the volar plate lies at the volar aspect. There are proper and accessory collateral ligaments at the radial and ulnar aspects of the IP joints and index through little-finger MCP joints (Figure 106.17). Injuries of any of these structures may occur leading to instability of the affected joint (Figure 106.18).

The UCL of the thumb MCP joint lies deep to the adductor pollicis tendon aponeurosis. Rupture of this ligament and slippage of the torn ligament end superficial to the adductor aponeurosis, is called a *Stener lesion*, whereas gamekeeper thumb comprises UCL tear without slippage outside the adductor aponeurosis (Figures 106.19 and 106.20).

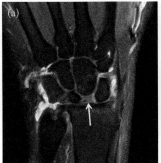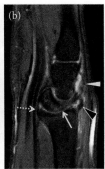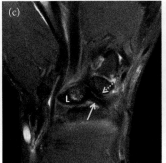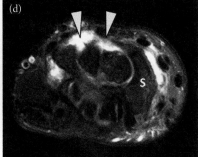

Figure 106.16. Scapholunate dissociation in a 37-year-old man status post fall. (*A*) Coronal PDW FS MR image of the wrist shows marked widening of the scapholunate joint/interval consistent with scapholunate dissociation (*arrow*). Note mildly increased synovial/fluid complexes in the radiocarpal and to a lesser extent midcarpal joints. (*B*) On the sagittal PDW FS image, note dorsal tilting of the lunate (*arrow*) in keeping with DISI deformity. Note high signal in the region of the torn dorsal intercarpal ligament (*white arrowhead*) and low signal in the normal short radiolunate (*dashed arrow*) and dorsal radiocarpal (*black arrowhead*) ligaments. (*C*) Coronal PDW FS MR image shows BME in the lunate (L) and normal low signal intensity of the visualized portions of the intact long radiolunate (*white arrow*) and radioscaphocapitate (*dashed white arrow*) palmar extrinsic wrist ligaments. (D) Axial T2W FS MR image shows disrupted dorsal intercarpal ligament (*arrowheads*). S = scaphoid.

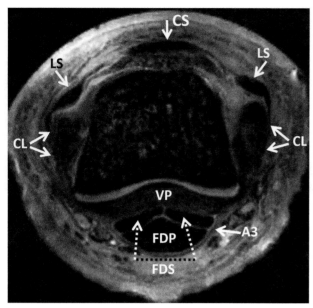

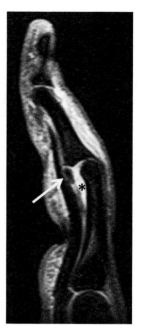

Figure 106.17. Normal anatomic structures of the PIP joint of a cadaveric finger. Axial GRE MR image of the PIP joint of a finger at the level of the proximal phalangeal head obtained on a 9.4 T research MRI machine shows normal central slip of the extensor tendon (CS), lateral slips of the extensor tendon (LS), proper and accessory collateral ligaments (CL), volar plate (VP), flexor digitorum superficialis (FDS) tendon, flexor digitorum profundus (FDP) tendon, and an A3 flexor pulley.

Figure 106.18. Volar subluxation of the middle finger PIP joint. Sagittal PDW FS MR image of the middle finger shows volar subluxation of the PIP joint with associated volar plate detachment from the proximal phalanx (*arrow*). Note lifting/bowstringing of the adjacent flexor tendon from the bony structures with subjacent high signal (*asterisk*) related to A3 and C1 pulley injuries.

These lesions should be suspected in cases with the *skier's thumb* with a small avulsion fracture at the ulnar aspect of the proximal phalangeal base. Soft tissue swelling makes clinical diagnosis difficult.

The extensor hood represents a triangular shape fibrous expansion at the dorsal aspect of the proximal phalanx of each digit with the base wrapped around the dorsal and lateral aspects of the MCP joints. The extensor digitorum longus or extensor pollicis longus tendons blend with these expansions. Sagittal bands and the interosseal and lumbrical muscle fibers contribute to the extensor hood. The central slips (bands) of

the extensor digitorum tendons attach to the dorsal aspect of the middle phalangeal base and the distally joined lateral bands (slips) at the distal phalangeal base (Figure 106.21). The extensor hood prevents subluxation/dislocation of the extensor tendons (Figure 106.22).

Imaging Strategy
- Imaging should start with wrist radiographs, which can demonstrate DISI and VISI, as well as SLAC wrist deformities.

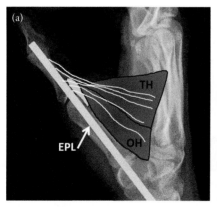

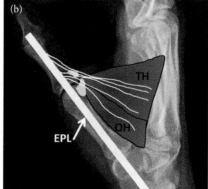

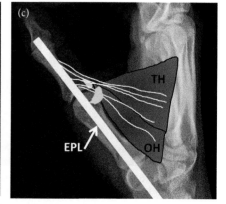

Figure 106.19. Diagram of the intact and torn UCL of the thumb MCP joint, superimposed on a hand radiograph. (*A*) The UCL (*green*) is seen underneath the adductor aponeurosis (*white lines*), which extends over the transverse (TH) and oblique (OH) heads of the adductor pollicis muscle and attaches onto the medial aspect of the proximal phalanx of the thumb. In (*B*), the UCL is completely torn but remains underneath the adductor aponeurosis. In (*C*), the UCL is torn with the proximal stump displaced beyond the adductor aponeurosis consistent with Stener lesion. EPL = extensor pollicis longus tendon.

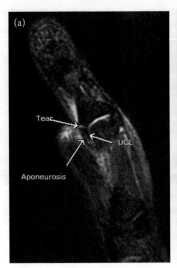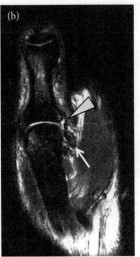

Figure 106.20. Gamekeeper thumb and Stener lesion. (*A*) Coronal PDW FS MR image of the thumb shows complete UCL tear at the proximal phalangeal side, which remains normally positioned underneath the adductor aponeurosis in keeping with gamekeeper thumb injury. (*B*) Coronal PDW FS image or the thumb shows a torn UCL (*arrow*) displaced beyond the adductor aponeurosis (*arrowhead*).The torn UCL has an appearance of yo-yo on string sign, which is consistent with a Stener lesion. (Courtesy of Kirkland Davis, MD)

- With suspected ligamentous injuries of the small joints of the hand and digits, imaging should start with dedicated radiographs.
- High-resolution T1W and fluid-sensitive FS 3T MRI with dedicated wrist coils and proper technique in 3 orthogonal planes, including thin submillimeter GRE sequences, is frequently sufficient in depicting normal anatomy and most of the intrinsic and extrinsic ligamentous injuries of the wrist, as well as ligamentous injuries of the small joints in the hand. MRA may improve visualization of the wrist ligaments.
- In most patients, US is able to evaluate the intrinsic and extrinsic wrist ligaments and the ligaments of the small joints of the hand and may be used if the proper expertise is available.

- With MRA of the wrist, a single injection in the radiocarpal joint is enough, provided that there is no symptomatology at the ulnar side of the wrist with possible undersurface TFC tears. In cases of contraindication for MRI, CTA shows excellent results in addition to fewer motion artifacts caused by fast acquisition of MR images. Articular distraction with only 3-kg loading may improve the quality of the MR images by means of widening the joint spaces and better delineating the articulate cartilage surface.
- Dynamic fluoroscopy under stress is widely applied in some centers with accurate results regarding SLL and LTL tears. These tests should be applied after excluding fractures from radiographs if persistent pain and swelling are present after acute trauma.
- A Stener lesion requires MRI or high-frequency US for accurate diagnosis.

Imaging Findings
- The PA radiograph in SLL disruption may show the *Terry Thomas* sign when the distance between the scaphoid and lunate is more than 3 mm. On the PA radiograph, the lunate may have a pie-shaped appearance caused by dorsal tilting. On the lateral radiograph, a scapholunate angle between 60 and 80 degrees is indeterminate. A scapholunate angle greater than 80 degrees is diagnostic for DISI. A capitolunate angle greater than 30 degrees is also suggestive of DISI. Measurements on MRI are not reliable in borderline cases.
- VISI is suggested on lateral radiographs when the scapholunate angle is less than 30 degrees and the capitolunate angle is more than 30 degrees. It is not as common as DISI. Radiographs show volar rotation of the lunate and dorsal rotation of the capitate and hamate.
- The dorsal SLL band shows homogenously low signal intensity on MRI. The other 2 bands show intermediate signal, resulting from the presence of fibrovascular components (Figure 106.13).

Figure 106.21. Artist drawing of the flexor and extensor tendons of the finger. FDP = flexor digitorum profundus; FDS = flexor digitorum superficialis; LM = lumbrical muscle; IM = interosseous muscle; ET = extensor tendon; DE = dorsal expansion; CL = collateral ligaments; CB = central band (slip); LB = lateral band; DI = distal phalangeal insertion of the terminal extensor tendon.

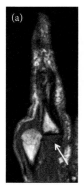
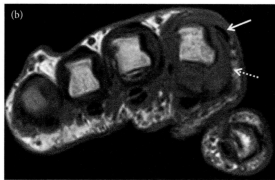
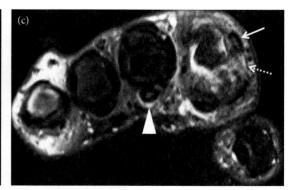

Figure 106.22. Dislocation of the second MCP joint with extensor hood injury in a 59-year-old man. (*A*) Sagittal T1W MR image shows volar dislocation of the second MCP joint with associated volar plate tear (*arrow*). Axial (*B*) T1W and (*C*) T2W FS MR images show radial dislocation of the common extensor tendon (*arrows*) secondary to extensor hood disruption (*dashed arrows*). Incidentally, in (*C*) note mildly increased synovial-fluid complex in the middle finger flexor tendon sheath and mild irregularity of the flexor tendons consistent with tenosynovitis.

- On routine MRI, the abnormal SLL may show irregular margins, fraying, increased signal on fluid-sensitive sequences, and discontinuity or absence of the fibers, with or without widening of the scapholunate distance.
- On axial images, heterogenous band-like signal is seen in the dorsal and volar components of an injured LTL.
- Depiction of a tear is much easier with MRA, which should include high-resolution axial or axial oblique images for evaluation of the dorsal band of the SLL and its attachments, particularly onto the lunate bone.

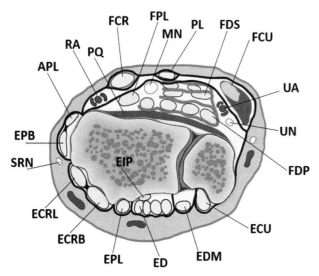

Figure 106.23. Artist drawing of the flexor and 6 extensor compartment tendons of the wrist at the level of the pronator quadratus (PQ) muscle. FCR = flexor carpi radialis; FPL = flexor pollicis longus; FDS = flexor digitorum superficialis; FDP = flexor digitorum profundus; PL = palmaris longus; FCU = flexor carpi ulnaris; first extensor compartment (APL = abductor pollicis longus; EPB = extensor pollicis brevis); second extensor compartment (ECRL = extensor carpi radialis longus; ECRB = extensor carpi radialis brevis); third extensor compartment (EPL = extensor pollicis longus); fourth extensor compartment (ED = extensor digitorum; EIP = extensor indicis proprius); fifth extensor compartment (EDM = extensor digiti minimi); sixth extensor compartment (ECU = extensor carpi ulnaris); MN = median nerve; UN = ulnar nerve; SRN = superficial radial nerve; RA = radial artery; UA = ulnar artery.

- The membranous components of both SLL and LTL are best depicted on coronal MRA and CTA images.
- Full-thickness tears of any of the SLL and LTL bands allow abnormal communication (contrast leak) between the radiocarpal and midcarpal joints (Figure 106.15*A*).
- It is important to mention that degenerative perforations of the central part of both SLL and LTL ligaments tend to increase with age and may remain asymptomatic.
- SLAC wrist may be depicted with either radiographs or MRI.
- Extrinsic wrist ligaments can be depicted with MRI and MRA, including 3D isotropic imaging, and have a striated appearance (Figure 106.16*C*). All imaging planes are used for their assessment.
- Injuries of extrinsic ligaments may coexist with injuries of intrinsic ligaments in carpal instability. The torn ligaments show discontinuity of the fibers, whereas the partially torn ligaments show irregularity of the fibers and/or increased signal on fluid-sensitive sequences.
- MRI of gamekeeper thumb injury shows discontinuity of the ligamentous fibers, usually from the proximal phalangeal attachment site with associated high signal intensity, but without extension of the torn ligament beyond adductor aponeurosis (Figure 106.20*A*). With the Stener lesion, the torn ligamentous fibers are flipped superficial to the adductor aponeurosis creating a yo-yo on the string sign (Figure 106.20*B*).

Treatment Options

Treatment options for patients with dissociative carpal instability depend on the degree of instability, the time elapsed from initial injury, the presence of OA, and daily functional demands.

- Partial-thickness SLL tears can be treated with arthroscopic debridement.
- Complete SLL tears with instability may be treated with debridement and percutaneous pinning with K-wires (Figure 106.15*C*).
- Failed repair or severe chronic lesions of the wrist ligaments, such as in SLAC wrist, may be treated with

proximal row carpectomy, indicated for patients older than 35 years, or scaphoid excision with 4-corner fusion (of capitate-hamate-lunate-triquetrum).

- Isolated LTL tears are treated conservatively with immobilization, NSAIDs, and steroid injections.
- Operative treatment of LTL tears is reserved for those with acute or chronic injuries showing a VISI deformity and include repair for acute injuries and ligament reconstruction (with ECU tendon) for chronic LTL instability, which has better outcome compared to arthrodesis.
- Surgery is the treatment of choice for a Stener lesion, whereas the gamekeeper thumb is typically treated conservatively.

Tendons and Muscles of the Wrist and Hand

Normal Anatomy

Normal anatomy of dorsal and volar wrist and hand tendons and muscles is complex. There are 6 extensor compartments at the dorsal aspect of the wrist under the extensor retinaculum that extend distally and attach onto the metacarpal bones and phalanges. Flexor tendons are situated at the volar aspect of the wrist and extend distally with the majority attaching onto the metacarpal bones and phalanges (Figure 106.23). The origin and the attachment sites of the wrist and hand muscles and tendons are described in Tables 106.3 and 106.4.

The carpal tunnel is an anatomic space at the volar aspect of the carpal bones under the thick flexor retinaculum (Figure 106.24). The radial margin of the carpal tunnel consists of the scaphoid bone, trapezium, and the flexor carpi radialis (FCR) tendon sheath, whereas the ulnar border consists of the hook of the hamate, triquetrum, and pisiform bones. The flexor retinaculum extends from the distal radius to the metacarpal bases and can be divided into 3 components, including the antebrachial fascia, transverse carpal ligament, and distal aponeurosis between the thenar and hypothenar muscles. This space contains 9 tendons including the 4 flexor digitorum superficialis and 4 flexor digitorum profundus tendons, all within the ulnar bursa, and the flexor pollicis longus tendon, which is located at the radial aspect lying within the radial bursa. The ulnar bursa is frequently in continuity with the fifth digit flexor tendon sheath, whereas the second through fourth digits have separate flexor tendon sheaths. The radial bursa is in continuity with the flexor pollicis longus tendon sheath at the volar aspect of the thumb. However, there are anatomic variations of the ulnar and radial bursae. The FCR tendon has its own osteofibrous tunnel and is separated from the carpal tunnel by the deep portion of the transverse carpal ligament that splits along its radial border, surrounding this tendon and bridging across the trapezium. The palmaris longus tendon is present in approximately 14% of the population and is located superficial to the flexor retinaculum. It inserts onto the central part of the flexor retinaculum and lower part of the palmar aponeurosis.

There are several muscles in the hand including the thenar musculature at the radial volar side, hypothenar musculature at the ulnar volar side, and the interosseous and lumbrical musculature between the metacarpals and proximal phalanges (Table 106.5).

Flexor tendons are secured to the volar aspect of the second through fifth fingers with 5 annular and 3 cruciate pulleys (Figure 106.25). It should be noted that pulley anatomy of the thumb is more variable and consists of A1, A2, oblique, and in some instances, variable pulleys. Injuries of the flexor pulleys may cause bowstringing of the flexor tendons (Figure 106.18).

In some individuals, additional accessory tendons and muscles may be present, which should not be mistaken for pathology. These on the palmar side include the accessory flexor digitorum superficialis indicis muscle, accessory hypothenar muscles, and FCR brevis vel profundus. On the dorsal side, the accessory muscles include extensor digitorum brevis manus and accessory extensor carpi radialis. One should be aware of additional common anatomic variants, such as septation of the first extensor compartment tendon sheath, supernumerary tendons in the first extensor compartment, and bifid ECU tendon, which should not be mistaken for pathology.

Pathophysiology and Clinical Findings

Tendinosis is a general term for tendon degeneration resulting from trauma, repetitive loading, or inflammatory disorder. *Tendinopathy* is the clinical counterpart of tendinosis with pain, swelling, and limited function of a specific tendon (Figure 106.26). Tendon tears (Figure 106.27) may result from acute trauma, chronic friction, systemic disease, and longstanding tendinosis and are associated with functional limitations during clinical examination. A small amount of fluid in the tendon sheath in a patient who has no history of trauma or symptoms is a normal finding. Tenosynovitis is characterized by synovial thickening of the tendon sheath and presence of excess fluid within it (Figure 106.28). The most common form of tenosynovitis is *de Quervain syndrome*, often seen bilaterally in middle-aged women, young mothers carrying babies, and athletes involved in racket sports (Figure 106.29). *De Quervain* tenosynovitis affects the first extensor compartment tendons; the abductor pollicis longus (APL) and extensor pollicis brevis (EPB). Clinically, pain and swelling are located over the radial styloid process. On physical examination, there is increased pain with thumb extension and abduction as well as with wide grasping. The ECU tendon disorders include tenosynovitis, tendinopathy, subluxation, or frank dislocation caused by sheath disruption and tendon rupture. Patients with RA commonly present with tenosynovitis and tendinopathy, but rarely tendon tears. Tenosynovitis in RA is often seen around the ECU tendon and other extensor and flexor tendons of the wrist and hand. Flexor tendons tenosynovitis may also be seen in psoriatic arthropathy. Tenosynovitis often occurs in athletes from overuse injuries, most commonly in racket sports and golf. ECU tendon subluxation usually follows an acute injury (Figure 106.30). Tenosynovitis of a finger flexor tendon, also known as *trigger finger*, results from abnormal thickening of the A1 pulley close to the MCP joint.

Intersection syndrome is an overuse, most commonly chronic, inflammatory condition that occurs at the dorsal radial aspect of the distal forearm, 4-5 cm proximal to the radiocarpal joint (Figure 106.31), at the crossing point of the first and second extensor compartment tendons, proximal to the more common condition of de Quervain tenosynovitis. Intersection syndrome results from repetitive friction, which can lead to tenosynovitis, stenosing tenosynovitis, and

FIRST EXTENSOR COMPARTMENT	ORIGIN	ATTACHMENT
Abductor pollicis longus	Middle one-third of the posterior surface of the radius, interosseous membrane, midportion of posterolateral ulna	Radial side of the base of the first metacarpal
Extensor pollicis brevis	Interosseous membrane and the posterior surface of the distal radius	Base of the proximal phalanx of the thumb
SECOND EXTENSOR COMPARTMENT	**ORIGIN**	**ATTACHMENT**
Extensor carpi radialis longus	Lower one-third of the lateral supracondylar ridge of the humerus	Dorsum of the second metacarpal base
Extensor carpi radialis brevis	Common extensor tendon (lateral epicondyle of the humerus)	Dorsum of the third metacarpal base
THIRD EXTENSOR COMPARTMENT	**ORIGIN**	**ATTACHMENT**
Extensor pollicis longus	Interosseous membrane and middle part of the posterolateral surface of the ulna	Dorsal aspect of the thumb distal phalangeal base
FOURTH EXTENSOR COMPARTMENT	**ORIGIN**	**ATTACHMENT**
Extensor indicis proprius	Interosseous membrane and the posterolateral surface of the distal ulna	Joins the tendon of the extensor digitorum to the second digit; both tendons insert into the extensor expansion
Extensor digitorum	Common extensor tendon (lateral epicondyle of the humerus)	Extensor expansion at the dorsal aspect of the second through fifth digits
FIFTH EXTENSOR COMPARTMENT	**ORIGIN**	**ATTACHMENT**
Extensor digiti minimi	Common extensor tendon (lateral epicondyle of the humerus)	Joins the extensor digitorum tendon of the fifth digit and inserts into the extensor expansion
SIXTH EXTENSOR COMPARTMENT	**ORIGIN**	**ATTACHMENT**
Extensor carpi ulnaris	Common extensor tendon and the middle one-half of the posterior border of the ulna	Ulnar side of fifth metacarpal base
OTHER	**ORIGIN**	**ATTACHMENT**
Brachioradialis	Upper two-thirds of the lateral supracondylar ridge of the humerus	Lateral side of the radial styloid process base

Table 106.3. Tendons at the Dorsal Aspect of the Wrist and Hand

sometimes formation of an adventitial bursa. This condition is commonly associated with rowing and racket sports. Less commonly, this condition results from direct trauma. Patients present with radial wrist or forearm pain exacerbated by flexion and extension. Swelling and tenderness may be present in the affected region.

Distal intersection syndrome comprises a friction tenosynovitis caused by the third extensor compartment tendon crossing the second compartment tendons just distal to Lister's tubercle. The second and third extensor compartments tendon sheaths communicate through a foramen that allows the spread of inflammation between them. This condition is most commonly associated with wrist trauma and may be prolonged. Predisposing conditions are various rheumatologic and degenerative diseases. Patients present with pain and swelling over Lister's tubercle and less commonly with local crepitus during thumb movements.

Imaging Strategy

- Frequently, US is the first-line examination for tendon disorders as it is fast; combines clinical examination with imaging findings; can show abnormalities, such

Table 106.4. Tendons at the Volar Aspect of the Wrist and Hand

TENDONS AT THE VOLAR ASPECT OF THE WRIST AND HAND	ORIGIN	ATTACHMENT
Flexor pollicis longus	Anterior surface of radius and interosseous membrane	Volar aspect of the thumb distal phalangeal base
Flexor carpi radialis	Common flexor tendon (medial epicondyle of the humerus)	Second and third metacarpal bases
Flexor digitorum superficialis	Humeroulnar head: common flexor tendon; radial head: middle third of radius	Radial and ulnar sides at the volar aspect of the middle phalangeal shafts of second through fifth digits
Flexor digitorum profundus	Posterior border of the ulna, proximal two-thirds of medial border of ulna, interosseous membrane	Volar aspect of the distal phalangeal bases of the second through fifth digits
Flexor carpi ulnaris	Common flexor tendon and (ulnar head) from medial border of olecranon and upper two-thirds of the posterior border of the ulna	Pisiform, hook of hamate, and fifth metacarpal base
Palmaris longus	Medial epicondyle of the humerus	Distal half of flexor retinaculum and palmar aponeurosis
Pronator quadratus	Medial side of the anterior surface of the distal one-fourth of the ulna	Anterior surface of the distal one-fourth of the radius

as subluxation, during dynamic maneuvers; and allows image-guided treatment.

■ Flexor and extensor tendons of the hand and wrist are best evaluated on axial T1W and fluid-sensitive MRI sequences.

Imaging Findings

■ Normal tendons should be of low signal intensity on all MR imaging pulse sequences.

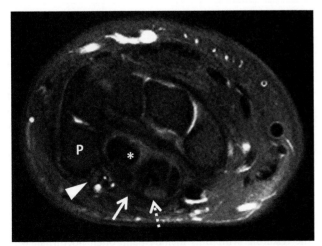

Figure 106.24. Normal carpal tunnel. Axial T2W FS MR image shows normal contents of the carpal tunnel under the flexor retinaculum (*arrow*) at the level of the pisiform bone (P). Note normal signal in the median nerve (*dashed arrow*), ulnar nerve (*arrowhead*), and flexor tendon (*asterisk*).

■ On MRI, tendinosis is characterized by a heterogeneous high signal intensity and thickening (Figure 106.26).

■ Partial-thickness tendon tears show attenuation of the affected tendons, whereas the full-thickness tears or tendon ruptures show complete discontinuity of the tendon fibers (106.11*B* and 106.27).

■ Active tenosynovitis-related inflammation shows enhancement on MRI (Figure 106.29).

■ Intersection syndrome: The main finding on MRI is peritendinous edema concentrically surrounding the second and first extensor compartments centered on the crossing point with variable distal extension (Figure 106.31). There may be fluid in the affected tendon sheaths or at the interval between the tendon sheaths at the intersection point. Tendinosis with increased intrasubstance signal within the affected tendon/s may also be present.

Treatment Options

■ Tendinosis is typically treated conservatively.

■ Tendon ruptures require direct repair and in cases with a gap greater than 3 cm, tendon grafting is the preferred technique.

■ Tenosynovitis and ECU tendon subluxation are initially treated with casting for several weeks. Persistent subluxation may require surgical reconstruction of the ulnar groove and the retinaculum.

■ Steroid injections have been used in de Quervain tenosynovitis, ECU tenosynovitis, and trigger finger. Surgery is reserved for failed conservative treatment, aiming at tendon lengthening and debridement.

Table 106.5. Intrinsic Muscles of the Hand

THENAR MUSCLES	ORIGIN	ATTACHMENT
Opponens pollicis	Trapezial tubercle and flexor retinaculum	Lateral margin and adjacent palmar surface of the first metacarpal
Abductor pollicis brevis	Scaphoid and trapezial tubercles and adjacent flexor retinaculum	Proximal phalanx and extensor hood of the thumb
Flexor pollicis brevis	Trapezial tubercle and flexor retinaculum	Proximal phalanx of the thumb
HYPOTHENAR MUSCLES	ORIGIN	ATTACHMENT
Opponens digiti minimi	Hook of the hamate and flexor retinaculum	Medial aspect of the fifth metacarpal
Abductor digiti minimi	Pisiform, pisohamate ligament, and flexor carpi ulnaris tendon	Fifth digit proximal phalanx
Flexor digiti minimi brevis	Hook of the hamate and flexor retinaculum	Fifth digit proximal phalanx
INTEROSSEI	ORIGIN	ATTACHMENT
Dorsal	Four muscles, each arising from 2 adjacent metacarpal shafts	Proximal phalangeal base and the extensor expansion on lateral side of the second digit, lateral and medial sides of the third digit, and medial side of the fourth digit
Palmar	Four muscles, arising from the palmar surface of the first, second, fourth, and fifth metacarpal shafts (the first palmar interosseous is often fused with the adductor pollicis muscle)	Proximal phalangeal base and extensor expansion of the medial side of the first and second digits, and lateral side of the fourth and fifth digits
LUMBRICAL	ORIGIN	ATTACHMENT
Four muscles	Flexor digitorum profundus tendons of the second through fifth digits	Extensor expansion on the radial side of the proximal phalanx of the second through fifth digits
Palmaris brevis	Palmar aponeurosis and flexor retinaculum	Skin at the medial margin of the hand
Adductor pollicis	Transverse head, third metacarpal; oblique head, capitate and second and third metacarpal bases	Proximal phalangeal base and extensor hood of the thumb

- Proximal intersection syndrome: Conservative management with immobilization, activity modification, NSAIDs, and/or local corticosteroid injection are usually sufficient. Surgical treatment is reserved for recalcitrant cases.
- Distal intersection syndrome: Usually nonoperative; for those with persistent pain, operative treatment may be considered.

Neuropathies/Nerve Entrapment in the Wrist and Hand Normal Anatomy, Pathophysiology, and Clinical Findings

Median Nerve

The median nerve is the most superficial structure at the radial aspect of the carpal tunnel (Figure 106.24). A bifid median nerve with persistent median artery is a common normal anatomic variant.

Carpal tunnel syndrome (CTS) is the most common nerve entrapment disorder in the upper limb. It may be idiopathic or occur when the median nerve is compressed by various causes including lunate dislocation, hematoma, and inflammation of the flexor tendons in the context of rheumatologic disorders. Other causes are obesity, diabetes, pregnancy, hypothyroidism, amyloid deposition, OA of the thumb carpometacarpal joint, and space-occupying lesions, both intraneural and extraneural. The median nerve is compressed between the carpal bones and flexor retinaculum and the resulting symptoms include pain, often nocturnal, with tingling and numbness in the thumb, index, and middle fingers. Atrophy and weakness of the thenar musculature along with disturbed sensation of the thumb to the lateral half of the fourth digit and intact sensation of the thenar eminence are often found. Clinically, a positive Tinel test (light percussion

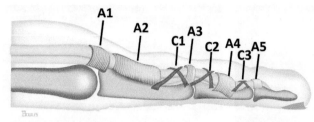

Figure 106.25. Artist drawing of the annular (A) and cruciate (C) flexor pulleys of the finger. Note normal anatomic location of the 5 annular (A1-A5) and 3 cruciate (C1-C3) flexor pulleys.

over the nerve that elicits a sensation of tingling or *pins and needles* in the distribution of the nerve), further supports the diagnosis.

Ulnar Nerve

The *ulnar nerve* lies within the *Guyon canal* (ulnar tunnel), an oblique fibroosseous tunnel formed by the flexor retinaculum and palmar carpal ligament, within the proximal part of the hypothenar eminence. The canal is approximately 4 cm long, begins at the proximal extent of the transverse carpal ligament at the level of the proximal pisiform, and ends at the aponeurotic arch of the hypothenar musculature at the level of the hamate hook.

Ulnar nerve compression may occur proximal to the Guyon canal (type I) or within the canal (type II), with isolated involvement of the superficial sensory branch. Compression may result from ganglion cysts, neuroma, and accessory muscles. Rarely, hypertrophy of the flexor carpi ulnaris tendon, ulnar artery pseudoaneurysm, OA of the pisotriquetral joint and hamate, or pisiform fractures may lead to ulnar nerve compression.

Clinically, fourth and fifth digit sensory loss with weakness of both may be present. On physical examination, sensory deficit of the little finger and ulnar half of the ring finger along with "claw" deformity of the ring and little fingers caused by weakness of the intrinsic muscles are found. Bilateral

neurapraxia may occur from external compression and repetitive microtrauma, such as in chronic use of forearm crutches or in cyclists.

Radial Nerve

Wartenberg syndrome (cheiralgia paresthetica), which results from isolated pathology of the superficial radial nerve, is rare. The patients present with pain over the dorsolateral aspect of the hand. The entrapment of the superficial radial nerve occurs between the brachioradialis and the extensor carpi radialis longus tendons.

Imaging Strategy

- In CTS, MRI may contribute to the diagnosis in patients with atypical symptoms and signs in the preoperative setting, in patients presenting with a palpable mass producing the CTS or in those with recurrent symptoms following surgical release.
- Newer MRI techniques, including diffusion tensor imaging with tractography, are increasingly applied for assessing the median nerve.
- MRI in Guyon canal and Wartenberg syndromes is valuable in detecting and characterizing any space-occupying lesions, which might compress the ulnar and superficial radial nerves, respectively.

Imaging Findings

- On MRI, the median nerve has an appearance of a rounded or slightly flattened structure of intermediate signal intensity with a rather constant caliber from the DRUJ up to the level of the hook of the hamate (Figure 106.28). Long-standing CTS may be associated with thinning and fibrosis of the median nerve.
- MRI findings in keeping with CTS (Figure 106.32) include increased signal within the median nerve, enlargement of the nerve at the level of the pisiform, and flattening at the level of the hook of the hamate.

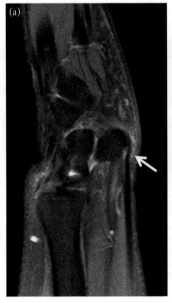
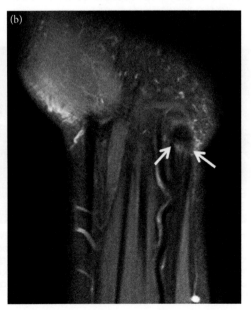

Figure 106.26. Tendinosis of the FCU tendon in a 41-year-old woman with volar ulnar-sided wrist pain. (*A*) Sagittal and (*B*) coronal PD FS MR images of the wrist show thickening, irregularity, and heterogeneous increased signal in the distal FCU tendon consistent with tendinosis (*arrows*).

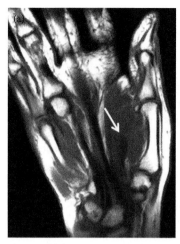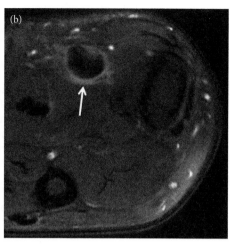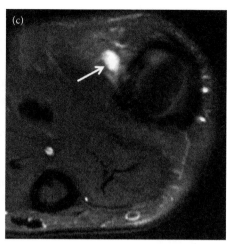

Figure 106.27. Laceration of the FPL tendon in a 42-year-old man. (*A*) Coronal T1W MR image of the hand shows rupture of the FPL tendon with proximal retraction of the tendon stump (*arrow*). (*B*) On the axial T2W FS MR image, note thickening of the FPL tendon stump with a small amount of fluid in the tendon sheath (*arrow*). (*C*) Axial T2W FS MR image at the level of the thumb MCP joint shows fluid in the FPL tendon sheath (arrow) with no tendon seen.

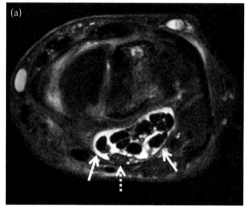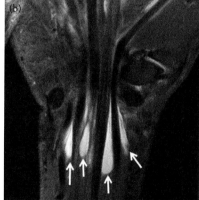

Figure 106.28. Tenosynovitis of the wrist flexor tendons in a 76-year-old man. (*A*) Axial T2W FS and (*B*) coronal PDW FS MR images of the wrist show moderately distended ulnar and radial bursae (*arrows*) about the flexor tendons at the volar aspect of the wrist in keeping with tenosynovitis. In (*A*), note normal appearance of the median nerve in the proximal carpal tunnel (*dashed arrow*).

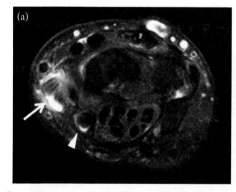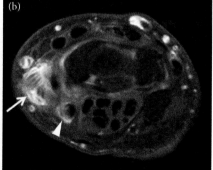

Figure 106.29. De Quervain syndrome in a 58-year-old woman. (*A*) Axial T2W FS MR image shows a markedly distended first extensor compartment tendon sheath (*arrow*) with indistinctness and increased signal in the APL and EPB tendons consistent with tenosynovitis/de Quervain syndrome. Note a small amount of fluid in the adjacent FCR tendon sheath with associated mild tendon thickening and signal heterogeneity consistent with tenosynovitis (*arrowhead*). (*B*) Axial T1W FS postcontrast MR image shows extensive heterogeneous synovial enhancement in the first extensor compartment tendon sheath (*arrow*) and incidentally additional synovial enhancement in the FCR tendon sheath (*arrowhead*).

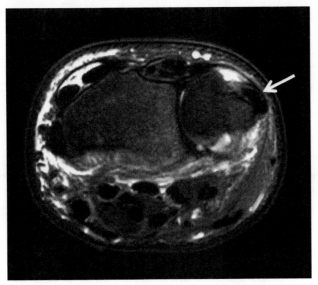

Figure 106.30. Tendinosis and posttraumatic subluxation of the ECU tendon. Axial T2W FS MRA image of the wrist in a patient with traumatic TFCC injury shows ulnar subluxation of the ECU (*arrow*). Note thickening and mild irregularity of the ECU consistent with tendinosis and high signal Gd-based contrast in the tendon sheath extending from the radiocarpal joint secondary to peripheral TFCC injury.

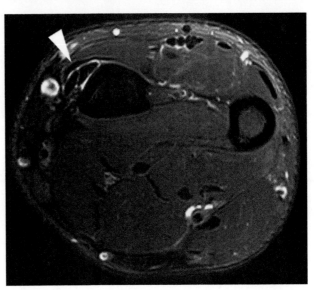

Figure 106.31. Intersection syndrome (proximal). Axial T2W FS MR image shows a small amount of fluid about the crossing point of the first and second extensor compartment tendons (*arrowhead*) at the dorsal radial aspect of the distal forearm consistent with intersection syndrome.

- Other MRI findings that are associated with CTS include thenar muscle denervation edema (Figure 106.32) and/or atrophy, reactive hypertrophy of the lumbrical muscles, palmar bowing of the flexor retinaculum, and median nerve enhancement, which is marked in edematous and reduced in ischemic nerves.
- Guyon canal syndrome is explored with MRI for assessing any lesion compressing the nerve. The ulnar nerve is swollen proximal to the canal and flattened within the canal with increased signal on fluid-sensitive sequences. Secondary signs of neuropathy are denervation edema of the hypothenar muscles, third/fourth lumbricals, and interosseous muscles, with or without atrophy.
- Common causes of Wartenberg syndrome are de Quervain syndrome and soft tissue ganglions, which can easily be detected with MRI.

Treatment Options
- Treatment for CTS is initially conservative. Persistent symptoms lead to surgical release of the flexor retinaculum either open or with endoscopy.
- Steroid injection around the median nerve may reduce inflammation.
- Soft tissue ganglia may be treated either with surgical excision or with image-guided aspiration and steroid injection.
- For ulnar nerve compression within Guyon canal, treatment aims at the underlying cause, that is, removal of a space-occupying lesion with simultaneous decompression of the tunnel.
- Treatment of Wartenberg syndrome aims at the primary cause of nerve compression (ie, de Quervain tenosynovitis or soft tissue ganglion).

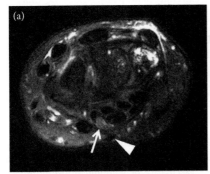
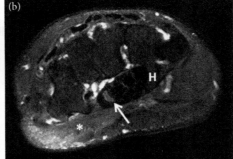

Figure 106.32. CTS in an 86-year-old woman. Axial T2WFS MR images of the wrist through the carpal tunnel show enlargement and minimal edema of the median nerve (*arrow*) in (*A*) at the level of the pisiform and flattening (*arrow*) in (*B*) at the level of the hamate hook (H) with minimal denervation edema in the thenar musculature (*asterisk*) consistent with CTS. In (*A*), incidentally noted is the palmaris longus tendon (*arrowhead*).

Key Points: Occult Fractures, and Osteonecrosis of the Scaphoid and Lunate

- Initial evaluation of scaphoid fractures and complications and Kienböck disease starts with radiographs. Increased sclerosis is suggestive of ON.
- CT is more sensitive in evaluation and quantification of solid bony bridging across the fracture side compared to radiographs.
- MRI is the study of choice in evaluation of scaphoid fracture nonunions and Kienböck disease.
- Contrast-enhanced MRI improves assessment of scaphoid nonunion with proximal pole ON in majority of cases.
- Scaphoid nonunions with viable proximal pole may be treated with nonvascularized bone grafting and screw fixation, whereas proximal pole ON requires vascularized bone grafting.
- Treatment options for Kienböck disease vary depending on the stage, associated findings, and the surgeon's expertise.

Key Points: Triangular Fibrocartilage Complex

- TFCC consists of the TFC, the dorsal and volar radioulnar ligaments, the ulnar collateral ligament, the meniscus homologue, and the ECU tendon sheath.
- Injuries of the TFCC may be acute or chronic and are classified according to the Palmer scheme.
- Management of TFCC injuries may be conservative and surgical, depending on clinical and imaging findings.

Key Points: Ligaments of the Wrist and Hand

- High-resolution 3T MRI is usually sufficient in depiction of normal anatomy and injuries of the intrinsic and extrinsic wrist ligaments and of the ligamentous structures of the hand, however, MRA is the imaging modality of choice for evaluation of wrist ligament injuries.
- CTA is a good alternative to MRA for evaluation of wrist ligaments.
- Partially injured ligaments show irregularity of the fibers with increased signal intensity, whereas full-thickness tears reveal discontinuity of the torn fibers.
- Surgery is the treatment of choice for a Stener lesion, whereas the gamekeeper thumb is typically treated conservatively.
- Carpal instability may result from combined injuries of the intrinsic and extrinsic wrist ligaments.
- In the acute setting, for wrist ligament injuries, conservative treatment is applied. In acute injuries recalcitrant to initial treatment and in chronic cases, surgical management is required.

Key Points: Tendons and Muscles of the Hand and Wrist

- Flexor and extensor tendons of the wrist can be affected with tendinosis/tendinopathy, tenosynovitis, and partial- and full-thickness tears. Commonly involved are the first extensor compartment tendons in de Quervain syndrome and the ECU tendon.
- Tendinopathy and tenosynovitis are initially treated conservatively.
- Tendon ruptures require surgical repair.

Key Points: Neuropathies/Nerve Entrapment in the Wrist and Hand

- CTS is the most common nerve entrapment disorder in the upper limb.
- MRI findings in keeping with CTS include increased signal within the median nerve, enlargement of the nerve at the level of the pisiform, and flattening at the level of the hook of the hamate. Denervation changes of the thenar musculature may be seen.
- In Guyon canal syndrome, the ulnar nerve is swollen proximal to the canal and flattened within the canal with increased signal on fluid-sensitive sequences.
- Common causes of Wartenberg syndrome are de Quervain syndrome and soft tissue ganglia, both of which can easily be detected with MRI.

Recommended Reading

Taljanovic MS, Karantanas A, Griffith JF, DeSilva GL, Rieke JD, Sheppard JE. Imaging and treatment of scaphoid fractures and their complications. *Semin Musculoskelet Radiol.* 2012;16(2):159–73. doi:10.1055/s-0032-1311767. Review.

Arnaizi J, Piedra T, Cerezal L, et al. Imaging of Kienböck disease. *AJR Am J Roentgenol.* 2014;203:131–39.

Cody ME, Nakamura DT, Small KM, Yoshioka H. MR imaging of the triangular fibrocartilage complex. *Magn Reson Imaging Clin N Am.* 2015;23;393–403.

Ringler MD, Murthy NS. MR imaging of wrist ligaments. *Magn Reson Imaging Clin N Am.* 2015;23(3):367–91. doi:10.1016/j.mric.2015.04.007. Review.

Clavero JA, Alomar X, Monill JM, et al. MR imaging of ligament and tendon injuries of the fingers. *Radiographics.* 2002;22(2):237–56. Review.

Davis KW, Blankenbaker DG. Imaging the ligaments and tendons in the wrist. *Semin Roentgenol.* 2010;45(3):193–217.

Chalian M, Hehzadi AH, Williams EH, Shores JT, Chhabra A. High-resolution magnetic resonance neurography in upper extremity neuropathy. *Neuroimag Clin N Am.* 2014;24:109–25.

References

1. Murthy NS, Ringler MD. MR imaging of carpal fractures. *Magn Reson Imaging Clin N Am.* 2015;23(3):405–16. doi:10.1016/j.mric.2015.04.006.
2. Syed MA, Raj V, Jeyapalan K. Current role of multidetector computed tomography in imaging of wrist injuries. *Curr Probl Diagn Radiol.* 2013;42(1)13–25.
3. Cerezal L, Abascal F, Canga A, et al. Usefulness of gadolinium-enhanced MR imaging in the evaluation of the vascularity of scaphoid non-unions. *AJR Am J Roentgenol.* 2000;174(1):141–49.
4. Donati OF, Zanetti M, Nagy L, Bode B, Schweizer A, Pfirrmann CW. Is dynamic gadolinium enhancement needed in MR imaging for the preoperative assessment of scaphoidal

viability in patients with scaphoid nonunion? *Radiology.* 2011;260(3):808–16.

5. Ng AW, Griffith JF, Taljanovic MS, Li A, Tse WL, Ho PC. Is dynamic contrast-enhanced MRI useful for assessing proximal fragment vascularity in scaphoid fracture delayed and non-union? *Skeletal Radiol.* 2013;42(7):983–2. doi:10.1007/s00256-013-1627-2.

6. Palmer AK. Triangular fibrocartilage complex lesions: a classification. *J Hand Surg.* 1989;14(4):594–606.

7. Lee RK, Ng AW, Toong CS, et al. Intrinsic ligament and triangular fibrocartilage complex tears of the wrist: comparison of MDCT arthrography, conventional 3-T MRI, and MR arthrography. *Skeletal Radiol.* 2013;42(9):1277–85.

8. Burns JE, Tanaka T, Ueno T, Nakamura T, Yoshioka H. Pitfalls that may mimic injuries of the triangular fibrocartilage and proximal intrinsic wrist ligaments at MR imaging. *Radiographics.* 2011;31(1):63–78. doi:10.1148/rg.311105114. Review.

9. Cerezal L, de Dios Berna-Mestre, Canga A, et al. MR and CT arthrography of the wrist. *Semin Musculoskelet Radiol.* 2012;16(1):27–41.

10. Moser T, Dosch JC, Moussaoui A, Dietemann JL. Wrist ligament tears: evaluation of MRI and combined MDCT and MR arthrography. *AJR Am J Roentgenol.* 2007;188:1278–86.

11. Taljanovic MS, Malan JJ, Sheppard JE. Normal anatomy of the extrinsic capsular wrist ligaments by 3-T MRI and high-resolution ultrasonography. *Semin Musculoskelet Radiol.* 2012;16(2):104–14. doi:10.1055/s-0032-1311762. Review.

12. Bateni CP, Bartolotta RJ, Richardson ML, Mulcahy H, Allan CH. Imaging key wrist ligaments: what the surgeon needs the radiologist to know. *AJR Am J Roentgenol.* 2013;200:1089–95.

13. Sookur PA, Naraghi AM, Bleakney RR, Jalan R, Chan O, White LM. Accessory muscles: anatomy, symptoms, and radiologic evaluation. *Radiographics.* 2008;28(2):481–99. doi:10.1148/rg.282075064. Review.

14. Steinberg DR. Surgical release of the carpal tunnel. *Hand Clin.* 2002;18(2):291–98. Review.

15. Bencardino JT. MR imaging of tendon lesions of the hand and wrist. *Magn Reson Imaging Clin N Am.* 2004;12:333–47.

16. Cockenpot E, Lefebvre G, Demondion X, Chantelot C, Cotten A. Imaging of sports-related hand and wrist injuries: sports imaging series. *Radiology.* 2016;279(3):674–92. doi:10.1148/radiol.2016150995.

17. Rotman MB, Donovan JP. Practical anatomy of the carpal tunnel. *Hand Clin.* 2002;18(2):219–30. Review.

18. Howe BM, Spinner RJ, Felmlee JP, Frick MA. MR imaging of the nerves of the upper extremity-elbow to wrist. *Magn Reson Imaging Clin N Am.* 2015;23:469–78.

CHAPTER 107

Internal Derangement of the Hip

Imran M. Omar

Introduction

Many osseous and soft tissue pathologies are occult on radiography. MRI is excellent in assessing hip internal derangement because it has superior contrast resolution. This allows better characterization of tissues, such as the acetabular labrum and articular cartilage, and improves detection of pathologic conditions. MRA of the hip is often helpful to detect and characterize labral and hyaline cartilage pathology. Conversely, US can be useful in identifying joint or bursal effusions and periarticular tendon injuries, as well as guiding intraarticular and periarticular procedures such as joint arthrocentesis or palliative injections into the hip joint or surrounding bursae.

General MRI Technique

- Many institutions combine smaller FOV imaging of the hip joint and larger FOV imaging of the entire pelvis to survey for additional potential sources of hip pain, such as from the pelvic bones in other locations, sacrum and coccyx, intrapelvic viscera, and surrounding soft tissues.
- If performed, large FOV imaging should include a fat-suppressed, fluid-sensitive sequence (often STIR) and a T1W nonfat-suppressed sequence, either in the coronal or axial planes.
- Small FOV images dedicated to the hip are most helpful in assessing the acetabular labrum and articular cartilage, the bone morphology, joint capsule and synovium, and the periarticular musculotendinous structures.
- Fluid-sensitive sequences, such as PDW or T2W imaging, are generally used to evaluate the labrum and articular cartilage. These may either be fat-suppressed or nonfat-suppressed depending on the institution.
- Because the femoral head and acetabulum are curved structures, imaging in any of the standard planes is susceptible to volume averaging as the imaged structure curves into the plane of imaging. Thus, a combination of pulse sequences in the 3 standard planes—axial, sagittal, and coronal—is recommended, especially if detailed assessment of the labrum and articular cartilage is needed.
  - The axial plane is particularly useful to assess the anterior and posterior segments of the labrum and articular cartilage, the joint recesses, periarticular bursae, and many of the surrounding tendons and muscles in cross-section.
  - The coronal plane is helpful in assessing the superior structures of the hip and can be useful in evaluating acetabular morphology for signs of dysplasia or excessive deepening.
  - The sagittal images are helpful to evaluate the anterosuperior, superior, and posterosuperior segments of the hip, including femoral head morphology, labrum, and articular cartilage.
- The axial oblique sequence is commonly used in the setting of femoroacetabular impingement and cam-type deformity of the femoral head and neck (Figure 107.1). The degree of cam deformity can be assessed on the axial oblique sequence by measuring the *alpha angle*. The normal value is between 50 and 55 degrees, and an alpha angle greater than 55 degrees is considered abnormal.
- In some cases, radial imaging may also be used to mitigate the impact of volume averaging and improve visualization of acetabular labral tears and articular cartilage loss (Figure 107.2).

Bones

Normal Anatomy
Refer to Figure 107.3.

The hip consists of the femoral head and acetabulum. The femoral head normally has a spheroid shape with a central concavity, called the *fovea*. The acetabulum is cup-shaped and developmentally derived from the 3 components of the innominate bone: the ilium, ischium, and pubis. Unlike the glenoid fossa in the shoulder, the acetabulum nearly completely covers the femoral head. Because of this greater congruence, the hip joint is intrinsically more stable than the shoulder, and the acetabular roof forms the weight-bearing region of the hip. On radiographs, this is seen as a smooth, curvilinear region of thickened subchondral bone, articulating with the superior femoral head. Medially within the acetabular fossa, there is a recessed region, called the *cotyloid fossa*, which contains extrasynovial fibrofatty connective tissue, called the *pulvinar*. On coronal imaging of the hip, the femoral neck forms an angle with the femoral shaft, called the *collo-diaphyseal angle*, which normally measures 125 degrees on average with a range between 120 and 135 degrees. An abnormally large angle is referred to as *coxa valga*, whereas an abnormally small angle is referred to as *coxa vara*. The acetabular fossa is normally slightly anteriorly directed, or anteverted, by 15 degrees on average.

Adult Osseous Pathology

Transient Osteoporosis of the Hip and Regional Migratory Osteoporosis

Pathophysiology and Clinical Presentation
Transient osteoporosis of the hip (TOH) was initially described in pregnant women in the third trimester, however, this is more commonly seen in middle-aged men. Patients

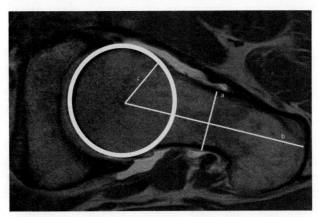

Figure 107.1. Alpha angle measured on an axial oblique MR sequence. Axial oblique PDW MR image along the axis of the femoral neck is used to measure the alpha angle. This is obtained by drawing a line along the short axis of the femoral neck *a* and a best-fit circle around the femoral head. Then, a second line, *b*, is drawn perpendicular to line *a* and through the center of the circle. Line *c* is drawn from the center of the circle to the anterior point when the femoral head cortex diverges from the drawn circle. The alpha angle is taken between lines *b* and *c*.

usually present with hip pain and without reported antecedent trauma. Regional migratory osteoporosis (RMO) represents a similar, self-limiting condition with episodic, migratory areas of BME around the joints in the lower extremities. It is not exclusively seen in the hip, and similar transient BME has been reported in other joints, such as the knee. It may represent a spectrum of injuries with TOH. These conditions are usually self-limiting, lasting approximately 6-12 months. The etiology is unknown; it may be related to decreased venous outflow in the femoral head resulting in congestion, or stress response from microtrabecular injury, in spectrum with subchondral insufficiency fracture (SIF).

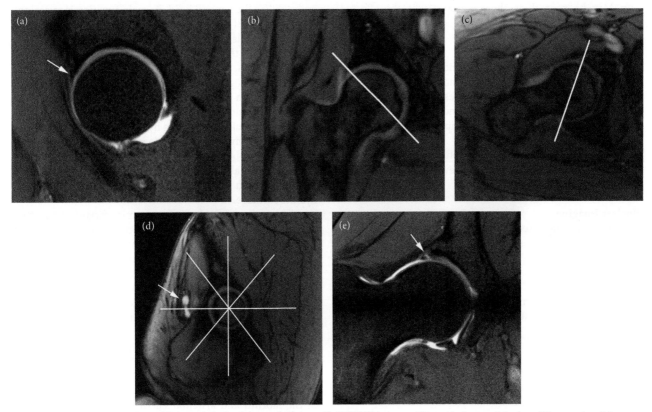

Figure 107.2. Radial imaging of the acetabular labrum. Initial sagittal T1W FS image of the anterior acetabulum (*A*) reveals mild labral irregularity (*arrow*) but no convincing tear. Radial imaging is obtained from images that look at the acetabular fossa en face as a double-oblique acquisition from initial scout images. The first oblique plane is planned on a coronal image and taken from a line connecting the superior acetabular rim and inferior margin of the medial acetabulum (*B*), whereas the second plane is planned from axial images with a line connecting the anterior and posterior acetabular rims (*C*). The acetabulum should appear circular on the resulting images. Radial images are obtained by planning image sections that connect points on the acetabular rim with the points 180 degrees away on the opposite sides, and the sections should intersect one another in the center of the acetabulum (*D*). The femoral vessels (*arrow*) indicate the anterior direction. In this case, radial imaging of the anterosuperior acetabular rim (*E*) clearly shows a labral tear (*arrow*).

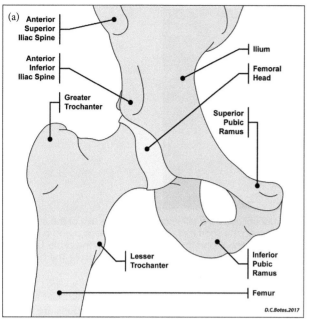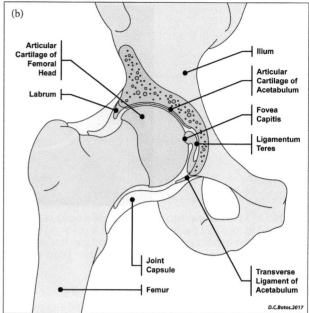

Figure 107.3. Frontal illustration of the hip (*A*) showing the normal osseous relationship of the femoral head and acetabulum. The second diagram (*B*) illustrates the normal intraarticular structures within the joint capsule that can lead to internal impingement.

Imaging Findings
Radiography
- May be normal or show osteopenia of the affected femoral head

Magnetic Resonance Imaging
- Florid femoral head BME on fluid-sensitive sequences, and possibly lower femoral head signal intensity on nonfat-suppressed T1W sequences
- Overlapping appearance of SIF and early ON
- MRI findings of RMO in the hip are similar to those of TOH.
- Follow-up MRI may be helpful to assess resolution of findings (TOH), the development of SIF, or findings of ON.

Nuclear Imaging
- May have increased radiotracer uptake within the femoral head on bone scintigraphy

Treatment Options
- Conservative measures, including rest and decreased weight-bearing, NSAIDs, and possibly bisphosphonates

---

Acetabular Labrum and Articular Cartilage

Normal Anatomy, Function, and Magnetic Resonance Imaging Appearance
The labrum is composed of fibrocartilage and has an inverted horseshoe shape along the anterior, superior, and posterior segments of the acetabular rim. The anterior and posterior margins are bridged inferiorly by the transverse acetabular ligament. Although it helps to deepen the acetabular fossa and stabilize the femoral head, its main function is to seal the lateral margin of the acetabular hyaline cartilage and prevent premature cartilage loss.

On MRI, the labrum usually has a triangular shape in cross-section, but it may be oval, flat, or round in older patients. It is slightly thicker posterosuperiorly than anteriorly. The labrum should have uniform, dark signal on all pulse sequences (Figure 107.4), and it may either attach directly onto the acetabular rim or onto hyaline cartilage overlying the acetabulum. If hyaline cartilage is interposed between the labrum and acetabular rim, there may be a smooth band of intermediate signal between labrum and acetabular rim that is continuous with and has the signal intensity of the adjacent hyaline cartilage.

There are a number of anatomic variants and other findings that can mimic labral tears. Intermediate signal within the labrum could represent magic angle artifact or intrasubstance degeneration. Additionally, there is a normal recess along the posteroinferior and anteroinferior labral margins where the labrum transitions to the transverse ligament. Fluid in this location should not be mistaken for paralabral cyst. The *sublabral sulcus* is a partial detachment involving the articular surface of the labrum at its junction with the hyaline cartilage. It occurs between the anterosuperior and posterosuperior regions of the acetabular rim. MRI findings of a sublabral sulcus include a smooth defect along the articular surface at the junction of the labrum and articular cartilage that does not penetrate more than 50% of the width of the labral base in cross-section. Additionally, this should not be associated with adjacent articular cartilage pathology. It is controversial whether this represents a real variant or a shallow undersurface tear.

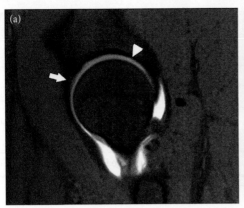 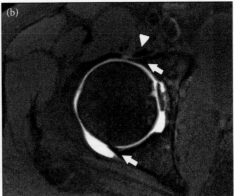

Figure 107.4. Appearance of normal acetabular labrum on MRA. Sagittal (*A*) and axial (*B*) T1W FS MR images of the hip show the normal morphology of the labrum as an intermediate signal intensity triangle that is darker than the adjacent articular cartilage and skeletal muscle with smooth margins (*arrows*). On the sagittal image, the femoral and acetabular hyaline cartilage is seen as smooth, intermediate signal intensity arcs between the weight-bearing regions of the femoral head and acetabulum (*arrowhead*). In this case the labrum attaches directly to the acetabular rim. However, in some cases the labrum may attach to hyaline cartilage, which may be interposed between the bone and the labrum. The intermediate signal of articular cartilage should not be mistaken for a labral detachment. On the axial image (*B*), the anterior and posterior segments of the labrum are similar in size. The iliopsoas tendon (*arrowhead*) courses just anterior to the anterior labrum. This should not be mistaken for a displaced labral fragment.

Labral Injuries
Pathophysiology and Clinical Presentation

Injuries of the acetabular labrum are common causes of hip pain, particularly in active patients. They may be separated into labral tears and detachments. Tears occur when a pathologic cleft is seen extending into the substance of the labrum, whereas detachments occur when the cleft occurs at the base of the labrum as it attaches onto the acetabular rim or hyaline cartilage. Although subtle, this distinction may have implications on surgical management, because labral tears are often debrided, whereas detachments are often repaired. The labrum is not felt to degenerate to the same degree as the menisci in the knee. Instead, most labral tears are felt to be related more commonly to acute trauma, repetitive impingement, called *femoroacetabular impingement* (FAI), or acetabular dysplasia. Although there have been some efforts to classify acetabular labral tears seen on MRI with findings noted on arthroscopy, such as the Czerny classification (Table 107.1), many institutions have elected to describe the location

and morphology of labral tears rather than assign a grade or stage when interpreting MRI findings.

FAI results from overdevelopment of the acetabulum or the femoral head/neck junction usually in the anterosuperior region, which leads to abnormal contact between these structures. This causes impingement on the labrum that worsens with hip flexion and internal rotation, with subsequent labral tears and adjacent acetabular cartilage loss. There are 2 main types: *cam-type* and *pincer-type* FAI. Overgrowth of the anterior or anterosuperior femoral head/neck junction is called a *cam deformity*. This distorts the normal spheroidal femoral head morphology. Some cam lesions may represent residual deformities in patients with prior SCFE.

Conversely, excessive deepening of the acetabular fossa is called a *pincer deformity*. This could be related to generalized acetabular deepening (coxa profunda). Another common cause of pincer deformity is *acetabular retroversion*, in which there is overgrowth of the anterosuperior acetabular rim and relative deficiency of the posterosuperior acetabular rim.

STAGE	MRA FINDINGS
Table 107.1. Czerny Classification of Acetabular Labral Tears on Magnetic Resonance Arthrography	
Stage 0	Normal
Stage 1A	Increased intrasubstance signal, triangular shape, perilabral recess
Stage 1B	Increased intrasubstance signal, thickened labrum, no perilabral recess
Stage 2A	Extension of contrast into the substance of the labrum without labral detachment, triangular shape, perilabral recess present
Stage 2B	Extension of contrast into substance of labrum without detachment, labrum thickened, no perilabral recess
Stage 3A	Labrum detached, triangular shape
Stage 3B	Labrum detached, labrum thickened

*Only stages 2A/2B and 3A/3B are considered labral tears

Table 107.2. Femoroacetabular Impingement: Pincer-Type Versus Cam-Type

PINCER-TYPE	CAM-TYPE
Middle-age, female	Young, male
Normal, spherical femoral head, normal alpha angle	Abnormal femoral sphericity, increased alpha angle
Acetabular labral tear/degeneration is anterosuperior	Acetabular labral tear/degeneration is anterosuperior
Smaller, focal cartilage defects	More extensive cartilage defects
Contrecoup cartilage injury roughly 180 degrees opposite of pincer deformity, usually along posterior acetabular rim	No contrecoup cartilage injury

Although the acetabular fossa is normally slightly anteverted (directed slightly anteriorly), instances in which the acetabulum is either directed completely laterally (neutral version) or slightly posteriorly (retroversion) can result in FAI. Most cases of FAI (85%) have mixed cam and pincer morphologies (Table 107.2).

Developmental dysplasia of the hip (DDH) represents an underdevelopment of acetabulum, causing the acetabulum to be shallow and widened. This results in excessive lateral femoral head undercoverage by the superior acetabular roof and subsequent instability. The acetabular labrum may become a load-bearing structure, which results in premature labral thickening and degeneration, with subsequent tearing and adjacent articular cartilage loss.

Magnetic Resonance Imaging Findings

- When describing labral tears on the MRI report, it is important to note the location of the tear. This is commonly done by indicating a region of the acetabular rim, such as anterior, anterosuperior, superior, posterosuperior, and posterior. Some imagers provide a clock-face description to more precisely localize the injured segment. Rather than using the standard clock-face orientation in which the assignment of the clock positions changes depending on whether the right or left hip is imaged, the superior margin of the rim is labeled as the 12 o'clock position, the anterior margin is usually the 3 o'clock position, and the posterior margin is the 9 o'clock position regardless of which hip is imaged (Figure 107.5). This may prevent errors in noting the location of tears when describing the pathology in either the right or left hip. The use of this system should be discussed with referring clinicians prior to study interpretation in order to avoid miscommunication of the location of labral and cartilage abnormalities.
- Labral tears
  - Look for surface irregularity or intrasubstance signal abnormalities on fluid-sensitive sequences. (Figure 107.6). If the abnormal signal is similar in intensity to fluid, the finding is more specific for tear.
  - In younger patients (younger than 30 years), blunted or irregular cross-sectional labral shapes should be considered tears.
  - Tears usually start in the anterosuperior region along the articular surface before extending anteriorly or superiorly.

  - Commonly associated with adjacent hyaline cartilage and subchondral bone injury
- Cam-type FAI (Figure 107.7)
  - Flattening or overgrowth of anterior or superior femoral head/neck junction
  - Bony protuberance is often best seen on frog-leg lateral radiograph of the hip, which depicts the anterosuperior femoral neck in profile.
  - Can be seen on axial oblique imaging along the anterior femoral neck
- Pincer-type FAI
  - Usually occurs in anterosuperior region
  - May be related to generalized overgrowth of acetabular rim (coxa profunda) or relative overgrowth of the anterosuperior acetabular rim compared to its posterosuperior segment (acetabular retroversion)
- DDH
  - The labrum may be abnormally thickened and globular (Figure 107.8).

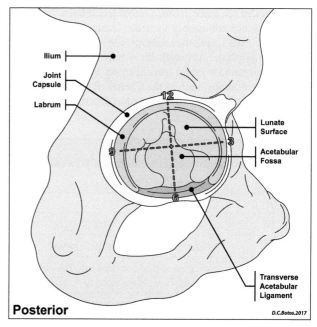

Figure 107.5. Acetabular clock face. Illustration of the acetabulum en face shows the position and orientation of the clock-face nomenclature. The 12 o'clock position is superior and the 3 o'clock position is anterior by convention. Lunate surface = articular surface of the acetabulum covered by articular cartilage.

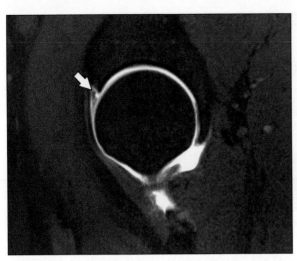

Figure 107.6. Anterior acetabular labral tear on MRA. Sagittal T1W FS MR image of the hip demonstrates bright signal from contrast separating the labrum and the underlying acetabular rim (*arrow*), called a *labral detachment*. There is also bright signal within the labral substance (labral tear). This is the most common region of acetabular labral pathology. The articular cartilage adjacent to this area should be closely examined because it is at greater risk for injury.

- Labrum often prematurely degenerates and tears.
- Associated with accelerated articular cartilage loss
- Often associated with thickening of the pulvinar within the cotyloid fossa
- Other findings that can be seen in FAI
  - Os acetabuli—ossification along the acetabular rim

- May represent an unfused ossification center, labral ossification, or sequela of acetabular fracture
- Reduces the space between the acetabular rim and the femoral neck
- Synovial herniation pit—round lucency with a thin sclerotic rim usually along the anterolateral femoral neck, which may arise from herniation of synovial tissue through a small cortical defect
  - Frequently incidental; however, if it is located along the anterosuperior femoral neck it may reflect repetitive FAI.

Treatment Options

- If limited or no symptoms, consider conservative treatments such as physical therapy, activity modification, or bracing.
- In more symptomatic patients, surgical repair/debridement is often recommended and usually performed arthroscopically.
- In cases of FAI, acetabular or femoral head/neck osteotomy is often performed to relieve impingement.
- In cases of DDH, periacetabular osteotomy may be advised to stabilize the hip joint.

Cartilage
Pathophysiology and Clinical Findings
Within the hip hyaline cartilage covers the femoral head except for the central fovea and the acetabulum except for the medial acetabular fossa. Cartilage loss often occurs adjacent to labral tears and is most commonly seen in anterosuperior and superior segments of acetabulum. The articular cartilage is usually thin

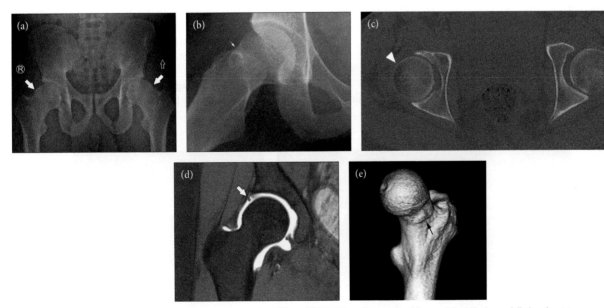

Figure 107.7. Findings of cam-type FAI on radiography, CT, and MRI. AP radiograph of the pelvis (*A*) shows bilateral osseous protuberances along the superior femoral head/neck junctions. The presence of extra bone in this area can reduce the space between the femoral neck and acetabulum during movement and result in labral injuries. A frog-leg lateral radiograph (*B*) demonstrates mild osseous protuberance along the anterosuperior femoral head/neck junction. In some cases, the cam deformity is only seen on the frog-leg lateral radiograph. Axial CT image of both femoral heads in a different patient (*C*) demonstrates an anterosuperior left femoral head/neck junction cam deformity (*arrow*). The contralateral right femoral head has a normal circular morphology (*arrowhead*). On a coronal T1W FS image of the hip in the same patient (*D*), there is an acetabular labral detachment (*arrow*). (*E*) A 3D reformatted image of the femur demonstrates a small anterior cam deformity (*arrow*). These images are frequently used by orthopedic surgeons for preoperative planning.

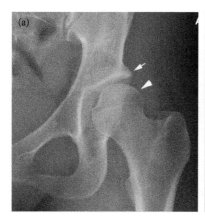
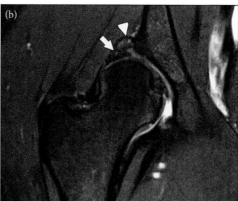

Figure 107.8. Findings of acetabular dysplasia in a 28-year-old woman with hip pain. On AP radiographs of the hip in skeletally mature patients, the acetabular roof should be nearly horizontal. In this patient (*A*), the roof is excessively sloped (*arrow*), indicating a shallow acetabulum. Additionally, the lateral femoral head is slightly excessively uncovered (*arrowhead*). Coronal T2W FS MR image of the same patient (*B*) reveals abnormal thickening of the labrum (*arrow*), which is often seen in cases of acetabular dysplasia, along with detachment of the labrum from the acetabular rim (*arrowhead*). The steep slope of the acetabular roof appears more pronounced on the MR image.

(<2 mm in thickness), which may make detection of articular cartilage injuries difficult. Two anatomic variants, the *supraacetabular fossa* and *stellate crease*, can be mistaken for an osteochondral injury. The supraacetabular fossa is a developmental notch of the superior acetabular subchondral bone plate at the 12 o'clock position (Figure 107.9). This may be completely or partially filled with articular cartilage and consequently may not be visible on arthroscopy. However, the surface of the articular cartilage should be smooth and should not be associated with abnormalities of the underlying subchondral bone. The stellate crease is a bare region of the hyaline cartilage in the superior acetabulum that is medial to the supraacetabular fossa. As with the supraacetabular fossa the location of the stellate crease is predictable and no associated subchondral bone abnormalities should be seen.

Magnetic Resonance Imaging Findings
Refer to Figure 107.10.

- MRI and MRA are current tests of choice to evaluate cartilage loss.

- On routine MRI, this is best detected on fluid-sensitive sequences with or without fat suppression.
- MRI findings range from cartilage heterogeneity indicating degeneration to partial- and full-thickness defects.
- Focally dark articular cartilage adjacent to a labral tear has been associated with cartilage delamination.

Paralabral Cysts
Pathophysiology and Clinical Findings
Paralabral cysts are loculated, fluid-filled lesions adjacent to the acetabular labrum and associated with labral tears in up to 90% of cases. They may occur when joint fluid extends through a labral tear into the surrounding soft tissues, similar to parameniscal cyst in the knee, and are most commonly seen anterosuperiorly and posterosuperiorly.

Magnetic Resonance Imaging Findings
- Fluid signal intensity lesions that often contain septations

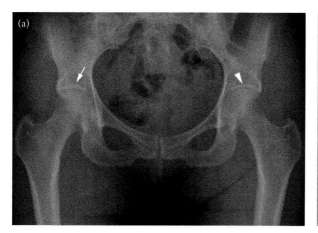
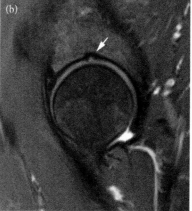

Figure 107.9. Supraacetabular fossa in a 52-year-old woman with hip pain. (*A*) AP pelvic radiograph demonstrates a small concavity along the superior right acetabular roof (*arrow*). The left acetabular roof is a smooth arc (*arrowhead*). (*B*) Sagittal T2W FS MR image of the mid left hip demonstrates a small concavity of the superior acetabular subchondral bone plate in the 12 o'clock position (*arrow*). The overlying hyaline cartilage is smooth, continuous with similar signal to the adjacent hyaline cartilage. Additionally, the underlying subchondral bone is normal in signal. This is an anatomic variant that should not be confused with an OCL.

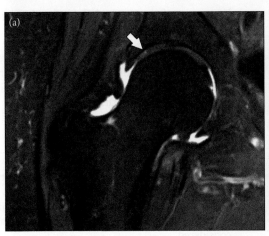
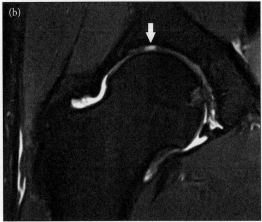

Figure 107.10. Cartilage pathology on MRI. Coronal T2W FS MR image of the hip (A) shows cartilage heterogeneity and partial thickness loss particularly on the acetabular side (arrow). The normal cartilage should be intermediate in signal intensity between the bright fluid and dark signal of the suppressed fat. It should be relatively uniform in thickness and signal intensity. Coronal T2W FS MR image of the hip (B) reveals a focal full-thickness cartilage defect in the superior acetabulum (arrow). The joint fluid enters the cartilage defect and outlines the margins.

- The neck of the cyst should communicate with labral tear, which confirms the diagnosis.
- Often extraosseous but can erode into the acetabular rim (intraosseous ganglion)
- May fill with dilute contrast on MRA or CTA, but this is not required for diagnosis

Synovium and Joint Capsule

Normal Anatomy

The joint capsule circumferentially encases the femoral head and helps to stabilize the hip by serving as a checkrein to movement. The capsule attaches along the acetabular rim to the base of femoral neck and is lined by synovium along its intraarticular surface. The paralabral recess is a small joint recess along the acetabular rim at the capsular attachment. Fluid trapped in this recess can mimic a paralabral cyst. Another anatomic structure, the *pectinofoveal fold*, can be seen on almost every MRI, especially in the setting of MRA or hip effusion. This is a thin fibrous band arising from the joint capsule, usually along the inferior/medial margin of the femoral neck and should not be mistaken for a pathologic structure (Figure 107.11).

Synovitis

- MRI findings are similar to those discussed elsewhere in chapters regarding synovial thickening and include smooth or irregular intermediate signal intensity tissue within the joint capsule on fluid-sensitive sequences (Figure 107.12).

Figure 107.11. Normal pectinofoveal fold and LT on MRI. On coronal T2W FS MR image of the hip the LT (arrow) is seen as a low signal curvilinear band of tissue extending from the fovea of the femoral head to the inferior medial acetabulum. Injuries to this structure have been associated with hip pain and sensation of instability. A second structure, the pectinofoveal fold, is seen as a thin curvilinear band along the inferior margin of the femoral neck (arrowhead). This is a normal structure and should not be confused for pathology.

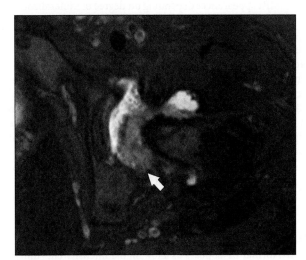

Figure 107.12. Synovitis on MRI. Axial T2W FS MR image through the femoral neck shows a joint effusion with irregular intermediate signal synovial proliferation (arrow). This was felt to be related to OA on additional images (not shown).

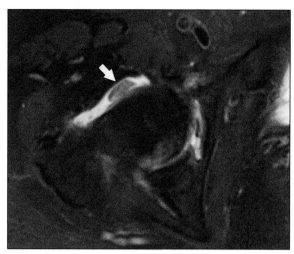

Figure 107.13. PVNS on MRI. Axial T2W FS MR image through the femoral neck shows a joint effusion with an oval-shaped intermediate signal lesion (*arrow*) in the anterior joint recess. This could be related to synovitis, retracted blood clot, or a developing intraarticular body. PVNS can be associated with hemarthrosis, which can lead to methemoglobin staining both the lesion and the inner lining of the joint capsule. As a result, it can produce dark foci on MRI that are often more pronounced on GRE imaging (blooming artifact). This patient did not have MRI evidence of prior hemarthrosis and was diagnosed with PVNS following resection.

- Enhancement on postcontrast imaging suggests active synovitis, whereas minimal or no enhancement suggests bland synovial proliferation.
- Frank osseous erosions or periarticular, subcortical marrow edema (osteitis) are seen with inflammatory arthropathies, such as RA or septic arthritis, or PVNS (Figure 107.13).

Intraarticular Bodies
- Occur as a result of displaced fragments of intraarticular tissues, such as cartilage, osteochondral or labral fragments
- Frequently undergo metaplasia and can have variable MRI appearances depending on degree of mineralization
- Look for cartilage or osteochondral donor site

Ligamentum Teres
Normal Anatomy, Pathophysiology, and Clinical Findings
The ligamentum teres (LT) is a fibrous band of tissue that extends from the fovea of the femoral head to the medial acetabular fossa (Figure 107.11). Although its true function is not completely understood, it may serve to stabilize the hip or contribute to hip proprioception. Chronic tears of the LT are seen in older patients and following surgical hip disarticulation. The role of LT tears in the development of hip pain is not well known. However, some authors have stated this is the third most common cause of hip pain in athletes.

Magnetic Resonance Imaging Findings
- Normal LT appears as a low signal intensity curvilinear band extending from the fovea to acetabular fossa and is best seen on fat-suppressed, fluid-sensitive sequences or MRA images.
- Frank fiber disruption or detachment of the ligament from its attachment sites indicates a ligament tear.
- Areas of ligament caliber change, including thickening and intermediate intrasubstance signal, or focal thinning may represent partial tearing.
- Diffuse thinning or absence of the LT may indicate a chronic injury.

Treatment Options
- Simple tears may be debrided.
- In cases of instability, surgical capsular tightening or LT reconstruction with synthetic graft or autograft can be considered.

Bursae Around the Hip

Background
Anatomic bursae are synovial-lined potential spaces generally located around tendons to reduce friction and tendon strain and are often positioned between tendons and bones. Any process that causes the synovium to secrete fluid or to become inflamed may result in pathologic bursal distention. MRI and occasionally US are the best imaging modalities to identify and characterize synovial pathology. In the hip, the main bursae are the iliopsoas bursa and the peritrochanteric bursae.

Iliopsoas Bursa
Refer to Figure 107.14*A*.

Normal Anatomy and Clinical Findings
The iliopsoas bursa is the largest bursa around the hip and in the body. It is located between the iliopsoas myotendinous junction and the iliopectineal eminence of the anterior innominate bone and extends cranially deep to the iliacus muscle along the iliacus fossa of the iliac wing. In 15% of people, it communicates with hip joint, and any cause of joint effusion in these patients can result in an iliopsoas bursal effusion. However, it may become primarily distended in patients with hip OA, RA, pyogenic infection (septic bursitis), and following hip arthroplasty among other causes.

Magnetic Resonance Imaging Findings
- Fluid signal intensity collection distending the bursa deep to the iliopsoas tendon on fluid-sensitive sequences
- May be best seen on axial sequences with 2 rounded fluid-filled recesses flanking the tendon medially and laterally. These recesses communicate with one another along the deep surface of the tendon.
- Intermediate signal may represent synovial proliferation, whereas enhancement on postcontrast imaging suggests active synovitis.
- Larger effusions often extend deep to the iliacus muscle.

Peritrochanteric Bursae
Refer to Figure 107.14*B*

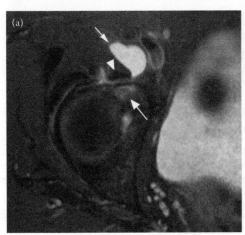 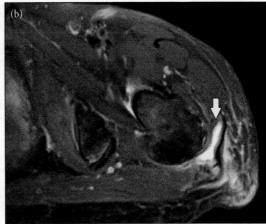

Figure 107.14. Examples of bursitis around the hip joint. Axial T2W FS MR image of the hip at the superior hip joint level in a 51-year-old patient with anterior hip pain (*A*) shows the iliopsoas tendon (*arrowhead*) along the anterior acetabulum flanked by fluid within the medial and lateral recesses of the iliopsoas bursa (*shorter arrow* points to the medial recess). Additionally, there is subtendinous BME in the anterior acetabulum that is probably reactive (*longer arrow*). In a 53-year-old patient presenting with lateral hip pain, an axial T2W FS MR image of the hip at the greater trochanter level (*B*) shows a bursal effusion (*arrow*) in the subgluteus maximus bursa between the iliotibial band and gluteus medius muscle.

Normal Anatomy and Clinical Findings

There are 3 main bursae around the greater trochanter: the *trochanteric (subgluteus maximus) bursa*, located between the gluteus maximus muscle and the posterior facet of the greater trochanter; the *subgluteus minimus bursa*, between the gluteus minimus muscle attachment and the anterior facet of the greater trochanter; and the *subgluteus medius bursa*, between the gluteus medius muscle attachment and the lateral facet of the greater trochanter. Peritrochanteric bursal effusions and bursitis are commonly associated with trochanteric pain syndrome and lateral hip pain and may be seen with gluteal tendinopathy and tendon tears. In addition, they are associated with obesity, trauma, and prior hip arthroplasty. However, trochanteric bursitis is a clinical diagnosis, and bursal effusions or synovial enhancement are frequently seen in asymptomatic patients.

Magnetic Resonance Imaging Findings

- Fluid signal intensity collection distending the bursa on fluid-sensitive sequences
- Synovial thickening, represented by intermediate signal on T1W and fluid-sensitive sequences
- Synovial enhancement on postcontrast imaging likely represents active synovitis.
- Commonly associated with adjacent gluteal tendinopathy or tendon tears

---

Muscles and Tendons

Background

There are a number of musculotendinous groups around the hip that allow a range of motions (Table 107.3). A complete discussion of these musculotendinous structures is beyond the scope of this chapter. However, review of the following conditions may be helpful because they often result in imaging studies.

Snapping Hip (Coxa Saltans)
Pathophysiology and Clinical Presentation

Patients with snapping hip experience an audible or palpable snap during certain movements, which is often associated with pain. This condition is more common in athletic patients, such as dancers, runners and weightlifters. It can be divided into *intraarticular* or *extraarticular* hip snapping. Causes of intraarticular snapping hip include anterior/superior labral tears, hip impingement, intraarticular bodies, and LT tears. Conversely, extraarticular snapping hip has internal (medial) and external (lateral) causes. In internal extraarticular snapping hip, the iliopsoas muscle may abruptly snap around the iliopsoas tendon and the iliopectineal eminence when moving the hip from flexion to extension. External extraarticular snapping hip is felt to occur when the gluteus maximus muscle, tensor fascia lata, or iliotibial band slide over the greater trochanter.

Imaging Findings

- MRI
  - Particularly helpful to detect cases of intraarticular snapping hip
  - May see labral tears, intraarticular bodies or cartilage loss
  - Often unrevealing in cases of extraarticular snapping hip
  - With medial extraarticular snapping hip, there may be iliopsoas tendinosis with tendon thickening or abnormal signal, or iliopsoas bursitis.
- US
  - Dynamic US may be helpful for cases of extraarticular snapping hip.
  - In external extraarticular snapping hip, there may be a sudden movement of the gluteus maximus or iliotibial band over the greater trochanter when moving the hip from flexion to extension.
  - Internal extraarticular snapping hip may occur when the iliopsoas muscle snaps under the tendon with hip

Table 107.3. Musculotendinous Attachments Around the Hip			
MUSCLE GROUP	**MUSCLE/TENDON**	**ATTACHMENT AROUND THE HIP**	**FUNCTION**
Gluteal			
	Minimus	Anterior facet of greater trochanter	Abduct and medially rotates hip
	Medius	Middle and posterior facets of greater trochanter	Abducts hip. Can either contribute to internal or external rotation depending on which fibers are activated
	Maximus	Iliotibial band and proximal posterior femoral diaphysis	Extends, laterally rotates and abducts hip
Hamstrings			
	Biceps femoris (long head)	Ischial tuberosity. Arises as a conjoint tendon along with the semitendinosus, medial and inferior to the semimembranosus	Extends hip. Flexes knee and laterally rotates tibia.
	Semitendinosus	Ischial tuberosity. Arises as a conjoint tendon along with the biceps femoris long head, medial and inferior to the semimembranosus	Extends hip. Flexes knee and medially rotates tibia
	Semimembranosus	Ischial tuberosity, superior/lateral to the conjoint tendon of biceps and semitendinosus	Extends hip and flexes knee. Rotates tibia medially
	Adductor magnus	Inferior pubic ramus and ischial tuberosity	Some fibers extend hip
Iliopsoas			
	Iliacus	Inserts along with the psoas tendon on the lesser trochanter	Flexes the hip and trunk
	Psoas	Inserts along with the iliacus tendon on the lesser trochanter	Flexes the hip and trunk
Adductor			
	Longus	Anterior pubic body	Adducts, flexes hip and laterally rotates hip
	Brevis	Anterior surface of inferior pubic ramus	Adducts, flexes and laterally rotates hip
	Magnus	Inferior pubic ramus and ischial tuberosity	Adducts hip and some fibers flex hip

flexion, or when the iliopsoas tendon snaps over the iliopectineal eminence.

Gluteal Tendons
Refer to Figure 107.15.

Normal Anatomy and Clinical Presentation
The gluteal tendons are the principle hip abductors and often referred to as the "rotator cuff of the hip." They consist of the *gluteus minimus*, the *gluteus medius*, and the *gluteus maximus*. Gluteal tendinopathy is one of the main causes of greater trochanteric pain syndrome. It is most common in middle-aged women and overweight patients.

Magnetic Resonance Imaging Findings
- May demonstrate tendon thickening and intermediate signal (tendinosis), or partial or complete tears on fluid-sensitive sequences

- Peritendinous edema may represent surrounding inflammation (peritendinitis) or may be asymptomatic.
- May see intratendinous mineralization from calcium hydroxyapatite deposition
- May see enthesophytes or subenthesial BME (enthesitis) at tendon insertion
- May see adjacent peritrochanteric bursal effusions and enhancement

Proximal Hamstring Tendons
Refer to Figure 107.16.

Normal Anatomy
The hamstring muscles are the main hip extensors and located in the posterior thigh muscular compartment. They arise from the ischial tuberosity, and the hamstring muscle complex origin consists of the *conjoined tendon*, which is formed by the long head of the biceps femoris and semitendinosus muscles; the *semimembranosus*; and a segment of *adductor magnus*. The semimembranosus tendon arises from a posterior, lateral, and superior position compared to the conjoined tendon.

Magnetic Resonance Imaging Findings
- Many similar findings are also seen on US.
- Ischial tuberosity enthesial spurring and enthesitis
- Tendinopathy—tendon thickening and globular intermediate signal on fluid-sensitive sequences
- Tendon tear—more sharply marginated bright signal on fluid-sensitive sequences either within the tendon or at the tendon attachment to ischial tuberosity (avulsion)
- Avulsions may be associated with avulsed osseous fragments, which can be seen on radiographs or US.
- In acute injuries, hamstring muscle and fascial edema is commonly seen on fluid-sensitive sequences.
- In chronic injuries, there may be muscle atrophy and fatty infiltration that is best seen on T1W nonfat-suppressed sequences.

- Hematoma—hemorrhagic fluid collection at the site of the tear that often has bright T1 and T2 signal

Adductor Tendons and Athletic Pubalgia
Refer to Figures 107.17 and 107.18.

Normal Anatomy, Pathophysiology, and Clinical Presentation
The 3 main adductor muscles from anterior to posterior are the *adductor longus*, the *adductor brevis*, and the *adductor magnus*. They originate from the ipsilateral pubic body and inferior pubic ramus. The adductor longus tendon merges with the rectus abdominis tendon cranially to form a common aponeurosis along the anterior pubic body. The adductor and rectus abdominis muscles are antagonists of one another, which helps stabilize the pubic symphysis.

Athletic pubalgia is a clinical diagnosis involving inguinal and peripubic pain, usually in athletes, which worsens with athletic activities such as twisting and side-to-side cutting. It represents a spectrum of injuries, including rectus abdominis/adductor aponeurotic injuries over the anterior pubic bodies, adductor tendinopathy/tendon tears, pubic symphyseal articular injury/osteitis pubis, and ilioinguinal nerve entrapment. It is much more common in male patients. Although more frequently unilateral, the findings may be bilateral in advanced cases.

The true cause of athletic pubalgia in a particular patient is frequently not diagnosed on physical examination and erroneously attributed to structures that may not be involved in the development of presenting symptoms. Furthermore, its clinical features may significantly overlap with other conditions, such as acetabular labral tears. MRI can be very helpful to better characterize the structures commonly responsible for athletic pubalgia and to avoid assigning pathology to uninjured structures.

Magnetic Resonance Imaging Findings
- MRI requires small FOV images centered on the pubic symphysis and its musculotendinous attachments,

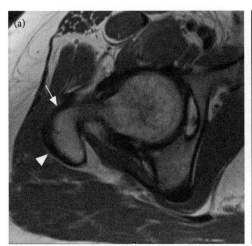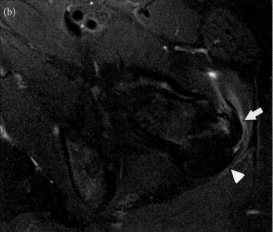

Figure 107.15. Normal gluteal tendon insertions and gluteal tendinopathy. (*A*) Axial PDW MR image of the hip at the level of the femoral greater trochanter shows the gluteus minimus tendon (*arrow*) and gluteus medius tendon (*arrowhead*) in short axis as they insert on the greater trochanter. (*B*) Axial T2W FS MR image of the hip at the greater trochanter level in a 48-year-old patient with lateral hip pain demonstrates thickening of the gluteus minimus tendon and surrounding peritendinous edema (*arrow*). There is BME in the greater trochanter where the tendon attaches to the bone (enthesitis). The gluteus medius tendon is normal (*arrowhead*).

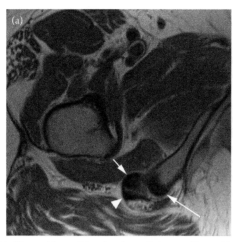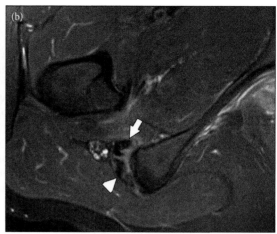

Figure 107.16. Normal hamstring tendon origins and hamstring tendinopathy. (*A*) Axial PDW MR image of the hip at the ischial tuberosity level demonstrates the normal hamstring tendons. The *arrowhead* indicates the conjoint tendon, consisting of the biceps femoris long head and semitendinosus tendons; the *short arrow* points at the semimembranosus tendon origin; and the *longer arrow* is directed toward a portion of the adductor magnus tendon. It should be noted that the semimembranosus tendon becomes more medial than the biceps tendon as the tendons course inferiorly. (*B*) Axial T2W FS MR image of the hip at the ischial tuberosity level shows abnormal intermediate signal in the hamstring tendon origin with surrounding peritendinous edema, suggesting peritendinitis. The *arrowhead* indicates the conjoint tendon, which is composed of the long head of the biceps femoris and the semitendinosus tendons, and the *arrow* points out the origin of the semimembranosus tendon.

as well as larger FOV imaging to assess surrounding structures such as the hips, which can result in similar symptoms.
- MRI is able to evaluate the bone, articular surfaces, and peripubic muscles and tendons.
- Detachment of the common rectus abdominis/adductor aponeurosis from the anterior pubic body ipsilateral to the symptomatic side may be seen as a near-fluid signal intensity curvilinear cleft along the anterior/inferior pubic body (*accessory cleft sign*).
- Adductor tendon thickening or tearing

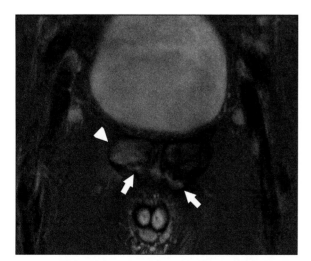

Figure 107.17. Findings of athletic pubalgia. Coronal T2W FS MR image of the pubic symphysis shows bilateral detachments (*arrows*) of the common aponeurosis between the rectus abdominis and adductor muscles with fluid clefts between the aponeurosis and anterior pubic bodies (often called the *accessory cleft sign*). There is pronounced right pubic body BME (*arrowhead*), which likely represents stress response, sometimes in the setting of developing osteitis pubis.

- Osteitis pubis—pubic symphyseal subchondral BME, irregularity, and possibly fracture. The findings may be bilateral.

Treatment Options for Tendon Injuries
- Treatment of tendon overuse injuries usually starts with conservative measures, such as activity modification, NSAIDs, physical therapy, and core strengthening.
- In cases of full-thickness tendon tears or in those cases that do not respond to conservative measures, tendon reattachment or debridement can be considered.
- In cases of athletic pubalgia, many patients, particularly elite athletes, fail these measures and require surgical management. This includes tendon debridement and reattachment.
  - Although hernia repair has been used to help stabilize the inguinal soft tissues, it does not address the underlying pathology in most instances and often fails.

Ischiofemoral Impingement
Pathophysiology and Clinical Presentation
Ischiofemoral impingement (IFI) represents impingement on the quadratus femoris muscle as it passes between the lesser trochanter of the femur and the ischial tuberosity, and can cause chronic hip, gluteal, or groin pain. It is most commonly seen in older women, and can be associated with hip arthroplasty.

Magnetic Resonance Imaging Findings
Refer to Figure 107.19.

- Focal quadratus femoris muscle edema, partial tearing, or fatty infiltration between the ischial tuberosity and the femoral lesser trochanter
- Narrowing of the ischiofemoral space that can result in mass effect on the muscle. The *ischiofemoral distance* is

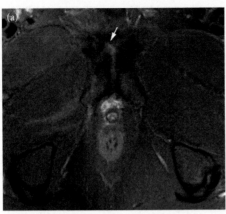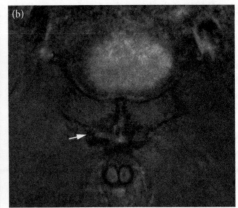

Figure 107.18. Athletic pubalgia in a 34-year-old man with right groin pain during exercise. (*A*) True axial T2W FS MR image of the pubic symphysis demonstrates bilateral common adductor tendon thickening, right greater than left, with a small fluid cleft extending toward the right (*arrow*). This may represent a small partial tear. (*B*) Axial oblique T2W FS MR image in the same patient better demonstrates the cleft extending along the deep fibers of the right common adductor tendon origin (*arrow*). This view is prescribed from a sagittal series that extends laterally to one side and included the apex of the femoral head as an axial stack of images that is obliqued a long the pelvic brim. The plane orientation demonstrates the adductor tendons in long axis and the rectus abdominis tendons in short axis and may be helpful to better visualize injuries to both sets of tendons.

measured between the ischial tuberosity and the lesser trochanter with the hip in neutral position and the patient supine. This distance should be greater than 15 mm. However, this measurement can significantly vary depending on patient positioning.

- Hamstring tendinopathy and partial tendon tears in 50% of patients

Treatment Options

- Start with conservative measures, such as stretching, avoidance of impinging positions, and NSAIDs.
- Can perform targeted US-guided steroid and local anesthetic injection into the ischiofemoral space
- In patients failing conservative therapies, resection of the femoral lesser trochanter can be considered.

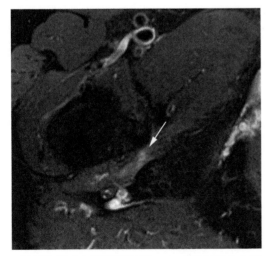

Figure 107.19. IFI. Axial T2W FS MR image of the hip in a 70-year-old man with gluteal pain shows narrowing of the space between the ischial tuberosity and the femoral lesser trochanter. There is focal edema in the quadratus femoris muscle (arrow) between these 2 osseous landmarks.

Key Points

- MRI of the hip using a combination of high-resolution small FOV fluid-sensitive sequences of the hip and larger FOV STIR and T1W nonfat-suppressed images of the entire pelvis provides a comprehensive assessment of the structures that most often contribute to hip pain.
- MRI is the best imaging technique to assess for radiographically occult osseous injuries of the hip, such as stress injuries, SIFs, TOH, and early bisphosphonate-related atypical fractures.
- FAI occurs when the anterosuperior acetabular labrum is impinged between the femoral head/neck junction and the acetabular rim. It is divided into cam-type and pincer-type impingement depending on whether the femoral head/neck junction or the acetabular rim are overgrown. However, most FAI cases have mixed features.
- In DDH, the labrum may become a partially load-bearing structure, which often leads to enlargement, degeneration, and tearing.
- Snapping hip has numerous causes and is divided by whether they are the result of intraarticular and extraarticular pathologies. Extraarticular causes are further divided into internal (medial) and external (lateral) etiologies.
- Athletic pubalgia represents a spectrum of pathologies, including articular, musculotendinous, and peripheral nerve causes.

Recommended Reading

Naraghi A, White LM. MRI of labral and chondral lesions of the hip. *AJR Am J Roentgenol.* 2015;205(3):479–90.

Thomas JD, Li Z, Agur AM, Robinson P. Imaging of the acetabular labrum. *Semin Musculoskelet Radiol.* 2013 Jul;17(3):248–57.

References

1. American College of Radiology. ACR–SPR–SSR practice parameter for the performance and interpretation of magnetic

resonance imaging (MRI) of the hip and pelvis for musculo-skeletal disorders. www.acr.org/~/media/fc429e5a40eb4513a6 934d8037445473.pdf. Accessed February 26, 2017.

2. Bancroft LW, Peterson JJ, Kransdorf MJ. MR imaging of tumors and tumor-like lesions of the hip. *Magn Reson Imaging Clin N Am*. 2005;13(4):757–74.

3. Beltran LS, Rosenberg ZS, Mayo JD, et al. Imaging evaluation of developmental hip dysplasia in the young adult. *AJR Am J Roentgenol*. 2013;200(5):1077–88.

4. Datir A, Xing M, Kang J, et al. Diagnostic utility of MRI and MR arthrography for detection of ligamentum teres tears: a retrospective analysis of 187 patients with hip pain. *AJR Am J Roentgenol*. 2014;203(2):418–23.

5. Gold SL, Burge AJ, Potter HG. MRI of hip cartilage: joint morphology, structure, and composition. *Clin Orthop Relat Res*. 2012;470(12):3321–31.

6. Heller A. Anatomy of the trochanteric bursae. *Radiology*. 2003;226(3):921.

7. Hodnett PA, Shelly MJ, MacMahon PJ, Kavanagh EC, Eustace SJ. MR imaging of overuse injuries of the hip. *Magn Reson Imaging Clin N Am*. 2009;17(4):667–79.

8. Hoffmann A, Pfirrmann CW. The hip abductors at MR imaging. *Eur J Radiol*. 2012;81(12):3755–62.

9. Jacobson JA, Khoury V, Brandon CJ. Ultrasound of the groin: techniques, pathology, and pitfalls. *AJR Am J Roentgenol*. 2015;205(3):513–23.

10. Klontzas ME, Vassalou EE, Zibis AH, Bintoudi AS, Karantanas AH. MR imaging of transient osteoporosis of the hip: an update on 155 hip joints. *Eur J Radiol*. 2015;84(3):431–36.

11. Koulouris G, Connell D. Hamstring muscle complex: an imaging review. *Radiographics*. 2005;25(3):571–86.

12. Nachtrab O, Cassar-Pullicino VN, Lalam R, Tins B, Tyrrell PN, Singh J. Role of MRI in hip fractures, including stress fractures, occult fractures, avulsion fractures. *Eur J Radiol*. 2012;81(12):3813–23.

13. Nguyen MS, Kheyfits V, Giordano BD, Dieudonne G, Monu JU. Hip anatomic variants that may mimic abnormalities at MRI: labral variants. *AJR Am J Roentgenol*. 2013;201(3):W394–400.

14. Omar IM, Zoga AC, Kavanagh EC, et al. Athletic pubalgia and "sports hernia": optimal MR imaging technique and findings. *Radiographics*. 2008;28(5):1415–38.

15. Riley GM, McWalter EJ, Stevens KJ, Safran MR, Lattanzi R, Gold GE. MRI of the hip for the evaluation of femoroacetabular impingement; past, present, and future. *J Magn Reson Imaging*. 2015;41(3):558–72.

16. Viana SL, Machado BB, Mendlovitz PS. MRI of subchondral fractures: a review. *Skeletal Radiol*. 2014;43(11):1515–27.

17. Wunderbaldinger P, Bremer C, Schellenberger E, Cejna M, Turetschek K, Kainberger F. Imaging features of iliopsoas bursitis. *Eur Radiol*. 2002;12(2):409–15.

CHAPTER 108

Internal Derangement of the Knee

Ankur Garg

Introduction

The knee is the most commonly imaged body part in musculo-skeletal MRI and is most often performed for pain, instability, decreased range of motion, or trauma. It is the test of choice to detect internal derangement, such as meniscal, ligament, and extensor mechanism and cartilage injuries, along with radiographically occult osseous injuries. Routine MRI of the knee is usually performed without contrast when evaluating for internal derangement. Standard protocols should contain a variety of fluid- and fat-sensitive sequences in various planes and are generally performed in fewer than 30 minutes. Furthermore, MRA and CTA of the knee can be especially useful in patients who have had prior knee surgery to detect meniscal re-tears or osteochondral injuries. MRI should always be evaluated in conjunction with radiographs of the knee. Initial radiographs are important to assess osseous alignment and mineralization and to detect intraarticular bodies, chondrocalcinosis, and vacuum phenomenon, which can produce MRI findings that overlap with other pathologies such as meniscal or cartilage injuries. Finally, clinical history can often assist in MRI interpretation and can direct the radiologist to clearly answer the referrer's questions.

General Magnetic Resonance Imaging Technique

Standard Musculoskeletal Magnetic Resonance Imaging Sequences

- MRI protocols vary depending on the institution; most protocols use combinations of 4 to 6 fluid- and fat-sensitive sequences (PDW, T2W, T1W) in 3 standard orthogonal planes: axial, coronal, and sagittal.
- Axial sequences are cross-sectional with respect to most structures in the knee and are most useful to look at patellofemoral cartilage, joint effusion, Baker cyst, and the proximal ACL, in addition to many other structures.
- Sagittal sequences are taken along the long axis of the femoral condyles and oriented in the anterior/posterior direction. These are most helpful to look at the extensor mechanism and cruciate ligaments, menisci, and articular cartilage.
- Coronal images are also oriented along the long axis of the femoral condyles, along the medial/lateral plane. These are best used for menisci, collateral ligaments, cruciate ligaments, and medial and lateral compartment articular cartilage.
- MRA and CTA of the knee can be useful in evaluating the postoperative knee, particularly following partial

meniscectomy or repair of osteochondral injury. In these cases, contrast extending into the meniscus (at least 6 months after surgery) increases specificity for tear detection.

- MRA can also be used to assess the integrity of articular cartilage repair and to assess for instability of an osteochondral fragment. MRA should include at least sagittal and coronal T1W FS sequences in addition to routine knee pulse sequences to better assess the menisci, whereas CTA should be performed in bone and soft tissue algorithms in all 3 planes. CTA is useful in detecting meniscal and cartilage injuries when MRI is contraindicated or when it has given equivocal results. However, CTA is relatively insensitive to other internal derangements, such as ligament or tendon injuries.

Bones

Normal Anatomy and Function

The knee joint is formed by the articulation of the medial and lateral condyles of the distal femur, the medial and lateral tibial plateau, and the dorsal patella as it articulates with the femoral trochlea. Because of the differences in forces acting on these regions, the joint is commonly divided into 3 functional compartments: *medial*, *lateral*, and *patellofemoral*. The knee primarily acts as a hinge joint, allowing flexion and extension during locomotion. However, there is a rotational component of movement as well. The medial compartment is larger than the lateral because approximately 70% of force is distributed to the medial compartment during weight-bearing. As a result, a greater number of injuries involve the medial compartment structures, such as the medial meniscus and articular cartilage. The patellofemoral compartment will be further discussed in the section describing the extensor mechanism. Finally, there is a smaller proximal tibiofibular joint that does not contribute significantly to load-bearing. However, this is seen on routine MRI of the knee and can contribute to lateral knee pain. Recent radiographs are of great value when evaluating osseous pathology to look for lesions, fractures, intraarticular bodies, and malalignment.

Adult Osseous Pathology

Osteochondral Lesions

Pathophysiology and Clinical Findings

OCLs are any injury to the articular cartilage and the underlying subchondral bone. They may be caused by repetitive microtrauma, acute traumatic injury, ON, or iatrogenic injury. In the setting of trauma, they may be related to axial load or shear injuries. In the knee, this is most common in the weight-bearing region of the femoral condyles in adults and the lateral margin of the medial femoral condyle in children. Patients are commonly active and present with localized joint pain, swelling, and decreased range of motion. They may also present with catching or locking sensations.

Magnetic Resonance Imaging Findings
- Articular cartilage findings can range from normal to full-thickness cartilage loss.
- Joint fluid may extend into the OCL through cartilage surface defects:
  - Joint fluid extending deep to the lesion is suggestive of instability on imaging.
- May have subchondral BME or cystlike lesions
  - Cystlike lesions might be a sign of developing instability.
- In unstable fragments, there may be a displaced osteochondral fragment.
- Can be associated with secondary OA
- Important to describe the size and location

Treatment Options
- Depends on size and location of the lesion as well as whether there are findings of OA
- For smaller lesions—arthroscopy may be performed to debride the lesion and drill the subchondral bone plate (microfracture).
- For larger lesions—osteochondral grafting may be needed to restore the articular surface contour.
- Arthroplasty may be advised in advanced disease.

Subchondral Insufficiency Fracture of the Knee
Pathophysiology and Clinical Findings
SIF was often formerly referred to as spontaneous ON of the knee (SONK). It is more common in middle-aged or elderly patients with demineralization and most commonly located in the weight-bearing region of the medial femoral condyle. It can present with acute onset of pain without antecedent trauma. SIF is often associated with cartilage loss and meniscal pathology or surgery, because meniscal pathology frequently transfers the load-bearing to the subchondral bone plate.

Magnetic Resonance Imaging Findings
- BME, typically in the medial femoral condyle, is seen in the acute and subacute phases.
- Subcortical hypointense fracture line can be seen, especially on T1W nonfat-suppressed (NFS) images, although these may be very small compared to the overall BME.
- Important to assess and describe if subchondral bone plate collapse is present
- Look for associated meniscal tears or signs of meniscectomy.

Osteophytes and Enthesophytes
Pathophysiology and Clinical Findings
Osteophytes are bone spurs that usually occur at the margins of the subchondral bone plate (marginal osteophytes).

Occasionally they can arise from the surface of the subchondral bone plate and protrude into the joint in the setting of overlying full- or partial-thickness cartilage loss (central osteophytes). Osteophytes are the result of cartilage metaplasia and are the hallmark of OA. They can enlarge and impair full range of movement or be edematous and contribute to joint pain.

The enthesis is the attachment site of the ligaments and tendons on the bone and is a frequent site of pain.

- *Enthesopathy* is the most general term that describes any abnormality at the enthesis.
- *Subenthesial edema* occurs when there is BME at the site of ligament or tendon attachment. It may be related to *enthesitis* in the setting of inflammatory arthropathies such as psoriatic arthritis. More commonly, it is related to repetitive ligamentous or tendinous traction on the bone.
- An *enthesophyte* represents osseous spurring that arises from the enthesis and is directed along the attaching ligament or tendon. It is most commonly related to repetitive traction and may be seen in the setting of prior ligament or tendon injury or tendinosis. DISH also commonly presents with bulky enthesophytes.

Fractures/Contusions
Pathophysiology and Magnetic Resonance Imaging Findings
Contusions represent localized direct trauma to the bone, almost always along the cortex or subchondral bone plate.

- On fluid-sensitive sequences, there is BME and possibly microtrabecular injury.
- No cortical or subchondral bone plate disruption is seen, and there is no visible fracture line.
- Healed contusions demonstrate resolution of BME on fluid-sensitive sequences, and T1W NFS images may reveal an area of darkened marrow that can be sclerotic on radiography.

Impaction is the result of direct trauma to the bone with depression or flattening of the cortex or subchondral bone plate. It is important to mention areas of significant depression particularly of the subchondral bone plate because this can alter the normal biomechanics and result in accelerated cartilage loss.

- T1W NFS sequences may be best at showing the degree of depression.
- A curvilinear fracture line deep to the area of cortical depression may represent underlying microtrabecular fracture.
- Fluid-sensitive sequences often show significant BME.

Finally, *fractures* commonly occur with frank disruption of the cortex. Fractures can be radiographically occult, but easily seen on MRI.

- The fracture line is often best seen on T1W NFS images as a linear or curvilinear low-signal intensity band. In cases of articular surface depression, T1W NFS images may allow quantification of articular surface step-off, which may help determine whether a patient will need surgical correction.

- On fluid-sensitive pulse sequences, there is often significant BME. If the fracture line is dark, it may become more conspicuous by the surrounding BME. Conversely, if it is bright, it may be masked by the BME.
- In healing fractures, the amount of BME decreases and the fracture line becomes less conspicuous, although this process can take many months to resolve on MRI.
- Although direct impact causes compressive forces on the bone with significant BME, many avulsion fractures, such as the Segond fracture along the lateral tibial epiphysis, produce significantly less or no BME. These fractures may be more difficult to detect, and the paucity of BME should not necessarily be taken as a sign of chronicity.

Cartilage

Anatomy and Function

Hyaline cartilage covers articulating surfaces in joints. Its structure allows it to resist compressive forces and disperse these forces over larger surface areas, preventing injuries to the underlying subchondral bone plate. Additionally, it forms a near-frictionless surface to allow smooth gliding of articulating surfaces.

It is mainly composed of type II collagen, proteoglycan matrix and water molecules, and it has a predictable ultrastructure that contributes to the MRI appearance. The basilar fibers are perpendicular to the subchondral bone plate and highly organized. This constricts the free movement of water molecules. The fibers closer to the articular surface are more parallel to the surface of the articular cartilage and randomly oriented. Thus, the movement of water molecules closer to the surface is less constricted. Please refer to Chapter 111, "Imaging of Articular Cartilage," for a more detailed discussion of the structure and pathology of hyaline cartilage.

The articular cartilage within the knee is generally thicker than in other joints because of the higher stresses in the knee experienced during weight-bearing and locomotion. As a result, the knee is a useful model of normal articular cartilage and cartilage pathology in imaging studies. The articular cartilage covers the dorsal surface of the patella, the femoral trochlea, and the surfaces of the femoral condyles and the medial and lateral tibial plateau, sparing the central tibial eminence.

Imaging Strategy

MRI and MRA are the current tests of choice to evaluate cartilage loss. PDW FS or T2W FS SE and 3D-GRE techniques are the most commonly used pulse sequences in clinical practice. The hyaline cartilage should have relatively uniform thickness and should demonstrate a subtle gradient of signal intensities with darker shades in the basal layer along the subchondral bone plate, caused by restriction in the movement of water molecules, and lighter shades along the articular surface. MRA can be used to assess surface lesions of the articular cartilage. This may be most helpful in patients who have had prior

cartilage augmentation procedures, such as microfracture, osteochondral grafting, and autologous chondrocyte implantation (ACI). CTA can be useful to assess articular cartilage when MRI is contraindicated.

Magnetic Resonance Imaging Findings

- Disruption of the normal gradient of signal intensities, or cartilage heterogeneity, often indicates degeneration. In many instances, the cartilage becomes brighter than expected on fluid-sensitive sequences and may be focally swollen.
- Cartilage defects may be divided into partial- or full-thickness defects.
  - Fluid signal on routine MRI or dilute Gd in the case of MRA, which extends to the subchondral bone plate, is compatible with a full-thickness defect.
  - In the setting of full-thickness defects, the knee joint recesses should be thoroughly examined for displaced cartilage fragments.
  - Focal cartilage thinning suggests partial-thickness cartilage loss.
  - Surface irregularity/fissuring (Figure 108.1): superficial versus deep fissuring
  - Delamination: separation of cartilage from subchondral bone plate or separation of chondral layers that parallels the subchondral bone plate
- Can use a grading system, such as the Outerbridge grading system, which is based on arthroscopic experience. However, MRI findings may not always

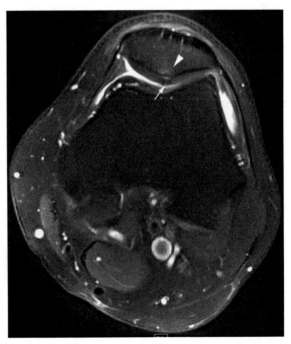

Figure 108.1. Chondral degeneration in a 46-year-old man with chronic anterior knee pain. Axial PD FS image demonstrates a full-thickness cartilage fissure at the patellar median ridge (*arrow*), associated with heterogeneous cartilage signal that indicates degeneration is also present. There is underlying subchondral BME (*arrowhead*), which is often seen adjacent to chondral loss.

accurately correspond to arthroscopic findings (see Chapter 111 for a description of the modified Outerbridge grading system), and many referrers and radiologists prefer description of the areas of abnormality rather than assigning grades.

- Cartilage loss is often associated with underlying subchondral bone marrow abnormalities such as cystlike changes, sclerosis (low signal on T1W NFS sequences), or BME on fluid-sensitive sequences.
- Recent chondral defects usually have a sharply marginated transition between the defect and normal-appearing cartilage (shouldered appearance).
- Chronic lesions tend to have a more gradually tapered transition between the defect and normal cartilage.
- Important MRI findings to report include location of cartilage loss/degeneration, depth of loss (full-thickness vs. partial-thickness), surface size of defect measured in 2 dimensions, and shape of chondral defect margins. When reporting the depth of a partial-thickness lesion, it should be noted whether the lesion is deep (>50% of the cartilage thickness) or shallow (involves ≤50% of the cartilage thickness).

Menisci

Anatomy and Function

The menisci are semilunar (C-shaped) fibrocartilage structures in the medial and lateral compartments of the knee (Figure 108.2). The medial meniscus (MM) is larger than the lateral meniscus (LM) because approximately 70% of the load in weight-bearing occurs in the medial compartment. They function to absorb axial loads, distribute forces across the articular surfaces, and are passive stabilizers of the knee. Overall, these functions serve to protect articular cartilage. Each meniscus

is divided into an *anterior horn, body,* and *posterior horn.* The anterior horn is tethered to the anterior tibial eminence by an *anterior root ligament,* and the posterior horn is attached to the posterior tibial eminence by a *posterior root ligament.* In short axis, the normal meniscus has a predictable isosceles triangular shape with longer superior and inferior articular surfaces and a shorter peripheral surface. The cross-section of the meniscus can be divided into thirds; the peripheral third of the meniscus is vascularized in adults, and often referred to in arthroscopic reports as the *red zone.* The middle third is partially vascularized and can be called the *pink zone.* The inner third is relatively avascular and often referred to as the *white zone.* Meniscal tears in more vascularized regions tend to heal better and are often more amenable to a desired surgical outcome. The central apex of the triangle is often called the *inner margin* or the *free edge.*

On routine MRI, the normal triangular meniscal shape is best seen on coronal and sagittal images; the meniscal body is best visualized on coronal planes, whereas sagittal imaging better depicts the anterior and posterior horns. Because menisci are mainly made of fibrocartilage, they are generally black or dark gray in signal intensity on all pulse sequences. Occasionally a normal meniscus may have intermediate peripheral signal that does not meet criteria for meniscal tear. In patients younger than 30 years, this signal may represent peripheral vascularity, whereas in older patients, it more likely represents intrasubstance degeneration. The posterior horn of the MM is larger than the anterior horn, which reflects generally greater axial loading on the posterior horn. The relative sizes of the anterior and posterior horns are best seen on sagittal imaging (Figure 108.3). Conversely, cross-sectional size of the LM posterior horn is equal to that of the anterior horn. Deviation in the relative sizes of the anterior and posterior horns in the absence of prior meniscal surgery may indicate a meniscal tear.

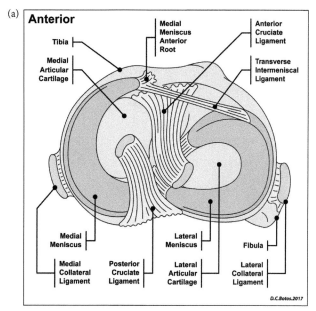
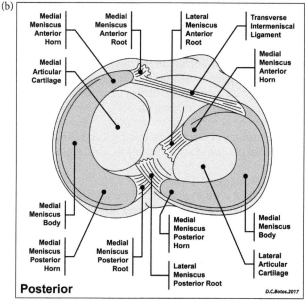

Figure 108.2. Diagrams of the menisci. (*A*) Birdseye (axial) view of the knee with the femur cut away shows the relationships of the cruciate and collateral ligaments with respect to the medial and lateral menisci. (*B*) The same view with the cruciate ligaments removed allows identification of the individual meniscal parts and depiction of the meniscal root ligaments.

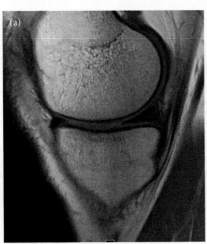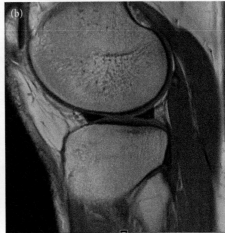

Figure 108.3. Normal menisci. (*A*) Sagittal PD NFS image demonstrates a normal MM. The meniscus is triangular in cross-section, the posterior horn is larger than the anterior horn, and meniscus demonstrates diffusely low signal. (*B*) Normal LM. Sagittal PD NFS image demonstrates a normal LM. The posterior horn is equal in size to the anterior horn.

Radiologists should be familiar with a number of structures supporting the menisci, such as the joint capsule and ligaments attaching on the menisci, not only to be able to properly identify when there are injuries of these structures, but also to avoid misdiagnosing meniscal pathology. For example, the meniscal root ligaments often have vertically oriented striations of alternating dark and intermediate signal as they attach onto the tibial eminence, which should not be mistaken for longitudinal meniscal tears.

The joint capsule attaches to the menisci (meniscocapsular attachment). The attachment involving the MM is tighter, preventing fluid from tracking along its periphery. The attachment is looser along the LM, allowing some fluid to track along its periphery. The meniscopopliteal fascicles are superior and inferior fibrous bands that attach to the LM. The anteroinferior and posterosuperior fascicles are usually seen on routine knee MRI, whereas the posteroinferior fascicle is variably seen. The LM posterior horn fascicles connect to the joint capsule and form the popliteus hiatus, which allows the passage of the popliteal tendon from within the joint capsule to an extraarticular position.

The meniscofemoral ligaments are variably visualized fibrous bands connecting the posterior horn of the LM to the lateral edge of the medial femoral condyle. If located anterior to the PCL, it is called a *ligament of Humphry*. If located posterior to the PCL, it is called a *ligament of Wrisberg*. Finally, the transverse intermeniscal ligament is a commonly seen fibrous band connecting the anterior horns of the medial and lateral menisci. A cleft of joint fluid can be seen as the ligament inserts onto the meniscal anterior horn that should not be mistaken for a meniscal tear. Oblique meniscomeniscal ligaments are seen in up to 5% of patients. The medial oblique meniscomeniscal ligament extends from the anterior horn of the medical meniscus to the posterior horn of the LM. The lateral oblique meniscomeniscal ligament extends from the anterior horn of the LM to the posterior horn of the medical meniscus.

Although the menisci usually have predictable shapes, there are a few variant morphologies that are important to note to avoid overcalling meniscal pathology. The most common variant is the *discoid meniscus* in which there is excessive meniscal tissue along the inner margin. This is most commonly seen on coronal imaging and can be diagnosed if the transverse width from the periphery of the meniscus to its inner margin is greater than approximately 13 mm. The Watanabe classification system divides discoid menisci into 3 types: *incomplete, complete,* and *Wrisberg-ligament variant* types. Incomplete discoid menisci are thicker and longer than normal menisci but do not fully cover the tibial plateau. Complete discoid menisci completely cover the tibial plateau. Finally, the Wrisberg-ligament variant type occurs when there is developmental absence of the meniscotibial (coronary) ligament, which allows the discoid meniscus to become hypermobile. The meniscus can migrate deeper into the femorotibial compartment and result in mechanical symptoms, such as locking and pain. The LM is 9 times more likely to have discoid morphology (Figures 108.4 and 108.5). Although this represents variant anatomy, it has a strong tendency for intrasubstance degeneration and meniscal tearing. Additionally, tears of discoid menisci do not follow the same strict criteria for diagnosis as tears in nondiscoid menisci, and a significant internal signal abnormality even if it does not extend to the meniscal surface may indicate a tear.

Meniscal flounce is a wavy appearance of the meniscal inner margin. Overwhelmingly this appearance represents an anatomic variation, and it should not be confused for a tear. On occasion, it can be associated with a meniscal tear, such as a radial tear, in which there is meniscal laxity.

Chondrocalcinosis and vacuum phenomenon are often seen in OA and can mimic other intraarticular pathology. For example, chondrocalcinosis can result in bright intrameniscal signal than can mimic a tear. Conversely, vacuum phenomenon occurs when there is focally trapped gas, usually within the medial or lateral compartments of the knee. This can result in focally dark signal, which can mimic a displaced meniscal fragment. A *meniscal ossicle* is a rare and usually asymptomatic finding. It is a small piece of bone that is most often located within the posterior horn of the MM. In these cases, radiographs can be helpful to confirm these findings and prevent erroneous diagnosis of meniscal pathology.

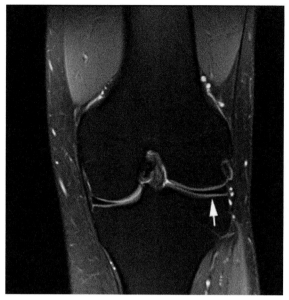

Figure 108.4. Incomplete discoid LM. Coronal PD FS image demonstrates a triangular-shaped discoid LM. The transverse meniscal body width measures 16 mm, which is enlarged (*arrow*).

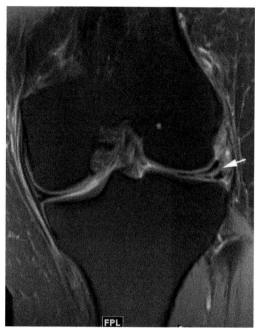

Figure 108.5. Incomplete discoid LM with a horizontal tear in a 42-year-old woman with medial knee pain and limited range of motion. Coronal PD FS image demonstrating a discoid medial meniscus with a complex but predominantly horizontal tear (*arrow*).

Meniscal Tears

Injuries to the menisci are one of the most common indications for knee MRI. They can be sources of knee pain and potentially contribute to accelerated articular cartilage loss. Therefore, accurate meniscal evaluation is one of the most important components of the MRI report. Meniscal tears are diagnosed either when there is signal abnormality contacting the superior and/or inferior articular surfaces or the free edge, abnormal morphology, or both. Tears are often categorized by their orientation: They may be horizontally or vertically oriented.

The International Society of Arthroscopy, Knee Surgery and Orthopaedic Sports Medicine (ISAKOS) arthroscopic tear classification system is a comprehensive method for evaluating and describing meniscal tears. The classification system includes *longitudinal-vertical, horizontal, radial, vertical flap, horizontal flap,* and *complex* tear patterns (Figure 108.6).

Horizontal tears include *cleavage tears*, in which the tear extends to the free edge (Figure 108.7), or *oblique tears,*

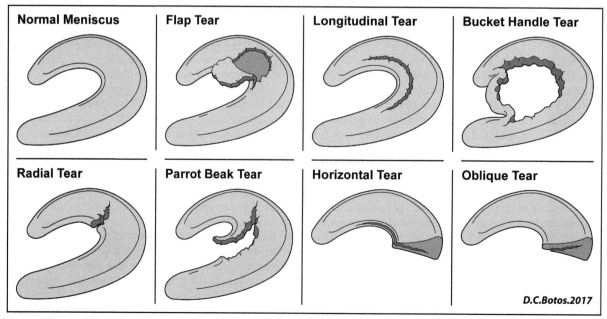

| Normal Meniscus | Flap Tear | Longitudinal Tear | Bucket Handle Tear |
| Radial Tear | Parrot Beak Tear | Horizontal Tear | Oblique Tear |

D.C.Botos.2017

Figure 108.6. Diagram showing the common types of meniscal tears.

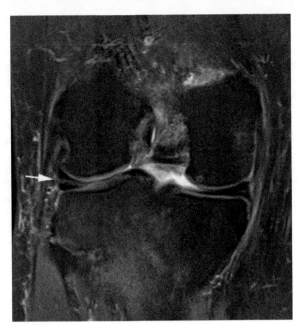

Figure 108.7. Lateral meniscal body horizontal tear in a 46-year-old man with lateral knee pain. Coronal PD FS image demonstrates a horizontal tear of the LM body extending to the inner margin (*arrow*).

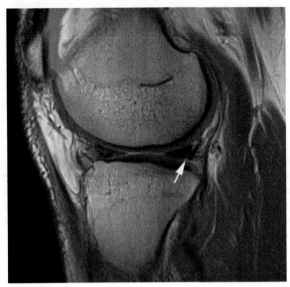

Figure 108.8. Lateral meniscal posterior horn longitudinal-vertical tear in a 53-year-old woman with worsening medial knee pain for 3 months. Sagittal PD NFS image demonstrates a peripheral vertically oriented longitudinal tear of the MM posterior horn (arrow). This cleft is lateral to the attachment of the meniscofemoral ligament, which can occasionally mimic a vertical longitudinal tear.

in which the tear extends to the superior articular surface or more commonly the inferior surface. These tears divide the meniscus into superior and inferior portions and are often degenerative. A portion of the inferior surface can become displaced, or flip, into the joint recess between the medial tibial plateau and the joint capsule.

Vertical tears extend from the superior surface to the inferior surface of the meniscus and may either be oriented along the long axis of the meniscus, known as a *vertical longitudinal tear* (Figure 108.8), or along the short axis, termed a *radial tear* (Figure 108.9). The orientation of a vertical longitudinal tear

parallels the collagen fibers along the long axis of meniscus. In a true vertical longitudinal tear, the tear has a relatively stable distance between the inner/outer meniscal surfaces along its length. This decouples the periphery and the inner margin and can lead to a bucket handle-type tear when the inner margin displaces centrally. Peripherally located nondisplaced tears have better surgical outcomes and may heal without surgical intervention. Occasionally, these tears may extend obliquely from the inner margin to the periphery and form what is often known as a *parrot beak-type tear*. These tears often contain radial and longitudinal components.

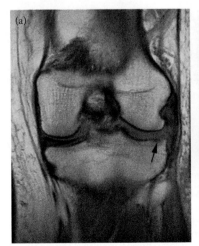
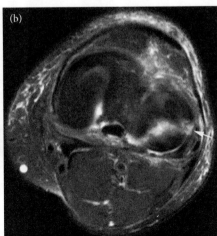
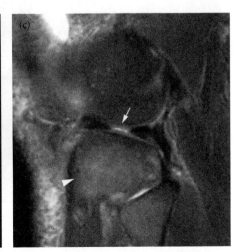

Figures 108.9. Lateral meniscal body radial tear in a 62-year-old woman with acute on chronic medial knee pain. Coronal PD NFS (*A*) and axial T2W FS (*B*) images demonstrates a full-thickness radial tear of the lateral meniscal body (*arrows*). Coronal image demonstrates the *absent meniscus sign (ghost meniscus)*. (*C*) Sagittal T2W FS image through the LM shows a fluid cleft through the meniscal body at the site of the radial tear (*arrow*). There is lateral tibial plateau BME that may represent associated stress response (*arrowhead*).

Radial tears are perpendicular to the long axis of the meniscus. They can be complete, extending from the inner margin to the periphery, or partial. These tears decouple the anterior and posterior meniscal segments and can allow the tear to displace further peripherally or extrude, especially during weight-bearing if the tear is full thickness. *Meniscal extrusion* is defined as the peripheral (outer) edge of the meniscal body located more than 3 mm peripherally from the tibial plateau peripheral surface. Extrusion significantly reduces the meniscal ability to withstand axial loading and can lead to accelerated cartilage loss. The MM posterior horn/root junction is a common place for a degenerative radial tear and may be overlooked unless this area is examined carefully. Radial tears are usually a result of higher forces, and surgical outcomes are not generally as favorable. The *marching cleft* sign describes a radial parrot beak-type tear that extends away from the free edge of the meniscus on contiguous images caused by an oblique orientation with respect to coronal/sagittal planes.

Complex or *multidirectional tears* are diagnosed when there is more than one type of tear. These are commonly degenerative and are more frequently associated with accelerated chondral loss and OA.

Magnetic Resonance Imaging Strategy and Findings
Native Meniscus

MRI is the best imaging study to detect and characterize meniscal pathology. Menisci should be evaluated on at least the coronal and sagittal planes. Because of its high SNR and generally high spatial resolution, the PDW SE sequence is the workhorse sequence for diagnosis of meniscal pathology. PDW sequences are more sensitive in detecting meniscal pathology, although many areas of signal alteration may not represent true meniscal tears. Conversely, although many meniscal tears are not visible on routine T2W images, T2W sequences are more specific. Therefore, any signal abnormality on T2W imaging that meets criteria for meniscal tear is more likely to represent a tear at arthroscopy. Fat saturation can be helpful to detect other pathologies, but is not usually helpful to diagnose meniscal tears.

- *Specific morphologic and signal criteria used to improve the specificity and accuracy of MRI in detecting meniscal tears*
  - The signal abnormality should clearly extend to the articular surface on 2 or more consecutive images in 1 imaging plane or at least 1 image in the same location on orthogonal planes.
  - Meniscal tears can also be diagnosed on seeing abnormal morphology, such as truncation of the free edge, on only 1 image.
- *MRI findings to report when describing meniscal tears*
  - Location of tear and which segment is involved
  - Whether the tear involves the periphery or the free edge
  - Which surface(s) the tear contacts; whether there is any meniscal extrusion; and in the case of a radial tear, the size of the meniscal gap
  - Size and location of any displaced meniscal fragments, because displaced fragments can result in mechanical symptoms, such as locking, clicking, and catching, and often require surgical debridement
- Bucket handle tears occur when there is a large, displaced inner meniscal fragment into the intercondylar notch, usually related to vertically oriented, longitudinal tears (Figure 108.10).
  - On sagittal MR images through the intercondylar notch, a *double PCL sign* represents a flipped meniscal fragment inferior to and paralleling the PCL.

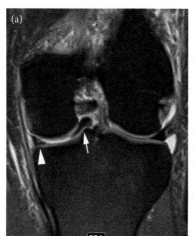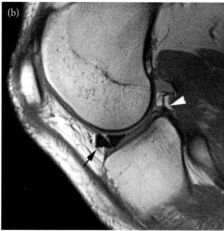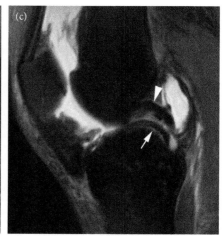

Figure 108.10. Medial meniscal bucket handle tears. (*A*) Coronal PD FS image in a 32-year-old woman with acute onset of knee pain and locking after injury demonstrates a bucket handle tear of the MM. Meniscal tissue is displaced into the intercondylar notch (*arrow*). The remnant medial meniscal tissue is smaller than normally encountered (*arrowhead*). (*B*) Sagittal PD NFS image of the LM in a 24-year-old woman who presented with a knee locked in 90 degrees of flexion shows 2 triangularly shaped meniscal segments (*black arrow*) in the anterior aspect of the lateral compartment. The more anterior segment is the anterior horn, whereas the more posterior segment is the flipped posterior horn. The *white arrowhead* indicates the absent posterior horn. The finding is called the *double anterior horn sign* or the *double delta sign*. (*C*) Sagittal T2W FS image of the knee in a 57-year-old woman demonstrates the double PCL sign, a common appearance of a bucket handle tear when the meniscal fragment (*arrow*) flips into the inter condylar notch. The fragment has a similar curvilinear orientation to the native PCL (*arrowhead*).

- If the bucket handle fragment arises from the posterior horn and is displaced anteriorly along the inner margin of the anterior horn, it may appear as a *double anterior horn sign*. In cross-section, the meniscal fragments are usually triangularly shaped, and the appearance has also been called the *double delta sign*.
- Meniscal root injuries are commonly missed because they are oblique to the standard imaging planes, which can lead to volume averaging. These are most common in the posterior horn of the MM and are associated with globular bright signal extending to an articular surface. Developing radial root tears may be associated with meniscal extrusion.
  - If the plane of imaging extends through the meniscal gap created by the radial tear, the meniscus will appear focally absent. Imaging slices on both sides of the tear that pass through the torn edges of meniscal tissue, and the meniscus will appear present in these images. The focal disappearance of the meniscus in the area of the radial tear has been called the *meniscal ghost sign*.
- Additional MRI findings associated with meniscal tears include parameniscal cysts (Figure 108.11). Approximately 90% of parameniscal cysts are associated with meniscal tears. These lesions are thought to occur when joint fluid extends through a meniscal tear into a lobulated cystlike structure. They have fluid-signal intensity on all pulse sequences and may have septations. They are most commonly associated with horizontal cleavage and oblique tears.
- *Meniscocapsular separation* occurs when there is detachment of the joint capsule from the periphery of the meniscus, allowing the meniscus to become unstable and potentially displaced. On MRI, abnormal fluid along the periphery of the meniscus, particularly the MM, is a sign of meniscocapsular injury.
- A complicated area to assess for meniscal tears is at the posterior surface of the LM posterior horn in the region of the meniscofemoral ligament of Wrisberg attachment. It is normal to have a smooth cleft of vertical signal at the attachment of the ligament to the LM posterior horn (Wrisberg pseudotear). If the vertical signal is irregular and/or extends further laterally into the meniscus, a peripheral vertical longitudinal tear of the LM posterior horn should be suspected (Wrisberg rip). The meniscofemoral ligament generally attaches to the lateral meniscal posterior horn within 14 mm from the lateral margin of the distal PCL, and any ligament attaching more than 14 mm from the PCL is a sign of a peripheral meniscal tear. These tears are commonly associated with ACL injuries.

Postoperative Meniscus

Symptomatic meniscal tears, including tears with flipped meniscal fragments, often require debridement of the unstable meniscal segment(s), called *partial meniscectomy*. In general, surgeons attempt to debride as little meniscal tissue as possible to maintain a stable margin of the remaining meniscal tissue. Abnormal signal of the residual meniscal tissue could represent intrasubstance degeneration or granulation tissue in the site of healed meniscal tearing. Debridement of a segment of the meniscus may allow signal abnormality that did not extend to an articular surface on preoperative imaging (representing intrasubstance degeneration) to appear to extend to the resected margin of the meniscus on postoperative imaging. In these cases, the signal abnormality may represent the original degenerative signal or a new meniscal tear. Thus, accurate detection and characterization of meniscal re-tears following meniscectomy can be challenging. Additionally, the meniscus may be smaller than expected, which may be caused by partial meniscectomy, flipped meniscal fragment, and meniscal maceration. It is very helpful to have prior imaging and/or an operative report in order to compare signal abnormalities and meniscal morphologies.

- *MRI findings to distinguish normal postoperative appearance from new meniscal tear or retear*
  - Comparison with preoperative imaging is critical.
  - Intermediate signal on PDW sequences could represent granulation tissue at the site of healed meniscal tear or new meniscal tear.
  - May use T2W sequence to look for fluid signal in the meniscus, which is a more specific finding for meniscal tear
  - Look for new or enlarging parameniscal cyst.
  - Look for new flipped fragment or meniscal signal not seen on prior studies.
  - MRA can be helpful for new tear identification.

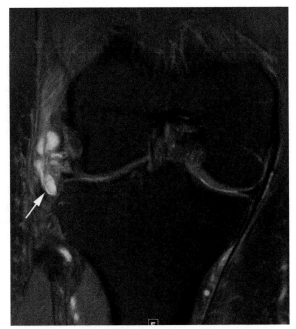

Figure 108.11. Lateral meniscal posterior horn horizontal tear with parameniscal cyst in a 59-year-old man with chronic generalized knee pain. Coronal PD FS image demonstrates a horizontal tear of the lateral meniscal posterior horn with an associated moderately sized parameniscal cyst (*arrow*).

Ligaments

Background

The major knee ligaments are the ACL and PCL, which are centrally located within the knee, and the medial and lateral collateral ligamentous complexes located along the periphery of the knee. Ligament injuries are called *sprains* and are commonly divided into 3 grades.

- *Grade 1 sprains* involve stretching of the ligament without discrete tearing. On MRI, there is periligamentous edema without discontinuity of the ligament.
- *Grade 2 sprains* are partial tears. MRI reveals ligament thickening and partial disruption in addition to periligamentous edema.
- *Grade 3 sprains* are the highest grade injures and involve complete tearing of ligament (Figure 108.12).

Cruciate Ligaments

Anterior Cruciate Ligament

Anatomy and Function

The ACL originates from the lateral femoral condyle in the intercondylar notch and extends inferiorly, anteriorly, and medially to insert on anterior intercondylar eminence of the tibia. It is composed of 2 bundles: the anteromedial bundle which is the stronger of the 2 bundles and taut in knee flexion; and the posterolateral bundle, which is taut in knee extension. Its major function is to prevent anterior tibial translation although it plays a minor role in resisting extension and rotational injuries as well. As a result, it is most commonly injured during hyperextension, valgus, and/or anterolateral rotary subluxation (pivot shift injury).

Imaging Strategy

The ACL is best evaluated on fluid-sensitive sequences, and fat saturation may help make soft tissue edema and fluid more conspicuous. Although sagittal imaging is often used to depict

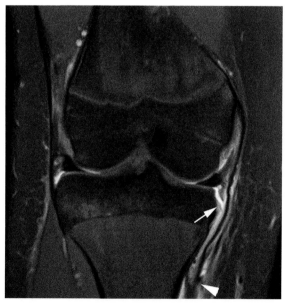

Figure 108.12. Grade 3 MCL sprain in a 33-year-old woman with acute onset of medial pain and swelling after injury. Coronal PD FS image demonstrates a grade 3 sprain of the distal MCL superficial (*arrowhead*) and deep (*arrow*) ligaments. Note the full-thickness tear of the distal superficial and the deep (meniscotibial) ligaments with surrounding edema.

the ligament in long axis, it may be difficult to detect some partial tears because of volume averaging. Standard coronal imaging provides visualization of the ligament that is more closely cross-sectional and reduces the impact of volume averaging. Axial imaging can also be helpful to examine the ACL origin and mid substance. However, the distal fibers may be difficult to differentiate from the tibial eminence in this plane. Whereas some institutions routinely image the ACL obliquely to depict the ligament either in true long or short axis, this may add time to the examination without significantly adding to diagnostic accuracy. In addition, these oblique planes may distort the remaining anatomy and make detection of additional pathology difficult.

Because of the dense collagen arrangement, the normal ligament fibers are low in signal intensity along the long axis of the ligament. On coronal and axial imaging, the anteromedial and posterolateral bundles are seen diverging from the femoral origin as they insert on the tibial eminence. There is usually intermediate signal distally within the ACL separating the dominant bundles, which should not be mistaken for an ACL injury.

Mucoid degeneration of the ACL is common and can be mistaken for partial or complete ligament tears. The natural history of mucoid degeneration has not been established, and it has not been convincingly associated with the development of ACL tears. In this condition, the ACL is thickened, and the fibers are splayed by intermediate and bright signal on fluid-sensitive sequences even though the fibers are intact. Intra- and extraligamentous ganglion cysts can form and may extend into the adjacent bone.

Magnetic Resonance Imaging Findings

- Majority of injuries (between 60 and 70%) are complete tears.
- Tears are associated with discontinuity of ligament fibers with ligament thickening and peri-ligamentous edema.
- Ligament is often wavy and may have an abnormal orientation.
- An *entrapped ACL stump* occurs when the distal ACL stump becomes interposed between the distal femoral intercondylar notch and the tibial eminence, which can block full extension. On MRI, it can appear nodular and resemble the cyclops lesion seen after ACL reconstruction.
- Secondary signs
  - Bone contusions/fractures
    - Pivot shift pattern of injuries (Figure 108.13) involves the anterior lateral femoral condyle and the posterior aspect of lateral tibial plateau, indicating a rotational component of the injury
      - *Deep sulcus sign* represents an impaction injury along the anterior weight-bearing region of the lateral femoral condyle along the sulcus terminalis. Normally this area of the bone is either flat or slightly concave. Impaction of this area may result in deepening of the sulcus. This is measured on a sagittal MR image or a true lateral radiograph by drawing a line connecting the anterior and posterior margins of

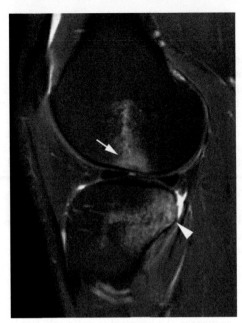

Figure 108.13. Pivot shift contusion pattern in the setting of ACL sprain in a 22-year-old woman with acute onset of knee pain after injury. Sagittal T2W FS image demonstrates the classic osseous contusions seen in the setting of a pivot shift injury resulting in an ACL sprain. Contusions involve the anterior lateral femoral condyle in the region of the terminal sulcus (*arrow*) and at the posterior lateral tibial plateau (*arrowhead*).

the sulcus and measuring the distance from that line to the greatest depth of the sulcus. A measurement greater than 1.5 mm is considered abnormal.

- May also see contusion of the posterior aspect of the medial tibial plateau
- Segond fracture (Figure 108.14)
  - Peripheral lateral tibial plateau chip fracture that is likely related to osseous avulsion. There is debate

in the literature about the structure responsible for this avulsion. Previous studies have implicated the lateral capsular ligament, the posterior bundle of the iliotibial band, an anterior bundle of the LCL, or fibers from the biceps femoris tendon that insert on the lateral tibial epiphysis. Most recently, however, some authors have suggested the anterolateral ligament (ALL), which arises from the lateral femoral condyle and travels anteriorly and obliquely to insert on the anterolateral tibial epiphysis, may be the most commonly involved structure.

- Nearly 100% associated with ACL injuries
- Often noted on initial radiographs, which can establish ACL injury
- Anterior tibial translation—on MRI, draw vertically oriented line parallel to the posterior cortex of the lateral femoral condyle and a second vertically oriented line parallel to the posterior cortex of the lateral tibial plateau. Anterior tibial translation is present if tibial line is greater than 7 mm anteriorly positioned relative to the lateral femoral condyle line (MRI anterior drawer sign).
- The O'Donoghue triad is a common injury pattern that includes ACL sprain, MM tear, and MCL sprain.
- LM tear is more commonly associated with ACL tear.
- Joint effusion
- Important findings to report include the type of tear: full- (Figure 108.15) or partial-thickness; location of tear in ligament: proximal, midsubstance, or distal; and orientation of torn ligament fragments. The MRI report should also include description of any associated cartilage injury.

Treatment Options

- Primary ACL repair has a poor outcome unless there is an avulsed osseous fragment that can be fixed.

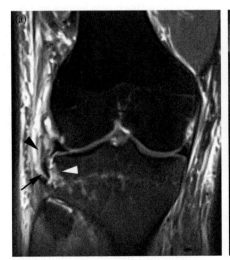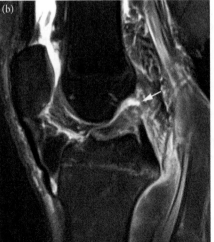

Figure 108.14. Segond fracture in a 53-year-old man. (*A*) Coronal T2W FS MR image of the knee shows a curvilinear low-signal focus representing a small avulsion fracture (*arrow*). There is a small cortical donor site with BME (*white arrowhead*). The anterior longitudinal ligament (*black arrowhead*) is seen attaching onto the avulsed fracture fragment. (*B*) Sagittal PDW MR image demonstrates a complete proximal ACL tear (*arrow*), which is commonly associated with Segond fractures.

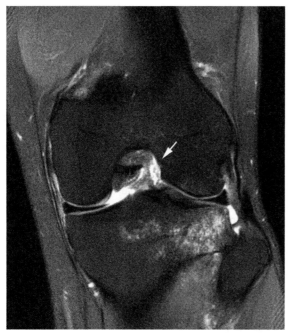

Figure 108.15. Grade 3 (full-thickness) ACL sprain in a 37-year-old woman with acute onset of pain and instability after injury. Coronal PD FS image demonstrates a full-thickness tear of the proximal ACL (grade 3 sprain). Absent ACL fibers along the lateral femoral condyle is known as the *empty notch sign* (*arrow*).

- Ligament reconstruction is preferred and most commonly performed with bone-patellar tendon-bone or hamstring autografts, or cadaveric allograft.
- Common complications after ACL reconstruction
  - Mucoid degeneration of the graft—mucoid (T2 hyperintense) material can be located within the graft and in the femoral/tibial tunnels. Tibial tunnel enlargement can occur. Mucoid material can also spill out in to the soft tissues anterior to the proximal tibia.
  - Tear of the graft—abrupt caliber decrease of graft or fiber discontinuity. Should be described in similar manner as native ACL tears
  - Tibial tunnel widening—abnormal bony resorption of the tibial tunnel that may be related to mechanical factors, such as graft motion, or biological factors, such as synovial fluid extension into the tunnel. This often occurs in the early postoperative period (within 3 months).
  - Arthrofibrosis—intermediate signal fibrous material that often forms anterior to the intraarticular segment of the graft (cyclops lesion). Can limit extension.
  - Distal femoral intercondylar notch osteophytes—can impinge on graft, particularly when knee is in terminal extension. May be best seen on sagittal imaging.
  - Roof impingement may also occur when the tibial tunnel is placed too far anterior on the tibial eminence. Normally, the tibial tunnel should be positioned posterior to a line drawn on a midsagittal image along the intercondylar notch as it intersects the anterior tibial eminence. If the tibial tunnel is positioned anterior to this line, the intercondylar notch may impinge on the graft particularly in terminal extension.

Posterior Cruciate Ligament
Anatomy and Function
The main function of the PCL is to prevent posterior translation of the tibia. It originates from the medial distal femoral intercondylar notch and extends posteriorly and inferiorly to insert on the posterior tibia. Anatomically, it has 2 bundles: the anterolateral and posteromedial bundles. However, these are not commonly distinctly visible on routine MRI, and determining whether an injury has occurred in one bundle versus another is often not possible.

Normal Magnetic Resonance Imaging Appearance and Magnetic Resonance Imaging Findings of Injuries
On imaging, the ligament is often divided into proximal, mid, and distal segments. The proximal segment is horizontally oriented, whereas the distal segment is more vertically oriented. The mid segment is angulated to accommodate the changing orientation from proximal to distal. On fluid-sensitive sequences, the ligament is uniformly low in signal and has a generally uniform caliber. It is often well seen in long axis on sagittal imaging, although coronal imaging may be helpful to visualize the proximal PCL in cross-section, whereas axial sequences may be helpful to assess the distal PCL.

Magnetic Resonance Imaging Findings
- Compared to the ACL, the PCL is less commonly torn, and PCL tears are more frequently partial tears.
- Ligament fiber disruption, abnormal caliber change, and periligamentous edema are signs of PCL tears.
- Describe whether the tear is partial or complete and location of tear.
- Rather than resulting in ligament tears, these injuries may result in osseous avulsion from the posterior tibial eminence.
- Often associated with injuries to the posterolateral stabilizing structures (posterolateral corner) of the knee, including the biceps femoris and popliteus tendons, LCL proper, and posterolateral joint capsule.
- *Reverse Segond fracture*, an avulsion fracture of the medial tibial plateau with valgus stress and external rotation, has most commonly been associated with PCL tears and medial meniscal injuries (Figure 108.16).
- PCL osseous avulsions can be seen either when there is posterior tibial translation with the knee flexed (dashboard injury) or with hyperextension (Figure 108.17). This injury usually occurs at the tibial attachment and can either occur in isolation or with multiligamentous injuries, including posterolateral corner injuries.

Treatment Options
- Generally, conservatively managed. Surgery is often not performed after isolated injury unless there is significant instability.
- For PCL osseous avulsion injuries, surgical fixation may be required if the avulsed fragment is displaced.

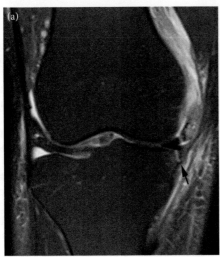
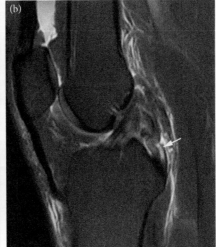

Figure 108.16. Reverse Segond fracture associated with a PCL tear in a 41-year-old man. (*A*) Coronal T2W FS MR image of the knee demonstrates a small avulsed osseous fragment from the medial tibial plateau associated with mild BME (*arrow*). (*C*) Sagittal T2W FS MR image of the knee shows a complete distal PCL tear (*arrow*).

Medial Supporting Structures

The medial supporting structures of the knee include the components of the MCL and the posteromedial corner structures. These structures include the posterior oblique ligament, oblique popliteal ligament, semimembranosus tendon, posteromedial capsule, and posterior horn of the MM. The *posterior oblique ligament* is formed from the capsule posterior to the superficial MCL fibers (Figure 108.18). Surgical repair may be indicated for high-grade posteromedial corner injuries.

Medial Collateral Ligament

Anatomy and Function

The MCL serves as the primary restraint to valgus force. It is made of 3 layers: the *superficial fascia*, which is the most superficial and difficult to see on routine MRI; the *superficial ligament*, which extends from the medial femoral condyle near the adductor tubercle to the proximal medial tibial diaphysis; and the *deep* or *coronary ligaments*, which consist of meniscofemoral and meniscotibial components and join the periphery of the menisci to the medial margins of the medial femoral condyle and medial tibial plateau.

Normal Magnetic Resonance Imaging Appearance and Magnetic Resonance Imaging Findings of Injuries

As with other ligaments, the MCL is best assessed on fluid-sensitive sequences, such as PDW or T2W sequences. The superficial ligament is the most easily seen and most commonly injured component. It should appear as a dark band of uniform thickness from the medial femoral condyle to the medial tibial diaphysis. In older patients, the proximal ligament may appear mildly thickened without disruption of the ligament fibers or periligamentous edema to suggest recent injury. This appearance may reflect chronic scarring caused by remote MCL injury or repetitive low-grade traction.

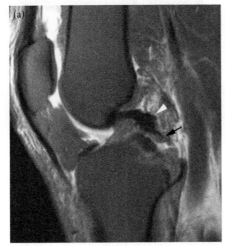
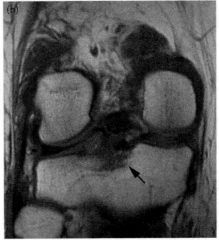

Figure 108.17. PCL osseous avulsion from the tibial eminence in a 29-year-old man following dashboard injury during a motor vehicle collision. (*A*) Sagittal T2W FS MR image of the knee shows the distal PCL is partially retracted (*arrowhead*) and attached onto a tibial eminence fracture fragment (*arrow*). (*B*) Coronal T1W MR image better depicts the low-signal intensity fracture line (*arrow*).

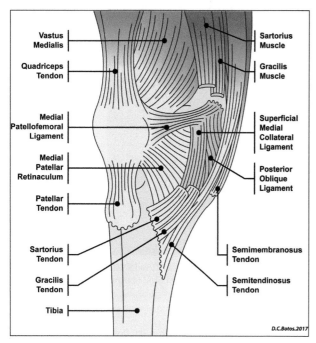

Figure 108.18. Diagram of the major medial stabilizing structures, including the MCL, medial patellar retinaculum with MPFL, and posterior oblique ligament.

- Important to describe where tear is located in the ligament and which components are involved
- Thickening of the proximal superficial ligament without periligamentous edema is seen commonly related to scarring from remote injury.
- Ossification of the proximal ligament on radiography is occasionally seen after remote injury (*Pellegrini-Stieda lesion*).
- Can be associated with injuries of the ACL and MM
- MCL bursal effusion may develop between the superficial and deep components.
- Valgus injuries are often associated with osseous contusions of the lateral femoral condyle and lateral tibial plateau.
- The MCL is intimately associated with the joint capsule and bowing of the MCL can occur as a result of meniscal or osseous pathology.
- Stener-like lesion of the MCL refers to a tear of the ligament with displacement of the fibers superficial to the pes anserine tendons that prevents adequate healing and often requires surgical management.

Treatment Options

- Isolated ligament tears often heal without surgery and are usually treated conservatively (except Stener-like lesion as described earlier) (Figure 108.20).

Magnetic Resonance Imaging Findings

- MCL injury most often occurs with valgus stress, and the same grading system is used as with other ligament injuries (Figure 108.19).

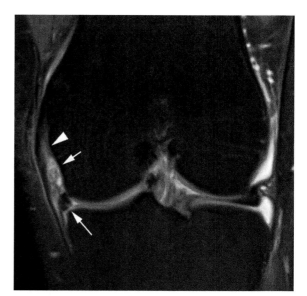

Figure 108.20. Grade 2 MCL sprain in a 26-year-old woman with medial pain after acute injury. Coronal PD FS image demonstrates a high-grade 2 sprain of the deep MCL ligament. Note the deep meniscofemoral ligament is markedly ill-defined and edematous with surrounding edema (*short arrow*). The superficial MCL ligament is mildly thickened and stripped away from the medial femoral condyle proximally with surrounding periligamentous edema (*arrowhead*), consistent with a lower grade partial tear. Additionally, the MM is truncated along its inner margin, and there is oblique signal extending to the inner margin, consistent with a complex tear with an oblique undersurface component (*long arrow*).

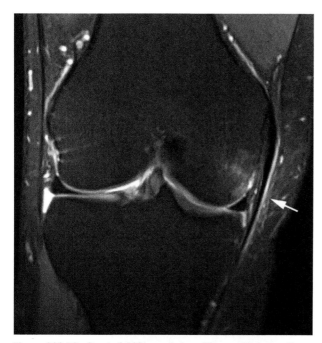

Figure 108.19. Grade 1 MCL sprain in a 39-year-old man with medial joint line pain after valgus injury. Coronal PD FS image demonstrates a grade 1 sprain of the MCL. Note the edema surrounding the intact ligament (*arrow*).

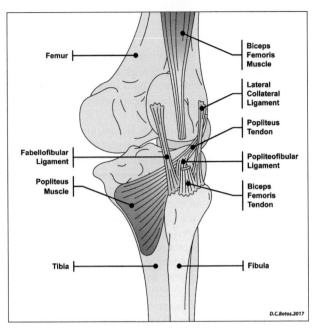

Figure 108.21. Diagram of the major posterolateral corner supporting structures. These include the LCL, biceps and popliteus tendons, and popliteofibular ligament. The tendons have been given a *light pink color*, whereas the ligaments are shown in *orange*.

Lateral Supporting Structures

The lateral supporting structures are divided into the lateral collateral ligamentous complex and the components of the posterolateral corner. Major structures seen on MRI examinations include dynamic stabilizers such as the biceps femoris and popliteus tendons and static stabilizers such as the lateral (fibular) collateral ligament and iliotibial band. Other less well seen structures of the posterolateral corner include the popliteofibular ligament, arcuate ligament, fabellofibular ligament, and lateral capsular ligaments (Figure 108.21).

A number of these structures can be injured with posterolateral corner injuries.

Posterolateral corner injuries commonly involve injury to other structures in the knee such as cruciate ligament sprains (PCL more commonly than ACL) and meniscal injuries. Mechanisms of injury include a direct blow to the anteromedial proximal tibia in extension, hyperextension injury to the externally rotated knee, and posterior/anterior rotary knee dislocations. Fibular head avulsion fractures (arcuate fractures) can be seen in the setting of posterolateral corner injuries; the location of the fracture can point to which structure might be injured (Figure 108.22). High-grade injuries of the posterolateral corner usually require reconstructive surgery (often along with cruciate ligament reconstruction). The common peroneal nerve is near the proximal fibula and can also be injured in posterolateral corner injures. Therefore, the nerve should be carefully evaluated on MRI in addition to the other structures.

Lateral (Fibular) Collateral Ligament
Anatomy and Function

The LCL functions as a posterolateral stabilizer and primarily serves to resist excessive varus stress. It extends from the lateral femoral condyle and most commonly blends with the biceps femoris tendon as it courses inferiorly and laterally to form a conjoined tendon that attaches to the fibular head. It can have variable insertion patterns, which are often best visualized on the axial images.

Pathophysiology and Clinical Presentation

The LCL is most commonly injured with varus stress. It rarely presents as an isolated injury and is commonly associated with injuries of the ACL and/or other lateral supporting structures.

Magnetic Resonance Imaging Findings

■ Same grading system used for other ligamentous injuries (Figure 108.23)

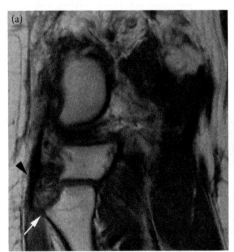
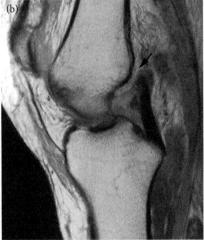

Figure 108.22. Arcuate sign in a 71-year-old woman with knee dislocation. (*A*) Coronal T1W MR image of the knee demonstrates a fracture of the fibular head (*arrow*) at the site of the biceps femoris/LCL conjoined tendon insertion (*arrowhead*). (*B*) Sagittal PDW MR image of the knee demonstrates a complete PCL origin tear (*arrow*), which is commonly associated with posterolateral corner injuries.

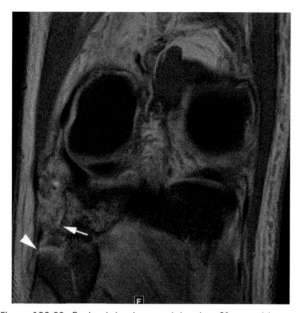

Figure 108.23. Posterolateral corner injury in a 31-year-old man with primarily lateral pain, swelling, and instability after twisting injury. Coronal PD FS image demonstrates a posterolateral corner injury. Note the near full-thickness tear of the distal biceps femoris tendon and LCL (*arrow*). Some fibers of the conjoined tendon remain attached to the fibular head. There is a nondisplaced fibular head fracture (*arcuate sign*) associated with BME as well (*arrowhead*). Note the associated extensive soft tissue edema as well as BME in the posterolateral tibial plateau.

- MRI report should include grade of sprain; location; size of ligament gap; location of any bone injuries, including the fibular head for an avulsion (arcuate) fracture.

Biceps Femoris Tendon

Anatomy and Function
The biceps tendon is the inferior continuation of the biceps femoris muscle. It often joins with the distal LCL to form a conjoined tendon that inserts onto the fibular head most commonly. Variations on the insertion pattern occur with fibers possibly inserting on the adjacent tibia. It primarily acts as a knee flexor, although it contributes to knee external rotation and hip extension as well.

Magnetic Resonance Imaging Findings
- Injuries to muscles and tendons are called *strains*. The grading system is similar to the one used to assess ligament injuries, with grade 1 strains representing low-grade injuries without muscle or tendon fiber disruption; grade 2 strains represent partial tears; grade 3 strains represent complete tears.
  - Grade 1 strains—there may be peritendinous edema without tendon caliber change or disruption
  - Grade 2 strains—partial tendon tearing with possible caliber change
  - Grade 3 strains—complete tendon disruption
- Often associated with biceps femoris muscle edema
- May note fibular head osseous avulsion; assess for associated fracture in conjunction with radiographs

Iliotibial Band

Anatomy and Function
The iliotibial band (ITB) is a thick fibrous band formed by the fascia from the gluteus maximus, gluteus medius, and tensor fascia lata. The ITB major insertion is on the Gerdy tubercle at the anterolateral proximal tibial metaphysis. In the knee, it primarily functions in lateral stabilization, and it moves anteriorly with extension and posteriorly with flexion. On MRI, it is a low-signal band of tissue along the lateral aspect of the knee overlying the lateral femoral condyle and inserting on the Gerdy tubercle.

Magnetic Resonance Imaging Findings
- Primary injury of the iliotibial band is uncommon. In the setting of acute injury, it may appear thickened or focally discontinuous and associated with intrasubstance signal abnormalities and surrounding soft tissue edema on fluid-sensitive sequences.
- *ITB friction syndrome*, an overuse condition, is more commonly seen.
  - Results from repetitive impingement of tissues between the ITB and the lateral femoral condyle
  - On MRI, there is edema deep to or surrounding the ITB, and possibly bursitis between the ITB and the lateral femoral condyle in the appropriate clinical scenario.
  - Caution should be exercised to not overcall the findings as joint fluid from the lateral recess can often extend into this region.

Popliteus Tendon and Popliteofibular Ligament
Anatomy and Function
The popliteus muscle has a broad distal attachment centered posterior to the proximal tibia. The tendon extends superiorly from the muscle and courses around the posterolateral region of the knee. It enters the joint capsule through the popliteus hiatus, formed by the meniscocapsular ligaments along the posterior horn of the LM, and attaches to the lateral surface of the lateral femoral condyle adjacent to the origin of the LCL. It helps to stabilize the knee during extension by slightly externally rotating the tibia. In addition, it partially attaches onto the LM and dynamically modulates the degree of anterior meniscal translation to prevent entrapment during knee flexion and extension. The popliteus tendon sheath communicates with the joint.

The *popliteofibular ligament* extends from the tendon to the fibular head. Although it is variably present, it can be seen in more than 90% of people on MRI. It is an important stabilizer of the posterolateral corner of the knee.

Magnetic Resonance Imaging Findings
- Popliteus tendon injuries are rarely isolated, and tendon degeneration/tendinosis is much more common. The tendon may appear thickened and contain intermediate signal on fluid-sensitive sequences.
- MRI reports should describe degree and location of tear(s) in the musculotendinous complex.
- Because the popliteus tendon sheath communicates with the joint and may actually represent a joint recess, fluid is often seen along the tendon, and any process affecting

the joint cavity can affect the popliteus tendon sheath. Commonly, intraarticular bodies can be seen within the tendon sheath.

- A bursa can form in the myotendinous region.
- The popliteofibular ligament is seen as a small, thin, low-signal intensity band between the fibular head and the popliteus tendon near the myotendinous junction.
  - Best seen on coronal and/or sagittal images
  - MRI findings of ligament injury are similar to those of other ligaments.
  - May see more extensive edema along the posterolateral joint capsule

Extensor Mechanism

Anatomy and Function

The extensor mechanism is primarily composed of the patella, which slides cranially and caudally along the distal femoral trochlear groove; and the quadriceps and patellar tendons. It stabilizes the anterior knee when the foot is placed on the ground and increases the mechanical advantage of the quadriceps musculature during knee extension, allowing greater movement with smaller forces generated. The quadriceps tendon is formed from 4 muscles: the rectus femoris, which gives the most anterior contribution to the tendon; the vastus intermedius, which forms the most posterior tendon fibers; the vastus medialis; and the vastus lateralis muscles. Slips of the quadriceps tendons insert on the superior patellar surface, whereas others continue along the anterior patellar surface to contribute to the patellar tendon. The patellar tendon originates from inferior surface of patella and inserts on the tibial tuberosity.

Additional structures of the extensor mechanism include patellar retinacula, peripatellar bursae, and fat pads. The medial and lateral retinacula are extensions of the fascia from the medial and lateral patellar borders that provide patellar support by serving as checkreins to excessive medial or lateral patellar movement during knee flexion and extension. An important component of the medial patellar retinaculum is the *medial patellofemoral ligament* (MPFL) (Figure 108.18), which is critical in preventing excessive lateral patellar displacement, particularly during the early phase of knee flexion from an extended position.

The *prepatellar bursa* is a synovial-lined space located anterior to the inferior segment of the patella and proximal patellar tendon, and the *superficial* and *deep infrapatellar bursae* are also lined with synovium and located adjacent to the distal patellar tendon. Bursal effusions can be reactive to adjacent tendinopathy or reflect isolated bursitis.

The 2 major anterior fat pads of the extensor mechanism are the *suprapatellar*, or *quadriceps fat pad*, and the *infrapatellar fat pad*, commonly referred to as the *Hoffa fat pad*. These fat pads help to cushion the extensor mechanism, and the infrapatellar fat pad may have a role in modulating local inflammatory responses.

Although not supporting structures of the extensor mechanism, the peripatellar plicae can also be a cause of anterior knee pain, and thorough assessment of the knee on MRI should include detection of these structures as well. They arise during embryological development of the knee joint when there is coalescence of different synovial compartments. The septae between these compartments normally resorb as development progresses. A plica forms if there is incomplete resorption of these septations. They have predictable locations, including medial, suprapatellar, infrapatellar, and rarely, lateral.

On fluid-sensitive sequences of routine MRI, the normal quadriceps tendon is relatively uniform in thickness and low in signal. As it inserts on the superior patella, the fibers divide and form a striated appearance of sharply marginated alternating dark and intermediate bands of similar widths. Sagittal images through the intermediate signal intensity segments can occasionally mimic tendinopathy. However, other findings of tendinopathy are absent on axial and coronal planes. Normal imaging findings of the patellar tendon are similar with a striated appearance often seen at both the tendon origin and insertion. There is often intermediate signal in the posterior proximal tendon that represents a common imaging variation and should not be mistaken for tendinopathy. In these patients, the tendon is not thickened, the intermediate signal is often triangularly shaped on sagittal imaging, and it is confined to the posterior half of the tendon.

Pathophysiology and Clinical Presentation

Pathology of the extensor mechanism is a major cause of anterior knee pain and can be seen in any age range. It can be divided into quadriceps and patellar tendinopathy, including tendinosis and tendon tears, and lateral patellar maltracking disorders, including patellar malalignment, soft tissue impingement, and patellofemoral cartilage loss and OA. Transient lateral patellar dislocation occurs when the patella is laterally displaced from the femoral trochlea as a result of excessive lateral force or insufficient medial restraints. In many cases, the femoral trochlear sulcus is shallow, or dysplastic, which can lower the force needed to displace the patella. The medial stabilizing structures, such as the MPFL, may be torn. Lateral patellar maltracking is commonly encountered in young and middle-aged women. Under the strong contractile force of the vastus lateralis muscle, there is a tendency for the patella to be pulled laterally, which can increase the axial and shear forces on the lateral patellofemoral cartilage. Over time, this can lead to progressive articular cartilage loss and lateral patellofemoral OA.

Some standard measurements are listed below when determining if anatomical factors could play a role in patellar maltracking (Figure 108.24):

- Normal trochlear groove depth is greater than 3 mm.
- Lateral trochlear inclination angle less than 11 degrees is abnormal.
- Patella alta—defined by the Insall-Salvati method as patellar tendon length to patellar height ratio greater than 1.3-1.5.
- Patella baja—defined by the Insall-Salvati method as patellar tendon length to patellar height ratio less than 0.8.
- Tibial tubercle—trochlear groove distance greater than 20 mm is abnormal.
- Trochlear sulcus angle—greater than 145 degrees usually considered abnormal

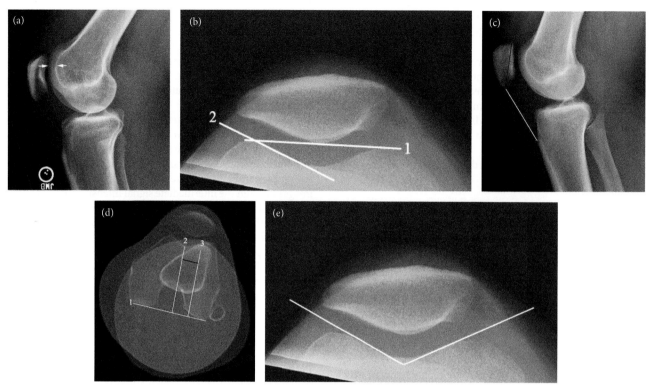

Figure 108.24. Measurements of patellofemoral alignment. (*A*) On a perfectly lateral radiograph, there are 2 nearly parallel arcs along the anterior distal femur that represent the anterior margin of the lateral femoral condyle (*anterior arrow*) and the deepest part of the trochlear sulcus (*posterior arrow*). The distance between the arrows represents the depth of the trochlear sulcus. A distance less than 3 mm, usually best seen superiorly, reflects trochlear dysplasia. (*B*) The lateral trochlear inclination angle is measured on a Merchant radiograph by drawing a line (1) that connects the anterior margins of the medial and lateral femoral condyles and another line (2) that is tangent to the lateral trochlear facet. On CT or MRI, line 1 is drawn by connecting the posterior margins of the medial and lateral femoral condyles. An excessively shallow, or dysplastic, trochlea measures less than 11 degrees. (*C*) Patellar height has been measured on a lateral radiograph of the knee in several ways. The most commonly used method is the Insall-Salvati method in which a ratio is made between the patellar tendon length from the inferior margin of the patella and the tibial tuberosity (*white line*) and the patellar height (*black line*). A ratio of greater than 1.3-1.5 is considered abnormally high (patella alta), whereas a ratio of less than 0.8 is considered low (patella baja). (*D*) The tibial tuberosity-trochlear groove (TT-TG) distance is determined by first drawing a line on an axial CT or MR image of the distal femur connecting the posterior margins of the femoral condyles. Then, a perpendicular line (2) is drawn through the central trochlear sulcus. On an image through the proximal tibia another line (line 3), which is parallel to line 2 and perpendicular to line 1, is drawn through the tibial tuberosity. Finally, the distance between lines 2 and 3 is measured (*black line*). A measurement greater than 2.0 cm is definitely abnormal. (*E*) The trochlear sulcus angle is measured on a Merchant view by drawing lines along the medial and lateral trochlear facets and measuring the resulting angle. A measurement greater than 145 degrees is abnormal.

Tendinopathy of the quadriceps tendon is usually related to repetitive overuse, whereas quadriceps tendon tears often occur with sudden forced muscle contraction. Patients taking steroids for chronic diseases, such as RA, are at increased risk for quadriceps tendinopathy and tendon tears.

Patellar tendon tears usually occur with knee flexion and sudden quadriceps contraction. They may be associated with chronic renal insufficiency, and collagen vascular diseases, such as SLE and RA. Conversely, proximal patellar tendinopathy, often known as jumper's knee, is a chronic overuse injury and most often seen in runners and activities requiring repetitive jumping.

In active adolescent patients, Sinding-Larsen-Johansson disease represents a repetitive traction injury at the junction of the inferior patella and proximal patellar tendon. Similarly, Osgood-Schlatter disease represents a traction injury affecting the distal patellar tendon in adolescents. These entities often resolve by skeletal maturity, although they occasionally can persist into adulthood.

Symptomatic plicae, in particular the medial patellar plica, can result either from repetitive impingement with synovitis or mass effect on the patellofemoral articular surfaces, causing damage to the articular cartilage. Suprapatellar and lateral patellar plicae may obstruct the flow of joint fluid, causing loculated fluid pockets that present with pain and a palpable abnormality.

Magnetic Resonance Imaging Findings
Transient Lateral Patellar Dislocation
Refer to Figure 108.25.

- Often see characteristic bony contusions/osteochondral injuries or impactions of the inferomedial patellar facet and anterolateral femoral condyle
- Cartilage or osteochondral defects of the patellar median ridge and medial facet are common.
- MPFL is commonly injured in the setting of lateral patellar dislocation.

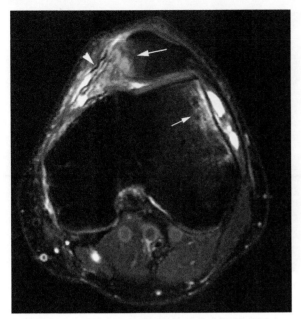

Figure 108.25. Transient lateral patellar dislocation in a 41-year-old man. Axial T2W FS MR image of the patellofemoral compartment of the knee shows a typical pattern of bone injuries seen in this condition. There is a lateral femoral condylar nonarticular contusion (*short arrow*) along with a contusion of the medial patellar facet (*long arrow*). In addition, there is high-grade partial tearing of the medial patellar retinaculum (*arrowhead*) at its patellar attachment.

- Strain of the distal fibers of the vastus medialis obliquus or VMO muscle
- Can be associated with a medial patellar osseous avulsion

Lateral Patellar Maltracking
- Lateral patellofemoral cartilage loss and OA
- Lateral patellar subluxation and/or tilt
- Patella alta
- Trochlear dysplasia (often hypoplastic medial trochlea)
- Proximal patellar tendinopathy
- Superolateral Hoffa fat pad edema related to repetitive impingement (patellar tendon lateral femoral condyle friction syndrome)

Quadriceps Tendinopathy
- Tendon thickening with globular intrasubstance signal—tendinosis
- Peritendinous edema
- Superior patellar traction enthesophytes and intratendinous mineralization
- Reactive quadriceps fat pad edema
- Tendon tear
  - If torn, the MRI description should include: whether tear is full or partial thickness; approximate percentage of tendon thickness involvement in partial tears; whether the tear is at the attachment or how far proximal to the attachment; which of the quadriceps tendons are involved, if it represents a partial-thickness tear; what the tendon gap is, particularly in cases of full-thickness tears; the quality of the torn tendon; any associated patellofemoral alignment abnormality

Patellar Tendinopathy
- Intermediate, globular intrasubstance signal and tendon thickening—tendinosis
- Peritendinous edema
- Hoffa fat pad edema
- Infrapatellar bursal effusions
- Sinding-Larsen-Johansson disease—proximal patellar tendinopathy with intratendinous ossification
  - In active disease, the inferior pole of the patella and patellar tendon may be edematous on fluid-sensitive sequences.
- Osgood-Schlatter disease—ossifications are commonly seen within or partially within the distal patellar tendon.
  - Often associated with irregularity of the tibial tuberosity
  - Active cases may be associated with BME in the tibial tuberosity and ossifications, tendinopathy, and peritendinous edema.

Patellar Tendon Tear
Refer to Figure 108.26.

- May be partial or complete
- Ill-defined tendon and focal caliber change
- Patella alta
- Avulsed inferior patellar fragment
- Effusion/hemarthrosis

Supporting Structures of the Extensor Mechanism
Hoffa Fad Pad
- Edema on fluid-sensitive sequences may be result of impingement between the distal femur and proximal tibia (called *Hoffa disease*), reactive to adjacent tendinopathy, or in patients with human immunodeficiency virus (HIV).
- Scarring is routinely seen on NFS pulse sequences in the infrapatellar fat pad after arthroscopy.
- *Patellar tendon/lateral femoral condyle friction syndrome*
  - Common cause of anterior knee pain that is likely associated with lateral patellar maltracking or malalignment
  - Focal edema on MRI in the superolateral aspect of Hoffa fat pad (Figure 108.27)

Peripatellar Plicae
- Medial patellar plica is a partial low-signal intensity septation projecting into the medial patellar joint recess best seen on fluid-sensitive sequences when there is a joint effusion.
- Can be associated with medial patellar and trochlear cartilage loss
- Suprapatellar plica often appears as a low-signal intensity, transverse or obliquely oriented structure in the suprapatellar recess. When obstructing, it may be complete or nearly complete and associated with loculated suprapatellar joint fluid.
- Infrapatellar plica (ligamentum mucosum) is a thin, curvilinear synovial fold that courses between the inferior pole of the patella and the inferior distal femoral intercondylar notch or the distal ACL. Some authors

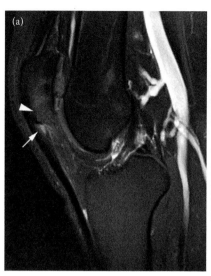
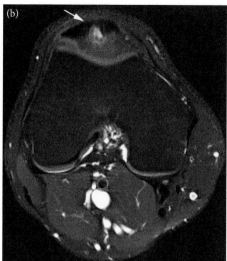

Figure 108.26. Grade 2 strain of the patellar tendon in a 27-year-old woman with chronic anterior knee pain below the patella. Sagittal (*A*) and axial (*B*) T2W FS images demonstrate a partial-thickness tear of the proximal patellar tendon involving the posterior surface (*arrow*). The tear involves greater than 50% of the tendon thickness and is superimposed on moderate tendon thickening. On the sagittal image, there is BME along the inferior pole of the patella (*arrowhead*) head that likely relates to enthesitis from repetitive traction.

have reported injuries and fibrosis of this structure that may be symptomatic in some patients.

Treatment Options
- Usually conservative, involving physical therapy and external support
- May perform patellar realignment procedures by releasing the lateral patellar retinaculum and vastus lateralis, or shifting the tibial tuberosity

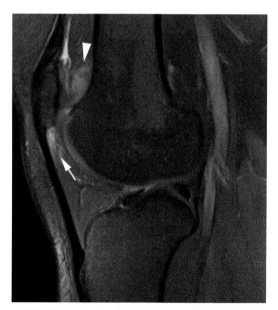

Figure 108.27. Patellar tendon/lateral femoral condyle friction syndrome in a 38-year-old man with intermittent anterior knee pain for many years. Sagittal T2W FS image demonstrates focal edema in the superolateral aspect of the Hoffa fat pad (*arrow*). This can be seen in the setting of patellar tendon/lateral femoral condyle friction syndrome. Additional lateral quadriceps fat pad edema (*arrowhead*) is also present.

Additional Medial Structures

Pes Anserine Tendons
Anatomy and Function
The pes anserinus represents 3 tendons that insert together on anteromedial aspect of the proximal tibia: the *sartorius*, which is the most anterior tendon; the *gracilis*, or the middle tendon; and the *semitendinosus*, which is the most posterior tendon. Tendinopathy is uncommon. A synovial-lined bursa between the tendons and the proximal medial tibial is called the *pes anserinus bursa*. Pes anserine bursitis can occur with repetitive irritation or acute injury. Patients often present with localized pain when ascending stairs and swelling over the medial proximal tibia.

Magnetic Resonance Imaging Findings
- Can see fluid distension of the bursa on fluid-sensitive sequences (Figure 108.28)

Semimembranosus
Anatomy and Function
The semimembranosus is one of the hamstring muscles and contributes to hip extension and knee flexion. The tendon has a number of fascicles that insert along the posteromedial aspect of the knee, with a dominant component inserting on the posteromedial aspect of the proximal tibia.

Magnetic Resonance Imaging Findings
- As with other tendons, tendon thickening and/or globular internal signal on fluid-sensitive sequences seen with tendinosis.
- Abrupt narrowing suggests tendon tear.
- Fatty replacement of the muscle is commonly seen.
- Semimembranosus-tibial (medial) collateral ligament bursal effusion- focal fluid along the semimembranosus tendon. The morphology and location (boomerang

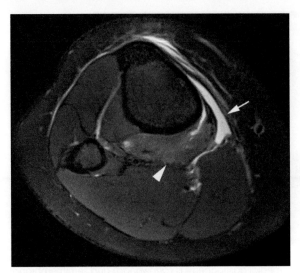

Figure 108.28. Pes anserine bursitis in a 34-year-old woman with mild medial-sided pain below the joint and no antecedent trauma. An axial T2W FS image demonstrates pes anserine bursitis, with fluid (*arrow*) distending the bursa deep to the pes anserine tendons, as well as soft tissue edema surrounding the pes anserine tendons. There is mild muscle edema in the popliteus muscle as well (*arrowhead*).

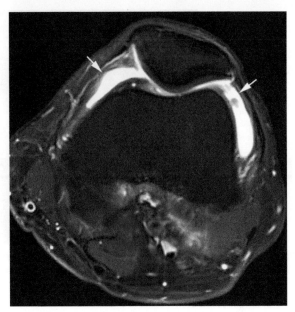

Figure 108.29. Joint effusion in a 61-year-old man who sustained an ACL tear following trauma (not shown). Axial T2W FS image of the suprapatellar joint recess shows a typical small to moderately sized joint effusion with fluid distending the joint recess (*arrows*).

shape, deep to the semimembranosus tendon) help differentiate the bursal effusion from a Baker cyst. May be misdiagnosed as parameniscal cyst.

Miscellaneous

Joint Effusion
Pathophysiology and Clinical Presentation
The knee joint is one of the most capacious joints in the body. Distension of the joint capsule with fluid is commonly seen with a variety of internal derangements, such as fractures, meniscal or ligament injuries (Figure 108.29), and acute cartilage damage, as well as with inflammatory conditions such as septic arthritis and RA.

Magnetic Resonance Imaging Findings
- Best seen on axial fluid-sensitive sequences in the medial and lateral peripatellar recesses, and on axial and sagittal fluid-sensitive sequences in the suprapatellar recess
- Should report approximate size (small, moderate, or large), complexity (whether it contains synovial thickening, hemorrhage, debris, or intraarticular bodies) and whether there is any internal loculation
- *Lipoma arborescens* is a condition in which there is frondlike, subsynovial fatty deposition, which is often seen in the setting of chronic joint effusions. Occasionally, this can mimic an intraarticular body or synovitis on MRI.

Baker (Popliteal) Cyst
Pathophysiology and Clinical Presentation
Baker cysts generally communicate with the joint and arise between the medial head of gastrocnemius and semimembranosus tendons. Cysts can rupture with adjacent soft tissue fluid inciting an inflammatory reaction that can mimic other pathology, such as cellulitis or meniscal tears. They may be difficult to treat and often recur after aspiration.

Magnetic Resonance Imaging Findings
Refer to Figure 108.30.

- A visible neck extending from the hiatus between these 2 tendons to the fluid collection is diagnostic of a Baker cyst. Cysts can become quite large and can be septated or multiloculated.
- Because it communicates with the joint, it can contain intraarticular bodies, debris, or synovial proliferation.

Treatment Options
- Because Baker cysts communicate with the joint, the primary treatment is treating intraarticular pathology that may lead to a joint effusion.
- Occasionally, aspiration to decompress a large Baker cyst followed by steroid injection may be helpful for palliative relief.

Synovitis
Pathophysiology and Clinical Presentation
The synovial lining can become inflamed and thickened during a number of conditions, such as OA, trauma, or inflammatory arthropathies, which ultimately can hinder joint function. Patients may present with decreased range of motion and joint swelling. In cases of active synovitis, they may present with warm and tender joints.

Magnetic Resonance Imaging Findings
- Curvilinear or frondlike synovial thickening within the joint capsule

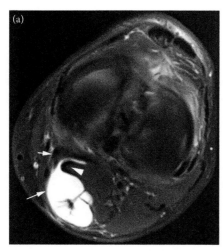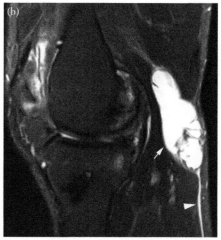

Figure 108.30. Baker cyst in a 57-year-old man with history of prior ACL reconstruction. (*A*) Axial T2W FS image demonstrates a Baker cyst (*long arrow*) with a focal fluid-filled structure extending between the medial gastrocnemius (*arrowhead*) and semimembranosus tendons (*short arrow*). (*B*) Sagittal STIR image shows the Baker cyst (*arrow*) along with fluid extending from the inferior margin of the cyst along the superficial fascia of the medial gastrocnemius muscle (*arrowhead*). This appearance is consistent with leaking or partial rupture of the cyst.

- Intermediate signal intensity on T1W and fluid-sensitive sequences
- Greater than the expected mild thin synovial enhancement on postcontrast imaging suggests active synovitis.
- Often associated with excess joint fluid
- Lamellated appearance has been described with septic arthritis
- Frank osseous erosions or BME (osteitis) is seen with inflammatory arthropathies such as RA, septic arthritis, or PVNS.

Intraarticular Bodies
Pathophysiology and Clinical Presentation
Intraarticular bodies, commonly referred to as loose bodies, occur as a result of displaced fragments of intraarticular tissues, such as cartilaginous, osseous, or meniscal fragments. They often adhere to the synovial lining and may enlarge or change shape. Over time, they may calcify or ossify, leading to variable appearances on imaging. Patients often present with knee pain and mechanical symptoms, such as locking and clicking.

Magnetic Resonance Imaging Findings
- When mineralized, they often become visible on radiography or CT as rounded or irregular radiopaque structures.
- Signal intensities on T1W and T2W MRI pulse sequences of intraarticular bodies vary depending on degree of mineralization.
- Recently displaced cartilage fragments have the signal intensity of hyaline cartilage and may have a linear or curvilinear morphology. The fragment may correspond to a cartilage defect that represents the donor site.
- They often occur in predictable locations, including the suprapatellar joint recess, the posterior joint recess, and the popliteus tendon sheath.

Key Points
- PDW sequences with or without fat-suppression are the most commonly used sequences for assessing meniscal pathology because of their high spatial resolution and high sensitivity for detecting tears.
- The normal menisci have predictable morphologies and signal intensities. The criteria for diagnosing meniscal tear include signal abnormalities unequivocally extending to an articular surface on 2 or more consecutive images from the same pulse sequence or in the same location on at least 1 image from orthogonal sequences, or any alteration in morphology on at least 1 image.
- T2W imaging is more specific for diagnosing meniscal tears. Therefore, T2W sequences may be helpful in diagnosing meniscal re-tears following partial meniscectomy.
- MRA and CTA may be helpful in diagnosing meniscal re-tears following partial meniscectomy, as well as cartilage defects.
- Although sagittal imaging can depict the ACL in long axis, it is prone to volume averaging. Coronal and axial images may be more useful in diagnosing and characterizing ACL injuries.
- Complications of ACL reconstruction include graft tear, graft impingement, arthrofibrosis, tibial tunnel widening, and mucoid degeneration.
- PCL tears are commonly associated with posterolateral corner injuries. In the setting of PCL tears, a thorough assessment of these structures should be made.
- The posterolateral corner includes the biceps femoris and popliteus tendons, LCL, popliteofibular ligament, arcuate ligament, and fabellofibular ligament.
- Extensor mechanism pathology, including lateral patellar maltracking, is a common cause of anterior knee pain and early OA. MRI can be helpful to assess the degree of abnormalities before the development of OA.

Recommended Reading

De Smet AA. How I diagnose meniscal tears on knee MRI. *AJR Am J Roentgenol*. 2012;199:481–99.

Mohankumar R, White LM, Naraghi A. Pitfalls and pearls in MRI of the knee. *AJR Am J Roentgenol*. 2014;203:516–30.

References

1. American College of Radiology. ACR–SPR–SSR practice parameter for the performance and interpretation of magnetic resonance imaging (MRI) of the knee. www.acr.org/~/media/4A4471FCA2B449059EFEB2DAB5421EB4.pdf. Accessed February 26, 2017.

2. Anderson MW. MR imaging of the meniscus. *Radiol Clin North Am*. 2002;40(5):1081–94.

3. "Knee." In: Manaster BJ, May DA, Disler DG, eds. *Musculoskeletal Imaging: The Requisites*. 3rd ed. Maryland Heights, MO: Mosby; 2007:224–48.

4. Bencardino JT, Rosenberg ZS, Brown RR, Hassankhani A, Lustrin ES, Beltran J. Traumatic musculotendinous injuries of the knee: diagnosis with MR imaging. *RadioGraphics*. 2000;20:S103–20.

5. Geiger D, Chang E, Pathria M, Chung CB. Posterolateral and posteromedial corner injuries of the knee. *Radiol Clin North Am*. 2013;51(3):413–32.

6. Magee T, Williams D. Detection of meniscal tears and marrow lesions using coronal MRI. *AJR Am J Roentgenol*. 2004;183:1469–73.

7. Nguyen JC, De Smet AA, Graf BK, et al. MR imaging-based diagnosis and classification of meniscal tears. *Radiographics*. 2014;34:981–99.

8. Recondo JA, Salvador E, Villanúa JA, Barrera MC, Gervás C, Alústiza JM. Lateral stabilizing structures of the knee: functional anatomy and injuries assessed with MR imaging. *Radiographics*. 2000;20:S91–102.

9. Sanders TG, Medynski MA, Feller JF, Lawhorn KW. Bone contusion patterns of the knee at MR imaging: footprint of the mechanism of injury. *Radiographics*. 2000;20:S135–51.

10. Vasilevska Nikodinovska V, Gimber LH, Hardy JC, Taljanovic MS. The collateral ligaments and posterolateral corner: what radiologists should know. *Semin Musculoskelet Radiol*. 2016;20(1):52–64.

CHAPTER 109

Internal Derangement of the Ankle and Foot

Laura W. Bancroft

Indications for Imaging

Clinical examination is always the first step in evaluating patients with suspected internal derangement of the ankle and foot, and radiography is the first study when imaging is warranted. However, MRI allows high spatial and contrast resolution of a variety of soft tissue and osseous pathology. Indications for ankle and foot MRI are outlined in the ACR Appropriateness Criteria and are based on acute or chronic symptoms. MRI is especially useful for evaluating patients with suspected tendon rupture or dislocation, ligamentous injury and/or ankle instability, ankle impingement syndromes, osteochondral defects identified on radiographs, suspected syndesmotic or Lisfranc injury, chronic ankle pain of uncertain etiology, and inflammatory arthritis.

Imaging Protocols

The current parameters for the performance of ankle, foot, and toe MRI are outlined by the ACR Practice Parameters. Foot and ankle MRI may be performed on 3T, 1.5T, or low field strength magnets with high-quality foot and ankle coils. Imaging should be performed in both short and long axes (ie, axial, coronal, sagittal planes) and should include both fluid-sensitive (T2W or STIR) and short-TE (T1W or PDW) sequences (Tables 109.1 and 109.2). Fat saturation (FS) on T2W sequences offers greater conspicuity of tendon/ligament tears and marrow lesions. Although FOV should generally be 16 cm or less, a sagittal larger FOV sequence may be helpful to assess the extent of a large Achilles tendon tear that extends beyond the standard ankle MRI FOV. Osteochondral defects may be better characterized on 12 cm or smaller FOV coronal images. Slice thickness should be 4 mm or less to minimize partial-volume effects, and phase and frequency encoding steps should be at least 192 × 256.

Ankle/Foot Tendons

Normal Magnetic Resonance Imaging Anatomy
- *Flexor tendons (medial ankle)*—posterior tibial (PTT), flexor digitorum longus (FDL), and flexor hallucis longus (FHL) (Figures 109.1 and 109.2)
- *Extensor tendons (anterior ankle)*—anterior tibialis (ATT), extensor hallucis longus (EHL) and extensor digitorum longus (EDL) (Figures 109.1 and 109.2)

- *Peroneal tendons (lateral ankle)*—peroneus brevis (PB), peroneus longus (PL), peroneus tertius, peroneus quartus, other accessory peroneal tendons (Figures 109.1 and 109.2)
- *Posterior ankle tendons*—Achilles, plantaris (Figures 109.1 and 109.2)

MRI is an excellent imaging modality for evaluating the tendons of the foot and ankle (Figures 109.3 through 109.5). Tendons are composed of dense connective tissue fascicles with parallel arrangements of collagen fibers and serve to connect muscles to bones. The ankle/foot tendons can be grouped into flexor (medial), extensor (anterior), peroneal (lateral), and posterior tendons.

The flexor tendons consist of the PTT, FDL, and FHL. The PTT is the far medial tendon that courses posterior to the medial tibia/malleolus and inserts mainly onto the navicular and medial cuneiform. The FDL tendon is located lateral to the PTT and inserts onto the plantar aspect of the distal phalangeal bases of the lesser toes. The FHL tendon lies posterolateral to the FDL tendon, courses under the sustentaculum tali, and inserts onto the plantar base of the distal phalanx of the hallux. The knot of Henry represents the crossing point of the FDL and FHL tendons at the plantar aspect of the navicular bone in the midfoot. Distal to the knot of Henry, there are additional connections between these 2 tendons.

The extensor tendons are composed of the ATT, EHL, and EDL. The ATT is the most medial extensor tendon and inserts onto the dorsal aspect of the medial cuneiform and hallux metatarsal base. The EHL tendon lies more lateral and inserts onto the dorsal base of the hallux distal phalanx. The EDL tendon is the most lateral extensor tendon and inserts onto the lesser toes.

The peroneal tendons serve to dorsiflex and evert the foot. They consist of the PB and PL tendons, with variable presence of multiple accessory peroneal tendons. The PB courses posterior to the peroneal/retromalleolar groove of the fibula/lateral malleolus and along the lateral aspect of the hindfoot and midfoot with distal attachment onto the fifth metatarsal base. The PL tendon courses posterior and lateral to the PB in the retromalleolar groove, at the lateral aspect of the hindfoot, through the cuboid groove and obliquely along the plantar aspect of the foot until its insertion onto the first metatarsal base and medial cuneiform. The *peroneus tertius* is commonly present, lies at the anterolateral aspect of the ankle, and inserts onto the dorsal aspect

Table 109.1. Sample Ankle Magnetic Resonance Imaging Protocol

PLANE	SEQUENCE	FOV (CM)	SLICE THICKNESS (MM)
Sagittal	FSE T1W	14	3
Sagittal	FSE PDW FS	14	3
Coronal	FSE PDW FS	12-14	3
Axial	FSE PDW	14	3
Axial	FSE T2W FS	14	3

of the fifth metatarsal base. The *peroneus quartus* is one of the more common accessory peroneal muscles/tendons, lies posteromedial to the other peroneal tendons, and inserts most often onto the retrotrochlear eminence of the calcaneus. In the retromalleolar groove, the peroneal tendons are secured by the superior peroneal retinaculum (SPR), which courses between the lateral malleolus and the posterior calcaneus. At the lateral aspect of the calcaneus, the peroneal tendons are secured to the bone by the inferior peroneal retinaculum. There are 2 bony protuberances at the lateral aspect of the calcaneus: the retrotrochlear eminence at the posterior aspect of the peroneal tendons and the peroneal tubercle between the peroneal tendons.

The *Achilles* (tendon of gastrocnemius and soleus muscles), which is the main plantar flexor of the foot, inserts on the posterior calcaneal tuberosity. This is the largest tendon in the human body and measures 10-15 cm in length. The soleus muscle lies deep to the medial and lateral heads of the gastrocnemius with fibers converging on a short tendon, which normally joins the deep surface of the Achilles tendon. The distal insertion of the soleus is variable. The Achilles tendon has a flat or oval shape with flat or slightly concave anterior surface. The *retrocalcaneal bursa* is located deep to the distal Achilles tendon within the posterior ankle fat pad (Kager fat pad) and may be distended in the setting of Achilles tendon pathology/injury. An adventitial bursa named the *retroachilles bursa* may be seen at the posterior aspect of the distal Achilles tendon. The *plantaris* is a thin and variably present tendon at the posterior aspect of the calf. It courses superolateral to inferomedial and can be seen along the medial aspect of the distal Achilles tendon with insertion onto the Achilles tendon or the medial aspect of the calcaneal tuberosity. Occasionally present, an accessory soleus muscle arises from the fibula and soleal line of the tibia and descends anterior or anteromedial to the Achilles tendon with variable distal insertion site onto the distal Achilles tendon or calcaneus.

- Normal tendons are relatively uniform in caliber and signal characteristics, being very low in signal intensity on MRI.
- Ankle and foot tendons (in particular the PTT and ATT) may have multiple insertions that should not be mistaken for longitudinal split tears.
- The Achilles tendon may have fibrofatty tissue between the joining gastrocnemius and soleus tendons, rendering a mixed linear high signal on T1W and GRE images.
- Although most tendons throughout the body have surrounding tendon sheaths that promote smooth, gliding tendon motion, the Achilles tendon lacks a tenosynovium. Instead, there is a surrounding paratenon at the posterior, medial, and lateral aspects of this tendon composed of fatty areolar tissue.

General Magnetic Resonance Imaging Findings of Common Ankle Tendon Pathology

Tendon unit pathology includes tenosynovitis, tendinosis, and partial- and full-thickness tears.

- Tenosynovitis is caused by chronic overuse, or inflammatory or infectious etiologies that will be evident on MRI as circumferential fluid greater than 3 mm in thickness and synovial thickening and may be associated with peritendinous edema or tendon thickening (Figure 109.4). Peritendinous enhancement is seen following IV Gd administration.

Table 109.2. Sample Forefoot/Toes Magnetic Resonance Imaging Protocol

PLANE	SEQUENCE	FOV (CM)	SLICE THICKNESS (MM)
Sagittal	FSE T1W	15	3
Axial	FSE T1W	13	3
Coronal	FSE T1W	15	3
Axial	FSE T2W FS	13	3
Sagittal	FSE IR (STIR)	15	3
Coronal	FSE T2W FS	15	3

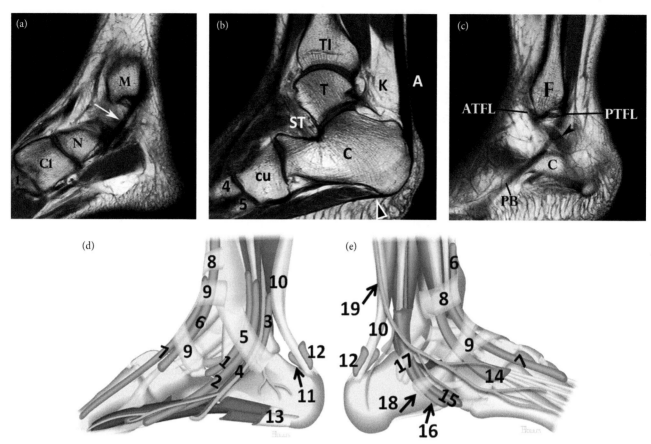

Figure 109.1. Sagittal T1W MRI and drawings of the normal ankle. (*A*) Image through the medial ankle shows the posterior tibial tendon (*arrow*) coursing posterior to the medial malleolus (M), with attachments onto the navicular and medial cuneiform (C1). 1 = first metatarsal. (*B*) Image through the more central aspect of the ankle shows the Achilles tendon (A) and subjacent Kager fat pad (K). The plantar fascia (*arrowhead*) originates from the plantar, posterior calcaneus (*C*). TI = tibia; T = talus; ST = sinus tarsi; Cu = cuboid; 4 = fourth metatarsal; 5 = fifth metatarsal. (*C*) Image through the far lateral ankle shows the ATFL and PTFL extending from the fibula (F). The SPR (*arrowhead*) extends over the peroneal tendons, with the PB extending toward its attachment onto the fifth metatarsal. C = calcaneus. Drawings of the medial (*D*) and lateral (*E*) ankle show normal anatomic structures. 1 = posterior tibialis tendon (PTT); 2 = flexor digitorum longus tendon (FDL); 3 = flexor hallucis longus tendon (FHL); 4 = posterior tibial artery (*red*) and nerve (*yellow*); 5 = flexor retinaculum; 6 = anterior tibialis tendon (ATT); 7 = extensor hallucis longus tendon (EHL); 8 = superior extensor retinaculum (SER); 9 = inferior extensor retinaculum (IER); 10 = Achilles tendon; 11 = retrocalcaneal bursa; 12 = retroachilles bursa; 13 = plantar fascia; 14 = extensor digitorum longus tendon (EDL); 15 = peroneus brevis tendon (PB); 16 = peroneus longus tendon (PL); 17 = superior peroneal retinaculum (SPR); 18 = inferior peroneal retinaculum (IPR); 19 = superficial peroneal nerve.

- Tenosynovitis may involve any of the ankle and foot tendons except the Achilles tendon, where a tendon sheath is absent.
- Tendinosis is a noninflammatory degenerative process that is caused by repetitive trauma or chronic disease such as inflammatory arthropathy, metabolic disorders, and diabetes.
  - Tendinosis is characterized by intermediate signal intensity within a tendon that persists on T2W images and globular tendon morphology. Care should be taken not to mistake magic angle effect for tendon pathology.
- Tendinosis and tendon tears may involve any tendon throughout the ankle and foot, but most commonly affect the Achilles (Figure 109.5), PTT (Figure 109.6), peroneal (Figure 109.7), FHL (Figure 109.8) and, much less commonly, the ATT (Figure 109.9).
- Tendon injury occurs at insertional stress, areas of relative hypovascularity, angulation, or repetitive friction adjacent to the malleoli.

- Tendons may demonstrate partial-thickness tearing (involving a portion of the cross-section of the tendon) or be completely ruptured.
  - Partial-thickness tears show partial discontinuity of the tendon fibers with increased or intermediate signal intensity on MRI.
  - Tendon ruptures show complete discontinuity of the tendon fibers.
- Partial-thickness tendon tears may involve the tendon surface and be visible on surgical inspection or may be concealed, intrasubstance tears detected on MRI (Figure 109.5).
- Furthermore, tendon tears in the ankle and foot may also extend along the longitudinal axis of the tendon as longitudinal split tears. Longitudinal split tears most commonly involve the PB (Figure 109.7) and PTT (Figure 109.6) at the malleolar and inframalleolar locations.
- Tendon ruptures are far less common than partial-thickness tears (Figures 109.5C and 109.8).

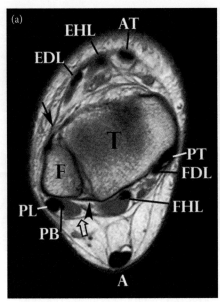 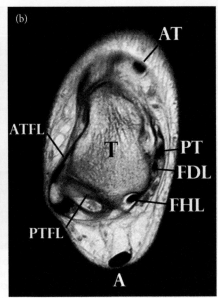 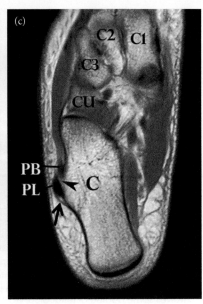

Figure 109.2. Axial T1W MRI of the normal ankle. (*A*) Image through the superior ankle shows the anterior inferior tibiofibular ligament (*arrow*) and posterior inferior tibiofibular ligament (*arrowhead*) connecting the tibia (T) and fibula (F). Note SPR (*open arrow*). PB = Peroneus brevis; PL = peroneus longus; A = Achilles; FHL = flexor hallucis longus; FDL = flexor digitorum longus; PT = posterior tibialis; AT = anterior tibialis; EHL = extensor hallucis longus; EDL = extensor digitorum longus tendons. (*B*) Image through the level of the lateral malleolus shows the ATFL and PTFL extending from the fibula onto the talus (T). (*C*) Image through the level of the peroneal tubercle of the calcaneus (*arrowhead*) shows the separation between the PL and PB tendons about the peroneal tubercle. Note inferior peroneal retinaculum (*arrow*). Cu = cuboid; C1 = medial cuneiform; C2 = middle cuneiform; C3 = lateral cuneiform.

- Ankle and foot tendons may also undergo subluxation or dislocation, most commonly seen with the peroneal tendons.

Several specific features of tendon pathology that occur in the ankle and foot are discussed in the following sections.

Achilles Tendon

- Pathology may occur at its insertion or in the less vascular critical zone, located approximately 4-6 cm proximal to its insertion (Figure 109.5).

Figure 109.3. Customized plane for evaluation of specific tendons. Oblique axial T1W MR image is aligned along the long axis of the distal plantar portion of the normal PL tendon (*arrows*). 1 MT = first metatarsal.

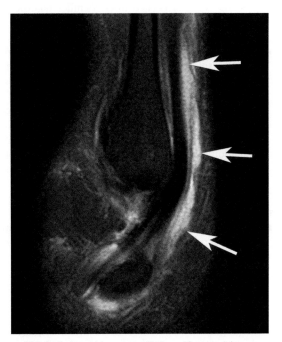

Figure 109.4. Peroneal tenosynovitis in a 49-year-old woman. Sagittal FSE PDW FS MR image through the right ankle demonstrates fluid (*arrows*) distending the peroneal tendon sheath and synovial thickening, consistent with tenosynovitis.

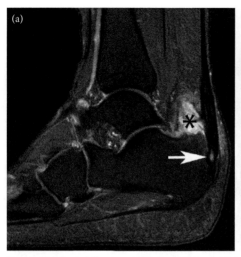 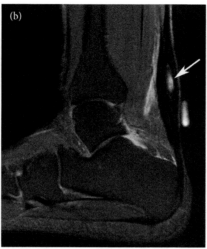 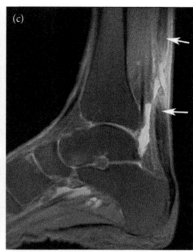

Figure 109.5. Achilles tendon tears. (*A*) Partial-thickness tear of the Achilles tendon in a 50-year-old woman. Sagittal FSE T2W FS MR image through the ankle demonstrates a partial-thickness intrasubstance tear of the Achilles insertion (*arrow*). Thickening and intermediate signal intensity in the more proximal Achilles tendon is consistent with tendinosis. Insertional Achilles tendinosis usually involves some degree of retrocalcaneal bursitis (*asterisk*), as shown in this case. (*B*) Sagittal FSE T2W FS MR image through the ankle in a different patient demonstrates a partial-thickness tear (*arrow*) within the critical zone of the Achilles tendon, with associated tendon thickening caused by underlying tendinosis. (*C*) Sagittal FSE T2W FS MR image through the ankle in another patient demonstrates Achilles tendon rupture involving the critical zone with retraction of the tendinous remnants (*arrows*).

- Because the Achilles tendon lacks a tendon sheath, there cannot be tenosynovitis. Instead, Achilles paratenonitis will be evident as peritendinous, edema-like signal changes at the medial, lateral, and posterior aspects of the tendon.
- Achilles tendon pathology may be associated with retrocalcaneal and retroachilles bursitis.
  - In particular, this may be seen in Haglund syndrome, which comprises the presence of a bony protuberance at the proximal calcaneal tuberosity (often called *pump bump*) with associated distal Achilles tendinopathy and bursitis (Figure 109.10). This abnormality may be associated with wearing of high-heel shoes.
- Partial avulsion of the medial head of the gastrocnemius from the soleus aponeurosis is a common injury of the posteromedial calf and is frequently termed *tennis leg injury*.
  - MRI shows edema and blood products at the medial head of gastrocnemius-soleus aponeurosis.
  - Similarly, the less frequently encountered plantaris tendon rupture demonstrates edema and blood products at the medial head of gastrocnemius-soleus aponeurosis.

Posterior Tibial Tendon
- Commonly injured in overweight, middle-aged women; additional risk factors include diabetes and hypertension.
- PTT dysfunction is the most common cause of asymmetric acquired adult flatfoot deformity. Patients typically present with gradual collapse of the longitudinal arch of the foot with hindfoot valgus and medial foot pain and swelling that is worse with activity.
- Imaging of PTT dysfunction can detect the progressive changes of tenosynovitis/tendinosis/tearing (Figure 109.6), flexible planovalgus, fixed/arthritic planovalgus with

progressive talar head uncoverage, and spring and deltoid ligament insufficiency. In advanced cases, subfibular impingement syndrome may be present with degenerative cystlike changes and BME in the distal lateral malleolus and adjacent lateral aspect of the talus and calcaneus.

Peroneal Tendons
Refer to Figure 109.7.

- The most frequent tear of the PB tendon is the longitudinal split (frequently the result of repetitive microtrauma that leads to tendon thinning and subsequent longitudinal split starting at the level of the retromalleolar groove).
- The PL tear most frequently occurs at the level of the cuboid bone (proximal or distal to the os peroneum or at the level of the os peroneum).
- With complete tear of the PL tendon, the os peroneum may be retracted, even to the lateral malleolus.
- Fractures of the os peroneum may lead to disruptions of the PL tendon.
- Both peroneal tendons are rarely torn simultaneously.
- Impingement (crowding) in the common peroneal sheath (in the retromalleolar groove) can be caused by a low-lying PB muscle belly or a peroneus quartus.
- Stenosing tenosynovitis occurs because of chronic friction of the peroneal tendons inside a narrowed inferior osteofibrous tunnel (facilitated by the hypertrophic peroneal tendons and usually associated with a thickened inferior peroneal retinaculum).
  - Tenosynovial fibrosis with synovial proliferation can prevent normal tendon excursion.
  - MRI shows irregular distension of the peroneal tendon sheath with multiple low signal intensity fibrous bands within the tendon sheath.

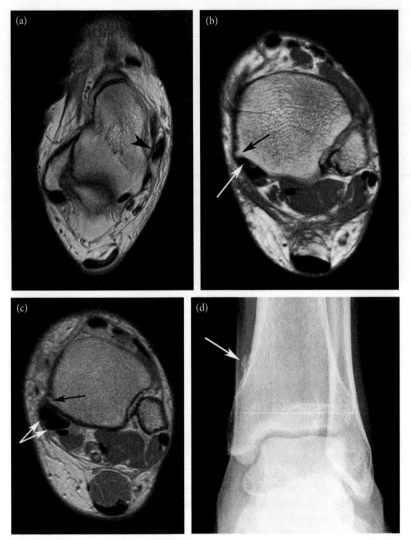

Figure 109.6. Posterior tibialis tendon (PTT) tears. (*A*) Axial PDW MR image through the ankle of a 78-year-old woman shows longitudinal split tearing (*arrowhead*) through the thickened PTT. (*B*) Axial PDW MR image in a different patient shows a markedly thinned PTT (*white arrow*) and adjacent reactive tibial spurring (*black arrow*). (*C*) Axial PDW MR image in another patient shows longitudinal split tearing of the markedly thickened PTT (*white arrows*) and reactive tibial spurring (*black arrow*). (*D*) Anteroposterior radiograph in a 59-year-old man shows reactive tibial spurring (*arrow*) associated with posterior tibial tendon dysfunction.

- Statistically significant correlations have been found between the presence of an os peroneum and PL pathology, an undulating peroneal groove and greater severity of PB tears, a boomerang-shaped PB tendon and peroneal tendon pathology, and a low-lying PB muscle belly and chronic injury of the SPR.
- The superior and inferior peroneal retinacula restrict tendon motion in the axial plane.
- When the SPR becomes partially or completely disrupted by chronic or acute trauma with a twisting mechanism, the peroneal tendons may subluxate or dislocate anteriorly from their normal retromalleolar location or may undergo intrasheath subluxation, with reversal of the PB and PL position in cross-section. Static MRI rarely documents subluxations/dislocations and cine MR images or dynamic US are more useful.

Treatment and Complications

- Symptomatic tenosynovitis and/or tendon tears are first treated conservatively with pain management, limitation of physical activities that exacerbate the pain, physical therapy, bracing and, in certain instances, steroid injections.
- Tendinosis that is unresponsive to conservative management may be treated with tenosynovectomy. Dry needling regions of tendinosis and injections with platelet-rich plasma (PRP) or whole blood have shown variable results in the literature.
- Low-grade partial-thickness tendon tears may be treated with debridement, repair, and tubulization for splayed or flattened tendons.
- High-grade tendon tears that are complex with multiple splits may be treated with debridement, tenodesis, and allograft reconstruction.

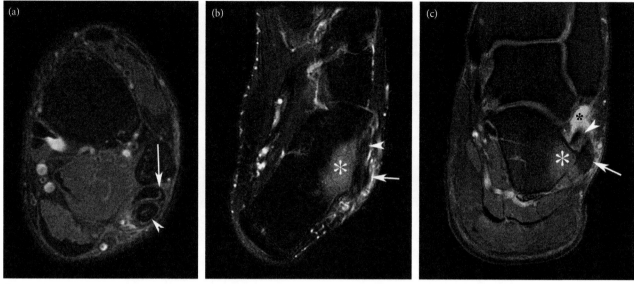

Figure 109.7. Peroneal tendon tears. (*A*) Axial FSE T2W FS MR image in a 64-year-old man shows longitudinal split tearing of the PB tendon (*arrow*) as well as thickening and intermediate signal intensity within the PL tendon (*arrowhead*), consistent with marked tendinosis. (*B, C*) Axial (*B*) and coronal (*C*) FSE T2W FS MR images in a 56-year-old woman show split tearing of the PB (*arrowheads*) and longus (*arrows*) tendons on a background of marked tendinopathy, with increased tendon sheath fluid (*black asterisk*) and adjacent reactive calcaneal BME (*white asterisks*).

- Patients with full-thickness, irreparable Achilles tendon tears may undergo FHL tendon transfer, with functional improvement.
- Acute subluxation/dislocation of the peroneal tendons may be treated with immobilization or surgery (SPR repair and retromalleolar groove-deepening procedures).
- Surgical options for the chronic peroneal tendon subluxations/dislocations include SPR repair, bone block procedures, reinforcement of the SPR with local tissue transfer, tendon rerouting, groove-deepening procedures, or a combination of these procedures. Hindfoot varus must be corrected prior to any SPR reconstructive procedure.
- Intrasheath subluxations of the peroneal tendons with an intact SPR may be treated with repair of the tendon

tears (if present) and a peroneal groove-deepening procedure.
- Complications of untreated or recurrent tendon tears include chronic ankle instability and early OA.

Ankle/Foot Ligaments, Plantar Fascia, Tarsal Tunnel, Sinus Tarsi, and Baxter's Neuropathy

Anatomy and Normal Magnetic Resonance Imaging Findings of the Ankle Ligaments

Ligaments are organized, fibrous structures that firmly connect bones and generally have low signal on all MRI sequences.

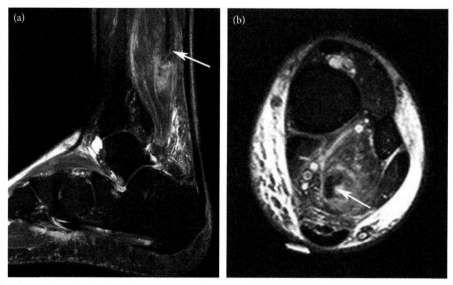

Figure 109.8. FHL tendon rupture in a 77-year-old man. (*A, B*) Sagittal (*A*) and axial (*B*) FSE T2W FS MR images show proximal retraction of the ruptured FHL tendon (*arrows*) to the level of the distal calf.

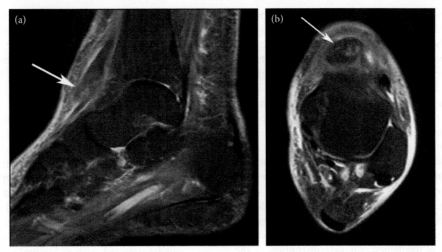

Figure 109.9. Anterior tibial tendon (ATT) tear and tendinosis. Sagittal (*A*) and axial (*B*) FSE T2W FS MR images show high-grade partial-thickness tearing of the thickened ATT tendon (*arrows*) at the level of the inferior extensor retinaculum.

Ankle ligaments may be divided into:

■ Syndesmotic: anterior inferior tibiofibular, posterior inferior tibiofibular, inferior transverse tibiofibular, and interosseous ligaments
■ Lateral: anterior talofibular (ATFL), calcaneofibular (CFL) and posterior talofibular ligaments (PTFL)
■ Medial: deltoid (superficial and deep portions) and spring (plantar calcaneonavicular) ligaments composed of 3 bands including the most important superomedial and less important medioplantar oblique and inferoplantar longitudinal.

There are numerous ligaments connecting the small bones of the foot. The ligaments comprising the Lisfranc joint include the intermetatarsal and tarsometatarsal ligaments, as well as the strong Lisfranc ligament complex (see Figure 24.1 in Chapter 24, "Foot Trauma"), which provides crucial support for the midfoot.

■ The Lisfranc ligament complex courses obliquely between the medial cuneiform and second metatarsal; is composed of several bands on MRI including the dorsal, interosseous and plantar bands; and appears striated with low to intermediate signal intensity on PDW sequences. The plantar band has 2 fascicles that extend to the second and third metatarsal bases.
■ Capsular ligaments of the MTP and interphalangeal (IP) joints of the toes can be delineated as focal thickening of the joint capsules on MRI.
■ The plantar plate is focal thickening of the plantar aspect of the MTP or IP joint capsule that serves to restrict hyperextension forces.

Pathophysiology and Magnetic Resonance Imaging Findings of Ankle and Foot Ligament Injuries

Ankle ligament sprains are one of the most common injuries of the musculoskeletal system. Furthermore, 85% of all ankle sprains involve the LCL complex. The lateral ankle ligaments are most commonly injured by an inversion mechanism sustained while stepping off a curb or sports activities.

■ Sprains may be evident on MRI as intermediate signal intensity within either thickened or thinned ligaments, with wavy or lax fibers.

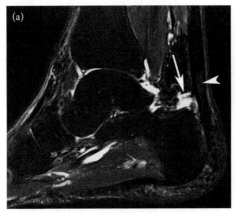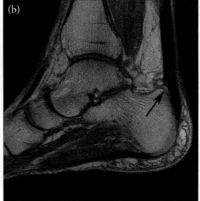

Figure 109.10. A 61-year-old man with Haglund syndrome. (*A*) Sagittal STIR MR image of the ankle shows mild thickening and increased signal within the distal Achilles tendon consistent with tendinosis (*arrowhead*) with moderate distension of the retrocalcaneal bursa (*arrow*). On T1W sagittal MR image (*B*) note bony protuberance of the proximal calcaneal tuberosity consistent with Haglund deformity (*arrow*).

- Rupture is evident by focal ligament disruption or diffuse absence of a ligament with intervening fluid.
- The ATFL is the most commonly torn ligament sustained during an inversion injury (Figure 109.11). Inversion forces may also lead to concomitant ligamentous injuries of the CFL and ultimately the PTFL.
- Abnormalities of the ATFL may be associated with talar cartilage lesions, synovitis, and anterior ankle impingement syndrome caused by osteophytes.
- Distal tibiofibular syndesmotic ligament injuries are most commonly caused by excessive external rotation and dorsiflexion.
- *High ankle sprain* is the term used for partial or complete disruption of the distal syndesmotic ligaments and commonly occurs in collision sports. MRI findings include increased T2 signal intensity or indistinctiveness of the abnormal ligaments, complete disruption of the ligaments, lateral fibular subluxation, and widening of the distal tibiofibular syndesmosis. Posterior inferior tibiofibular ligament tears tend to broadly delaminate from the posterior malleolus; posterior ligament ruptures uncommonly involve the intrasubstance portion of the ligament.
- Medial ankle sprains are more common in male athletes, and may be associated with distal tibiofibular syndesmotic and lateral collateral ligamentous injuries.
- Deltoid ligament sprains are caused by eversion forces and are less common than lateral ligament injuries.
- Because the deltoid ligament is stronger than bone, medial malleolar fractures typically occur before deltoid ligament injuries do.
- Failure of the spring ligament complex on MRI has been shown to occur concurrently with PTT dysfunction, often resulting in symptomatic flatfoot.

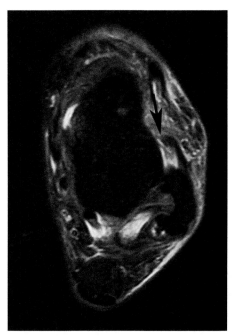

Figure 109.11. Rupture of the ATFL at the talar insertion in a 57-year-old woman. Axial FSE T2W FS MR image shows the retracted margin *(arrow)* of the avulsed ATFL.

- Spring (calcaneonavicular) ligament complex sprains may be evident as focal thickening or thinning on MRI (normal thickness of ~3 mm for superomedial and medioplantar oblique and ~4 mm for inferoplantar longitudinal ligaments), as well as loss of the normal striation.

Midfoot sprains typically occur with low-impact forces injuring the Lisfranc ligament complex (more commonly in athletes), whereas Lisfranc fracture subluxations/dislocations occur with high-impact forces. Injuries to the Lisfranc joint and, specifically, the Lisfranc ligament complex are important to detect because undetected or untreated injuries may result in chronic midfoot pain, dysfunction, and OA.

- Lisfranc injuries may lead to diastasis/malalignment that can be detected with radiographs. If the radiographic alignment is normal and there is continued concern for Lisfranc ligament complex injury, weight-bearing and follow-up radiographs can be considered.
- MRI is usually performed in patients with suspected Lisfranc injury and inability to tolerate weight-bearing radiographs.

Plantar plate injuries in the forefoot occur most commonly with a hyperextension mechanism of injury.

- Sprain of the plantar plate will be reflected as increased T2 signal intensity within the thickened, central plantar portion of the joint capsule, whereas focal tearing will show fluid within the gap.
- Plantar plate injuries of the hallux MTP joint (*turf toe*) may be accompanied by hallux sesamoid ligament injury and sesamoid dislocation, traumatic hallux valgus, hallux MTP joint dislocation, and OCLs of the adjacent bones.

Treatment and Complications
- Low-grade ligamentous sprains are treated conservatively with pain management and functional rehabilitation (strengthening exercises and motion restoration), and sometimes bracing and resistive walking boots.
- Severe sprains are usually treated nonsurgically, although surgical repair may be considered if conservative treatment fails, there is persistent ankle instability, or a patient has high performance needs.
- There is generally a lower threshold for considering surgical fixation of Lisfranc joint injuries because of the poor prognosis of inadequately treated injuries.
- Most patients with forefoot sprains are treated nonsurgically with conservative management.
- Mild turf toe injuries are treated with gentle range of motion exercises, stiff-soled shoes, or bracing. Moderate turf toe injuries are treated with walking boots or crutches. Severe injuries may be treated with reconstructive surgery of the involved plantar plate and/or hallux sesamoid complex.

Ankle Impingement Syndromes
Ankle impingements represent entrapment of anatomic structures that lead to pain and decreased range of motion.

They are divided into the anterolateral, anterior, anteromedial, posteromedial, and posterior. Ankle impingement syndromes are classified as either soft tissue or osseous and limit full range of movement with symptoms related to compression of soft tissues or osseous structures during particular movements. MRI is the most useful imaging modality in evaluating suspected soft tissue impingement.

Plantar Fascia

The plantar fascia is a thick connective tissue aponeurosis that supports the plantar arch and extends from the calcaneal tuberosity onto the metatarsal heads. *Plantar fasciitis* will be clinically evident with heel pain, especially with the first few steps after awakening and after exercise. Plantar fascial tearing is more commonly partial thickness (Figure 109.12) but may progress to complete rupture with sustained overuse, inflammation, or in patients taking corticosteroids or fluoroquinolones. *Plantar fibromatosis* is a benign entity with nodule formation, usually along the central and medial bands of the fascia.

Magnetic Resonance Imaging Findings

- Normal MRI appearance shows low signal intensity within the individual central (largest), medial, and lateral bands of the plantar fascia, measuring 3-4 mm in thickness.
- *Plantar fasciitis* is evident on MRI when there is intermediate or high signal intensity within and/or surrounding the thickened (≥5-6 mm) plantar fascia, with or without adjacent calcaneal BME.
- Partial-thickness tears show partial discontinuity (Figure 109.12), whereas the full-thickness tears show complete discontinuity of the plantar fascia in the affected region with associated increased signal intensity.

Tarsal Tunnel

The tarsal tunnel is a canal housing the tibial neurovascular structures, located between the medial malleolus of the ankle and flexor retinaculum. Compression on the neurovascular structures (posterior tibial nerve) within the confined compartment may be caused by mass effect from ganglia (Figure 109.13), hematoma, nerve sheath tumors, accessory muscles, varicose veins, or other etiologies. Patients with tarsal tunnel syndrome may experience sensory deficits, numbness and/or pain in the bottom of the foot, and ankle weakness. Resection of the inciting cause and/or tarsal tunnel release may be indicated.

Sinus Tarsi Syndrome

The sinus tarsi is a hollow space at the lateral aspect of the hindfoot bordered by the neck of the talus and anterosuperior aspect of the calcaneus. It opens medially, posterior to the sustentaculum tali as a funnel-shape and separates the anterior and posterior subtalar joints. The sinus tarsi contains several ligaments including the lateral cervical ligament, medial talocalcaneal interosseous (ligament of sinus tarsi) as well as the medial, intermediate, and lateral roots of the inferior extensor retinaculum. It also contains fat, blood vessels, and nerves. Patients with sinus tarsi syndrome present with pain and tenderness on the lateral side of the hindfoot originating from the area of the sinus tarsi.

Magnetic Resonance Imaging Findings

- MRI is probably the best test to show changes in the soft tissues of the sinus tarsi including inflammation, scar tissue formation or ligamentous injuries. Look for high signal intensity edema on fluid-sensitive sequences and low signal intensity fibrosis on the T1W sequences with fat replacement and disruption of the ligaments (Figure 109.14).
- Of note, the bursa of Gruberi is a fluid-filled structure located beneath the EDL tendon and the dorsolateral talus and should not be mistaken for a soft tissue ganglion.

Baxter's Neuropathy

The inferior calcaneal nerve is most commonly a branch of the lateral plantar nerve, but its origin may vary. The nerve

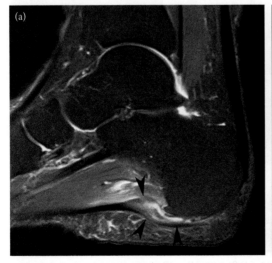
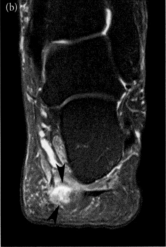

Figure 109.12. Plantar fascial tear in a 61-year-old woman. Sagittal (*A*) and coronal (*B*) FSE PDW FS MR images through the left ankle show high-grade partial-thickness tearing of the proximal central band of the plantar fascia (*arrowheads*), with small amount of adjacent fluid and small calcaneal spur.

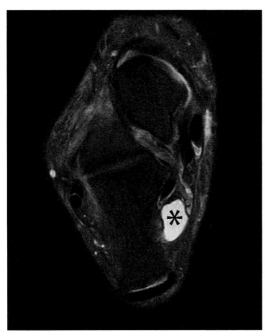

Figure 109.13. Ganglion in the tarsal tunnel in a 42-year-old man. Axial FSE T2W FS MR image through the right ankle shows a high signal intensity well-circumscribed cystic mass (*asterisk*) in the tarsal tunnel, consistent with ganglion.

courses along the plantar aspect of the calcaneal tuberosity, deep to the plantar fascia and flexor digitorum brevis muscle complex and superficial to the quadratus plantae muscle. The inferior calcaneal nerve provides motor innervation to the abductor digiti minimi muscle and sensory innervation to the anterior aspect of the calcaneus. At the plantar aspect of the heel, it may be compressed by calcaneal enthesophytes, plantar fasciitis, or varicose veins, which may result in pain and denervation changes of the abductor digiti minimi muscle, termed *Baxter's neuropathy*, which

can produce symptoms indistinguishable from plantar fasciitis. This entity accounts for up to 20% of heel pain. The initial treatment of Baxter's neuropathy is conservative. If conservative treatment fails, operative intervention may be performed.

Magnetic Resonance Imaging Findings
Refer to Figure 109.15.

- Edema with high signal intensity in the abductor digiti minimi muscle on fluid-sensitive sequences
- Fatty infiltration/atrophy of the abductor digiti minimi muscle in chronic cases is best seen on the coronal T1W MR images.

Normal Cartilage and Posttraumatic Osteochondral Lesions/Defects

Normal Magnetic Resonance Imaging Anatomy of Cartilage and Underlying Bone

The MRI appearance of normal hyaline cartilage of the foot and ankle depends on the sequence used and magnetic field and coil strength, with higher resolution systems rendering a more organized and zonal cartilage pattern. Cartilage sequences are constantly developing, but commonly used sequences in clinical practice are 2D PDW FSE with or without FS and 3D water-excited (WE) T1W spoiled gradient recalled acquisition in the steady state (SPGR). Ankle and foot cartilage should be uniform in thickness along the central portions, taper along the joint margins, and be hyperintense on PDW images. The mineralized portion of the deep cartilage and the underlying cortex should show low signal on all sequences, and there should not be any subchondral BME. Quantitative T2 mapping, *delayed gadolinium enhanced MRI of cartilage* (dGEMRIC), and investigative sequences such as ultrashort TE (UTE) pulse sequence

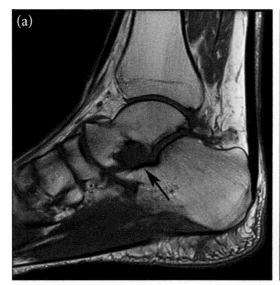
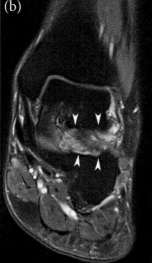

Figure 109.14. A 44-year-old man with sinus tarsi syndrome. (*A*) Sagittal T1W MR image shows intermediate signal intensity within the sinus tarsi with fat replacement and nonvisualization of ligaments consistent with sinus tarsi syndrome (*arrow*). (*B*) On the coronal PDW FS MR image, note high signal intensity edema within the sinus tarsi with ill-defined/disrupted ligaments (*arrowheads*).

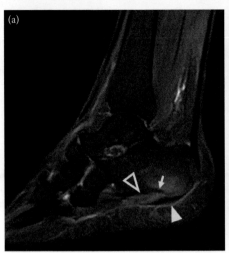 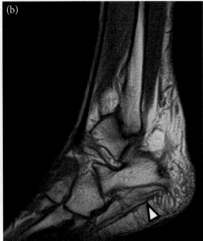

Figure 109.15. Baxter's neuropathy with denervation changes of the abductor digiti minimi muscle in a 60-year-old woman with 3-month history of plantar fasciitis. (*A*) Sagittal STIR MR image of the ankle shows high signal intensity BME involving the inferior aspect of the calcaneal tuberosity with associated thickening of the proximal central limb of the plantar fascia and perifascial edema (*white arrowhead*). Note edema with high signal intensity of the abductor digiti minimi muscle (*open arrowhead*). Arrow is pointing to the inferior calcaneal nerve. In (*B*) sagittal T1W MR image note diffuse increased signal of the abductor digiti minimi muscle consistent with marked fatty atrophy (*arrowhead*).

have proven useful, but require additional scan time and post processing (see Chapter 111, "Imaging of Articular Cartilage" for further discussion).

Pathophysiology and Imaging Findings of Posttraumatic Osteochondral Lesions/Defects

Posttraumatic OCLs/defects in the ankle and foot most commonly involve the talar dome, but can occur in the lateral talar

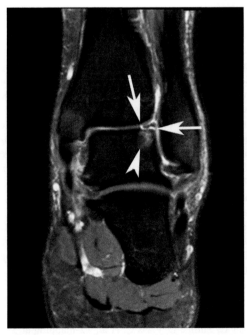

Figure 109.16. Unstable osteochondral defect of the lateral talar dome in an 18-year-old man. Coronal FSE PDW FS MR image through the ankle shows joint fluid (*arrows*) extending entirely beneath the unstable, nondisplaced osteochondral defect in the lateral talar dome. Note the BME subjacent to the defect (*arrowhead*), as well as mild BME within the medial and lateral malleoli.

process, tibial plafond, and less commonly, metatarsal heads. They are often symptomatic in the acute stage, but may be discovered incidentally when chronic. Depending on the location, talar dome OCLs result in pain in the ipsilateral side of the ankle. In the setting of an unstable ankle, OCLs will be larger (compared to patients with stable ankles), and additional chondral lesions may involve the medial malleolar tip and tibial plafond.

Magnetic Resonance Imaging Findings

- MRI has proven to be sensitive for the characterization of OCLs and can help differentiate stable from unstable lesions. Classification of the osteochondral talar lesions is described in Chapter 23, "Ankle Trauma."
- MRI is useful in determining OCL size, subchondral compression, incomplete separation of a fragment, formation of subchondral cystlike changes, and the detection of unattached or displaced fragments.
- Instability is suggested when there is a fluid-filled cleft partially or completely extending between the OCL and viable bone (Figure 109.16), cystlike changes beneath the OCL, or large lesion size. A high signal intensity line surrounding the OCL/defect on MRI is considered most predictive of instability, and highly suggests a loosened or completely detached osteochondral fragment.
- Inverted orientation of an osteochondral fragment can occur with twisting injuries and is pathognomonic for an unstable lesion.

Treatment and Complications

Patient treatment depends on their symptoms and performance demands. If left untreated, some talar osteochondral defects can be a source of persistent ankle pain, OA, and disability.

- Surgical treatment includes debridement and microfracture of the OCL, osteochondral plug transfer, and autologous chondrocyte implantation.

- Microfracture is recommended as a first-line treatment, and has shown good-to-excellent results, especially with small OCLs.
- Concomitant correction of lateral ankle ligamentous complex pathology must be performed for patients with chronic lateral ankle instability.

Postoperative Magnetic Resonance Imaging Appearance of the Talar Osteochondral Lesion Repair

- The MRI MOCART (magnetic resonance observation of cartilage repair tissue) evaluation of repaired OCLs consists of degree of defect infill, integration to the border zone, surface of the repaired tissue, structure of the repaired tissue, signal intensity of the repaired tissue, intact subchondral lamina and subchondral bone, and the presence of any adhesions and joint effusion.
- The reduction of BME has shown to correlate with improved patient clinical outcome after surgical treatment.

Key Points

- Tendinosis and tendon tears occur most commonly in the Achilles, posterior tibial, and peroneal tendons.
- Tenosynovitis may occur anywhere except where a tendon sheath is absent, namely the Achilles tendon.
- Peroneal tendons may subluxate or dislocate with peroneal retinacular disruption or may undergo intrasheath subluxation with reversal of the PB and longus positions.
- The ATFL is the most commonly torn ligament caused by an inversion injury.
- *High ankle sprain* is the term used for partial or complete disruption of the distal anterior and/or posterior tibiofibular (syndesmotic) ligaments.
- Deltoid ligament sprains are caused by eversion forces and are less common than lateral ligament complex injuries.
- Lisfranc ligament complex injuries are well-delineated by MRI and are important findings to detect because midfoot dysfunction may progress to medial midfoot arch collapse and OA.
- Plantar plate injuries of the hallux MTP joint (*turf toe*) caused by hyperextension may be accompanied by hallux sesamoid ligament injury and sesamoid dislocation, traumatic hallux valgus, hallux MTP joint dislocation, and OCLs.
- Plantar fasciitis is evident on MRI as intermediate or high signal intensity within and/or surrounding the thickened (≥5-6 mm) plantar fascia, with or without adjacent calcaneal subenthesial BME.
- Tarsal tunnel syndrome may be caused by ganglia, hematoma, or nerve sheath tumors. Patients may experience sensory deficits, numbness, and/or pain in the bottom of the foot and ankle weakness.
- Sinus tarsi syndrome presents with pain and tenderness at the lateral aspect of the hindfoot. MRI shows high signal intensity edema on the fluid-sensitive sequences and low signal intensity fibrosis on T1W sequences with disruption of the ligaments.

- Entrapment of the inferior calcaneal nerve at the plantar aspect of the heel may result in Baxter's neuropathy with denervation changes of the abductor digiti minimi muscle.
- OCLs/defects in the ankle and foot most commonly involve the talar dome, but can occur in the lateral talar process, tibial plafond, and metatarsal heads.
- A high signal intensity line surrounding the OCL on MRI is considered most predictive of instability and highly suggests a loosened or completely detached osteochondral fragment.
- Surgical treatment options for OCLs include debridement and microfracture, osteochondral plug transfer, and autologous chondrocyte implantation.

Recommended Reading

Taljanovic MS, Alcala JN, Gimber LH, et al. High-resolution US and MR imaging of peroneal tendon injuries. *Radiographics.* 2015;35(1):179–99.

Chhabra A, Soldatos T, Chalian M, et al. Current concepts review: 3T magnetic resonance imaging of the ankle and foot. *Foot Ankle Int.* 2012;33(2):164–71.

Hodgson RJ, O'Connor PJ, Grainger AJ. Tendon and ligament imaging. *Br J Radiol.* 2012;85(1016):1157–72.

Gallo RA, Mosher TJ. Imaging of cartilage and osteochondral injuries: a case-based review. *Clin Sports Med.* 2013;32(3):477–505.

Nazarenko A, Beltran LS, Bencardino JT. Imaging evaluation of traumatic ligamentous injuries of the ankle and foot. *Radiol Clin North Am.* 2013;51(3):455–78.

Ngai SS, Tafur M, Chang EY, et al. Magnetic resonance imaging of ankle ligaments. *Can Assoc Radiol J.* 2016;67(1):60–68.

References

1. American College of Radiology. ACR–SPR–SSR practice parameter for the performance and interpretation of magnetic resonance imaging (MRI) of the ankle and hindfoot. www.acr.org/-/media/ACR/Files/Practice-Parameters/MR-AnkleHindFoot.pdf. Accessed March 18, 2018.
2. American College of Radiology. ACR-SPR-SSR Practice parameter for the performance and interpretation of magnetic resonance imaging (MRI) of the fingers and toes. www.acr.org/-/media/ACR/Files/Practice-Parameters/mr-finger-toes.pdf?la=en. Accessed March 18, 2018.
3. Arnoldner MA, Gruber M, Syré S, et al. Imaging of posterior tibial tendon dysfunction—Comparison of high-resolution ultrasound and 3T MRI. *Eur J Radiol.* 2015;84(9):1777–81.
4. Bancroft LW, Anderson RB. Radiologic case study. Traumatic dislocation of the tibial sesamoid of the hallux. *Orthopedics.* 2010;33(9):618, 690–93.
5. Bancroft LW, Kransdorf MJ, Adler R, et al. ACR appropriateness criteria acute trauma to the foot. *J Am Coll Radiol.* 2015;12(6):575–81.
6. Becher C, Zühlke D, Plaas C, et al. T2-mapping at 3 T after microfracture in the treatment of osteochondral defects of the talus at an average follow-up of 8 years. *Knee Surg Sports Traumatol Arthrosc.* 2015;23(8):2406–12.
7. Brodsky JW, Toppins A. Postsurgical imaging of the peroneal tendons. *Semin Musculoskelet Radiol.* 2012;16(3):233–40.

8. Castro M, Melao L, Carnella C, et al. Lisfranc ligamentous complex: MRI with anatomic correlation in cadavers. *AJR Am J Roentgenol.* 2010;195:W447–55.

9. Cha SD, Kim HS, Chung ST, et al. Intra-articular lesions in chronic lateral ankle instability: comparison of arthroscopy with magnetic resonance imaging findings. *Clin Orthop Surg.* 2012;4(4):293–99.

10. Chhabra A, Soldatos T, Chalian M, et al. Current concepts review: 3T magnetic resonance imaging of the ankle and foot. *Foot Ankle Int.* 2012;33(2):164–71.

11. Clanton TO, Chacko AK, Matheny LM, et al. Magnetic resonance imaging findings of snowboarding osteochondral injuries to the middle talocalcaneal articulation. *Sports Health.* 2013;5(5):470–75.

12. de César PC, Avila EM, de Abreu MR. Comparison of magnetic resonance imaging to physical examination for syndesmotic injury after lateral ankle sprain. *Foot Ankle Int.* 2011;32(12):1110–14.

13. Dunlap BJ, Ferkel RD, Applegate GR. The "LIFT" lesion: lateral inverted osteochondral fracture of the talus. *Arthroscopy.* 2013;29(11):1826–33.

14. Espinosa N, Maurer MA. Peroneal tendon dislocation. *Eur J Trauma Emerg Surg.* 2015;41(6):631–37. doi:10.1007/s00068-015-0590-0. Epub November 12, 2015.

15. Galli MM, Protzman NM, Mandelker EM, et al. Examining the relation of osteochondral lesions of the talus to ligamentous and lateral ankle tendinous pathologic features: a comprehensive MRI review in an asymptomatic lateral ankle population. *J Foot Ankle Surg.* 201;53(4):429–33.

16. Galli MM, Protzman NM, Mandelker EM, et al. An examination of anatomic variants and incidental peroneal tendon pathologic features: a comprehensive MRI review of asymptomatic lateral ankles. *J Foot Ankle Surg.* 2015;54(2):164–72.

17. Gatlin CC, Matheny LM, Ho CP, et al. Diagnostic accuracy of 3.0 tesla magnetic resonance imaging for the detection of articular cartilage lesions of the talus. *Foot Ankle Int.* 2015;36(3):288–92.

18. Ghahremani S, Griggs R, Hall T, et al. Osteochondral lesions in pediatric and adolescent patients. *Semin Musculoskelet Radiol.* 2014;18(5):505–12.

19. Haleem AM, Ross KA, Smyth NA, et al. Double-plug autologous osteochondral transplantation shows equal functional outcomes compared with single-plug procedures in lesions of the talar dome: a minimum 5-year clinical follow-up. *Am J Sports Med.* 2014;42(8):1888–95.

20. Haverkamp D, Hoornenborg D, Maas M, et al. A new snowboard injury caused by "FLOW" bindings: a complete deltoid ligament and anterior talofibular ankle ligament rupture. *J Am Podiatr Med Assoc.* 2014;104(3):287–90.

21. Hunt KJ, Githens M, Riley GM, et al. Foot and ankle injuries in sport: imaging correlation with arthroscopic and surgical findings. *Clin Sports Med.* 2013;32(3):525–57.

22. Gianakos AL, Hannon CP, Ross KA, et al. Anterolateral tibial osteotomy for accessing osteochondral lesions of the talus in autologous osteochondral transplantation: functional and T2 MRI analysis. *Foot Ankle Int.* 2015;36(5):531–38.

23. Kitsukawa K, Hirano T, Niki H, et al. MR Imaging evaluation of the Lisfranc ligament in cadaveric feet and patients with acute to chronic Lisfranc injury. *Foot Ankle Int.* 2015;36(12):1483–92. doi:10.1177/1071100715596746. Epub August 7, 2015.

24. Klammer G, Maquieira GJ, Spahn S, et al. Natural history of nonoperatively treated osteochondral lesions of the talus. *Foot Ankle Int.* 2015;36(1):24–31.

25. Kolodenker G, Esformes I, Napoli R. Isolated chronic anteroinferior tibiofibular ligament rupture repair. *J Foot Ankle Surg.* 2012;51(6):787–89.

26. Kwak SK, Kern BS, Ferkel RD, et al. Autologous chondrocyte implantation of the ankle: 2- to 10-year results. *Am J Sports Med.* 2014;42(9):2156–64.

27. Kwon DG, Sung KH, Chung CY, et al. Associations between MRI findings and symptoms in patients with chronic ankle sprain. *J Foot Ankle Surg.* 2014;53(4):411–14.

28. Lee M, Kwon JW, Choi WJ, et al. Comparison of outcomes for osteochondral lesions of the talus with and without chronic lateral ankle instability. *Foot Ankle Int.* 2015;36(9):1050–57.

29. Lee SJ, Jacobson JA, Kim SM, et al. Ultrasound and MRI of the peroneal tendons and associated pathology. *Skeletal Radiol.* 2013;42(9):1191–200.

30. Lektrakul N, Chung CB, Lai Y, et al. Tarsal sinus: arthrographic MR imaging, MR arthrographic, and pathologic findings in cadavers and retrospective study data in patients with sinus tarsi syndrome. *Radiographics.* 2001;219:802–10.

31. Luchs JS, Flug JA, Weissman BN, et al. ACR appropriateness criteria chronic ankle pain. https://acsearch.acr.org/docs/69422/Narrative. Accessed December 30, 2015.

32. Mosher TJ, Kransdorf MJ, Adler R, et al. ACR appropriateness criteria acute trauma to the ankle. *J Am Coll Radiol.* 2015;12(3):221–27.

33. Murawski CD, Smyth NA, Newman H, et al. A single platelet-rich plasma injection for chronic midsubstance Achilles tendinopathy: a retrospective preliminary analysis. *Foot Ankle Spec.* 2014;7(5):372–76.

34. Othman MI, Chew KM, Peh WC. Variants and pitfalls in MR imaging of foot and ankle injuries. *Semin Musculoskelet Radiol.* 2014;18(1):54–62.

35. Roemer FW, Jomaah N, Niu J, et al. Ligamentous injuries and the risk of associated tissue damage in acute ankle sprains in athletes: a cross-sectional MRI study. *Am J Sports Med.* 2014;42(7):1549–57.

36. Ross KA, Hannon CP, Deyer TW, et al. Functional and MRI outcomes after arthroscopic microfracture for treatment of osteochondral lesions of the distal tibial plafond. *J Bone Joint Surg Am.* 2014;96(20):1708–15.

37. Russo A, Zappia M, Reginelli A, et al. Ankle impingement: a review of multimodality imaging approach. *Musculoskelet Surg.* 2013;97(suppl 2):S161–68.

38. Shang XL, Tao HY, Chen SY, et al. Clinical and MRI outcomes of HA injection following arthroscopic microfracture for osteochondral lesions of the talus. *Knee Surg Sports Traumatol Arthrosc.* 2016;24(4):1243–49. doi:10.1007/s00167-015-3575-y. Epub March 13, 2015.

39. Sikka RS, Fetzer GB, Sugarman E, et al. Correlating MRI findings with disability in syndesmotic sprains of NFL players. *Foot Ankle Int.* 2012;33(5):371–78.

40. Slaughter AJ, Reynolds KA, Jambhekar K, et al. Clinical orthopedic examination findings in the lower extremity: correlation with imaging studies and diagnostic efficacy. *Radiographics.* 2014;34(2):e41–55.

41. Sookur PA, Naraghi AM, Bleakney RR, Jalan R, Chan O, White LM. Accessory muscles: anatomy, symptoms, and radiologic evaluation. *Radiographics*. 2008;28(2):481–99.

42. Tao H, Shang X, Lu R, et al. Quantitative magnetic resonance imaging (MRI) evaluation of cartilage repair after microfracture (MF) treatment for adult unstable osteochondritis dissecans (OCD) in the ankle: correlations with clinical outcome. *Eur Radiol*. 2014;24(8):1758–67.

43. Warner SJ, Garner MR, Schottel PC, et al. Analysis of PITFL injuries in rotationally unstable ankle fractures. *Foot Ankle Int*. 2015;36(4):377–82.

44. Williams G, Widnall J, Evans P, et al. Could failure of the spring ligament complex be the driving force behind the development of the adult flatfoot deformity? *J Foot Ankle Surg*. 2014;53(2):152–55.

45. Williams G, Widnall J, Evans P, et al. MRI features most often associated with surgically proven tears of the spring ligament complex. *Skeletal Radiol*. 2013;42(7):969–73.

46. Wise JN, Weissman BN, Appel M, et al. ACR appropriateness criteria chronic foot pain. https://acsearch.acr.org/docs/69424/Narrative. Accessed December 30, 2015.

47. van Putte-Katier N, van Ochten JM, van Middelkoop M, et al. Magnetic resonance imaging abnormalities after lateral ankle trauma in injured and contralateral ankles. *Eur J Radiol*. 2015;84(12):2586–92. doi:10.1016/j.ejrad.2015.09.028. Epub October 8, 2015.

48. Yasui Y, Takao M, Miyamoto W, et al. Simultaneous surgery for chronic lateral ankle instability accompanied by only subchondral bone lesion of talus. *Arch Orthop Trauma Surg*. 2014;134(6):821–27.

CHAPTER 110

Internal Derangement of the Temporomandibular Joints

Josephina A. Vossen

Introduction

The temporomandibular joints (TMJs) play a crucial role in mastication, jaw mobility, and verbal and emotional expression. Temporomandibular disorders (TMDs) include several entities that can lead to orofacial pain symptoms. Prevalence of chronic TMJ pain ranges from 5 to 12%, with an incidence of first time pain of 4% per year. In a recent U.S. National Health Interview Survey including 189,977 people, 4.6% of the people had experienced TMJ and muscle disorders. The incidence of TMD peaks in the second to fourth decade of life. The annual cost of managing TMD is estimated at $4 billion. Common symptoms include jaw pain, jaw dysfunction, earache, headache, and facial pain. Multiple risk factors have been implicated, including trauma, anatomical factors, pathophysiological factors, and psychosocial factors. There is a higher prevalence of TMD in females than males with ratios ranging from 2:1 to 8:1.

Indications for Imaging and Protocols

TMJ radiographic examinations include transcranial (oblique lateral view), transmaxillary (modified AP view), transpharyngeal (oblique lateral view), and submental vertex radiographs. Cross-sectional imaging is usually indicated in cases where malocclusion or intraarticular abnormalities are suspected. CT is most useful for evaluation of the osseous components. In the setting of trauma, CT is the primary imaging modality. CT is also particularly valuable for planning of surgical reconstruction, in the evaluation of calcified loose bodies, and in some cases of inflammatory, infectious or oncologic entities. Cone-beam computed tomography (CBCT) has shown comparable osseous detail to CT, with the advantage of decreased radiation dose. MRI is the best modality for evaluation of intraarticular processes. Given the high MRI contrast resolution of the soft tissues, it is currently the gold standard for the diagnosis of disc disorders. The standard MR imaging protocol consists of oblique sagittal and oblique coronal images of the TMJ, which are obtained perpendicular or parallel to the long axis of the mandibular condyle, to visualize disc position and morphology as well as the bone structures. T1W/PDW MRI sequences in both closed- and open-mouth positions are often obtained. Open-mouth imaging can be facilitated by using a mechanical mouth opener, such as a bite block or gauze-wrapped syringe in the patient's mouth. T2W images are useful for detecting degenerative periarticular changes and the presence of a joint effusion. Gd contrast is not used routinely, but would be indicated for cases in which infection or inflammatory arthropathy is suspected.

Cine GRE images depict disc movement and can be used to evaluate condylar translation. New dynamic techniques, such as a half-Fourier acquired single-shot turbo SE or a balanced steady-state free precession sequence, appear to further contribute to the evaluation of the disc movement and functionality. Because of higher SNRs, 3T MRI magnets have the advantage of depicting improved anatomic and pathologic details of the TMJ as compared with 1.5T MRI magnets.

Normal Magnetic Resonance Imaging Anatomy of the Temporomandibular Joints

The TMJ is a synovial joint between the temporal bone and the mandibular condyle (Figure 110.1). The central anatomic structure of the TMJ is the articular disc, or meniscus. The disc is a fibrocartilaginous structure that divides the joint into superior and inferior compartments. The disc is round to oval, with a thin center (intermediate zone), giving the disc a biconcave appearance on sagittal MR images. The posterior aspect of the disc, or band, is thicker than the anterior band. The anterior and posterior bands are longer in the mediolateral than the anteroposterior dimension. The posterior margin of the posterior band is termed the *bilaminar zone*, a rich neurovascular structure, which is composed of superior and inferior layers. These retrodiscal layers serve as posterior attachments blending with the joint capsule and temporal bone. The lateral attachments of the disc blend with the capsule and insert into the condylar neck. Anteriorly, the attachments of the disc are variable and called the *disc-capsular complex*. There can be fibers of the lateral pterygoid muscle and tendon attaching to the anterior band of the disc complex. The normal position of the disc is evaluated by the location of the intermediate zone and posterior band, which should be located superiorly between the condyle and temporal bone on the sagittal MR images. The medial and lateral corners of the disc align with the condylar borders and should not bulge medially or laterally.

The motion of the mandibular condyle has 2 components. The condyle first rotates and then translates anteriorly with respect to the temporal bone as the mouth is opened. The lateral pterygoid muscle contributes to jaw opening and the medial pterygoid, masseter, and temporalis muscles facilitate jaw closure. As the condyle translates anteriorly, the disc should move into a position in between the condyle and the articular eminence with full contact of the intermediate zone. The disc should not change position in the coronal plane during mouth opening. Variation in meniscus position can be may be due

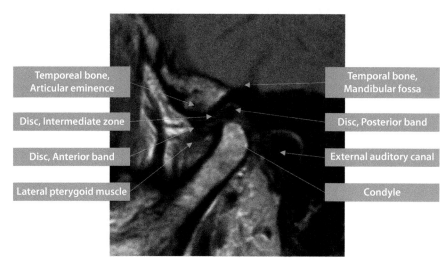

Figure 110.1. TMJ anatomy. Normal anatomic structures are marked on the sagittal oblique PDW MR image of the TMJ in closed-mouth position.

to suboptimal mouth opening resulting in incomplete condyle rotation and translation.

Imaging Findings of Temporomandibular Disorders

TMDs are a heterogeneous group of conditions involving the temporomandibular joint complex, surrounding musculature, and osseous components. *Internal derangement* is a general orthopedic term implying a mechanical interference of the smooth joint movement. Internal derangement is a functional diagnosis, and for the TMJ the most common cause of internal derangement is displacement of the disc (Figures 110.2 through 110.4).

Common findings associated with internal derangement

- Joint sounds (clicking and popping), crepitus, or joint locking
- Disc displacement of the TMJ is considered to have 4 clinical stages:
  - Stage I: The articular disc is displaced in closed-mouth position and reduces to normal relationship in open-mouth position. This is referred to as *disc recapture* (Figure 110.3A,B).
- Stage II: The disc is displaced in closed-mouth position and intermittently locks in open-mouth position.
- Stage III: The disc is displaced in closed-mouth position and does not reduce to normal contact in open-mouth position (Figure 110.4).
- Stage IV: The disc is displaced and does not reduce, with perforation of the disc or posterior attachment tissues.
  - A *stuck disc* remains in a fixed position in both the open- and closed-mouth positions, likely related to the formation of adhesions.
- Although most disc displacement occurs anteriorly, 30% of cases are medial or lateral.
  - Posterior disc displacement is rare.
- A commonly used classification of TMJ disc displacement using clinical and radiographic findings was described by Wilkes (Table 110.1).
- Disc degeneration is seen as loss of T1 and T2 signal and normal biconcave shape (Figure 110.4).

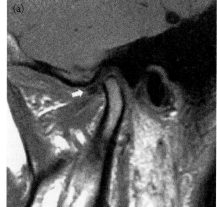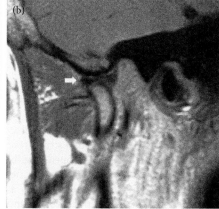

Figure 110.2. Normal TMJ on MR imaging. (*A, B*) Sagittal oblique PDW MR images obtained in the (*A*) closed- and (*B*) open-mouth positions show the normal position of the TMJ disc (*thick arrow*). The anterior and posterior bands are thick, and the intermediate zone is thin, creating the biconcave disc shape.

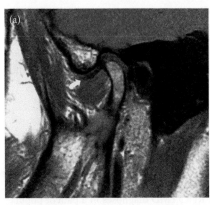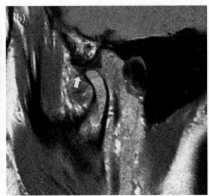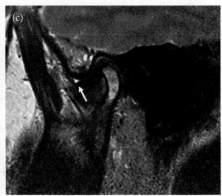

Figure 110.3. Abnormal disc with reduction. (*A, B*) Sagittal oblique PDW MR images obtained in the (*A*) closed- and (*B*) open-mouth positions show an abnormally anterior displaced TMJ disc on the closed-mouth image. Recapture of the disc into a normal position between the condyle and the temporal bone is seen on the open-mouth image. (*C*) Sagittal oblique, closed-mouth T2W MR image demonstrates a small anterior joint effusion (*thin arrow*).

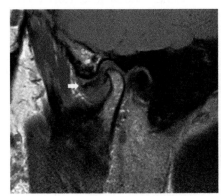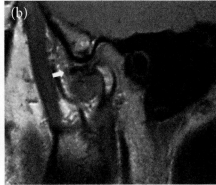

Figure 110.4. Abnormal disc without reduction. (*A, B*) Sagittal oblique PDW MR images obtained in the closed- and open-mouth position show an anterior displaced disc on both the (*A*) closed- and (*B*) open-mouth images. Intermediate signal, especially of the posterior band, with a loss of biconcave architecture is present.

Table 110.1. Clinical and Radiologic Findings According to Wilkes Classification for Temporomandibular Joint Internal Derangement

STAGE	CLINICAL FINDINGS	RADIOLOGIC FINDINGS
I	No significant mechanical symptoms, no pain or limitation of motion	Slight forward displacement and good anatomic contour of TMJ disc
II	First few episodes of pain, occasional joint tenderness and related temporal headaches, increase in intensity of clicking, joint sounds later in opening movement, beginning transient subluxations or joint locking	Slight forward displacement and beginning anatomic deformity of TMJ disc, slight thickening of posterior edge of disc
III	Multiple episodes of pain, joint tenderness, temporal headaches, locking, closed locks, restriction of motion, difficulty (pain) with function	Anterior displacement with significant anatomic deformity/prolapse of TMJ disc, moderate to marked thickening of posterior edge of disc, no hard tissue changes
IV	Characterized by chronicity with variable and episodic pain, headaches, variable restriction of motion, and undulating course	Increase in severity over intermediate stage, early to moderate degenerative TMJ disc remodeling, hard tissue changes
V	Crepitus on examination, scraping, grating, grinding symptoms, variable and episodic pain, chronic restriction of motion, difficulty with function	Gross anatomic deformity of TMJ disc and hard tissue, essentially degenerative arthritic changes, osteophytic deformity, subcortical cystlike formation

Degenerative OA or degenerative joint disease (DJD) is the second most common TMJ pathology, with higher prevalence in older age populations.

Common findings associated with DJD

- Pain during chewing
- Articular surface cortical bone irregularity, erosion, and osteophyte formation
- Joint effusion: best seen on a T2W MR images, commonly seen surrounding the anterior band (Figure 110.3C)

Other pathologies involving the TMJ include trauma, inflammatory arthritis (RA, psoriatic arthritis, and AS), synovial chondromatosis, CPPD, PVNS, tumors, infection, and ON.

Treatment Options

Management of TMJ OA may be divided into noninvasive (conservative), minimally invasive, and invasive or surgical modalities. Usually, therapy is performed in a stepwise manner with minimally invasive or invasive techniques only considered after failing of conservative management.

- Conservative management includes:
  - Occlusal splints
  - Physical therapy
  - Pharmacotherapy (NSAIDs and muscle relaxants)

- Minimally invasive management includes:
  - Intraarticular injections (hyaluronic acid, corticosteroids)
  - Arthrocentesis/arthroscopy with lavage and lysis; in patients with acute or subacute closed lock of the TMJ and for disc displacement without reduction of less than 3 months evolution

- Invasive management includes:
  - Arthroplasty (disc repositioning, disc repair, discectomy with or without graft replacement); in patients with chronic closed lock of the TMJ (>3 months evolution) and for internal derangement of the TMJ, mainly Wilkes stages II, III, and IV
  - Total joint replacement; in patients with ankylosis or severely damaged joints that have failed all other more conservative treatment modalities

Key Points

- MRI is the imaging modality of choice for evaluation of disc position and internal derangement of the TMJ.
- CT scan can be useful for evaluation of bony anatomy and changes.
- Understanding of the TMJ anatomy and biomechanics is important to accurately recognize various pathologies.

Recommended Reading

Tomas X, Pomes J, Berenguer J, et al. MR imaging of temporomandibular joint dysfunction: a pictorial review. *Radiographics*. 2006;26(3):765–81.

Morales H, Cornelius R. Imaging approach to temporomandibular joint disorders. *Clin Neuroradiol*. 2016;26(1):5–22.

References

1. Liu F, Steinkeler A. Epidemiology, diagnosis, and treatment of temporomandibular disorders. *Dent Clin North Am*. 2013;57(3):465–79.
2. Manfredini D, Piccotti F, Ferronato G, Guarda-nardini L. Age peaks of different RDC/TMD diagnoses in a patient population. *J Dent*. 2010;38(5):392–99.
3. Schiffman E, Ohrbach R, Truelove E, et al. Diagnostic criteria for temporomandibular disorders (DC/TMD) for clinical and research applications: recommendations of the International RDC/TMD Consortium Network and Orofacial Pain Special Interest Group. *J Oral Facial Pain Headache*. 2014;28(1):6–27.
4. Plesh O, Adams SH, Gansky SA. Temporomandibular joint and muscle disorder-type pain and comorbid pains in a national US sample. *J Orofac Pain*. 2011;25(3):190–98.
5. Larheim TA. Role of magnetic resonance imaging in the clinical diagnosis of the temporomandibular joint. *Cells Tissues Organs*. 2005;180(1):6–21.
6. Larheim TA, Westesson PL, Sano T. MR grading of temporomandibular joint fluid: association with disk displacement categories, condyle marrow abnormalities and pain. *Int J Oral Maxillofac Surg*. 2001;30(2):104–12.
7. Ahmad M, Schiffman EL. Temporomandibular joint disorders and orofacial pain. *Dent Clin North Am*. 2016;60(1):105–24.
8. Carrasco R. Juvenile idiopathic arthritis overview and involvement of the temporomandibular joint: prevalence, systemic therapy. *Oral Maxillofac Surg Clin North Am*. 2015;27(1):1–10.
9. Morales H, Cornelius R. Imaging approach to temporomandibular joint disorders. *Clin Neuroradiol*. 2016;26(1):5–22.
10. Mercuri LG. Osteoarthritis, osteoarthrosis, and idiopathic condylar resorption. *Oral Maxillofac Surg Clin North Am*. 2008;20(2):169–83, v–vi.
11. González-García R. The current role and the future of minimally invasive temporomandibular joint surgery. *Oral Maxillofac Surg Clin North Am*. 2015;27(1):69–84.
12. Li C, Su N, Yang X, Yang X, Shi Z, Li L. Ultrasonography for detection of disc displacement of temporomandibular joint: a systematic review and meta-analysis. *J Oral Maxillofac Surg*. 2012;70(6):1300–309.
13. Tsiklakis K. Cone beam computed tomographic findings in temporomandibular joint disorders. *Alpha Omegan*. 2010;103(2):68–78.
14. Wilkes CH. Internal derangements of the temporomandibular joint. Pathological variations. *Arch Otolaryngol Head Neck Surg*. 1989;115(4):469–77.

CHAPTER 111

Imaging of Articular Cartilage

Kevin B. Hoover

Introduction

Cartilage loss is inferred on radiographs and CT images by the presence of joint space loss, altered alignment, and subchondral bone changes. Direct cartilage imaging using specific pulse sequences is a standard part of all musculoskeletal MRI joint protocols. The importance of cartilage in normal joint function and the development of therapeutic techniques to treat osteochondral injury necessitates the use of high-resolution sequences for cartilage assessment. Anatomic (morphologic) and compositional (biochemical) imaging are the 2 main types of cartilage MRI.

Normal Magnetic Resonance Imaging Anatomy of the Examined Structures

Adult hyaline articular cartilage is an avascular, hypocellular tissue with nutrients supplied by diffusion primarily from the synovial fluid. It is composed of a complex extracellular matrix consisting largely of proteoglycans arranged in a network of collagen. Proteoglycans provide compressive strength to the cartilage. Collagen fibers provide tensile and shear strength.

Articular cartilage has 4 structural/functional zones (Figure 111.1). The superficial or tangential *gliding* zone makes up 10-20% of total cartilage thickness. It has the highest collagen content, which is oriented parallel to surface. Deep to the superficial layer is the middle or transitional zone, which makes up 40-60% of the cartilage thickness. It has a more random collagen orientation, which distributes stress. The deep or radial zone makes up 30% of the thickness with radially oriented anchoring collagen fibers crossing from noncalcified to calcified cartilage. The calcified zone is the deepest, which is separated from the radial zone by the tidemark, which may act as a shear plane.

Visualization of the cartilage zones is dependent on cartilage thickness and MRI field strength. Cartilage thickness varies by bone, joint, and specific articulating surface. For example, in the lower extremities of cadavers, the knee tibial and femoroarticular surfaces have the thickest cartilage (1.69-2.55 mm). The acetabular and femoral head cartilage is next thickest (1.35-2.0 mm) followed by the ankle (1.0-1.62 mm). It is the cartilage of the tibial plateaus and the patella where the different structural zones are most apparent. In general, the higher the field strength, the more apparent the different zones become with the transitional and radial zone apparent on 1.5T and the calcified zone more apparent at 3.0T. The superficial zone is not apparent at either field strength.

Indications for Imaging and Protocols

Radiography and Computed Tomography

Radiographs are the first-line imaging modality to evaluate adult joint pain. The radiographic changes encountered from cartilage loss in OA were described previously (see Chapter 44, "Osteoarthritis of the Upper and Lower Extremity Joints"). CT is not routinely acquired to evaluate cartilage injuries, but demonstrates with greater sensitivity the secondary bone changes from overlying cartilage loss. CTA is highly sensitive in detecting cartilage defects.

Anatomic Magnetic Resonance Imaging

Anatomic imaging requires contrast resolution to distinguish articular hyaline cartilage from fibrocartilage, underlying bone, and synovial fluid. This is routinely acquired at 1.5T and 3.0T with active research into the clinical utility of 7.0T. The 3.0T field strength allows for faster image acquisition and a higher SNR. However, negatives of the higher field strength include chemical shift artifact, increased specific absorption rate (SAR), or power absorbed by tissue, greater susceptibility, and pulsation artifacts.

The most commonly used cartilage imaging sequence is a 2D FSE PDW pulse sequence (Figure 111.2) with a repetition time (TR) of 3500-5000 msec, a TE of 30-34 msec, 3-4 mm slice thickness with an in-plane resolution of 250-350 microns. This is acquired without or with fat saturation (FS). This sequence is also useful to evaluate other structures such as tendons, ligaments, fibrocartilage, and bone marrow, especially with the use of FS. It is typically acquired in 3 planes (axial, coronal, and sagittal) to evaluate these structures and the cartilage. The sensitivity of this sequence in detecting cartilage injury compares well with arthroscopy findings both with and without FS.

A commonly used 3D volume acquisition sequence is the 3D spoiled gradient recalled acquisition in the steady state (SPGR) echo sequence. This sequence has excellent spatial resolution and isotropic (cubic) voxels with comparable accuracy for cartilage lesion detection to arthroscopy. However, the acquisition is longer than 2D FSE sequences with inferior evaluation of subchondral bone, ligaments, and tendons and greater metal artifact susceptibility. Similar 3D sequences include fast low-angle shot (FLASH), DEFT, DESS, and 3D bSSFP including True FISP, FIESTA, and balanced FFE. Less well validated are 3D FSE and SPACE/CUBE sequences that use parallel imaging.

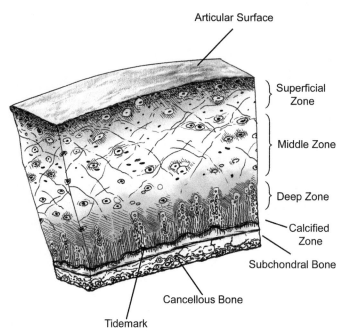

Figure 111.1. Drawing of hyaline cartilage structure. Four layers of articular cartilage visualized in cross-section from superficial (*top*) to deep (*bottom*): superficial zone, middle zone, deep zone, and calcified zone. Artist Sydney Leighton.

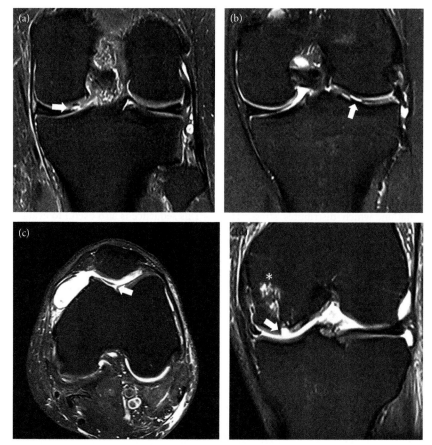

Figure 111.2. Chondral defect grading on MRI. (*A*) A coronal PDW FS MR image demonstrates a grade 2 defect (modified Outerbridge classification) of the lateral aspect of the medial femoral condyle (*thick arrow*) involving less than 50% of cartilage thickness. (*B*) A coronal PDW FS MR image demonstrates a grade 3 cartilage defect of the lateral tibial plateau (*thick arrow*) extending to the calcified (*dark*) cartilage layer. (*C*) An axial PDW FS MR image demonstrates a large full-thickness, grade 3 cartilage flap extending from the central into the lateral femoral trochlea (*thick arrow*) without involvement of the subchondral bone plate. (*D*) Full-thickness cartilage defect in same patient as (*C*) extending through the subchondral bone plate of the medial femoral condyle (*thick arrow*) with subjacent BME (*asterisk*).

Compositional Magnetic Resonance Imaging

Compositional imaging sequences use image post-processing to determine the integrity of articular cartilage. These are used primarily in clinical research and drug trials to evaluate OA treatments in the knee joint. Three of these sequences are T2 mapping, delayed gadolinium enhanced MRI of cartilage (dGEMRIC), and T1ρ (rho) imaging.

T2 mapping is a technique that uses a standard T2 FSE sequence to measure collagen organization within the cartilage (Figure 111.3C). The T2 relaxation time is the rate constant of dephasing in the transverse plane after application of an RF pulse. Cartilage T2 relaxation time reflects water content, collagen content, and collagen fiber orientation in the extracellular matrix. Water protons that are embedded within organized collagen demonstrate less signal than those outside collagen or in a less organized collagen network. Thus, there is increased signal and higher values on the T2 map from cartilage that is damaged and disorganized. Long acquisition times are necessary.

dGEMRIC is a more complicated technique than T2 mapping. It is a T1 relaxation time (spin-lattice relaxation) measurement technique performed using 3D SPGR or bSSFP sequences. IV Gd dimeglumine (Gd-DTPA^{2-}) is administered at double or triple the standard dose, followed by approximately 10 minutes of knee joint exercise. Approximately 90 minutes after the injection, the MRI is acquired. This technique provides an assessment of proteoglycan content and cartilage integrity. The negatively charged Gd is normally repelled by the negatively charged proteoglycans. Thus, the greater the T1 signal caused by Gd, the more disorganized or destroyed the cartilage structure is.

The third compositional technique, T1ρ, has greater accuracy in detecting cartilage degeneration than T2 mapping (Figure 111.4). T1ρ evaluates the spin-lattice (T1) relaxation in the rotating frame. This requires an additional RF pulse after the magnetization is tipped into the transverse plane. Similar to T2 mapping, T1ρ relies on interaction of water molecules with surrounding macromolecules, especially proteoglycans. T1ρ signal processing is time consuming and requires special acquisition pulse sequences, which are not routinely available outside research institutions. Other compositional techniques used primarily for research are diffusion-weighted imaging and sodium imaging.

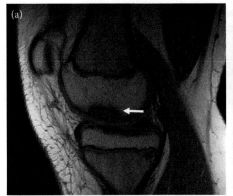 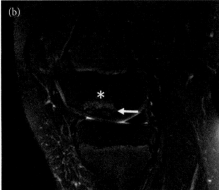 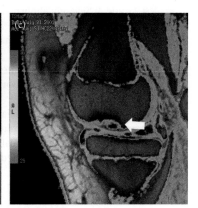

Figure 111.3. OCD incidentally detected in a 14 year-old boy. (*A*) Sagittal PDW and (*B*) PDW FS MR images demonstrate an OCD lesion of the medial femoral condyle with a low signal line (*thin arrow*) separating an osseous fragment from the subjacent femoral condyle with mild BME (*asterisk*) in (*B*). (*C*) A sagittal T2 map MR image demonstrates cartilage signal extending around the base of the osteochondral defect (thick arrow) with absence of bony bridging. Images courtesy of Dr. Jie Nguyen.

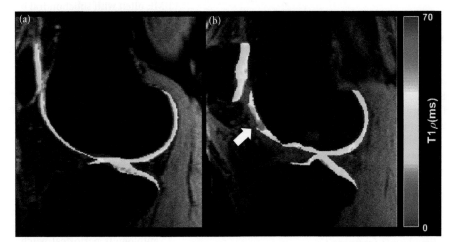

Figure 111.4. T1ρ imaging. Sagittal T1ρ map MR images in (*A*) healthy volunteer and (*B*) patient with patellofemoral compartment cartilage repair (microfracture). In (*B*), the T1ρ values are elevated in the anterior lateral femoral cartilage (*thick arrow*) with associated increased red signal. Images courtesy of Drs. Ravinder Regatte, Azadeh Sharafitafreshimoghaddam, and Gregory Chang.

Imaging Findings of Different Traumatic/Pathologic Conditions

Osteochondral Injury

- Cartilage injury is caused by a wide variety of mechanisms including acute trauma, chronic microtrauma, inflammatory arthritis, septic arthritis, and hemophilia
- Cartilage injuries can present as
  - Early edema with cartilage swelling and increased signal on PDW
  - Blistering
  - Fissuring, including extensive fissuring with a *crab meat* appearance
  - Delaminating flaps
  - Partial or complete cartilage defects or gaps
- Cartilage is routinely graded using the Modified Outerbridge/International Cartilage Repair Society system:
  - Grade 0: Normal
  - Grade 1: Nearly normal with superficial defects, difficult to detect
  - Grade 2: Defects less than 50% overall thickness (Figure 111.2*A*)
  - Grade 3: Severely abnormal with defects greater than 50% thickness (Figure 111.2*B,C*)
  - Grade 4: Severely abnormal into subchondral bone (Figure 111.2*D*)
- Defects can be focal or diffuse, with sharp, shouldered margins when acute or more rounded and tapering when chronic.
- Grade 4 defects can be associated with a displaced fragment with an attached T1 high signal (trabecular) and T1 and PD low signal (cortical) bone fragment.
  - Donor site can be detected by an absent low signal subchondral bone plate.

Osteochondritis Dissecans

- Osteochondritis dissecans (OCD) is a common source of pain and dysfunction in children and young adults.
- Repetitive microtrauma is thought to be the primary mechanism with other possible causes including acute trauma, ischemia, ossification abnormalities, and genetic factors.
- OCD affects the knee in approximately 75% of cases, however, it is also common in the talus and the capitellum.
- OCD of the knee is classically divided into the juvenile type with open physes (Figure 111.3) and the adult type with closed physes.
  - Adult OCD more commonly represents an incompletely healed previously asymptomatic juvenile lesion.
  - Juvenile OCD has better prognosis than adult OCD with higher rates of healing after conservative therapy.
- Lesion stability is a critical feature with 4 findings on fluid-sensitive sequences (PDW and T2W) suggesting instability:
  1. High signal line deep to fragment
  2. High signal line extending through the cartilage
  3. Fluid-filled defect
  4. Larger than 5 mm cyst deep to lesion
- Presence of all 4 findings are highly sensitive for instability in juvenile and adult OCD.
- Adult OCD: each of 4 findings highly specific
- Juvenile OCD: both high signal extending through the cartilage and fluid-filled defect highly specific

Osteoarthritis

- Acute (posttraumatic) and chronic OA are defined by chronic and progressive cartilage loss in addition to other findings including subchondral bone remodeling and BME.
- See Chapter 44, "Osteoarthritis of the Upper and Lower Extremity Joints."

Treatment and Complications

- Treatment of cartilage injury has been primarily described and used for the knee joint.
- Microfracture chondroplasty for small osteochondral defects, commonly of less than 1 cm^2 in patients younger than 40 years
  - Performed arthroscopically using an awl to create 4-mm deep holes in subchondral plate
  - Results in formation of less resilient fibrocartilage containing type I collagen rather than the original, type II collagen
  - Heterogeneous fibrocartilage signal on PDW and 3D SPGR
  - Increased signal on T2 map
- Osteochondral autografts/allografts used for larger defects
  - Autografts for osteochondral defects less than 2.5 cm^2 in patients younger than 50 years but can be performed for larger lesions
    - Harvested from nonweight-bearing articular surfaces
  - Cadaveric allografts sometimes used, especially for defects larger than 4 cm^2
  - Early MRI signal: hyperintense fluid signal fibrocartilage with subchondral BME
  - Late MRI signal: decrease in cartilage fluid signal and BME often with subchondral bone overgrowth
  - It is important to assess the following graft characteristics on follow-up MRI:
    - Presence and size of residual, unfilled defect
    - Morphology of graft including radius of curvature relative to adjacent cartilage and integration with peripheral cartilage and underlying bone
    - Evidence for cartilage delamination
    - Graft displacement
- Autologous chondrocyte implantation (ACI) used for large, full-thickness defects greater than 2 cm^2 in 15- to 60-year-old patients
  - Two-step procedure
    - Initial arthroscopic cartilage harvest usually from intercondylar notch with culture of chondrocytes
    - Second arthroscopy to debride defect, place either autologous periosteal patch or synthetic collagen membrane and inject cultured chondrocytes under the patch

- Early MRI appearance
  - Hyperintense fluid signal cartilage and cover
  - Subchondral BME
  - Cover hypertrophy
- Late appearance
  - Decreased cartilage fluid signal
  - Decreased BME
  - Important to evaluate graft characteristics as described for osteochondral grafts

Key Points

- MRI allows the direct imaging of the structure and composition of cartilage in situ.
- 2D FSE PDW and 3D SPGR sequences are routinely used for multiplanar cartilage imaging.
- The precise description of cartilage defects including the size and grade is important for treatment planning.
- Posttreatment imaging is acquired to evaluate fibrocartilage or graft integrity with signal characteristics that evolve over time.
- Compositional imaging is primarily investigational, but is a promising means to assess the response to current and future therapies.

Recommended Reading

Crema MD, Roemer FW, Marra MD, et al. Articular cartilage in the knee: current MR imaging techniques and applications in clinical practice and research. *Radiographics.* 2011;31:37–61.

Guermazi A, Roemer FW, Alizai H, et al. State of the art: MR imaging after knee cartilage repair surgery. *Radiology.* 2015;277:23–43.

References

1. Alizai H, Chang G, Regatte RR. MRI of the musculoskeletal system: advanced applications using high and ultrahigh field MRI. *Semin Musculoskelet Radiol.* 2015;19:363–74.
2. Apprich S, Welsch GH, Mamisch TC, et al. Detection of degenerative cartilage disease: comparison of high-resolution morphological MR and quantitative T2 mapping at 3.0 tesla. *Osteoarthritis Cartilage.* 2010;18:1211–17.
3. Choi YS, Potter HG, Chun TJ. MR imaging of cartilage repair in the knee and ankle. *Radiographics.* 2008;28:1043–59.
4. Choi YS, Potter HG, Chun TJ. MR imaging of cartilage repair in the knee and ankle. *Radiographics.* 2008;28:1043–59.
5. Crema MD, Roemer FW, Marra MD, et al. Articular cartilage in the knee: current MR imaging techniques and applications in clinical practice and research. *Radiographics.* 2011;31:37–61.
6. De Smet AA, Ilahi OA, Graf BK. Untreated osteochondritis dissecans of the femoral condyles: prediction of patient outcome using radiographic and MR findings. *Skeletal Radiol.* 1997;26:463–67.
7. Goodwin DW, Wadghiri YZ, Zhu H, Vinton CJ, Smith ED, Dunn JF. Macroscopic structure of articular cartilage of the tibial plateau: influence of a characteristic matrix architecture on MRI appearance. *AJR Am J Roentgenol.* 2004;182:311–18.
8. Guermazi A, Roemer FW, Alizai H, et al. State of the art: MR imaging after knee cartilage repair surgery. *Radiology.* 2015;277:23–43.
9. Hughes RJ, Houlihan-Burne DG. Clinical and MRI considerations in sports-related knee joint cartilage injury and cartilage repair. *Semin Musculoskelet Radiol.* 2011;15:69–88.
10. Jazrawi LM, Alaia MJ, Chang G, Fitzgerald EF, Recht MP. Advances in magnetic resonance imaging of articular cartilage. *J Am Acad Orthop Surg.* 2011;19:420–29.
11. Kijowski R, Blankenbaker DG, Shinki K, Fine JP, Graf BK, De Smet AA. Juvenile versus adult osteochondritis dissecans of the knee: appropriate MR imaging criteria for instability. *Radiology.* 2008;248:571–78.
12. Kladny B, Bail H, Swoboda B, Schiwy-Bochat H, Beyer WF, Weseloh G. Cartilage thickness measurement in magnetic resonance imaging. *Osteoarthritis Cartilage.* 1996;4:181–86.
13. Shepherd DE, Seedhom BB. Thickness of human articular cartilage in joints of the lower limb. *Ann Rheum Dis.* 1999;58:27–34.
14. Welsch GH, Mamisch TC, Hughes T, Domayer S, Marlovits S, Trattnig S. Advanced morphological and biochemical magnetic resonance imaging of cartilage repair procedures in the knee joint at 3 tesla. *Semin Musculoskelet Radiol.* 2008;12:196–211.
15. Yao K, Troupis JM. Diffusion-weighted imaging and the skeletal system: a literature review. *Clin Radiol.* 2016;71:1071–82.

Section Eight

Congenital and Developmental Diseases

Edited by Mihra S. Taljanovic and Tyson S. Chadaz

CHAPTER 112

Developmental Hip Dysplasia

Dorothy L. Gilbertson-Dahdal

Introduction

DDH includes a spectrum of abnormalities ranging from a stable hip with a mildly dysplastic acetabulum to complete hip dislocation formerly known as congenital hip dislocation. It is relatively common with an incidence in the United States of approximately 1.5 of 1,000 live births in whites. It occurs bilaterally in approximately 25% of these infants. It is important to differentiate true DDH from physiologic immaturity, caused by the circulating maternal hormone, relaxin, which causes mild instability in the first few weeks of life and is normal. Therefore, screening US for presence of DDH should not be performed before 4 weeks of age.

Screening US is performed on infants with predisposing risk factors such as family history of DDH, breech presentation, or hip click on physical examination. It is 4-8 times more common in female infants and 3 times more common in the left hip than the right. The occurrence in the left hip is because of the normal left occiput anterior position in utero with the infant's left hip against the mother's spine, limiting abduction.

The pathophysiology is multifactorial including mechanical, genetic, and hormonal factors. Mechanical factors are encountered in cases of oligohydramnios and breech presentation in which the knee is in extension. The growth of the femoral head and acetabulum are interdependent. The lack of a femoral head in the acetabular fossa during growth causes the acetabulum to assume a flattened shape, whereas femoral head presence results in a normal concave acetabulum. Outcome is quite variable with many cases resolving spontaneously without treatment whereas others stabilize with acetabular dysplasia. Some will progress to further subluxation or even dislocation.

Pathophysiology and Clinical Findings

- Approximately 60-80% of abnormalities identified by physical examination and more than 90% identified by US resolve spontaneously.
- Untreated subluxated and dislocated hips can lead to leg length discrepancy, early degenerative joint disease (DJD), and OA as early as adolescence.
- Clinical examination recommended by the American Academy of Pediatrics (well-baby visit at 1-2 weeks and at 2, 4, 6, 9, and 12 months of age) includes evaluation for DDH.
- Physical examination findings suggestive of DDH
  - Asymmetric skin folds in the proximal thigh
  - Shortening of the thigh on the dislocated side

- Physical examination confirmatory tests: Barlow and Ortolani
  - Barlow test—the unstable hip can be passively dislocated by hip adduction and placing mild pressure on the knee while directing the force posteriorly (Figure 112.1A).
  - Ortolani test—performed following the Barlow test to determine if the hip is dislocated; reduction is performed by hip abduction and pushing the thigh anteriorly (positive if a palpable, audible clunk is heard from the hip being reduced) (Figure 112.1B).

Imaging Strategy

- US examination (Figure 112.2)
  - Performed with 7.5-15 MHz linear-array transducer; hip in 90 degrees of flexion and in neutral (hips slightly flexed) position in coronal and transverse planes
  - Imaging study of choice in an infant 6 months or younger; in older infants, ossification of the femoral head/epiphysis precludes US examination (radiography is performed)
  - Dynamic evaluation (Harcke); imaging during stress maneuvers used for physical examination; flexed hip is moved between abduction and adduction to assess for stability; stress applied during adduction is equivalent to the Barlow test; the dislocated femoral head can relocate while in abduction (US equivalent of Ortolani test)
  - Per Graf's method, 2 angles are measured. The *baseline* is drawn along the ilium (iliac line) (Figure 112.3):
    - The *alpha* (α) angle is formed by the bony acetabular roof line and the iliac line ($\alpha > 60$ degrees in a mature infant hip is considered normal).
    - The *beta* (β) angle is formed by the iliac line and the fibrocartilaginous roof line (inclination line) through the main echo of the acetabular labrum intersecting the other 2 lines ($\beta < 55$ degrees in a mature infant hip is considered normal).
    - Greater than 50% of the femoral head should be below the baseline or iliac line when normal.

Imaging Findings

- US classification system for DDH combining both alpha (α) and beta (β) angles (Graf)

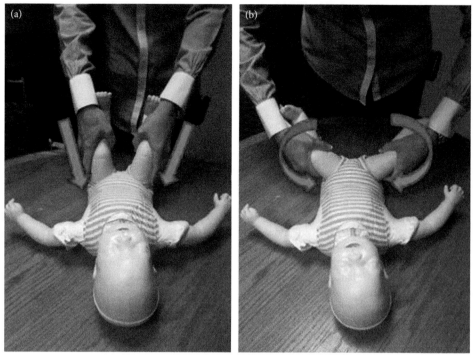

Figure 112.1. Barlow and Ortolani tests. (*A*) Photograph demonstrating Barlow test on a doll. The unstable hip can be passively dislocated by hip adduction and placing mild pressure on the knee while directing the force posteriorly. (*B*) Photograph demonstrating Ortolani test on a doll. This is performed following the Barlow test to determine if the hip is dislocated; reduction is performed by hip abduction and pushing the thigh anteriorly (positive if a palpable, audible clunk is heard from the hip being reduced).

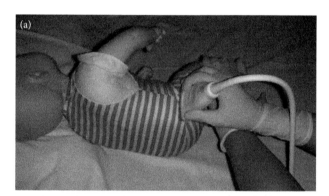

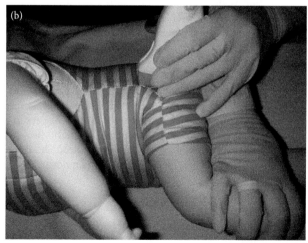

Figure 112.2. Positioning of the US probe for imaging the neonatal hip (*A*) in transverse and (*B*) longitudinal planes.

- Type I: α angle > 60 degrees (normal); superior acetabular rim— sharp; > 50% femoral head acetabular bony coverage (Figure 112.4)
  - Type Ia: β angle less than 55 degrees
  - Type Ib: β angle greater than 55 degrees

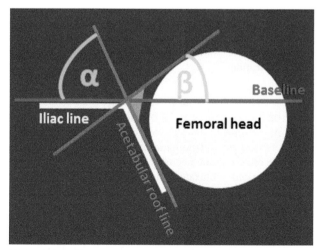

Figure 112.3. Measurements of α and β angles. Drawing demonstrates measurements of normal α angle with lines drawn along the acetabular roof (*orange*) and lateral iliac line (*red*) and normal β angle with lines drawn at the lateral iliac line and acetabular labral line (*tan*). An α angle >60 degrees and β angle <55 degrees in a mature infant hip should be considered normal (Graf R. *Arch Orthop Trauma Surg.* 1980;97(2):117-33.)

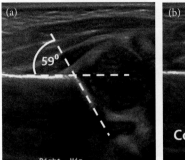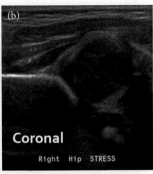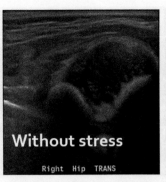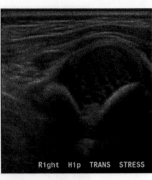

Figure 112.4. US of the normal neonatal hip. (*A*) Coronal US image of a normal neonatal hip in a 2-month-old boy with hip click; family history of hip dislocation. Right hip α angle = 59 degrees, >50% femoral head coverage by the bony acetabulum. (*B*) Coronal and transverse images of the same hip with applied stress show no subluxation or dislocation.

- Type II: superior acetabular rim—round; 40-50% femoral head acetabular bony coverage
  - Type IIa (<3 months old): α angle 50-59 degrees
  - Type IIb (>3 months old): α angle 50-59 degrees
  - Type IIc (critical zone dysplasia): α angle 43-49 degrees
  - For all β angle less than 77 degrees
- Type D (*about to decenter*)
  - α angle 43-49 degrees
  - β angle greater than 77 degrees
- Type III: α angle less than 43 degrees (severe dysplasia/subluxation); superior acetabular rim—round; less than 40% femoral head acetabular bony coverage
  - Types IIIa and IIIb distinguished on the grounds of structural alteration of the cartilaginous roof
- Type IV: superior acetabular rim—round; 0% femoral head acetabular bony coverage
  - α angle less than 43 degrees
  - Dislocated hip with labrum interposed between the femoral head and acetabulum (Figure 112.5)
- Evaluation for DDH should be performed at age 5-6 weeks.

- A decreased α angle with less than 50% coverage of the hips is a normal finding in a 2-week-old infant because of circulating maternal hormones (Figure 112.6).
- Radiographs performed in children older than 6 months (Figure 112.7)
  - *Hilgenreiner line*: Drawn horizontally through the inferior aspect of both triradiate cartilages; mainly a reference line
  - *Perkin line*: Drawn perpendicular to the Hilgenreiner line, intersecting the lateral most aspect of the acetabular roof. The femoral epiphysis should be in the inferomedial quadrant.
  - *Acetabular angle*: Formed by intersection between the line drawn parallel to the acetabular roof and Hilgenreiner line, forming an acute angle. Normal angle measures less than 30 degrees at 4 months and decreases until it reaches 20 degrees or less, which applies for pediatric patients.
  - *Shenton line*: Drawn along the inferior border of the superior pubic ramus and continues laterally along the inferomedial aspect of the proximal femur as a smooth arc. With DDH, the line is discontinuous.

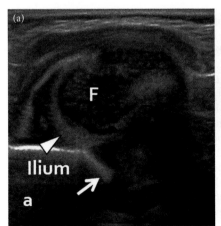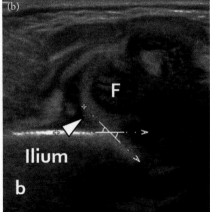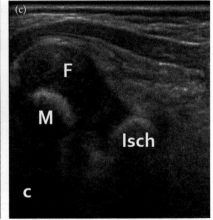

Figure 112.5. Coronal US images of an abnormal neonatal hip in a 2-month-old boy (same patient as in Figure 112.4) with hip click and family history of hip dislocation. (*A, B*) Left hip: α angle = 43 degrees, the bony acetabulum is poorly formed (*arrow*), the labrum and cartilaginous rim are displaced (*arrowheads*) by the dislocated left femoral head (F). (*C*) Transverse image of the left hip in the same patient shows lateral dislocation of the femoral head (F). Isch = ischium; M = femoral metaphysis.

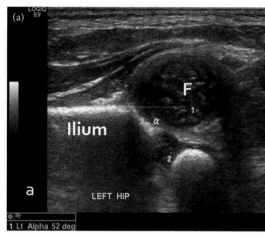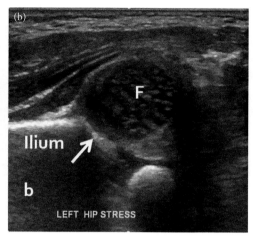

Figure 112.6. Coronal US images of a neonatal hip in a 2-week-old female infant with breech position. (*A*) Decreased α angles with less than 50% coverage of both hips is a normal finding in a 2-week-old infant because of circulating maternal hormones. (*B*) There is no evidence of additional subluxation with the stress maneuver. Evaluation for DDH should be performed at age 5-6 weeks. F = femoral head; *arrow* = acetabulum.

- Role of MRI
  - MRI is generally used as a problem-solving modality. It is excellent to delineate soft tissue structures without ionizing radiation. It is often used in the postoperative patient, after spica cast placement to ensure that the femoral head is in the acetabular fossa.

Treatment Options

- Subluxation/dislocation treated with immobilization in a soft (Pavlik) harness with flexion-abduction and external rotation of the hips. For patients younger than age 6 months.
  - Follow up with serial US examinations in harness; no stress maneuvers should be performed apart from passive abduction and adduction of the hips.

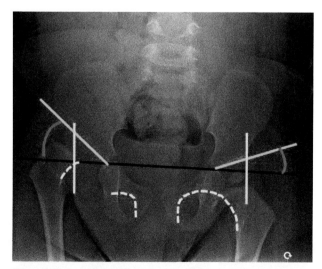

Figure 112.7. A 15-month-old child with neglected congenital right hip dislocation. AP pelvic radiograph with superimposed lines was performed for assessment of right hip dislocation. Acetabular angle (*red*) is normal on the left and abnormal on the right. Hilgenreiner line (*black*); Perkin line (*green*); Shenton line (*yellow*); acetabular roof (*blue*).

- The α angle and femoral head acetabular bony coverage should improve over time.
- Irreducible dislocations or delayed presentation after 6 months may require surgical treatment/reduction.

Key Points

- US is the imaging modality of choice for both diagnosis and follow-up of DDH in infants younger than 6 months old, as it enables direct visualization of the cartilaginous femoral head and acetabulum.
- Older patients will require radiographs.
- MRI for problem solving in postoperative patient

Recommended Reading

Starr V, Ha BY. Imaging update on developmental dysplasia of the hip with the role of MRI. *AJR Am J Roentgenol.* 2014;203(6):1324–35. doi:10.2214/AJR.13.12449. Review.

References

1. Bracken J, Ditchfield M. Ultrasonography in developmental dysplasia of the hip: what have we learned? *Pediatr Radiol.* 2012;42(12):1418–31. doi:10.1007/s00247-012-2429-8. Review.
2. Bell DJ, Gillard F, et al. Developmental dysplasia of the hip. Radiopaedia. https://radiopaedia.org/articles/developmental-dysplasia-of-the-hip. Accessed April 14, 2018.
3. Graf R. The diagnosis of congenital hip-joint dislocation by the ultrasonic Combound treatment. *Arch Orthop Trauma Surg.* 1980;97(2):117–33.
4. Kotlarsky P, Haber R, Bialik V, Eidelman M. Developmental dysplasia of the hip: what has changed in the last 20 years? *World J Orthop.* 2015;6(11):886–901. doi:10.5312/wjo.v6.i11.886. Review.
5. Starr V, Ha BY. Imaging update on developmental dysplasia of the hip with the role of MRI. *AJR Am J Roentgenol.* 2014;203(6):1324–35. doi:10.2214/AJR.13.12449. Review.

CHAPTER 113

Scoliosis

Dorothy L. Gilbertson-Dahdal

Introduction

Scoliosis consists of the presence of one or more lateral and rotatory curves of the spine. The curve should be at least 10 degrees and is described in direction by the convexity of the curve. Scoliosis can be acquired (during adolescent growth spurt), which is more common, or it can be congenital and associated with numerous other anomalies including vertebral anomalies. Degenerative scoliosis also occurs secondary to degenerative disc or facet disease in elderly adults.

- Mild scoliosis is defined as a curve ranging from 10 to 25 degrees.
- Moderate scoliosis is defined as a curve ranging from 26 to 40 degrees.
- Severe scoliosis is defined as a curve greater than 40 degrees.

Pathophysiology and Clinical Findings

- Lateral curvature of the spine with a Cobb angle of 10 degrees or greater (Figure 113.1)
  - A rotational component may also be present.
- Most often idiopathic: Primary (80%), occurs at periods of rapid growth:
  - Healthy individuals age 10-18 years
  - Affects 2-4% of population, 10 times more common in female patients
- Other causes: secondary
  - Congenital: second most common (10%), hemivertebrae, fused vertebrae, wedge vertebrae, tethered cord, Chiari malformation
  - Developmental: achondroplasia, neurofibromatosis, osteogenesis imperfecta
  - Neuromuscular: cerebral palsy, muscular dystrophy
  - Tumor associated: osteoid osteoma, osteoblastoma, neurofibroma, astrocytoma
  - Adult degenerative: caused by disc degeneration, facet joint arthritis, collapse and wedging of the vertebral bodies
- Two stages: curve initiation and progression
  - Curves greater than 20 degrees are much more likely to progress and should be monitored more closely.

Imaging Strategy

Whether the examination is performed PA or AP, breast and gonadal shielding should be used.

- Radiography (should be primary study)
  - Standardized technique reduces error, obtained in standing position
  - PA/AP upright radiograph of the thoracic and lumbar spine includes the cervical spine superiorly and pelvis inferiorly
  - Two PA/AP digital radiographs are usually stitched together
- MRI indicated if underlying osseous or neurologic pathology is suspected or
  - Age younger than 10 years
  - Rapid progression
  - Pain
  - Unusual pattern of curvature such as thoracic levoscoliosis, especially in male patients
  - Short segment curve

Imaging Findings

- Identify the apex vertebrae that is farthest deviated from the center of the vertebral column.
- Identify the end vertebrae that demonstrate the maximum tilt toward the apex of the curve and are used to generate the Cobb angle.
- *Cobb angle*: does not take rotation into account, yet remains standard for diagnosis and treatment planning
  - Technique: A line is drawn at the superior endplate of the superior end vertebra and a line is drawn at the inferior endplate of the inferior end vertebra. Their intersection forms the Cobb angle. A Cobb angle less than 10 degrees is termed a *mild curvature* and is not clinically significant. To be qualified as mild scoliosis, the curvature needs to measure at least 10 degrees, such as in Figure 113.1.
  - Figure 113.2 is an example of typical appearance of idiopathic scoliosis.
  - The same end vertebrae should be used on follow-up imaging.
- *Sagittal balance*: the relationship of the head to the pelvis in sagittal plane, also called the *sagittal vertical axis*.
  - Technique: A line is drawn on the lateral standing radiograph from the center of C7 vertically down, the plumb line. A line is drawn from the posterior aspect of the superior endplate of the S1 vertebra, the sacral landmark, to the vertical line. When the plumb line is anterior to the S1 superior endplate, the measurement is positive (positive sagittal balance) and when posterior the line is negative (negative sagittal balance).

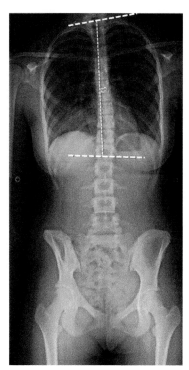

Figure 113.1. AP standing radiograph of the thoracolumbar spine for scoliosis measurements. Note minimal/mild levoconvex scoliosis of the thoracic spine measuring 10 degrees.

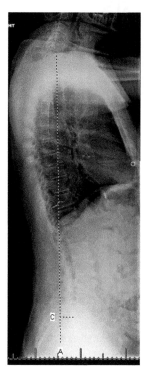

Figure 113.3. Lateral standing radiograph of the entire spine for sagittal balance assessment. Line C demonstrates 3 cm of negative sagittal balance. This is the distance between the vertical plumb line drawn from mid C7 (line A) and the posterior superior aspect of the S1 vertebral body. For normal reference, this distance can measure up to 2 cm.

For normal reference, this distance can measure up to 2 cm.
- In Figure 113.3: Line C demonstrates 3 cm of negative sagittal balance.

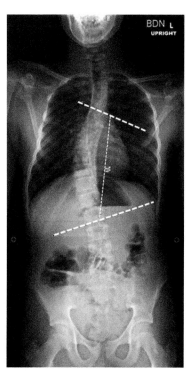

Figure 113.2. Scoliosis measurements on standing AP radiograph of the thoracolumbar spine. A line is drawn at the superior endplate of the superior end vertebra and a line is drawn at the inferior endplate of the inferior end vertebra. Their virtual intersection of these lines forms the Cobb angle.

Treatment Options
- Progression depends on the magnitude of scoliosis and skeletal maturity. Skeletally immature patients are more likely to progress with initial curves greater than 20 degrees.
- Patients with greater than 50 degrees of curvature more frequently have back pain.
- Treatment options include observation, bracing, or surgery:
  - Based on curve severity, likelihood of progression and patient perception
  - Observation if Cobb angle is less than 20 degrees in a skeletally immature patient with idiopathic scoliosis or in a skeletally mature patient with Cobb angle less than 30 degrees.
  - Bracing used for adolescent idiopathic scoliosis with Cobb angle 20-45 degrees. Bracing is not used for adult idiopathic scoliosis.
  - Surgery is used to prevent curve progression and stabilize the spine with solid bone fusion of involved segments. In children, the goal of curve correction is to restore seated balance, pain control, and ease wheelchair use as well as improve respiratory function. This

is most often seen in the setting of neuromuscular scoliosis.

Recommended Reading

Malfair D, Flemming AK, Dvorak MF, et al. Radiographic evaluation of scoliosis: review. *AJR Am J Roentgenol.* 2010;194(3 suppl): S8–22.

References

1. Malfair D, Flemming AK, Dvorak MF, et al. Radiographic evaluation of scoliosis: review. *AJR Am J Roentgenol.* 2010;194(3 suppl): S8–22.
2. Kim H, Kim HS, Moon ES, et al. Scoliosis imaging: what radiologists should know. *Radiographics* 2010;30(7):1823–42.

CHAPTER 114

Common Congenital Syndromes

Dorothy L. Gilbertson-Dahdal

Introduction

Achondroplasia

Achondroplasia is the most common cause of short stature/dwarfism. It is caused by a mutation in the FGFR3 gene. Individuals display short arms and legs with a large head and frontal bossing. Life expectancy and intelligence are near normal.

Mucopolysaccharidoses

Mucopolysaccharidoses are represented by Hurler, Hunter, and Morquio syndromes (see Chapter 84, "Mucopolysaccharidoses"). These are lysosomal storage disorders that occur when there is a lack of the enzyme required to break down glycosaminoglycans (GAGs).

Hurler syndrome (mucopolysaccharidosis type I) is autosomal recessive and caused by a mutation on 4p16.3, which results in a deficiency of the alpha-L-iduronidase enzyme. Patients appear normal at birth and develop clinical manifestations such as corneal clouding and cardiac valvular disease within the first 2 years of life. Life expectancy is approximately 10 years.

Morquio syndrome (mucopolysaccharidosis type IV) is caused by mutations in 2 genes, 16q24.3 and 3p21.33, causing types IVa and IVb, respectively. Patients are usually diagnosed in the first or second year of life with an enlarged skull, chest deformities, and dorsolumbar kyphosis. Intelligence may be normal and patients may live to adulthood.

Hunter syndrome (mucopolysaccharidosis type II) results in deficiency of the enzyme iduronate sulfatase. Patients display dysostosis multiplex, organomegaly, and short stature with a life expectancy of 15 years.

Osteogenesis Imperfecta

Osteogenesis imperfecta (OI) is caused by mutation in either the COL1A1 or COL1A2 gene resulting in abnormalities in type I cartilage. OI is characterized by bones that break easily, often from little or no apparent cause. It is most commonly inherited autosomal dominantly but can be autosomal recessive or spontaneous, with a wide range of clinical presentations from mild to severe, depending on the subtype of OI. The most severe form is usually diagnosed on prenatal US with fractures and other abnormalities of the femora, humeri, skull, or ribs. Less severe forms may go unnoticed and may present with

blue sclerae (type I) or yellow teeth called dentinogenesis imperfecta (type III).

Thanatophoric Dysplasia

Thanatophoric dysplasia is caused by a mutation in the FGFR3 gene. There are 2 types, with type I displaying micromelia with bowed femora. Type II is characterized by micromelia with straight femora and the characteristic cloverleaf skull deformity. Both types show short ribs, narrow thorax, and macrocephaly, and are lethal in the perinatal period.

General Imaging Strategy for Skeletal Dysplasias
- Many are detected on prenatal US.
- Family history, physical examination, and molecular and genetic testing are also used in diagnosis.
- Skeletal survey including skull AP and lateral, thoracolumbar spine AP and lateral and AP views of the chest, pelvis, upper limbs, and lower limbs

Achondroplasia

Pathophysiology and Clinical Findings
- Most common nonlethal skeletal dysplasia
- Rhizomelic (proximal limb) dwarfism
- Autosomal dominant inheritance but 80% occur sporadically, associated with increased paternal age
- Typical features seen at birth
  - Exaggerated lumbar lordosis; prone to severe spinal stenosis
  - Mid face sunken with depressed nasal bones
  - Frontal bossing

Imaging Findings
- Symmetric shortening of long bones, with proximal portions being more affected (rhizomelia) (Figure 114.1)
- Metacarpals and phalanges appear thick and tubular with widely separated second and third digits giving appearance of trident hand
- Metaphyseal splaying with normal epiphyses (Figure 114.2)
- Pelvic cavity is short and broad with squaring of iliac wings and rounding of corners on a frontal projection (ping-pong paddle–shaped iliac wings). The roofs of the acetabula are flat and horizontal (Figures 114.1 and 114.3).

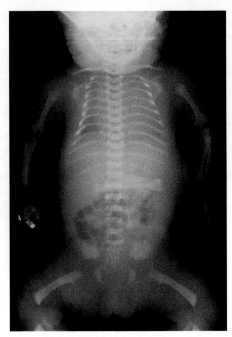

Figure 114.1. Achondroplasia. The pelvic cavity is short and broad with squaring of the iliac wings and rounding of the corners on frontal projection (ping-pong paddle–shaped iliac wings). The roofs of the acetabula are flat and horizontal.

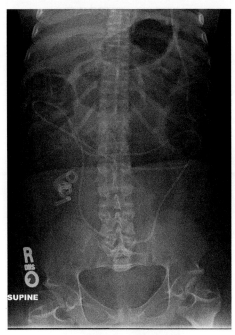

Figure 114.3. Achondroplasia. There is decreased intrapedicular distance of the inferior vertebrae compared to superior. Note bilateral hip dysplasia and iliac wing squaring.

- Progressive decrease in the interpedicular distance in the lumbar spine (Figure 114.3)
- Posterior scalloping of vertebral bodies; rounded anteriorly to give a bullet shape (Figure 114.4)
- Narrowed skull base with narrowing of foramen magnum

Treatment Options
- Ventriculoperitoneal shunt may be required for increased intracranial pressure.
- Aggressive management of middle-ear dysfunction

- Evaluation by orthopedics if bowing of the legs occurs
- Surgery to correct spinal stenosis in symptomatic adults
- Avoidance of activities that may injure the craniocervical junction, such as collision sports, trampoline, diving,

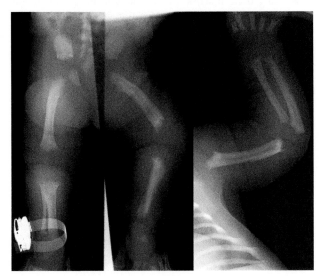

Figure 114.2. Achondroplasia. Note flaring and splaying of the metaphyses of the upper and lower extremities.

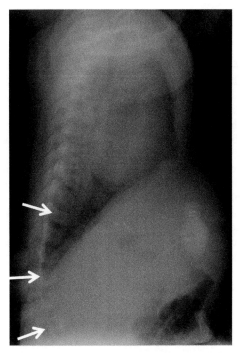

Figure 114.4. Achondroplasia. Note posterior scalloping of the vertebral bodies, which are rounded anteriorly to give a bullet shape (*arrows*).

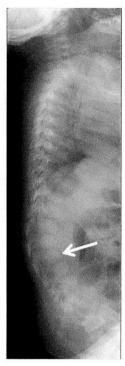

Figure 114.5. Hurler syndrome. There is anterior beaking of the lumbar vertebral bodies (*arrow*).

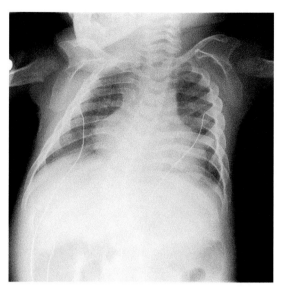

Figure 114.6. Hurler syndrome: Note canoe paddle ribs, which are thin posteriorly and broad anteriorly.

vaulting in gymnastics, and hanging upside down from the knees or feet on playground equipment
- Pregnant women with achondroplasia must undergo cesarean section delivery because of small pelvic size.
- Genetic counseling

Mucopolysaccharidoses (Lysosomal Storage Disorders)

Hurler and Morquio Syndromes
Pathophysiology and Clinical Findings
- Absence of lysosomal enzymes required for degradation of GAG or mucopolysaccharides
- Deposition of GAG in various tissues causing coarse facies, mental retardation, and hepatosplenomegaly
- Subsets of mucopolysaccharidoses include Hurler and Morquio syndromes.
- Hurler and Morquio syndromes are autosomal recessive disorders.

Imaging Findings of Lysosomal Storage Disorders
- Epiphyseal abnormalities
- Proximal pointed metacarpals
- Beaking of lumbar vertebral bodies (Figure 114.5)

Imaging Findings of Hurler Syndrome
- Macrocephalic skull with frontal bossing and J-shaped sella

- Canoe paddle ribs, which are thin posteriorly and broad anteriorly (Figure 114.6)
- Lateral ends of clavicles are hypoplastic with small scapulae.
- Tubular bones of the hands are typically short and wide. Metacarpals appear broad distally and tapered proximally (Figure 114.7).

Imaging Findings of Morquio Syndrome
- Enlarged skull
- Dorsolumbar kyphosis
- Platyspondyly with central beaking

Treatment Options for Mucopolysaccharidoses
- Therapy is mainly focused on correction of enzyme activity
- Using bone marrow transplantation, peripheral blood hematopoietic cell transplantation, and umbilical cord blood transplantation
- Alternatively, enzyme-replacement therapy

Osteogenesis Imperfecta

Pathophysiology and Clinical Findings
- Autosomal dominantly or recessively inherited genetic disorder
- Characterized by decreased bone density and increased bone fragility
- Severity varies widely from perinatal lethality (type II) to milder forms with minimal fractures
- Extraskeletal manifestations include blue sclerae, dentinogenesis imperfecta, and deafness.
- Eight subtypes have been described.

Imaging Findings of OI
- Diffuse osteopenia, pencil-thin cortices, and multiple fractures (Figure 114.8)

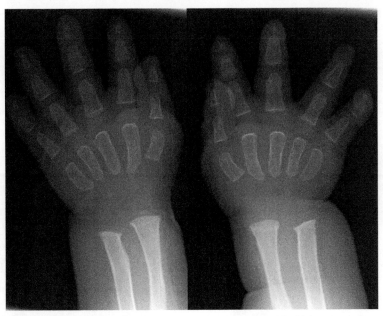

Figure 114.7. Hurler syndrome: Tubular bones of the hands are typically short and wide. Metacarpals appear broad distally and tapered proximally.

- Fractures heal with exuberant callus formation giving rise to *pseudotumor* formation.
- Vertebrae have a biconcave appearance with areas of collapse (Figure 114.9).
- Skull shows multiple wormian bones and lucent calvarium (Figure 114.10).
- Pelvis with deformities such as protrusio acetabuli and *shepherd crook* femora (Figure 114.11)

Treatment Options

Treatment varies based on the disease severity and the age of the patient.

- Nonsurgical
  - Decrease fracture risk and increase bone density with medication such as IV and oral bisphosphonates and vitamin D and calcium supplements.

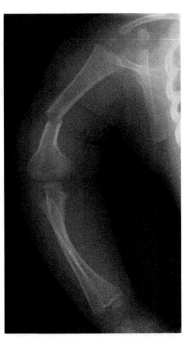

Figure 114.8. Osteogenesis imperfecta. There are diffuse osteopenia, thin cortices, and associated fractures. Note, transverse fracture of the humeral shaft.

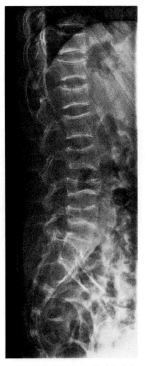

Figure 114.9. Osteogenesis imperfecta. Vertebrae have a biconcave appearance with central areas of collapse.

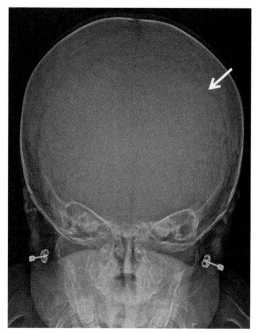

Figure 114.10. Osteogenesis imperfecta. The skull shows multiple wormian bones along the parietal sutures (*arrow*) and a lucent calvarium with poor visualization of the inner table.

- ■ Physical therapy to build muscle strength
- ■ Casting/splinting fractures
- ■ Dental care because of fragile teeth
- ■ Hearing screening
  - ■ Surgical: Intramedullary rod placement
  - ■ Pharmacological: Increase vitamin D, calcium, bisphosphonates and sometimes growth hormone.

Thanatophoric Dysplasia

Pathophysiology and Clinical Findings:
- ■ Thanatophoric dysplasia is a short-limb dwarfism syndrome that is usually lethal in the perinatal period.

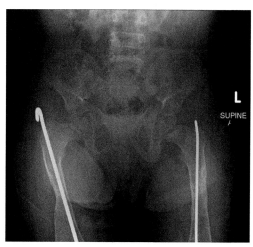

Figure 114.11. Osteogenesis imperfecta. The pelvis demonstrates deformities such as protrusio acetabuli and *shepherd crook* femurs. Note intramedullary nail fixation of both femora.

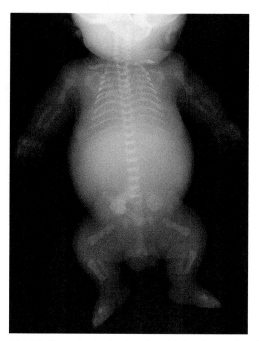

Figure 114.12. Thanatophoric dwarfism: Note micromelia with straight femurs, short ribs, and a narrow thorax.

- ■ Two subtypes
  - ■ Type I demonstrates micromelia with bowed femora.
  - ■ Type II demonstrates micromelia with straight femora and moderate to severe cloverleaf skull deformity.
- ■ Both subtypes demonstrate short ribs, narrow thorax, macrocephaly, distinctive facial features, brachydactyly, and hypotonia.
- ■ Most infants die of respiratory insufficiency shortly after birth.

Imaging Findings
- ■ Rhizomelic (proximal limb) shortening of long bones (Figure 114.12)
- ■ Irregular long bone metaphyses
- ■ Small foramen magnum with brain stem compression
- ■ Platyspondyly (Figure 114.12)
- ■ Bowed femora
- ■ Cloverleaf skull (Figure 114.13)

Treatment Options
- ■ Management focuses on the parents' wishes for comfort care for the newborn. Newborns require aggressive respiratory support (with tracheostomy and ventilation) to survive and generally have a very poor long-term prognosis.
- ■ Genetic counseling: Most patients have de novo mutations. Risk of recurrence for parents who have had 1 affected child is not significantly increased above the general population.

Recommended Reading
Panda A, Gamanagatti S, Jana M, Gupta AK. Skeletal dysplasias: a radiographic approach and review of common non-lethal skeletal dysplasias. *World J Radiol.* 2014;6(10):808–25. doi:10.4329/wjr.v6.i10.808.

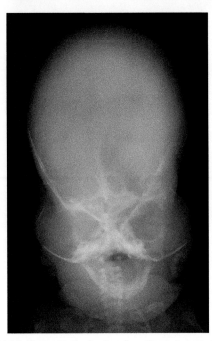

Figure 114.13. Thanatophoric dwarfism. There is a severe cloverleaf skull deformity.

References

1. Karczeski B, Cutting GR. Thanatophoric dysplasia. In: Pagon RA, Adam MP, Ardinger HH, et al., ed. *GeneReviews*. Seattle: University of Washington; 2004. www.ncbi.nlm.nih.gov/books/NBK1366/. Updated September 12, 2013.

2. Monti E, Mottes M, Fraschini P, et al. Current and emerging treatments for the management of osteogenesis imperfecta. *Ther Clin Risk Manag*. 2010;6:367–81.

3. Panda A, Gamanagatti S, Jana M, Gupta AK. Skeletal dysplasias: a radiographic approach and review of common non-lethal skeletal dysplasias. *World J Radiol*. 2014;6(10):808–25. doi:10.4329/wjr.v6.i10.808.

4. Palmucci S, Attinà G, Lanza ML, et al. Imaging findings of mucopolysaccharidoses: a pictorial review. *Insights Imaging*. 2013;4(4):443–59. doi:10.1007/s13244-013-0246-8.

5. Pauli RM. Achondroplasia. In: Pagon RA, Adam MP, Ardinger HH, et al., ed. *GeneReviews*. Seattle: University of Washington; 1998. www.ncbi.nlm.nih.gov/books/NBK1152/. Updated February 16, 2012.

6. Rasalkar DD, Chu WCW, Hui J, Chu C-M, Paunipagar BK, Li C-K. Pictorial review of mucopolysaccharidosis with emphasis on MRI features of brain and spine. *Br J Radiol*. 2011;84(1001):469–77. doi:10.1259/bjr/59197814.

7. Renaud A, Aucourt J, Weill J, et al. Radiographic features of osteogenesis imperfecta. *Insights Imaging*. 2013;4(4):417–29. doi:10.1007/s13244-013-0258-4.

Miscellaneous

Edited by Mihra S. Taljanovic and Tyson S. Chadaz

CHAPTER 115

Osteonecroses and Osteochondroses

Winnie A. Mar

Pathophysiology and Clinical Findings

Osteonecroses

ON occurs from an ischemic insult to bone with subsequent death of the hematopoietic, osteoblastic, osteoclastic, and fat cells. By convention, ON describes necrosis of the subchondral epiphyseal bone, and bone infarct describes necrosis in the metaphysis or diaphysis. Patients may present with insidious or abrupt pain, or they may be asymptomatic. The primary cause of ON is trauma, and the second most common cause is corticosteroid therapy. The most common and important clinical site of ON is the femoral head, with bilateral involvement in 50% of cases (Figures 115.1 and 115.2). Men are affected 4 times as often as women. Other common locations of ON are the humeral head and the femoral condyles, and after fracture, the proximal pole of the scaphoid bone and talar dome. Additional common etiologies of ON include alcoholism, sickle cell disease and idiopathic, with less common etiologies including lupus, pancreatitis, radiation, and Gaucher and caisson diseases (decompression syndrome). Complications include secondary OA, septic arthritis, pathologic fracture, and sarcomatous transformation.

The stages of ON are ischemia, revascularization, repair, deformity, and osteoarthrosis. In the revascularization phase, reparative granulation tissue attempts to heal the necrotic bone, which is intrinsically weaker, and thus susceptible to subchondral fracture.

The pathophysiology depends on the etiology. In trauma, the blood supply is directly disrupted. Increased intraosseous pressure may result in vessel compression, such as with steroids where there is fat cell hypertrophy or Gaucher disease caused by crowding of marrow by Gaucher cells. ON from alcoholism is thought to be a result of fat embolism. In the case of hemoglobinopathies, bone ischemia results from sludging of blood in small blood vessels or from thromboembolism and collagen vascular diseases by vasospasm. Embolism from nitrogen in the case of caisson disease may occur because of rapid depressurization in divers. Radiation is directly toxic to the vasculature.

Bone infarcts tend to be multiple and are usually asymptomatic. Malignant transformation of bone infarcts, although rare, is mostly by MFH (pleomorphic undifferentiated high grade sarcoma; see Chapter 57, "Malignant Fibrous Lesions of the Bone").

Kienböck disease is ON of the lunate and is associated with trauma and ulnar negative variance. It predominantly affects men ages 20–40. Patients present with dorsal wrist pain and decreased grip strength (see Chapter 106, "Internal Derangements of the Wrist and Hand").

Osteochondroses

Osteochondroses comprise a variety of diseases involving epiphyses or apophyses in children with epiphyseal or apophyseal fragmentation and increased sclerosis. Some may be caused by ischemia, and others are thought to be caused by repetitive microtrauma. Most of these are associated with an eponym.

Legg-Calvé-Perthes disease is idiopathic ON of the femoral head presenting in children usually between ages 4 and 8 with a much greater incidence in boys (Figure 115.3). Patients usually present with knee or hip pain and a limp. In 10% of cases, there is bilateral involvement. The majority heal spontaneously. The most common complication is premature degenerative joint disease.

Osteochondritis dissecans (OCD) usually affects adolescents who are active in sports, likely because of repetitive micro-trauma and is the result of a subchondral fracture. Common locations are the knee, talar dome, and capitellum. In the knee, the most common location is the lateral aspect of the medial femoral condyle (Figure 115.4) (see Chapter 109, "Internal Derangements of the Ankle and Foot").

Osteochondrosis of the capitellum (Panner disease) is also likely caused by repetitive trauma. In contrast to OCD, it occurs in younger patients in their first decade. Patients present with lateral elbow pain and inability to fully extend the elbow (see Chapter 105, "Internal Derangements of the Elbow").

Blount disease, also known as *tibia vara*, has a male predominance and affects the posteromedial portion of the proximal tibial physis (Figure 115.5). The infantile form affects boys and girls equally, ages 1-3, and is most often bilateral and symmetric, which should not be confused with physiologic bowing in which a medial tibial physeal beak is seen with thickening of the medial tibial and medial femoral cortex. The later or adolescent form affects children ages 7-14. It more commonly affects overweight boys of African ancestry. It is thought to be caused by abnormal enchondral ossification from abnormal pressure on the proximal tibial physis.

Osgood-Schlatter disease (Figure 115.6) and Sinding-Larsen-Johansson syndrome or disease are osteochondroses of the tibial tuberosity and the distal patellar pole, respectively, affecting children ages 8-15. They are thought to be caused by repetitive microtrauma and are often seen in children who play basketball or do other activities involving jumping. Sinding-Larsen-Johansson syndrome is also called *jumper's knee*.

Freiberg infraction represents subchondral collapse of the second metatarsal head classically seen in teenage girls (Figure 115.7). It may be caused by abnormal pressure from wearing high heels. This may less commonly affect other lesser metatarsal heads.

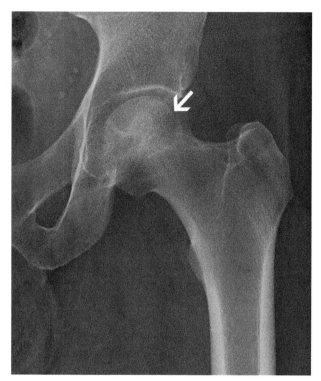

Figure 115.1. Femoral head ON. Frontal radiograph of the hip shows a linear sclerotic line in the femoral head (*arrow*) consistent with ON.

Köhler disease affects toddlers with fragmentation of the tarsal navicular and is sometimes a normal variant. Patients favor weight-bearing on the lateral aspect of the foot.

Scheuermann disease is an osteochondrosis of the vertebral body ring apophyses resulting in a kyphosis, disc space narrowing, and Schmorl nodes. This typically presents between ages 8 and 12; girls and boys are equally affected. Patients often present with kyphosis rather than pain. The etiology is unknown, but repetitive axial loading of the spine has been postulated, and there is a possible autosomal dominant association.

Imaging Strategy

Initial evaluation for ON and osteochondrosis is typically with radiographs. MRI is the study of choice when radiographic findings are not diagnostic as MRI is more sensitive for detecting early ON. Contrast is not typically needed in the routine assessment of ON, but dynamic contrast enhancement has been shown experimentally to be able to detect early ON.

Bone scintigraphy may be used in lieu of MRI, and shows decreased uptake in early ON and Legg-Calvé-Perthes disease and increased activity in the later revascularization and reparative phases. MRI is not necessary in the late stages of ON.

Dystrophic calcification of the fatty marrow within a bone infarct can simulate a cartilage matrix tumor. The serpiginous sclerotic line at the periphery can help to confirm a bone infarct.

Radiographs are helpful in identifying OCD, however, MRI should be performed to evaluate stability of the lesion. The other osteochondroses are usually well depicted radiographically.

Imaging Findings

Osteonecrosis

- Radiographs may be normal in early stages. Later stages are characterized by sclerosis (Figure 115.1), subchondral lucency/fracture, collapse, and secondary OA. Peripheral sclerotic line corresponds to reactive bone remodeling at the junction of viable and necrotic bone. Subchondral linear crescent sign of the femoral head corresponds to a subchondral fracture, which is frequently best seen on frog leg lateral radiograph of the hip.
- The Ficat radiographic staging system for ON is the most commonly used (Table 115.1):
  - Stage 0—normal
  - Stage I—normal with pain
  - Stage II—trabecular changes without collapse (look for geographic areas of medullary subchondral sclerosis)
  - Stage III—subchondral fracture/collapse
  - Stage IV—associated OA
- CT shows sclerotic serpiginous geographic lesion.
- With MRI, early ON is uncommonly seen, but characterized by BME. Later stages of ON are characterized by linear serpiginous geographic lesion *peripheral double line sign*, representing the reactive interface with the dark line corresponding to necrotic bone

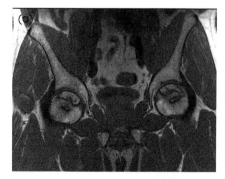
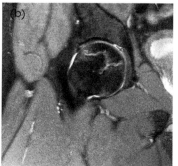

Figure 115.2. Bilateral femoral head ON. (*A*) Coronal T1W MR image shows geographic lesions with T1 hypointense serpiginous linear areas in the bilateral femoral heads consistent with femoral head ON. (*B*) Coronal PDW FS smaller FOV MR image of the right hip shows a hyperintense serpiginous line consistent with granulation tissue.

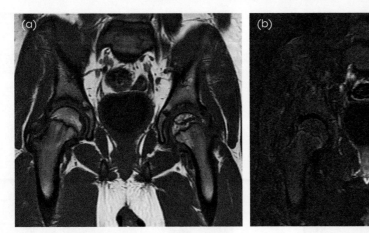

Figure 115.3. Coronal T1W (*A*) and T1W FS postcontrast (*B*) MR images of both hips show a geographic lesion with peripheral linear hypointense signal involving the flattened left capital femoral epiphysis seen on the precontrast image with corresponding nonenhancement of the entire epiphysis on the postcontrast image consistent with Legg-Calvé-Perthes disease.

and the hyperintense line corresponding to granulation tissue (Figure 115.2). This sign may also be partially caused by chemical shift misregistration artifact.

- Nuclear medicine: Bone scan with ^{99m}Tc-methylene diphosphonate shows lack of uptake centrally surrounded by an area of increased uptake in early ON, with increased uptake in later stages.
- Several different ways of estimating the degree of femoral head involvement exist, with one method using visual estimation of the percentage of involvement of the weight-bearing surface (one option is to draw a horizontal line bisecting the femoral head on the coronal view at the mid hip and estimate the percentage of involvement). Other imaging planes can help with this estimation. Collapse is more likely if greater than 50% of the femoral head weight-bearing surface is involved.

Bone Infarct
- With radiography and CT, calcified bone infarcts may be visible as sclerotic serpiginous linear geographic areas in the medullary cavity.
- MRI shows irregular serpiginous hypointense border on T1 and fluid-sensitive sequences. Acute or subacute infarcts have a surrounding T2 hyperintense linear area corresponding to granulation tissue from revascularization and remodeling.
- Malignant degeneration is associated with lytic lesion and soft tissue mass.

Kienböck Disease
- Radiography and CT—appearance ranging from normal to sclerosis, flattening and fragmentation of the lunate
- MRI—early stage T2 hyperintense and T1 hypointense; late stage T2 and T1 hypointense; enhancement may be

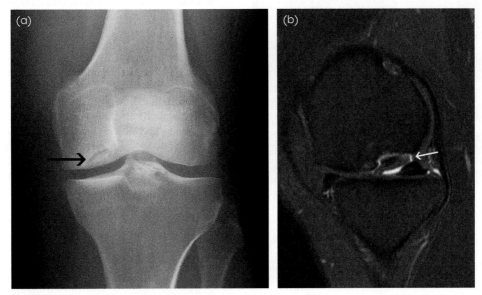

Figure 115.4. Osteochondritis dissecans (OCD) of the medial femoral condyle of the knee. Frontal radiograph of the knee (*A*) shows OCD in the lateral aspect of the medial femoral condyle (*arrow*). (*B*) Sagittal T2W FS MR image of the knee shows fluid signal undermining the osteochondral fragment (*arrow*), consistent with an unstable lesion.

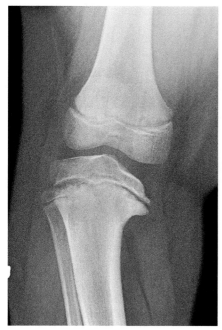

Figure 115.5. Blount disease. Frontal radiograph of the knee shows beaking and depression of the proximal medial tibial physis, resulting in varus angulation of the knee.

present early and absent in later stages (see Chapter 106, "Internal Derangements of the Wrist and Hand")

Legg-Calvé-Perthes Disease
Refer to Figure 115.3.

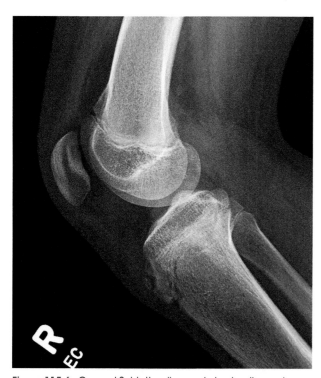

Figure 115.6. Osgood-Schlatter disease. Lateral radiograph of the knee shows fragmentation of the tibial tuberosity with overlying soft tissue thickening and edema in the Hoffa fat pad.

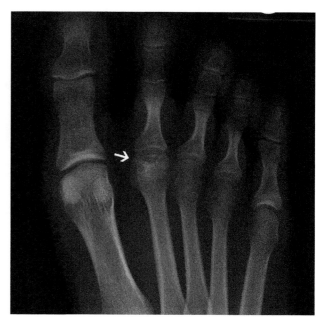

Figure 115.7. Freiberg infraction. Coned-in frontal radiograph of the foot shows flattening and irregularity of the second metatarsal head with a subchondral lucency (*arrow*), consistent with Freiberg infraction.

Initial Ischemic Phase
- Radiography—small femoral epiphysis, widened joint space and subchondral crescent sign
- MRI—edema of the capital femoral epiphysis on fluid-sensitive sequences with decreased enhancement on postcontrast sequences

Revascularization Phase
- Fragmented sclerotic femoral epiphysis; subchondral collapse

Reparative and Reossification Phase
- Broad short femoral neck (coxa magna), widened and irregular physis and metaphyseal cysts

Healed Phase
- Flattened femoral head, short femoral neck, and degenerative joint disease; minority of hips may appear normal

Osteochondritis Dissecans
- Radiography shows subchondral lucency with surrounding sclerosis (Figure 115.4*A*) and possible intraarticular body from displaced fragment.
- MRI shows BME and a subchondral hypointense line. It is important to evaluate the overlying cartilage, which may be disrupted. If there is fluid undermining the cartilage or bone, the fragment is unstable, and surgery may be indicated (Figure 115.4*B*) (see Chapter 109, "Internal Derangements of the Ankle and Foot").

Panner Disease
(Also see Chapter 105, "Internal Derangements of the Elbow.")
- Radiography—sclerosis and collapse of the capitellum
- MRI—BME of the capitellum on fluid-sensitive sequences

Table 115.1. Ficat Radiographic Staging System for Femoral Head Osteonecrosis

STAGE	RADIOGRAPHIC FINDINGS
1	Normal or slight osteopenia
2	Mixed sclerosis and lucency, typically sclerosis surrounding an osteopenic area
3	Femoral head collapse from subchondral fracture (subchondral crescent sign)
4	Femoral head collapse and joint-space narrowing with associated osteoarthritis

Blount Disease
Refer to Figure 115.5.

- Infantile form presents with proximal medial tibial epiphyseal sloping and fragmentation, beaking of the metaphysis, and physeal widening.
- Adolescent form presents with proximal medial tibial physis beaking, irregularity, depression, narrowing or fusion of the medial tibial physis, and widening of the lateral physis.
- MRI may depict a physeal bar (bony bridge crossing the physis resulting from partial premature physeal arrest) and enlargement of the MM with associated intermediate signal related to degeneration.

Osgood-Schlatter Disease
Refer to Figure 115.6.

- Radiography and MRI show fragmentation of the tibial tuberosity accompanied by edema in the Hoffa fat pad and thickening of the inferior patellar tendon.

Sinding-Larsen-Johansson Disease
- Radiography—fragmentation of the inferior patellar pole
- MRI—edema involving the inferior patellar pole, proximal patellar tendon, and adjacent soft tissues

Freiberg Infraction
Refer to Figure 115.7.

- Flattening and possible fragmentation of the second metatarsal head (other lesser metatarsal heads are less commonly affected)

Köhler Disease
- Radiography shows sclerosis, flattening, and fragmentation of the tarsal navicular.

Scheuermann Disease
- Kyphosis with multilevel Schmorl nodes, endplate irregularity, and disc space narrowing
- Mild anterior wedging of 3 or more consecutive vertebrae
- Increased vertebral body AP diameter

Treatment Options

Osteonecrosis
- Core decompression for early stages of ON
- Hip replacement for late stages of ON
- Bone infarct—no treatment necessary
- Kienböck disease—bracing, radial shortening osteotomy, and revascularization procedures for earlier stages with salvage procedures (proximal row carpectomy or partial or total wrist fusion) for later stages

Osteochondroses
- Osteochondroses typically spontaneously heal and conservative treatment (rest and activity modification) is initially performed.
- Legg-Calvé-Perthes: Goal to reduce stress on the femoral head and maintain the femoral head within the acetabulum. Bracing with an abducted hip, physical therapy, core decompression, femoral varus derotation osteotomy, or innominate osteotomy. If more than 50% of the femoral head is involved, surgery will be more likely indicated.
- OCD: Conservative therapy with stable fragment. Surgery may be performed for unstable fragment or the presence of loose bodies.
- Panner disease: Usually heals with bracing.
- Blount disease: Tibial osteotomy for severe cases
- Osgood-Schlatter and Sinding-Larsen-Johansson disease: Almost always resolve with conservative treatment, which includes physical therapy.
- Freiberg infraction: Conservative treatment with padding of the MTP joint
- Köhler disease: Almost always spontaneously resolves. Conservative treatment includes arch supports and rest.
- Scheuermann disease: Bracing and physical therapy. Surgery if kyphosis greater than 75 degrees

Key Points
- The imaging hallmark of ON is a geographic lesion with peripheral serpiginous sclerotic line.
- ON of the hip is commonly bilateral.
- Trauma and corticosteroids are the most common causes of ON.
- Osteochondroses have a typical radiologic appearance of epiphyseal or apophyseal fragmentation and sclerosis, and most heal with conservative treatment.

Recommended Reading
Murphey MD, Foreman KL, Klassen-Fischer MK, Fox MG, Chung EM, Kransdorf MJ. From the radiologic pathology archives imaging of osteonecrosis: radiologic-pathologic correlation. *Radiographics*. 2014;34:1003–28.

Malizos KN, Karantanas AH, Varitimidis SE, Dailiana ZH, Bargiotas K, Maris T. Osteonecrosis of the femoral head: etiology, imaging and treatment. *Eur J Radiol*. 2007;63:16–28.

Developmental and congenital conditions. In: Chew FS, ed. *The Core Curriculum: Musculoskeletal Imaging*. Philadelphia, PA: Lippincott Williams & Wilkins; 2003:444–47.

References

1. Arnaiz J, Piedra T, Cerezal L, et al. Imaging of Kienbock disease. *AJR Am J Roentgenol.* 2014;203:131–39.

2. Dillman JR, Hernandez RJ. MRI of Legg-Calve-Perthes disease. *AJR Am J Roentgenol.* 2009;193:1394–407.

3. Doyle SM, Monahan A. Osteochondroses: a clinical review for the pediatrician. *Curr Opin. Pediatr.* 2010;22:41–46.

4. Dupuis CS, Westra SJ, Makris J, Wallace EC. Injuries and conditions of the extensor mechanism of the pediatric knee. *Radiographics.* 2009;29:877–86.

5. Ejindu VC, Hine AL, Mashayekhi M, Shorvon PJ, Misra RR. Musculoskeletal manifestations of sickle cell disease. *Radiographics.* 2007;27:1005–21.

6. Gillespie H. Osteochondroses and apophyseal injuries of the foot in the young athlete. *Curr Sports Med Rep.* 2010;9:265–68.

7. Imhof H, Breitenseher M, Trattnig S, et al. Imaging of avascular necrosis of bone. *Eur Radiol.* 1997;7:180–86.

8. Siegel MS, Coley B, ed. *The Core Curriculum: Pediatric Imaging.* Philadelphia, PA: Lippincott Williams & Wilkins; 2006:405–553.

9. Stacy GS, Lo R, Montag A. Infarct-associated bone sarcomas: multimodality imaging findings. *AJR Am J Roentgenol.* 2015;205:W432–41.

10. Talusan PG, Diaz-Collado PJ, Reach JS, Jr. Freiberg's infraction: diagnosis and treatment. *Foot Ankle Spec.* 2014;7:52–56.

11. Watson RM, Roach NA, Dalinka MK. Avascular necrosis and bone marrow edema syndrome. *Radiol Clin North Am.* 2004;42:207–19.

CHAPTER 116

Hypervitaminoses, Hypovitaminoses, Fluorosis, and Lead Poisoning

Winnie A. Mar and Eléonore Blondieux

Pathophysiology and Clinical Findings

Hypervitaminosis A

Vitamin A is fat soluble and has many functions including impact on vision, bone growth, cell division, and cell differentiation. Hypervitaminosis A may result from overingestion of vitamin A or treatment with retinoids, synthetic vitamin A derivatives, for severe acne, psoriasis, ichthyosis, or burns. Acute vitamin A poisoning results from ingestion of several hundred thousand IU. Children are particularly sensitive to vitamin A, with doses of only 1500 IU per day reported to result in toxicity. Symptoms include vague musculoskeletal pain, anorexia, pseudotumor cerebri, hair loss, hepatosplenomegaly, and skin desquamation. Growth retardation and delayed physeal closure with limb length discrepancy may occur. Increased intracranial pressure can result from both hypervitaminosis A and hypovitaminosis A.

In the musculoskeletal system, too much vitamin A results in osteoclastic activation and interferes with vitamin D, resulting in osteopenia. Additionally, vitamin A decreases type 2 collagen, which affects cartilage-specific proteoglycan, resulting in an abnormal matrix produced by metaphyseal chondrocytes that cannot be absorbed. This results in wavy periostitis or enthesopathy that occurs at the insertions of muscles and ligaments (Figure 116.1). Bone changes of hypervitaminosis A are typically seen in children 1 year or older and less commonly in adults. The differential diagnosis includes Caffey disease that usually occurs in infants 6 months or younger, which causes self-limiting HOA or periostitis.

Hypervitaminosis D

Vitamin D plays an important role in bone mineral metabolism and calcium homeostasis. Hypervitaminosis D typically results from the overingestion of vitamin D and can be seen in patients being treated with vitamin D for Paget disease, psoriasis, renal osteodystrophy, or rickets. Symptoms are the result of hypercalcemia and include nausea and vomiting, polyuria, and polydipsia. Metastatic calcifications made of calcium hydroxyapatite are seen. The differential diagnosis includes calcinosis from milk alkali syndrome, hyperparathyroidism, or collagen vascular disease.

In children, there is increased calcification of the proliferative cartilage at the physis, resulting in dense metaphyseal bands. An adjacent lucent metaphyseal band is also seen. There may also be cortical thickening caused by periosteal apposition in some areas, with cortical thinning in other areas.

Scurvy

Vitamin C is needed for collagen synthesis. Scurvy results from a vitamin C deficiency, resulting in a propensity for capillary hemorrhage and is currently rarely seen (Figure 116.2). It may be seen in people with a developmental delay or psychiatric disorder, alcoholics, and in infants older than 6 months fed on boiled pasteurized milk, which denatures the vitamin C. It may be seen in malnourished adults as well. Collagen is a key component of bone matrix. In children, scurvy affects the tubular bones and costochondral junctions, with changes of the endochondral bone where bone proliferation is most active, because cellular activity becomes suppressed. The differential diagnosis includes leukemia and neuroblastoma, which also have radiolucent metaphyseal bands.

Fluorosis

Fluorosis occurs after chronic ingestion of water with high levels of fluoride greater than 4 parts per million in endemic areas; fluoride-containing medications such as voriconazole; or from occupational exposure (Figure 116.3). Symptoms include bone and joint pain. Fluoride stimulates new bone formation, but the bone is imperfectly mineralized.

Lead Poisoning

Lead toxicity impairs resorption of the primary spongiosa bone, resulting in dense metaphyseal bands as new bone continues to be laid down (Figure 116.4). In children, it most commonly occurs from ingestion of lead from paint or from certain ceramics. Manifestations are most commonly seen in rapidly growing sites such as the knee and wrist. Lead poisoning can also result from bullet fragments, resulting in synovitis. Other heavy metals, such as phosphorus or bismuth, have a similar effect on bone. Symptoms include abdominal pain, peripheral neuropathy, neurologic dysfunction, and mild anemia. Porphyrin can be detected in the urine.

Imaging Strategy

Radiographs are the mainstay of imaging for these disorders. In hypervitaminosis A, hyperostosis is most commonly seen in the ulna, metatarsals, clavicle, tibia, and fibula. It can also be diagnosed on bone scan. Yearly radiographic monitoring may be considered for patients on retinoid therapy.

With scurvy, MRI is more sensitive for detection of disease and may show findings in the setting of normal radiographs.

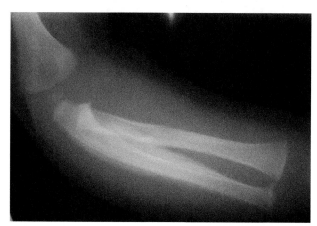

Figure 116.1. Hypervitaminosis A. Lateral radiograph of the forearm shows periosteal reaction of the ulna with fraying of the distal metaphysis secondary to hypervitaminosis A. Image courtesy of Dr. William Schey.

The MRI differential diagnosis includes osteomyelitis and leukemia.

Imaging Findings

Hypervitaminosis A
Refer to Figure 116.1.

- Diaphyseal periosteal reaction, hyperostosis, and cortical thickening, which may be wavy and often underlies areas of soft tissue nodules

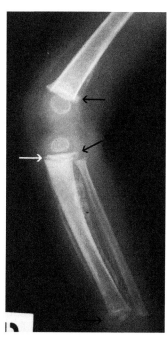

Figure 116.2. Scurvy in a 1-year-old child. Note metaphyseal fractures (*black arrows*) and periosteal elevation. The epiphyses of the distal femur and proximal tibia have a sclerotic rim (Wimberger sign). There is a lucent band of the metaphysis (*white arrow*) with adjacent increased sclerosis at the physis.

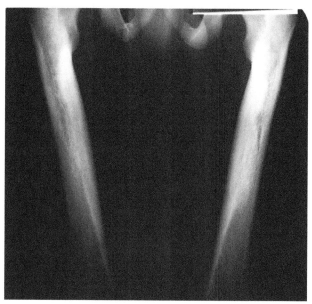

Figure 116.3. Fluorosis. Frontal radiograph of the femurs shows increased sclerosis and cortical thickening related to fluorosis.

- Fraying and cupping of metaphyses with invagination of the epiphysis into the metaphysis with narrowing and premature closure of physes
  - Ulna and metatarsals most commonly affected
  - In contrast to Caffey disease, mandible uncommonly involved
  - Enthesopathy commonly about the spine, which can mimic DISH
  - Osteopenia
  - Bulging fontanelle and cranial suture widening
  - Increased uptake along long bones on ^{99m}Tc-methylene diphosphonate bone scan

Hypervitaminosis D
- Metastatic calcium deposits in joint capsules, bursae, and periarticular soft tissues
- In children, alternating dense and lucent metaphyseal bands
- Osteopenia or dense bones

Pediatric Scurvy
Refer to Figure 116.2.

- Lower extremities more commonly involved with the knee most commonly involved
- Periosteal elevation from subperiosteal hemorrhage
- Metaphyseal beak from a metaphyseal fracture
- Sclerotic line directly adjacent to the physis caused by thickening of the provisional zone of calcification
- Lucent line at the metaphysis caused by unorganized osteoid; scurvy line or Trümmerfeld zone
- Wimberger sign—sclerosis surrounding the epiphysis caused by thickening of the provisional zone of calcification with increased epiphyseal lucency centrally
- On MRI, increased metaphyseal T2 signal intensity and decreased T1 signal intensity
- May have subperiosteal hemorrhage

Adult Scurvy
- Hemarthrosis
- Osteoporosis

Fluorosis
Refer to Figure 116.3.

- Increased bony sclerosis and hyperostosis of the axial skeleton
- Enthesopathy and nodular periostitis

Lead Poisoning
Refer to Figure 116.4.

- Dense metaphyseal bands
- Knees and wrists most commonly affected
- A dense metaphyseal band in the fibula helpful to confirm diagnosis

Treatment Options
- For hypervitaminoses A and D, stop the administration of vitamin A or D.
- For hypervitaminosis D, treat with IV fluid, diuretics, and calcitonin.
- For scurvy, administer vitamin C.
- For fluorosis, stop ingestion of fluoride and find an alternative medication if voriconazole is the offending agent.
- For lead poisoning, prevention of lead ingestion is best with blood screening of children at high risk.

Key Points
- Although rare, hypervitaminoses and hypovitaminoses should be considered with the appropriate clinical and radiographic findings; the radiologist may be the first to suggest these diagnoses.
- Hypervitaminosis A shows periostitis and enthesopathy.
- Hypervitaminosis D shows metastatic calcifications.
- Scurvy shows metaphyseal lucency with dense physeal lines, metaphyseal fractures, and periosteal elevation.
- Fluorosis shows increased bone density and periostitis.
- Lead poisoning shows dense metaphyseal bands.

Recommended Reading
Resnick D. Hypervitaminosis and hypovitaminosis. In: Resnick D, ed. *Diagnosis of Bone and Joint Disorders*. 3rd ed. Philadelphia, PA: Saunders; 2005:1022–27.

References
1. Bansal RK, Tyagi P, Sharma P, et al. Iatrogenic hypervitaminosis D as an unusual cause of persistent vomiting: a case report. *J Med Case Rep.* 2014;8:74.

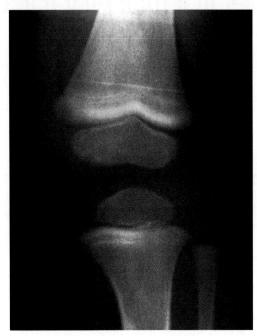

Figure 116.4. Lead poisoning. Frontal radiograph of the knee shows dense metaphyseal bands secondary to lead poisoning.

2. Chen L, Mulligan ME. Medication-induced periostitis in lung transplant patients: periostitis deformans revisited. *Skeletal Radiol.* 2011;40:143–48.
3. Flora G, Gupta D, Tiwari A. Toxicity of lead: a review with recent updates. *Interdiscip Toxicol.* 2012;5:47–58.
4. Gulko E, Collins LK, Murphy RC, Thornhill BA, Taragin BH. MRI findings in pediatric patients with scurvy. *Skeletal Radiol.* 2015;44:291–97.
5. Holman CB. Roentgenologic manifestations of vitamin D intoxication. *Radiology.* 1952;59:805–16.
6. Miller JH, Hayon, II. Bone scintigraphy in hypervitaminosis A. *AJR Am J Roentgenol.* 1985;144:767–68.
7. Polat AV, Bekci T, Say F, Bolukbas E, Selcuk MB. Osteoskeletal manifestations of scurvy: MRI and ultrasound findings. *Skeletal Radiol.* 2015;44:1161–64.
8. Rothenberg AB, Berdon WE, Woodard JC, Cowles RA. Hypervitaminosis A-induced premature closure of epiphyses (physeal obliteration) in humans and calves (hyena disease): a historical review of the human and veterinary literature. *Pediatr Radiol.* 2007;37:1264–67.
9. Sidhu HS, Venkatanarasimha N, Bhatnagar G, Vardhanabhuti V, Fox BM, Suresh SP. Imaging features of therapeutic drug-induced musculoskeletal abnormalities. *Radiographics.* 2012;32:105–27.
10. Ved N, Haller JO. Periosteal reaction with normal-appearing underlying bone: a child abuse mimicker. *Emerg Radiol.* 2002;9:278–82.

CHAPTER 117

Medication-Induced Musculoskeletal Changes

Winnie A. Mar

Pathophysiology and Clinical Findings

Osteoporosis and Osteomalacia

Osteoporosis can be caused by multiple medications, most commonly by corticosteroids, but also by selective serotonin reuptake inhibitors (SSRIs), proton pump inhibitors (PPIs), and antiepileptic medications. Corticosteroids decrease osteoblastic activity, stimulate bone resorption, and decrease intestinal absorption of calcium. Antiepileptic medications cause osteomalacia by inducing P450 cytochrome enzymes.

Other Corticosteroid Effects

Approximately 2% of ON is caused by corticosteroid therapy, most commonly affecting the hip, humeral head, or knee (Figure 117.1). The exact pathophysiology is unclear; several hypotheses exist, including fat cell hypertrophy with vessel compression, fat embolism, vessel thrombosis, or osteocyte apoptosis.

High doses of corticosteroids may also increase cartilage degeneration by altering chondrocyte expression of matrix proteins. There have also been reports of rapid chondrolysis of the glenohumeral joint after pain pump infusion of local anesthetic.

Bisphosphonates

Bisphosphonates are used to treat osteoporosis, but also Paget disease, metastatic bone disease, and multiple myeloma. They cause decreased osteoclastic activity, resulting in increased bone mineralization, although increasing bone brittleness. Atypical femoral fractures are insufficiency fractures associated with long-term bisphosphonate use and occur most commonly in the subtrochanteric region, proximal third of the femur, but may also occur elsewhere along the lateral aspect of the femoral diaphysis (Figure 117.2). They occur without trauma or with low-impact trauma such as falling from a standing height or less. Prodromal symptoms include thigh pain or weakness.

ON of the jaw is a rare complication with oral bisphosphonate therapy and is more common with IV bisphosphonate therapy usually for cancer treatment (Figure 117.3). There is an association with tooth extraction or other major dental work. An association with *Actinomyces* has been postulated. The pathophysiology is thought to be microtrauma and oversuppression of bone turnover. The clinical diagnosis is made when exposed bone is seen. Biopsy may worsen the condition and should be avoided, thus imaging should be performed if there is any clinical doubt.

Myopathy and Tendinopathy

Multiple different medications can cause myopathy. One of the most common medications, statins used for lowering cholesterol, have been known to rarely cause myopathy ranging from myalgias to rhabdomyolysis. Corticosteroids can also cause a symmetric painless proximal myopathy, particularly in the pelvic girdle.

Tendinopathy and tendon tears are a rare complication of fluoroquinolone therapy for community-acquired infections. The Achilles tendon is most commonly involved, although other tendons may also be involved.

Fluorosis

Voriconazole is an antifungal medication commonly used in immunocompromised patients that contains a high amount of fluoride, and can result in fluoride toxicity (see Figure 116.3 in Chapter 116, "Hypervitaminoses, Hypovitaminoses, Fluorosis, and Lead Poisoning"). Patients present with bone pain, and fluoride levels are generally elevated. The differential diagnosis includes HOA or medication-induced periostitis from prostaglandin, vitamin A, or fluoride treatment. In contrast to HOA, alkaline phosphatase levels are elevated, and there is no clubbing.

Imaging Strategy

For osteoporosis, DXA scan is the gold standard and is indicated in patients on long-term corticosteroid therapy. Radiographs are less sensitive.

Patients who may be at risk for a bisphosphonate-related atypical femoral fracture should have screening with radiography. If periosteal and cortical thickening is seen without a fracture line on radiography, MRI should be performed to evaluate for a fracture line or significant BME. In those with a fracture on one side, the contralateral femur should be screened with radiography, MRI, CT, or bone scan, as the incidence of a bilateral abnormality is high. In patients treated conservatively, follow-up with MRI or bone scan should be performed to evaluate for resolution of BME or increased radiotracer uptake.

In evaluation for ON of the jaw, CT is the preferred imaging modality, with findings easily seen on MRI. Radiographs are less sensitive but can demonstrate findings.

Radiography is usually the first imaging modality performed in patients on voriconazole therapy who

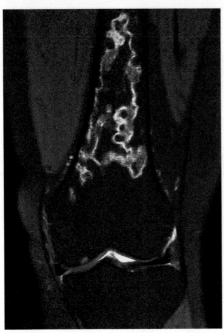

Figure 117.1. Steroid-induced bone infarct. Coronal T2W FS MR image of the knee shows a serpiginous hyperintense linear area in the distal femoral diametaphysis consistent with a bone infarct.

present with pain. In the initial presentation, association with voriconazole is usually not recognized clinically.

Imaging Findings

Osteoporosis or Osteomalacia
(See Chapter 71, "Osteoporosis.")

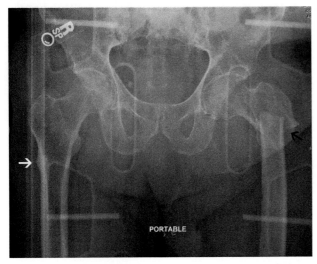

Figure 117.2. Bisphosphonate-related atypical femoral fracture and stress reaction. Frontal radiograph of the pelvis in a patient on long-term bisphosphonate therapy and an atypical femoral fracture shows a transverse left femoral subtrochanteric fracture (*black arrow*) with cortical thickening and beaking of the lateral fracture site. Right femoral subtrochanteric lateral cortical thickening from stress reaction is also seen (*white arrow*).

- Secondary osteoporosis caused by medications is radiographically indistinguishable from primary osteoporosis and results in diminished bone mineralization.
- DXA is the gold standard. A T score of or less than −2.5 corresponds to osteoporosis. A T score between −1.0 and −2.4 corresponds to osteopenia in postmenopausal women and men older than 50 years.
- Radiography (CR) and CT show decreased bone density, cortical thinning, and decreased bone trabeculae.
- Insufficiency fractures are possible, most commonly in the spine, sacrum, and hip.

Osteonecrosis and Bone Infarct
(See Chapter 115, "Osteonecroses and Osteochondroses.")
- CR—Radiographs may be normal in early stages. In later stages, linear or patchy sclerosis is seen. Subchondral lucency, collapse, and secondary OA may be seen.
- CT shows sclerotic serpiginous lines.
- On MRI, in early ON, BME is seen. In late ON, linear serpiginous areas *double line sign* (Figure 117.1) is seen.
- With nuclear medicine (NM), bone scan with ^{99m}Tc-methylene diphosphonate shows lack of uptake centrally surrounded by an area of increased uptake in early ON, with increased uptake later.

Atypical Femur Fractures
Refer to Figure 117.2.
- CR shows lateral cortex periosteal stress reaction with possible incomplete transverse fracture with cortical thickening and lateral beak or spike.
- Complete fractures are transverse and with minimal, if any, comminution.
- MRI shows lateral cortical thickening and BME with or without fracture line.

Osteonecrosis of the Mandible
- CR shows increased sclerosis, decreased corticomedullary differentiation, possible periosteal reaction, and persistent socket after tooth extraction.
- CT shows sclerosis, fragmentation, and lysis. Cortical erosion, sequestrum, or pathologic fracture may also be present (Figure 117.3).
- On MRI, in early ON, T2 signal is isointense or slightly hyperintense; in late ON, both T2 and T1 signal are hypointense. Heterogeneous enhancement of the affected mandible and surrounded tissue with nonenhancement of the necrotic region is seen.
- NM shows increased radiotracer uptake, unless there is sequestrum, which may have decreased central uptake.

Voriconazole
- Diffuse, dense, symmetric, irregular periosteal reaction (Figure 117.4)
- Increased periosteal radiotracer uptake on bone scan

Myositis
- MRI shows nonspecific muscle edema in the acute phase.
- If advanced to rhabdomyolysis and muscle ischemia or infarct, hyperenhancement or hypoenhancement are seen on MRI.

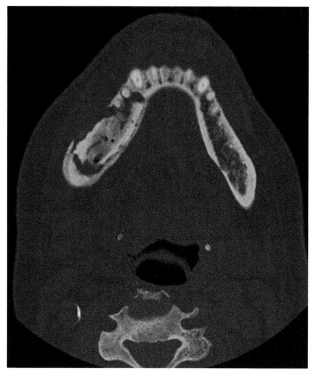

Figure 117.3. Bisphosphonate-related ON of the mandible. Axial CT image of the mandible shows late-stage ON of the jaw in a patient with prostate cancer treated with IV bisphosphonates, with periosteal reaction, fragmentation, and sequestrum. Image courtesy of Dr. Edward Michals.

- Fatty muscle atrophy is seen in the chronic phase.

Treatment Options

Medication-Induced Osteoporosis
- Calcium and vitamin D supplementation
- Using the minimal amount of causative medication as necessary or discontinuing the medication if possible

Osteonecrosis
- Core decompression or a vascularized fibular graft for early stages
- Joint replacement for late stages

Atypical Femoral Fractures
- Conservative treatment
  - Can be considered when a fracture line is not present and there is minimal to no pain
  - Withdrawing bisphosphonate therapy
  - Supplementation with calcium and vitamin D and decreasing weight-bearing
- Surgical treatment
  - Intramedullary nailing for patients with incomplete and complete fractures and pain

Osteonecrosis of the Jaw
- Antibiotics; recontouring if needed, with avoiding more extensive surgery
- Prevention; avoiding tooth extraction or implants; good dental hygiene

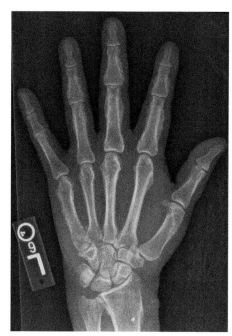

Figure 117.4. Voriconazole-related periostitis. Frontal radiograph of the hand shows thick irregular periostitis about the phalanges, metacarpals, and distal radius in this renal transplant patient on chronic voriconazole therapy for *Aspergillus* infection.

Voriconazole
- Cessation of voriconazole treatment results in resolution of pain and radiologic findings.

Key Points
- Medication-related musculoskeletal disorders are becoming increasingly frequent and should be recognized by the radiologist.
- The index of suspicion for ON/bone infarcts and osteoporosis should be increased in those on corticosteroids. Additionally, these are usually multiple and often bilateral.
- If an atypical femoral fracture is detected, one should correlate with history of bisphosphonate therapy and have a high clinical suspicion for involvement of the contralateral side.
- Patients with fluoride toxicity related to voriconazole use have painful, dense, irregular periostitis.

Recommended Reading
Sidhu HS, Venkatanarasimha N, Bhatnagar G, Vardhanabhuti V, Fox BM, Suresh SP. Imaging features of therapeutic drug-induced musculoskeletal abnormalities. *Radiographics.* 2012;32:105–27.

References
1. Bannwarth B. Drug-induced musculoskeletal disorders. *Drug Safety.* 2007;30:27–46.
2. Chan KL, Mok CC. Glucocorticoid-induced avascular bone necrosis: diagnosis and management. *Open Orthop J.* 2012;6:449–57.

3. Chen L, Mulligan ME. Medication-induced periostitis in lung transplant patients: periostitis deformans revisited. *Skeletal Radiol.* 2011;40:143–48.

4. Hasan SS, Fleckenstein CM. Glenohumeral chondrolysis: part I—clinical presentation and predictors of disease progression. *Arthroscopy.* 2013;29:1135–41.

5. Krishnan A, Arslanoglu A, Yildirm N, Silbergleit R, Aygun N. Imaging findings of bisphosphonate-related osteonecrosis of the jaw with emphasis on early magnetic resonance imaging findings. *J Comput Assist Tomogr.* 2009;33:298–304.

6. Mirza F, Canalis E. Management of endocrine disease: secondary osteoporosis: pathophysiology and management. *Eur J Endocrinol.* 2015;173:R131–51.

7. Morag Y, Morag-Hezroni M, Jamadar DA, et al. Bisphosphonate-related osteonecrosis of the jaw: a pictorial review. *Radiographics.* 2009;29:1971–84.

8. Neviaser AS, Lane JM, Lenart BA, Edobor-Osula F, Lorich DG. Low-energy femoral shaft fractures associated with alendronate use. *J Orthop Trauma.* 2008;22:346–50.

9. Shane E, Burr D, Abrahamsen B, et al. Atypical subtrochanteric and diaphyseal femoral fractures: second report of a task force of the American Society for Bone and Mineral Research. *J Bone Miner Res.* 2014;29:1–23.

10. Wise SM, Wilson MA. A case of periostitis secondary to voriconazole therapy in a heart transplant recipient. *Clin Nucl Med.* 2011;36:242–44.

Musculoskeletal Ultrasound

Edited by Mihra S. Taljanovic and Tyson S. Chadaz

CHAPTER 118

An Introduction to Musculoskeletal Ultrasound

James F. Griffith

Getting Started: Ultrasound Machine and Transducers

The range of US machines has grown tremendously over the past 15 years, which has led to improvements in the quality of the images produced. US machines now vary from high-end departmental systems to portable point-of-care devices that in some cases simply involve connecting transducers to smartphones to generate diagnostic imaging.

For musculoskeletal (MSK) US, one should have a high-resolution transducer. High-resolution transducers range from approximately 10 to 20 MHz and are ideal for examining the superficial soft tissues. The relationship between increasing US transducer frequency and resolution is not linear. Most MSK US examinations can be performed with a linear transducer in the 10-12 MHz range. Moving from a 12- to an 18-MHz transducer will improve resolution to a mild degree but usually does not change diagnostic capability. Thus, access to 1 high-frequency transducer is usually enough to begin MSK US. High-resolution transducers have limited depth penetration so that for deeper areas, such as the gluteal region, a lower frequency transducer, such as a 7.5-MHz transducer, is also necessary.

The transducer is a delicate and expensive piece of equipment and must be handled with care. The transducer contains an interlinked array of piezoelectric crystals. These piezoelectric crystals convert an electrical signal into an US wave and vice versa. The same array of piezoelectric crystals emits and receives the US signal. The transducer sends signal, or "calls out," to the tissues and then "listens" for the returning sound wave or echo. This calling and listening happens many thousands of times a second (*pulse repetition frequency*). To improve sound wave transmission and allow the transducer to glide more freely over the skin, US gel is applied between the skin and the transducer. Sound waves pass from the transducer through the US gel to the skin and into the deeper tissues.

Three main factors affect the strength of the returning echoes. These are (a) the acoustic impedance of the tissues, (b) the smoothness of the reflective surface, and (c) the sound absorption of the tissues encountered. Acoustic impedance is the ability of tissues to transmit sound waves. At tissue interfaces where there is a large difference in acoustic impedance (such as soft tissue–bone interface), most sound waves are reflected back to the transducer (producing a relatively bright echo). At interfaces where there is little or no difference in the acoustic impedance of the tissues (such as muscle–muscle interface), most sound waves will be transmitted and will not be reflected back to the transducer (producing a relatively dark echo). As expected, most sound waves that contact an interface parallel to the transducer face will be reflected back to the transducer. Sound waves impacting an irregular surface will be reflected away from the transducer (refraction). Sound wave attenuation also occurs when sound waves are absorbed by the tissues encountered, and this is greater in tissues of higher viscosity.

Scanning Method

When performing the US examination, the examiner should have sufficient time and be undistracted and attentive to the examination that he or she is performing. The examiner and the patient should be in comfortable positions, and the area to be examined should be optimally exposed and positioned. This applies especially to areas such as the shoulder, the cubital tunnel, or the peroneal tendons, where there are particular maneuvers one can do to optimize examination of the specific structures. Before starting the examination, the examiner should ask the patient about his or her symptoms. For example, knowing the location of the patient's pain and whether has there been any history of trauma can help greatly narrow the differential diagnosis, which in turn makes the overall US examination more focused and saves examination time.

The examiner should grasp the transducer lightly between his or her fingertips and thumb. When scanning, the examiner's little finger or hypothenar eminence should maintain contact with the patient's skin (Figure 118.1). This will allow the examiner to apply only light pressure to the transducer without pressing down too hard on the skin surface. This is particularly important when (a) examining color flow in superficial structures; (b) assessing vascular malformations for slow flow; (c) trying to detect movement of tissues, such as subluxations or clicks; and (d) assessing muscle, groin, or abdominal wall hernias. When assessing superficial vasculature, the imager should apply copious amounts of gel and actively lift the transducer from the skin so as not to blanch any vasculature. That said, applying some downward pressure can occasionally be helpful to gauge the firmness and compressibility of any area being examined.

One should develop a schematic examination method for each joint. The freely downloadable European Society of Musculoskeletal Radiology (ESSR) MSK US guidelines are an excellent source in this respect. Concentrate first on that area where symptoms are most prominent. MSK US is most

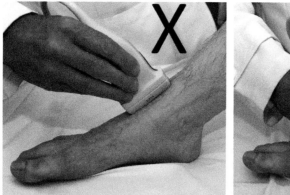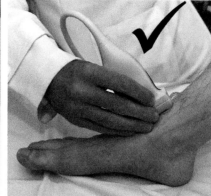

Figure 118.1. Transducer positioning. The correct way to hold an US transducer is to have the little and ring fingers in contact with the patient's skin.

helpful in those patients who can point quite precisely to the site of pain or symptoms. For example, if there are symptoms on the medial side of the ankle, the examiner should concentrate most of his or her efforts on examination of the medial ankle structures, which will help ensure that the US findings correspond to the patient's symptoms. One could, in this situation, also check the anterior ankle for signs of an ankle joint effusion, but there will be little additional benefit to be gained from examining the lateral ankle if there are no signs/ symptoms related to this side. Of course, each patient should be approached on a case-by-case basis, though in general, for time efficiency, it is better to have a more thorough examination of the symptomatic area. In children or uncooperative patients, full examination may not be possible, and an approach of concentrating on the most critical area prior to examining the rest of joint or region should be adopted. Sedation is not usually necessary or beneficial in children or uncooperative patients.

Understanding proper US machine setup is crucial to conducting high-quality US. It is important before and during scanning to optimize image quality. It is helpful to routinely first examine the contralateral normal side as this may allow the examiner to (a) familiarize himself or herself with normal US anatomy and (b) set up the machine properly for the region under examination. The initial setup, however, will usually need frequent readjustment during the course of the US examination.

All lesions should be properly documented and labeled because US is a once-off examination with any subsequent review, being entirely dependent on the quality of the images obtained initially. It is better to take a few high-quality images than many suboptimal images. By convention, the examiner should orient the image so that the proximal end is on the left side of the screen and the distal end on the right side. Copious coupling gel should be used to make sure there is no shadowing artifact from too little gel at the sides of the image. The depth should be adjusted to include the relevant area only. The image can be zoomed within reason to better depict the target tissues, and the focal zone and US gain should be optimized to improve image quality. Cine clips of any pertinent findings, particularly during dynamic maneuvers, may be helpful to confirm abnormalities that may only be seen with movement.

During scanning, the tissues can be compressed by the transducer to broadly gauge their stiffness. This dynamic capability of US is also helpful when differentiating between fluid and soft tissue in suspected abscess or hematoma or between synovial proliferation and effusion. The dynamic capability of US can also be used to assess tendon or muscle tears, tendon or nerve subluxation, tendon movement restriction, or shoulder impingement. Snaps or clicks are common reasons for dynamic US examination, although it is not always possible to demonstrate the causes of these sensations because of (a) inaccessibility of the responsible tissues, (b) inability to recognize the abnormal movement, or (c) failure of the click to occur during scanning.

When following nerves or tendons, it is best to scan them in the transverse rather than the longitudinal plane. The examiner should follow only 1 tendon or nerve at a time. It is very difficult to follow 2 structures simultaneously and not overlook subtle abnormalities.

Color and/or power Doppler imaging are used routinely in the assessment of soft tissue inflammation or infection, disease activity, synovitis, and soft tissue masses or lymph nodes. Doppler frequency shift relates to a change in sound frequency depending on whether an object is moving toward or away from a fixed point of reference. The relative sensitivity of color or power Doppler does vary from machine to machine. Color Doppler is flow-direction sensitive, whereas power Doppler is not flow-direction sensitive and overall is considered more sensitive for detecting slow flow and flow in small vessels. Slow venous flow is often best seen with grayscale rather than color or power Doppler imaging. This is because the rouleaux-like aggregation of slow-flowing red blood cells will provide a finely speckled appearance on grayscale imaging even though there is no significant Doppler shift on color imaging.

Supplementary Imaging Techniques

With conventional US imaging, the transducer emits and receives a sound pulse of a specific frequency at a single angle of insonation. The returning signal is of the same frequency though weaker, and the transducer normally listens specifically for that frequency. Several techniques, over and above standard grayscale imaging, are available to enhance image resolution, depiction, and interrogation. *Spatial compound*

US combines sonographic data from several different angles of insonation into a single image. By averaging image data from multiple angles of insonation, spatial compound imaging helps to improve definition of soft tissue planes, reduce speckle and other noise, and improve overall image detail. With *tissue harmonic imaging*, the transducer listens for not only the returning signals of the transmitted frequency but also returning signals of harmonic frequencies (generated by passage of the sound wave through tissue). The benefits of tissue harmonic imaging are most apparent in the midfield region helping to improve tissue visibility such as the edge of soft tissue masses or tendon tears. *Extended FOV imaging* allows one to build up a panoramic image, which is helpful for (a) measuring large masses, (b) comparing tissue thickness or echogenicity in confluent areas, and (c) perceiving the anatomical relationship of any abnormality.

Normal Anatomy Appearances

The *epidermis* is seen as a thin echogenic line immediately deep to the transducer surface. The epidermis is thicker on the palms and the soles. In some instances, the skin can significantly attenuate the US beam. For example, the thick skin of manual workers can have considerable US beam attenuation.

The *subcutaneous layer* is seen on US as a hypoechoic tissue with fine echogenic strands. These fine echogenic strands represent the fibrous interlobular septae separating the subcutaneous fat lobules. Normally the subcutaneous tissues show very little venous or arterial flow except for some perforating vessels on color Doppler imaging. Increased flow is seen in subcutaneous inflammation because of infection or panniculitis. The lymphatic channels are not visible on US. The more superficial aspect of the subcutaneous tissues can be referred to as the *subdermal tissues*. The deeper subcutaneous tissues overlie the investing fascia.

The *muscle layer* is a relatively hypoechoic tissue containing linear strands of fibroadipose tissue surrounded by a thin layer of echogenic connective fibrous tissue known as the *perimysium*. The fibroadipose strands within muscle can be seen as fine echogenic lines on longitudinal (long axis) imaging and fine echogenic dots on transverse (short axis) imaging (Figure 118.2). These intramuscular fibroadipose septae correspond to the internal muscle architecture, which may be fusiform, unipennate, bipennate, or multipennate in type. They converge onto the central tendon, which becomes the main tendon of the muscle. Individual muscles can be recognized by their locations, but one can follow the muscle in a transverse direction more distally to its main tendon to confirm its identity. Nerves and blood vessels can be recognized in the connective tissue between muscles (Figure 118.2). The attachment of muscle to bone may be purely muscular, musculoaponeurotic, or tendinous.

Nerves are normally followed in transverse axis more easily than in long axis. On short-axis imaging, nerves have a distinctive honeycomb-like pattern with the hypoechoic fascicles interspersed between hyperechoic perifascicular perineurium (Figure 118.3). Commonly, nerves are identified on US at specific sites and then followed either proximally or distally to the point of interest. The epineurium surrounding the nerve is difficult to distinguish from the perineural fat.

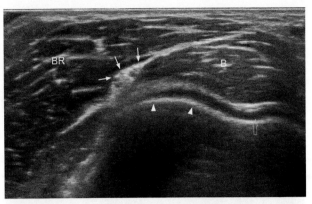

Figure 118.2. Normal muscle, normal cortical bone, and normal articular cartilage. Short-axis US image at the anterolateral aspect of the elbow. The normal radial nerve (*arrows*) can be seen lying between the brachioradialis (Br) and brachialis muscles (B). Note the normal hypoechoic appearance of the muscles on transverse section, normal smooth appearance of the hyperechoic cortical bone at the capitellum (*arrowheads*), and normal appearance of the overlying hyaline articular cartilage (*open arrow*).

On long-axis imaging, nerves have a tramlike appearance with multiple hypoechoic parallel, linear fascicles separated by hyperechoic interfascicular perineurium. Nerves are quite malleable and can change their shape with compression. Nerves are often accompanied by arteries and veins. Veins are easily compressible, and the examiner needs to actively lift the transducer off of the skin to see them properly.

Tendons have a highly ordered structure with parallel collagen bundles giving rise to fine linear echoes on longitudinal US scanning and a stippled echogenic pattern on transverse imaging (Figure 118.4). This highly ordered infrastructure makes tendons particularly prone to anisotropy such that regular 90-degree transducer angulation is necessary during scanning. Movement of tendons can be readily appreciated on dynamic imaging. Tendons around the wrist, hand, ankles, and feet have tendon sheaths and as such are prone to tenosynovitis. Many tendons, such as the Achilles tendon, do not

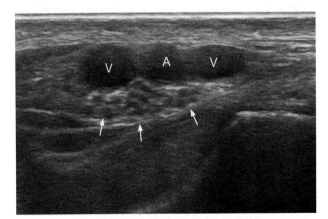

Figure 118.3. Normal nerve. Short-axis US image of the medial aspect of the ankle shows the normal posterior tibial neurovascular bundle. The posterior tibial artery (A) is interposed between the 2 accompanying posterior tibial veins (V). Deep to these vascular structures lies the posterior tibial nerve (*arrows*).

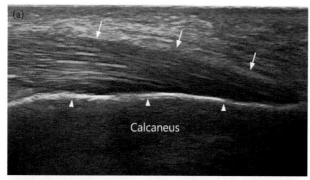

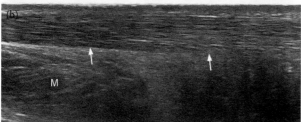

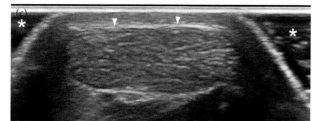

Figure 118.4. Normal Achilles tendon. (*A*) Long-axis US image of a normal Achilles tendon at its insertion onto the calcaneal tuberosity (*arrowheads*). Note the normal tapering appearance of the Achilles tendon at its insertion (*arrows*) as well as the normal smooth bony contour. (*B*) Long-axis US image at the proximal end and mid-third of the normal Achilles tendon. Note the normal fine fibrillar echotexture of the Achilles tendon (*arrows*). Superficial to the Achilles tendon lies the subcutaneous fat and deep to the Achilles tendon lies the flexor hallucis longus muscle (M). (*C*) Short-axis US image of mid-third of the Achilles tendon. The normal speckled echotexture of the tendon on transverse section can be appreciated. The thin echogenic line that covers the dorsal aspect and also the sides of the Achilles tendon is the Achilles paratenon (*arrowheads*). To allow best appreciation of the overall configuration of the tendon on transverse section, copious amounts of gel should be used to fill up the lateral recesses between the leg and the transducer (*asterisks*).

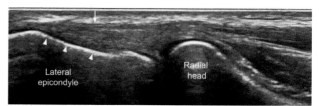

Figure 118.5. Sharpy fibers at the tendon attachment onto the bone enthesis. Long-axis US image showing a normal common extensor tendon origin at the elbow. The conjoint insertion of the common extensor tendons into the lateral humeral epicondyle (*arrowheads*) is shown. Note the thin hypoechoic line at the tendon insertion into the bone cortex caused by Sharpy fibers. This is a normal appearance. Note the normal straight superficial contour of this tendon (*arrow*) and the normal smooth contour of the bone at the insertion area. The radial head is also shown.

closely apposed to the tendon and attach to the bone on either side. Retinacula should not be mistaken for tendon sheath thickening. Occasionally, these retinacula may compress the underlying tendon, giving rise to a stenosing tenosynovitis. The classic examples, brought on by de Quervain disease, involve the first extensor compartment tendons of the wrist and trigger finger. The A1 pulley, which focally encircles the flexor tendons at the MCP joints, is typically involved.

The ankle and knee *ligaments* as well as some of the wrist ligaments are readily accessible to US examination. Normal ligaments are seen as bandlike structures with a fine, linear echogenic echotexture connecting to bony surfaces in typical locations (Figure 118.7). The most commonly assessed ligaments with US are the anterior talofibular, the

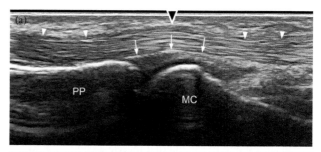

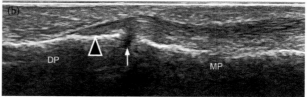

Figure 118.6. A1 pulley and normal flexor tendons and joints of the finger. (*A*) Long-axis US image of the palmar aspect of the finger at the level of the MCP joint. The flexor tendons (superficialis and profundus) are clearly seen (*white arrowheads*). They pass deep to the A1 pulley (*black arrowhead*). The volar plate on the palmar aspect of the MCP joint is also shown (*arrows*) as are the bony contours of the metacarpal (MC) and proximal phalanx (PP). (*B*) Long-axis US image of the palmar aspect of the finger at the level of the DIP joint. The DIP joint can be clearly seen (*arrow*) between the middle phalanx (MP) and the distal phalanx (DP). Note the insertion of the flexor digitorum profundus tendon into the volar aspect of the DP (*arrowhead*).

have tendon sheaths and cannot develop tenosynovitis. All tendons can potentially be affected by tendon degeneration or tendinosis, though typically this tends to affect those tendon areas where tendons curve around bony structures or where they insert onto their bony attachments. Tendons often tend to splay out slightly and become more hypoechoic at their insertion into bone. There is also a thin hypoechoic zone typically present at the insertion of tendon into bone caused by Sharpey fibers or fibrocartilage (Figure 118.5). This thin hypoechoic band should not be taken for an avulsive-type tear.

At certain areas, particularly at the wrist, the fingers, and around the ankle joint, there are fibrous retinacula and pulleys present, which serve to keep the tendon closely apposed to the underlying bone during joint movement (Figure 118.6). These retinacula and pulleys are seen as thin echogenic fibrous bands

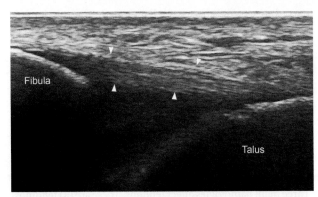

Figure 118.7. Normal ligament. Long-axis US image along the normal anterior talofibular ligament (ATFL) (*arrowheads*) extending between the distal fibula and the talus. The ATFL is the most commonly torn ankle ligament.

calcaneofibular, and the anterior tibiofibular ligaments of the ankle, and the MCL of the elbow.

Although the US beam does not penetrate the surface of the *bone* well and cannot characterize the marrow cavity, the outer margin of bone can be seen as a well-defined thick echogenic line, which is curved on axial imaging (Figure 118.8). Dense acoustic shadowing is present deep to bone surface. The normal periosteum cannot be seen, although reactive periostitis is seen as a mildly hyperechoic rim around bone. This periosteal reaction can be seen on US before it is visible radiographically as radiography requires mineralization to occur prior to visualization. Nutrient channels can be readily seen on bone as can physiological cortical irregularity at the insertional sites of muscle and intermuscular fibrous septae.

Unossified hyaline cartilage is visible as hypoechoic tissue on US with a mildly echogenic surface. Cartilage does not significantly attenuate the US beam, allowing one to appreciate structures deep to the cartilage such as in the hip joint when the proximal femur is unossified or the pleura deep to the costal cartilages. Normal fibrocartilage appears hyperechoic on US images. This includes the menisci of the knee, glenoid and acetabular labra, and the TFC of the wrist.

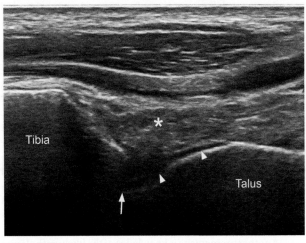

Figure 118.9. Normal ankle joint. Long-axis US image at anterior aspect of the ankle joint (*arrow*). The distal tibia as well as the talus can be appreciated. The hypoechoic cartilage on the anterior aspect of the talar dome can be appreciated (*arrowheads*). A fat pad (*asterisk*) lies between the joint and the anterior ankle capsule.

The *joint* capsule, joint synovium, and the degree of distension of most joints can be readily assessed with US examination (Figures 118.9 and 118.10). If a joint effusion is present, it can be readily aspirated under US guidance. Similarly, if no joint effusion is present and either infection or synovial tumor is suspected, then synovial biopsy can be performed. It may sometimes be difficult to distinguish between hyperechoic synovial fluid and hypoechoic synovial proliferation on US examination. Demonstrating hyperemia within the thickened synovium can be helpful to differentiate these possibilities, although hyperemia is not always readily appreciable in thickened synovium, particularly in the hip joint and in the shoulder joint.

For the most part, US does not allow full examination of intraarticular structures such as the articular cartilage, menisci, labra, cruciate ligaments, and the articular disc of the triangular fibrocartilaginous complex. MRI examination provides a better assessment of these structures. Similarly, when one wants to assess the degree of inflammation in relatively inaccessible joints such as the SI joints, it is best to proceed to MRI

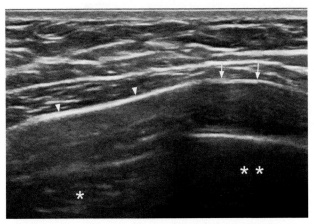

Figure 118.8. Normal rib. Long-axis US image through the anterior aspect of the rib. The osseous portion of the rib (*arrowheads*), which shows acoustic shadowing (*asterisk*), is clearly identified from the cartilaginous portion of the rib (*arrows*), which shows acoustic transmission (*double asterisk*).

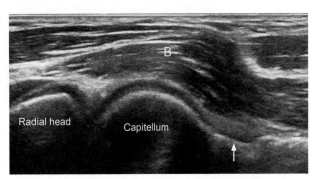

Figure 118.10. Normal elbow joint. Long-axis US image along the anterolateral aspect of the normal elbow. The radial head and the capitellum can be seen covered by hypoechoic articular cartilage. Anteriorly is the brachialis muscle (B). Just proximal to the capitellum is part of the anterior fat pad (*arrow*).

examination as US cannot assess features such as subchondral BME and inflammation.

Recognizing Pathology

Good-quality MSK US is dependent on a good understanding of MSK anatomy. As mentioned, it is helpful to be familiar with normal anatomy on the asymptomatic side before examining the symptomatic side. It should be remembered that the normal side may not always serve as an internal reference of normality. Tendinosis and nerve entrapment, in particular, are often asymptomatic, and US often shows abnormal findings (to a comparable or lesser degree) on the asymptomatic side. Therefore, one needs to have a good idea as to what the normal appearances or values are before proceeding to diagnose tendon or nerve pathology.

Another prerequisite is knowledge of the likely pathologies that occur in specific areas. Most MSK pathology is site specific. Tissue-specific pathology has a similar appearance irrespective of location. For example, tendinosis, tendon tears, or tenosynovitis appear similar irrespective of location. Tendons, nerves, and ligaments are prone to anisotropy, so frequent transducer angulation is necessary to view all portions. This is the most commonly encountered artifact. To overcome this artifact, frequent transducer realignment to examine different areas of curved structures is necessary. For example, the anterior, mid, and posterior fibers of the supraspinatus tendon as well as the medial and lateral aspects usually need to be assessed independently. For soft tissue masses, one should evaluate location, extent, internal structure, consistency, vascularity, relationship to adjacent critical structures, surrounding tissues, and if sarcoma is suspected, the regional nodes.

Common Pathologies

Tendon

Three main pathologies affect tendons. These are (a) tendinosis that relates to degeneration of the tendon substance (Figure 118.11); (b) tenosynovitis, which is inflammation of the tendon sheath surrounding the tendon (Figure 118.12); and calcific tendinitis/tendinosis, which is the result of calcium hydroxyapatite deposition within the tendon substance, inducing tendon inflammation (Figure 118.13).

Tendinosis is by far the most common tendon pathology that one will encounter. It can potentially affect any tendon, although certain tendon areas are particularly prone to developing tendinosis. These include the supraspinatus tendon, the biceps tendon at the upper end of the bicipital groove, and the subscapularis tendon. Other tendons prone to tendinosis

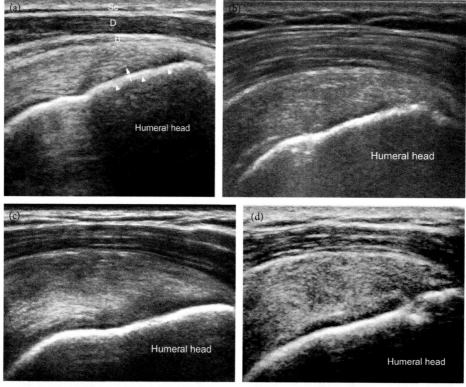

Figure 118.11. Normal supraspinatus tendon and tendinopathy (mild, moderate, severe). (*A*) Long-axis US image showing normal supraspinatus tendon (*arrow*). Note the normal thickness and fibrillar echotexture of this tendon. The supraspinatus tendon inserts onto the greater tuberosity (*arrowheads*). There is a normal thin hypoechoic layer at the insertional region caused by Sharpey fibers. Overlying the supraspinatus tendon is the peribursal fat surrounding the subacromial-subdeltoid bursa (B). Above this is the deltoid muscle (D) and the subcutaneous fat (SC). (*B*) Mild supraspinatus tendinosis. Note how the tendon is diffusely and mildly thickened with mild reduction in clarity of the fibrillar echotexture. (*C*) Moderate supraspinatus tendinosis. The tendon is moderately thickened with moderate loss in clarity of the fibrillar echotexture. (*D*) Severe supraspinatus tendinosis. There is marked diffuse swelling of the supraspinatus tendon with near complete loss of the underlying fibrillar echotexture.

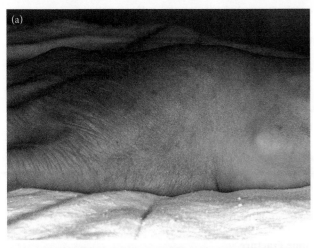

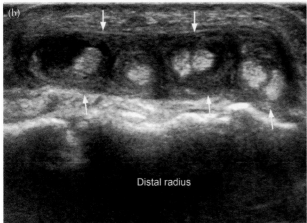

Figure 118.12. Tenosynovitis of the extensor digitorum tendons. (*A*) Localized soft tissue swelling and erythema on the dorsum of the hand in an elderly female patient with tenosynovitis. (*B*) Corresponding short-axis US image on the dorsal aspect of the distal radius shows moderate extensor digitorum tenosynovitis. Note how the tendon sheath around the extensor tendons on the dorsum of the wrist is moderately thickened (*arrows*), whereas there is only mild thickening of the echogenic extensor digitorum tendons.

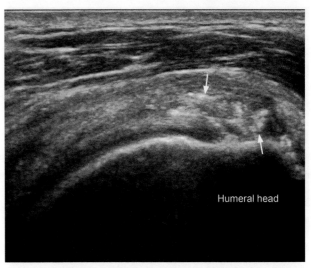

Figure 118.13. Calcific tendinitis of the supraspinatus tendon. Long-axis US image shows moderate calcific tendinosis with irregular calcific deposition (*arrows*) within the more lateral fibers of the supraspinatus tendon just proximal to the insertional area.

are of the common extensor tendon origin at the elbow, the first and sixth extensor compartment tendons at the wrist, the adductor and hamstring tendons at their pelvic attachments, the patellar and Achilles tendons, as well as the posterior tibialis tendon.

It is very important to grade the severity of tendinosis present into mild, moderate, or severe (Figure 118.11). This grading is mainly based on the degree of (a) tendon thickening, (b) disruption of the normal fibrillar echotexture, (c) tendon hypoechogenicity, and (d) intrinsic vascularity. Tendon tears are uncommon in normal tendons, though they occur with increasing frequency in more severe degrees of tendinosis.

Muscle

Muscle tears can occur either within the substance of the muscle or at the myotendinous junction. The most common muscle tear encountered is at the distal end of the medial belly of the gastrocnemius muscle (Figure 118.14A). Myotendinous tears at this location manifest as loss of the normal arrowhead

configuration (Figure 118.14*B*). These myotendinous tears can be very small, and one should closely look at this area in patients presenting with *tennis leg*.

Ligament

Most ligament tears can be readily assessed with US. Ligament tears can be complete or partial. A partial tear is diagnosed when overall ligament continuity is maintained; either a discrete partial tear is seen or there is diffuse ligamentous swelling in the absence of any discrete localized tear. The most commonly torn ligament is the anterior talofibular ligament of the ankle (Figure 118.15). This can be readily appreciated with US as can attached avulsion fractures. One should routinely also assess the calcaneofibular and the anterior talofibular ligaments when examining the posttraumatic ankle.

Nerve Entrapment

US is increasingly used to assess nerve entrapment, particularly at the carpal and cubital tunnels. The main US criterion used to determine nerve entrapment is localized nerve swelling (Figure 118.16) proximal to the site of entrapment and narrowing at the entrapment site.

Bursa

Most bursae can be readily assessed with US. Appearances vary from a hypoechoic fluid-filled mass to a more solid-looking appearance as seen in olecranon bursitis (Figure 118.17). Hyperemia on color/power Doppler imaging may indicate active inflammation.

Cysts

Other than ganglion cysts, the most common cyst encountered is a popliteal/Baker cyst. This cyst originates from a capsular recess on the posteromedial aspect of the knee. It extends in a soap-bubble configuration between the medial belly of the gastrocnemius and the adjacent semimembranosus/semitendinosus tendons (Figure 118.18A). Because they are in

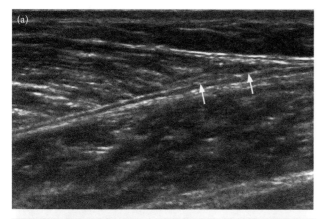

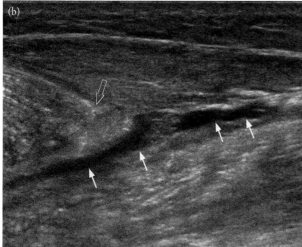

Figure 118.14. Normal medial head of gastrocnemius-soleus aponeurosis and muscle tear (tennis leg). (*A*) Long-axis US image of the distal end of the medial belly of the gastrocnemius muscle shows the normal arrowhead configuration of the muscle belly at the myotendinous junction (*arrows*). (*B*) Long-axis US image of the distal end of the medial belly of the gastrocnemius muscle in a patient with calf muscle tear (tennis leg) shows a tear at the myotendinous junction (*arrows*). The tear is filled with fluid. Note the more rounded appearance of the retracted medial belly of the gastrocnemius muscle (*open arrow*).

continuity, pathologic processes affecting the knee synovium, such as synovitis; osseous/chondral fragments; and synovial tumors, such as PVNS may extend into the bursa (Figure 118.18*B*). One should always assess Baker cysts for signs of peribursal fluid leakage or internal hemorrhage (Figure 118.18*C*).

Synovitis and Erosions

US is used frequently to assess for the presence, severity, and activity of synovial proliferation. The wrist and small joints of the hand are most commonly assessed (Figure 118.19). Synovitis is usually graded semiquantitatively as mild, moderate, or severe, based on the degree of synovial proliferation and vascularity. US is approximately 6 times more sensitive than radiography at detecting bone erosions (Figure 118.20).

Bone Fracture

Some bone fractures are radiographically occult, and some of these fractures can be readily appreciated with US. The classic example are rib fractures. Only approximately 15% of acute rib fractures are visible radiographically even with dedicated rib views. US over the painful area will demonstrate close to 100% of these fractures and can also discriminate between acute fractures and healing chronic fractures (Figure 118.21).

Soft Tissue Masses

US is very useful for assessing superficial soft tissue masses. Based on the US appearances, one can determine the nature of superficial masses with a high degree of accuracy (Figures 118.22 and 118.23). In experienced hands, the overall accuracy in this aspect is more than 80%.

Clinical Implications

US is the best first-line investigation for most soft tissue pathologies. An explanation for patient symptoms can often be obtained with US examination. MSK US is most useful when symptoms are localized to specific area, for example, point tenderness. US is much less useful when symptoms are not localizable or poorly localized, for example, pain related to the entire knee or the entire ankle joint. One should try to grade every abnormality encountered. For example, rather than mentioning that there is supraspinatus tendinosis present, it

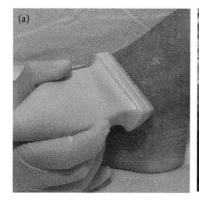

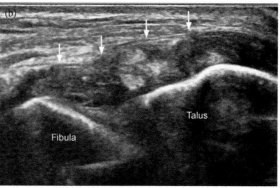

Figure 118.15. ATFL tear. (*A*) Positioning of the transducer over the ATFL. (*B*) Long-axis US image shows a complete tear of the ATFL between the fibula and the talus. The intervening gap is partially filled with hematoma (*arrows*).

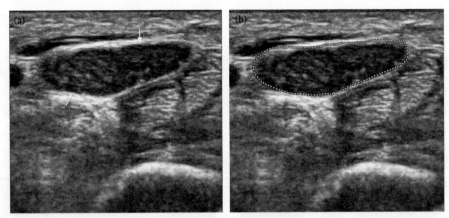

Figure 118.16. Thickened median nerve in CTS. (*A*) Short-axis US image of the wrist shows a thickened median nerve just proximal to the carpal tunnel inlet (*arrows*). The transverse carpal ligament is not visible on this image, which is located just proximal to the tunnel inlet. (*B*) Tracing around the margin of the nerve using electronic calipers shows the cross-sectional area of the median nerve to be 17 mm2. The normal cross-sectional area of the nerve in the carpal tunnel should be <11 mm². The larger the cross-sectional area of the median nerve at the carpal tunnel, the more likely the patient has CTS.

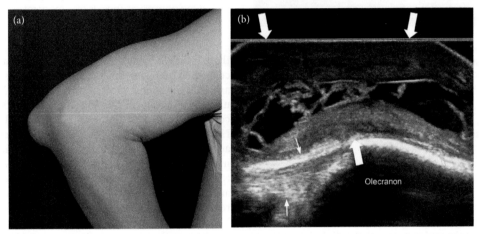

Figure 118.17. Olecranon bursitis. (*A*) Clinical image of patient with olecranon bursitis. (*B*) Long-axis US image of the same patient as previous image shows a markedly thickened septated fluid-filled complex olecranon bursa that blends with subcutaneous fat, consistent with olecranon bursitis (*block arrows*). Note the triceps tendon (*arrows*) inserting onto the tip of the olecranon process.

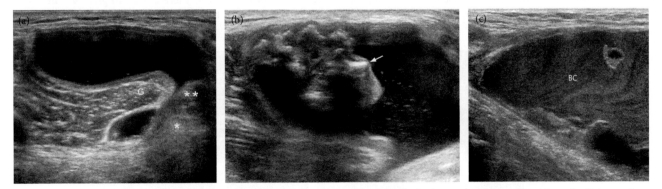

Figure 118.18. Baker cyst. (*A*) Short-axis US image of the popliteal fossa shows the typical *soap-bubble* configuration of a Baker cyst. The neck of the cyst extends between the medial belly of the gastrocnemius (G) and the adjacent semimembranosus (*asterisk*) and semitendinosus (*double asterisk*) tendons. The cyst is filled with anechoic fluid. (*B*) Short-axis US image of the popliteal fossa shows a partially calcified body within the popliteal (Baker) cyst (*arrow*). Osteochondral bodies from the knee can displace into a Baker cyst where they can enlarge and ossify similar to those seen within the knee joint. (*C*) Longitudinal oblique US image of popliteal fossa shows a distended Baker cyst (BC) that is filled with echogenic fluid from spontaneous internal hemorrhage.

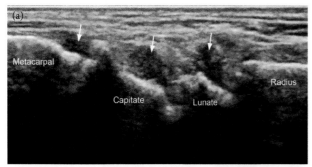

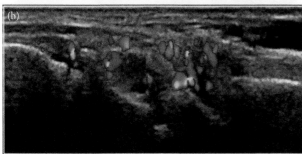

Figure 118.19. Synovitis in the wrist. (*A*) Long-axis US image of the dorsal aspect of the wrist showing moderate synovial proliferation at the radiolunate, lunocapitate, and carpometacarpal articulations (*arrows*). (*B*) Color Doppler image (US) of the same area shows moderate hyperemia compatible with moderate synovitis. When assessing color Doppler in this situation, the transducer should be actively lifted off the skin while using copious amounts of gel to minimize any transducer pressure.

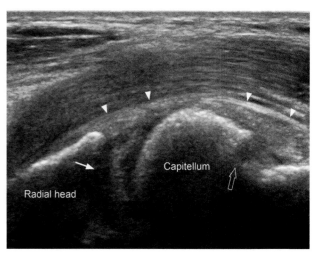

Figure 118.20. RA of the elbow. Long-axis US image in a patient with long-standing RA shows severe synovial proliferation on the anterior aspect of the elbow joint (*arrowheads*) with a moderate-sized discrete erosion (*open arrow*) at the proximal end of the capitellum. There is also moderate subchondral reabsorption of the radial head (*arrow*).

is important to describe whether the abnormality is minimal, mild, moderate, or severe.

US diagnosis is based not just on a single US sign, but on multiple US findings according to their relative strengths and known specificities in conjunction with the clinical symptoms. If the findings are indeterminate, one can either follow up with repeat US; proceed to an alternative investigation, such as MRI; or proceed to US-guided biopsy (or fine-needle aspiration).

Similarly, if satisfactory explanations for other symptoms are not found on US examination, it is usually best to proceed to further investigation, usually MRI. Generally,

there is little benefit to be gained from repeating the US, except when following the longitudinal progress of disease. US and MRI are complementary investigations. MRI has particular advantages over US, and in these situations either proceed directly to MRI (or perform MRI after US assessment). However, MRI is particularly useful for assessing areas not accessible to US (eg, intraarticular or intraosseous abnormality). MRI allows improved perception of large objects (particularly those with deep margins, ill-defined lesions, and large tumors) and provides a clear anatomical surgical roadmap. MRI allows more reliable volume assessment of ill-defined structures (eg, synovial volume) and is more sensitive at depicting soft tissue edema. US should ideally precede MRI for most soft tissue problems. MRI examination can then be tailored to answer only those specific questions not answered by US. For example, there is no need to examine regional lymph nodes if US assessment was already performed, nor is there a need to give IV contrast if tumor vascularity has been determined by US, unless the

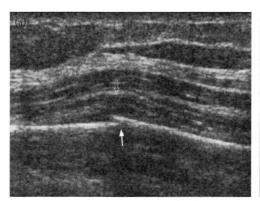

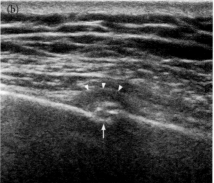

Figure 118.21. Radiographically occult rib fracture on US. (*A*) Transverse US image of the chest wall shows a mildly angulated acute rib fracture (*arrow*) along the anterior axillary line with mild overlying soft tissue swelling (*open arrow*). The radiograph (*not shown*) was normal. (*B*) Transverse US image of the chest wall shows a healing rib fracture (*arrow*) in the mid-axillary line. There is a rim of hypoechoic callus (*arrowheads*) surrounding the fracture with partial echogenic mineralization of this callus.

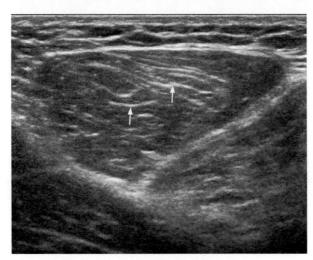

Figure 118.22. Soft tissue lipoma. Transverse US image of the groin shows a well-defined lipoma lying within the subcutaneous tissue. Lipomas are typically well marginated, of similar echogenicity to the surrounding fat, and contain fine echogenic lines (*arrows*) aligned along the long axis of the tumor.

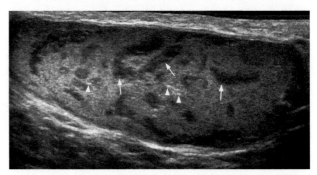

Figure 118.23. Epidermoid inclusion cyst. Transverse extended FOV US image of the gluteal region shows a well-defined subcutaneous epidermoid cyst. Epidermoid cysts are typically well-defined with hypoechoic areas caused by myxoid accumulation (*arrows*) as well as echogenic linear clefts caused by keratin deposition (*arrowheads*). Although not apparent in this image, a small tract extending from the cyst to the skin surface may occasionally be seen.

contrast-enhanced MRI is used as a baseline prior to therapy for follow-up studies.

Newer Ultrasound Techniques

3D US imaging acquires volumetric US data, which can be reconstructed along any plane. This has been used to evaluate rotator cuff tears, soft tissues masses, and synovial proliferation. *Fusion imaging* allows real-time US imaging to be superimposed onto preloaded CT or MRI and viewed simultaneously on the US screen. Fusion imaging has been used to assist with needle guidance for bone biopsy or SI joint injection. It generally tends to be used by practitioners less familiar with US. *US elastography* is a technique that measures and displays tissue elasticity using US. There are 2 types of US elastography. *Strain elastography* involves gentle manual compression of the tissues by the transducer, which causes axial tissue displacement (strain) that is measured by comparing echo datasets before and after compression. The measure is a ratio of normal-to-abnormal tissue. *Shear wave elastography* is based on a different physical principle and requires a specially modified transducer that produces high-intensity acoustic pulses (push pulses). These acoustic push pulses induce shear waves, the velocities of which are then tracked by diagnostic impulses. The measure is a quantifiable. Elastography has been used to study tendons, muscles, and soft tissue masses and seems to be able to detect tendon abnormality before grayscale imaging. Although elastography is a potentially useful technical development in US, it does require (a) standardization to provide consistency in clinical application and allow comparison between studies and (b) recognition of those areas where elastography is likely to provide added value over standard US imaging. Microbubble-based US contrast imaging significantly improves the detection of synovial vascularity, helping to grade the degree of synovial activity.

References

1. Arend CF. Top ten pitfalls to avoid when performing musculoskeletal sonography: what you should know before entering the examination room. *Eur J Radiol.* 2013;82(11):1933–39.
2. Barr RG. Elastography in clinical practice. *Radiol Clin North Am.* 2014;52(6):1145–62.
3. Carra BJ, Bui-Mansfield LT, O'Brien SD, Chen DC. Sonography of musculoskeletal soft-tissue masses: techniques, pearls, and pitfalls. *AJR Am J Roentgenol.* 2014;202(6):1281–90.
4. Corazza A, Orlandi D, Fabbro E, et al. Dynamic high-resolution ultrasound of the shoulder: how we do it. *Eur J Radiol.* 2015;84(2):266–77.
5. Gimber LH, Melville DM, Klauser AS, Witte RS, Arif-Tiwari H, Taljanovic MS. Artifacts at musculoskeletal US: resident and fellow education feature. *Radiographics.* 2016;36(2):479–80.
6. Griffith JF, Rainer TH, Ching AS, Law KL, Cocks RA, Metreweli C. Sonography compared with radiography in revealing acute rib fracture. *AJR Am J Roentgenol.* 1999;173(6):1603–609.
7. Gupta H, Robinson P. Normal shoulder ultrasound: anatomy and technique. *Semin Musculoskelet Radiol.* 2015;19(3):203–11.
8. Tagliafico AS, Bignotti B, Martinoli C. Elbow US: anatomy, variants, and scanning technique. *Radiology.* 2015;275(3):636–50.
9. Hung EH, Griffith JF, Ng AW, Lee RK, Lau DT, Leung JC. Ultrasound of musculoskeletal soft-tissue tumors superficial to the investing fascia. *AJR Am J Roentgenol.* 2014;202(6):W532–40.
10. Klauser AS, Miyamoto H, Bellmann-Weiler R, Feuchtner GM, Wick MC, Jaschke WR. Sonoelastography: musculoskeletal applications. *Radiology.* 2014;272(3):622–33.
11. Taljanovic MS, Alcala JN, Gimber LH, Rieke JD, Chilvers MM, Latt LD. High-resolution US and MR imaging of peroneal tendon injuries. *Radiographics.* 2015;35(1):179–99.
12. Taljanovic MS, Melville DM, Scalcione LR, Gimber LH, Lorenz EJ, Witte RS. Artifacts in musculoskeletal ultrasonography. *Semin Musculoskelet Radiol.* 2014;18(1):3–11.
13. Taljanovic MS, Melville DM, Gimber LH, et al. High-resolution US of rheumatologic diseases. *Radiographics.* 2015;35(7):2026–48.

14. Sofka CM. Ultrasound of the hand and wrist. *Ultrasound Q.* 2014;30(3):184–92.

15. Taljanovic MS, Goldberg MR, Sheppard JE, Rogers LF. US of the intrinsic and extrinsic wrist ligaments and triangular fibrocartilage complex—normal anatomy and imaging technique. *Radiographics.* 2011;31(1):e44.

16. Yablon CM, Lee KS, Jacobson JA. Musculoskeletal ultrasonography: starting your practice. *Semin Roentgenol.* 2013;48(2):167–77.

17. Wong SM, Griffith JF, Hui AC, Lo SK, Fu M, Wong KS. Carpal tunnel syndrome: diagnostic usefulness of sonography. *Radiology.* 2004;232(1):93–9.

CHAPTER 119

Imaging Artifacts in Musculoskeletal Ultrasound

Lana H. Gimber

Introduction

US artifacts can be seen with B-mode grayscale and Doppler imaging. These artifacts occur when the US beam deviates from ideal physical beam assumptions. Recognizing artifacts helps to differentiate them from true pathology.

Grayscale Artifacts

Artifacts Related to Intrinsic Characteristics of the Ultrasound Beam

Side Lobe Artifact
Refer to Figure 119.1.

- Side lobes are much weaker secondary US lobes outside the main beam.
- Produced: When a side lobe interacts with an object outside the main US path, the object is incorrectly recorded as if located along the main US beam path.
- Appearance: multiple needle paths and echoes or reflections within cystic or solid structures
- Minimize: Use alternate scanning planes.

Beam-Width Artifact
Refer to Figure 119.1.

- The main US beam narrows to a focal zone and then fans out distally.
- Produced: When an object is located outside the margin of the transducer but inside the distal widened beam, the object is recorded at an incorrect location.
- Appearance: spurious echoes within cystic structures or reduced contrast at a lesion border
- Minimize: Adjust the focal zone to the level of the structure of interest.

Anisotropy
Refer to Figure 119.2.

- The US beam should be perpendicular to an imaged structure to create maximum sound wave reflection.
- Produced: when the transducer is not perpendicular to an imaged structure and many returning echoes are not recorded

- Appearance: hypoechogenicity that can mimic tears in tendons and ligaments
- Minimize: Use the heel-toe maneuver of the transducer.

Artifacts Related to Errors in Velocity
Refraction

- Sound travels through different materials or tissues at different speeds.
- Produced: when US beam changes direction as it reaches an interface between 2 materials at different speeds of sound, creating an echo that is recorded in an incorrect location
- Appearance: widened or misplaced structure on the US image
- Minimize: Use multiple scan planes.

Speed Displacement
Refer to Figure 119.3.

- The depth of an object is not always related to the time it takes the echo to return to the US transducer.
- Produced: When the US beam in 1 region travels slower than in the other regions, the echo in the slower region is recorded later than the surrounding echoes, causing this portion to appear as if it is located farther away.
- Appearance: biopsy needle with an area of focal displacement or discontinuity

Artifacts Related to Errors in Attenuation
Increased Through Transmission or Posterior Acoustic Enhancement
Refer to Figure 119.4.

- Some sound waves are absorbed in the examined tissues.
- Produced: when a weak attenuator, such as a cyst, attenuates the US beam to a lesser extent than the surrounding tissues causing the soft tissues deep to the lesion to appear hyperechogenic compared to the surrounding soft tissues
- Appearance: Tissues deep to a lesion appear hyperechoic compared to surrounding tissues.
- Benefit: helps to differentiate a cystic lesion from a solid lesion
- Pitfall: Some solid lesions such as peripheral nerve sheath tumor or lymphoma may produce this artifact.

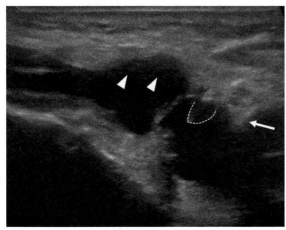

Figure 119.1. Side lobe and beam-width artifact. Long-axis grayscale US image at the posterior aspect of the knee shows a Baker cyst. A low-level echo (*delineated with a dotted line*) is seen within the cystic structure secondary to a side lobe beam interacting with an off-axis, highly reflective acoustic surface (*arrow*), which is erroneously recorded as if along the main US beam path, consistent with side lobe artifact. Also seen are spurious echoes within the cyst (*arrowheads*), which are generated by objects located outside the margin of the transducer but inside the distal widened beam consistent with beam-width artifact.

Posterior Acoustic Shadowing
Refer to Figures 119.5 and 119.6.

- Produced: when the US beam is reflected, absorbed, or refracted by a strongly attenuating object (eg, bone, calcification, foreign body, gas). Echoes deep to the object are lower in intensity when compared to surrounding tissues.
- Appearance: anechoic or hypoechoic area deep to a structure
- Clean posterior acoustic shadowing: anechoic region deep to an object with a small radius of curvature or rough surface

- Dirty posterior acoustic shadowing: heterogeneous hypoechoic region deep to an object with a large radius of curvature or smooth surface

Artifacts Related to Multiple Echo Paths
Posterior Reverberation Artifact
Refer to Figure 119.7.

- A reflector can produce more than 1 echo.
- Produced: when there are 2 parallel strong reflectors and an echo is repeatedly reflected back and forth between them before returning to the transducer. Each returning echo will take longer and longer to reach the transducer and will erroneously be displayed as deeper to the echo before it.
- Appearance: can be seen with biopsy needles where there are multiple echoes at regularly spaced intervals located deep to the actual needle

Comet-Tail Artifact
Refer to Figure 119.8.

- Produced: a form of posterior reverberation artifact, often caused by metal or calcium
- Appearance: decreased amplitude of distal echoes and appearance of trailing off of echoes deep to a structure. It may be impossible to discern individual echoes from one another because they are closely spaced.

Ring Down Artifact
Refer to Figure 119.9.

- Produced: resonant vibrations caused by fluid trapped between air bubbles
- Appearance: similar to posterior reverberation and comet-tail artifact

Mirror Image Artifact
Refer to Figure 119.10.

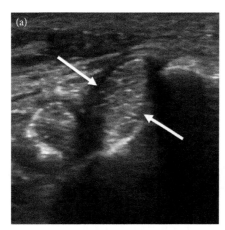
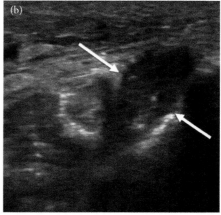

Figure 119.2. Anisotropy. (*A*) Short-axis grayscale US image of the posterior tibial tendon at the level of the ankle shows a normal echogenic tendon (*arrows*). (*B*) The tendon appears hypoechoic (*arrows*), which can mimic a tendon tear, caused by anisotropy when the transducer is not perpendicular to the imaged structure.

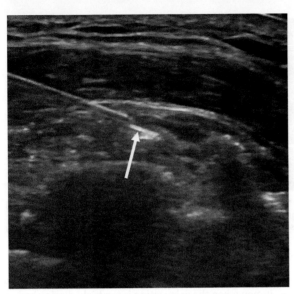

Figure 119.3. Speed displacement. Grayscale US image during calcium lavage for calcific tendinosis shows a lavage needle with a focally displaced region (*arrow*) caused by increased travel time of the US sound waves through the soft tissues superficial to this region.

- Produced: when there is a strong reflector (eg, bone) deep to an imaged object. An US echo bounces off the strong reflector and object of interest before returning to the transducer. The delay in echo return causes an image to be recorded as if it is deep to the strong reflector.
- Appearance: an erroneous duplicate image appearing deep and equidistant to a strong reflective interface

---

Artifacts Related to Doppler Imaging

Transducer Pressure
Refer to Figure 119.11.

- Produced: when vascular flow is blocked by excessive transducer pressure

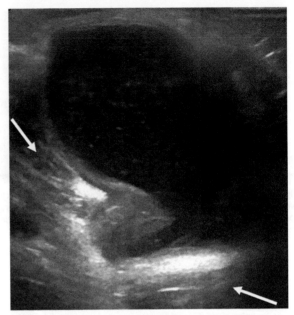

Figure 119.4. Increased through transmission or posterior acoustic enhancement. Grayscale US image of a Baker cyst at the posterior aspect of the knee shows a hyperechoic appearance of the soft tissues deep to this lesion (*arrows*) caused by less attenuation of US waves by the cyst compared to the adjacent soft tissues.

- Appearance: erroneously low or lack of blood flow within a structure
- Minimize: Avoid excessive transducer pressure and use copious amounts of US gel on the skin.

Motion Artifact
Refer to Figure 119.12.

- Produced: by motion of the transducer or patient
- Appearance: erroneous areas of vascularity and flashes of color on Doppler imaging
- Minimize: Reduce motion and use of high-pass wall filters.

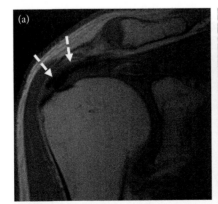
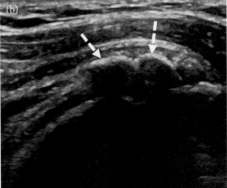

Figure 119.5. Clean posterior acoustic shadowing. (*A*) T1W coronal MR image of the right shoulder demonstrates calcific tendinitis (*dashed arrows*) within the distal supraspinatus tendon. (*B*) Long-axis grayscale US image of the same region in the right shoulder shows an anechoic appearance deep to the small radius calcifications, which is consistent with clean posterior acoustic shadowing (*dashed arrows*).

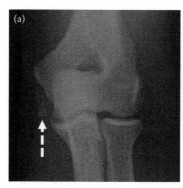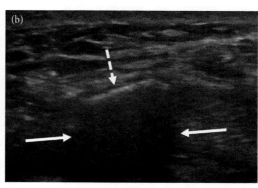

Figure 119.6. Dirty posterior acoustic shadowing. (*A*) AP radiograph of the elbow shows a radiopaque foreign body (*dashed arrow*) within the soft tissues at the medial aspect of the elbow. (*B*) Long-axis grayscale US image in this region demonstrates the same foreign body (*dashed arrow*) with dirty posterior acoustic shadowing (*solid arrows*) within the soft tissues deep to this site caused by the smooth surface of the object.

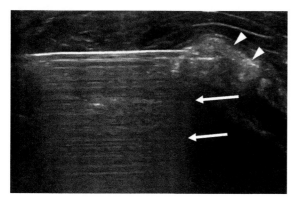

Figure 119.7. Posterior reverberation. Grayscale US image during calcium lavage for calcific tendinosis (*arrowheads*) of the right subscapularis tendon shows a lavage needle with multiple echoes (*arrows*) at regularly spaced intervals located deep to the actual needle.

Blooming
Refer to Figure 119.13.

- Produced: when there is inappropriate gain setting on the US machine

- Appearance: *bleeding* of color outside the true vessel lumen when the gain setting is too high; diminished caliber of the vessel when the gain setting is too low
- Minimize: Select an appropriate gain setting.

Background Noise
Refer to Figure 119.14.

- Produced: when the gain setting is set too high on the US machine
- Appearance: With color Doppler, the background noise appears as a speckled pattern of colors; with power Doppler, the background noise appears as a uniform color as it does not show direction of the flow.
- Minimize: Set the gain to a level where there is almost no background noise.

Mirror Image Artifact
Refer to Figure 119.15.

- Produced: by similar mechanism as with grayscale mirror image artifact
- Appearance: erroneous duplicate vessel that is equidistant and deep to a strong reflector

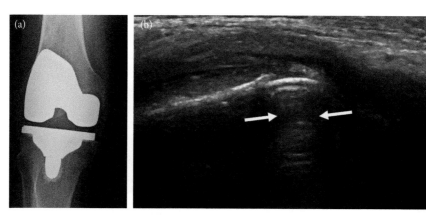

Figure 119.8. Comet-tail artifact. (*A*) External oblique radiograph of the right knee demonstrates a total knee arthroplasty. (*B*) Long-axis grayscale US image of this region shows multiple echoes (*arrows*) deep to the highly reflective metal surface that appear to trail off.

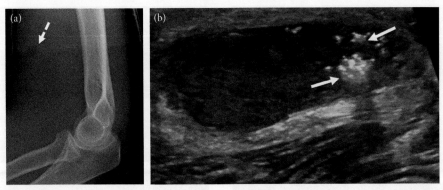

Figure 119.9. Ring down artifact. (*A*) Lateral radiograph of the elbow in a patient with history of IV drug abuse demonstrates a focus of air (*dashed arrow*) within the soft tissues at the anterior aspect of the distal upper arm. (*B*) Long-axis grayscale US image of the same region demonstrates a hypoechoic fluid collection containing foci of air (*arrows*) with multiple trailing echoes deep to the foci of air, which is created by resonant vibrations of fluid trapped between air bubbles.

Aliasing

Refer to Figure 119.16.

- The maximum velocity scale is limited by the pulse repetition frequency (PRF), which is the number of US pulses per second that can be transmitted and received by the transducer. For proper US imaging, the maximum velocity scale must be at least twice the Nyquist limit, which is the maximum frequency shift. Directional flow velocity information is only provided with color Doppler imaging and not with power Doppler imaging.
- Produced: occurs when the velocity scale is less than twice the Nyquist limit and the measured velocities exceed the scale available to display it
- Appearance: only seen with color Doppler imaging as multiple adjacent colors within a vessel
- Minimize: Raise the PRF, change the baseline, or use power Doppler imaging.

Twinkle Artifact

Refer to Figure 119.17.

- Produced: caused by intrinsic machine noise called *phase* (or clock) jitter

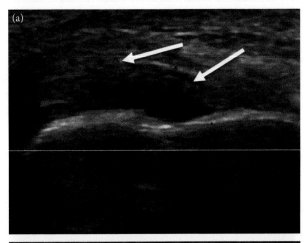

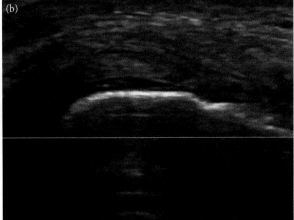

Figure 119.11. Transducer pressure. (*A*) Long-axis power Doppler US image of the great toe extensor tendon at the level of the metatarsal head shows mildly increased vascularity (*arrows*) in this region. (*B*) Excessive transducer pressure applied in the same region blocks vascular flow and gives the appearance of no vascularity to this region.

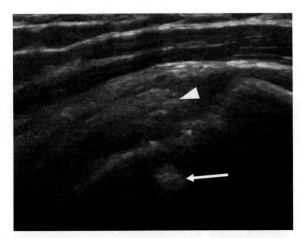

Figure 119.10. Mirror image artifact. Long-axis grayscale US image of the infraspinatus tendon shows an echogenic focus of calcium hydroxyapatite (*arrowhead*). An erroneous duplicated lesion appears deep and equidistant to the humeral cortex, which acts as a highly reflective interface (*arrow*).

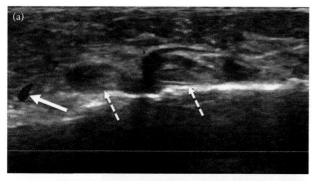

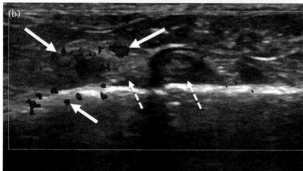

Figure 119.12. Motion artifact. (*A*) Short-axis power Doppler US image of the peroneus longus and peroneus brevis tendons (*dashed arrows*) at the lateral aspect of the ankle shows minimal peripheral vascularity (*arrow*). (*B*) With transducer motion, there are increased random flashes of color (*arrows*).

- Appearance: color signal related to a strongly reflecting interface (eg, calcifications, calculi, bones, foreign bodies) that does not have intrinsic real flow or movement
- Benefit: can be used to verify presence of calcifications, stones, or foreign bodies

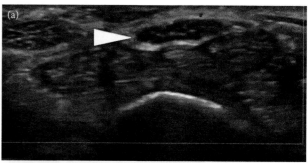

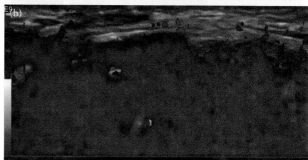

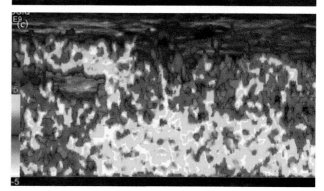

Figure 119.14. Background noise. (*A*) Short-axis power Doppler image shows the median nerve (*arrowhead*) at the level of the carpal tunnel. (*B*) Power Doppler image with the gain set too high shows uniform background color because power Doppler does not provide directional information of flow. (*C*) Color Doppler image with the gain set too high shows a speckled pattern of background colors.

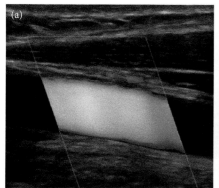
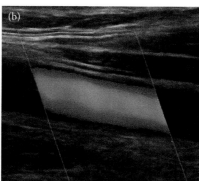
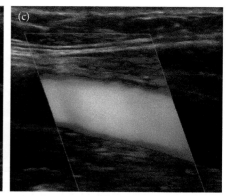

Figure 119.13. Blooming artifact. (*A*) Long-axis power Doppler US image of the femoral artery shows normal caliber of the vessel. (*B*) When the gain is set too low, the caliber of the vessel appears diminished. (*C*) When the gain is set too high, there is extensive *bleeding* of color outside the true vessel lumen.

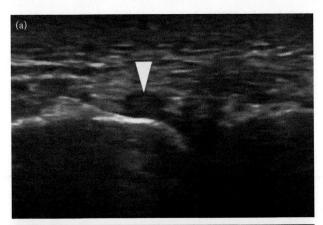

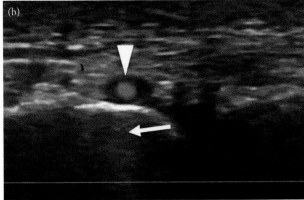

Figure 119.15. Mirror image artifact with Doppler imaging. (*A*) Short-axis grayscale US image of the dorsalis pedis artery shows the hypoechogenic vessel (*arrowhead*). (*B*) Power Doppler image in the same region demonstrates the red-colored dorsalis pedis artery (*arrowhead*) with a deeper erroneous duplicate vessel (*arrow*) secondary to the highly reflective surface of the bone.

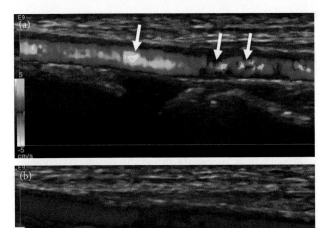

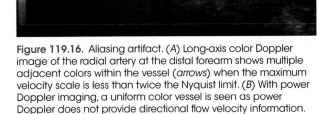

Figure 119.16. Aliasing artifact. (*A*) Long-axis color Doppler image of the radial artery at the distal forearm shows multiple adjacent colors within the vessel (*arrows*) when the maximum velocity scale is less than twice the Nyquist limit. (*B*) With power Doppler imaging, a uniform color vessel is seen as power Doppler does not provide directional flow velocity information.

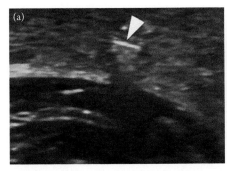

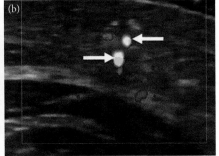

Figure 119.17. Twinkle artifact. (*A*) Short-axis grayscale US image of the soft tissues at the dorsal aspect of the mid forearm shows a linear echogenicity corresponding to 1 of the foreign bodies (*arrowhead*). (*B*) Color Doppler US image in this region show spurious Doppler signal (*arrows*) in the areas of the foreign bodies.

Key Points

- US artifacts occur with both B-mode grayscale and Doppler imaging when evaluating the MSK system.
- It is important for radiologists to have an understanding of these artifacts in order to distinguish them from pathology.

Recommended Reading

Gimber LH, Melville DM, Klauser AS, Witte RS, Arif-Tiwari H, Taljanovic MS. Artifacts at musculoskeletal US: resident and fellow education feature. *Radiographics*. 2016 Mar-Apr;36(2):479–80

References

1. Feldman MK, Katyal S, Blackwood MS. US artifacts. *Radiographics.* 2009;29(4):1179–89.
2. Kamaya A, Tuthill T, Rubin JM. Twinkling artifact on color Doppler sonography: dependence on machine parameters and underlying cause. *AJR Am J Roentgenol.* 2003;180(1):215–22.
3. Nilsson A. Artefacts in sonography and Doppler. *Eur Radiol.* 2001;11(8):1308–15.
4. Pozniak MA, Zagzebski JA, Scanlan KA. Spectral and color Doppler artifacts. *Radiographics.* 1992;12(1):35–44.
5. Reynolds DL Jr., Jacobson JA, Inampudi P, Jamadar DA, Ebrahim FS, Hayes CW. Sonographic characteristics of peripheral nerve sheath tumors. *AJR Am J Roentgenol.* 2004;182(3):741–44.
6. Rubens DJ, Bhatt S, Nedelka S, Cullinan J. Doppler artifacts and pitfalls. *Radiol Clin North Am.* 2006;44(6):805–35.
7. Rubin JM, Adler RS, Bude RO, Fowlkes JB, Carson PL. Clean and dirty shadowing at US: a reappraisal. *Radiology.* 1991;181(1):231–36.
8. Scanlan KA. Sonographic artifacts and their origins. *AJR Am J Roentgenol.* 1991;156(6):1267–72.
9. Taljanovic MS, Melville DM, Scalcione LR, Gimber LH, Lorenz EJ, Witte RS. Artifacts in musculoskeletal ultrasonography. *Semin Musculoskelet Radiol.* 2014;18(1): 3–11.
10. Teh J. Applications of Doppler imaging in the musculoskeletal system. *Curr Probl Diagn Radiol.* 2006;35(1):22–34.

CHAPTER 120

Ultrasound of the Shoulder

Corrie M. Yablon

Background

Shoulder soft tissue injuries in the United States most commonly occur because of chronic overuse and repetitive microtrauma, rather than acute trauma. Rotator cuff injury is the most common indication for US of the shoulder. US provides equal accuracy to MRI in the diagnosis of full-thickness and partial-thickness rotator cuff tears. US has several advantages over MRI: higher resolution, portability, lower cost, and the capacity to perform dynamic imaging. Less common indications for shoulder US include the evaluation of pathology of the long head of the biceps tendon (LHBT), subacromial-subdeltoid bursa, postsurgical rotator cuff, and AC joint. US is less useful for the evaluation of bone or deep intraarticular structures such as the glenoid labrum, because the sound beam is attenuated by bone. If labral, ligamentous, glenohumeral joint, or osseous abnormalities are suspected, MRI is the preferred examination. US should be the first-line modality in the evaluation of shoulder pain in patients older than 40 years, as the incidence of rotator cuff disease increases with patient age. In patients younger than 40 years with shoulder pain, MRI should be the modality of choice, as labral pathology is much more common than rotator cuff disease in this age group.

Ultrasound Examination of the Shoulder

There are many excellent textbooks and articles that describe in detail how to perform an US examination of the shoulder, which is beyond the scope of this review. US examination of the shoulder should be performed according to a defined protocol evaluating the rotator cuff and surrounding structures (Table 120.1). High-frequency linear transducers of at least 12 MHz provide high-resolution images of the rotator cuff. Rotator cuff tendons should be evaluated in both the long and short axis planes.

Tendon Pathology

- *Tendinosis* is caused by mucoid degeneration of the tendon and not by inflammation:
  - *Tendinitis* is an inappropriate term as there is no inflammation.
  - In older patients, most rotator cuff and LHBT injuries in the shoulder are caused by repetitive motion, causing tendon degeneration, which may lead to tendon rupture.
  - In younger patients, rotator cuff injury is most often caused by acute trauma or by overhead-throwing sports.
  - Tendinosis may cause pain even in the absence of associated tears.
- *Tendon rupture* or avulsion infrequently occurs because of acute trauma or because of systemic disease such as RA, lupus, or diabetes.
- *Partial-thickness tendon tear*
  - Occurs in patients of all ages
  - Most commonly seen in the supraspinatus tendon
  - May eventually progress to full-thickness tear
  - Both anteroposterior and medial-lateral dimensions of the tear should be reported, in addition to the percentage of the tendon thickness involved with partial tears.
  - Conservative therapy is generally reserved for partial-thickness tears involving less than 50% of the tendon thickness.
  - Debridement may be performed for partial-thickness tears exceeding 50% of the tendon thickness.
- *Calcific tendinosis* (calcium hydroxyapatite deposition)
  - Occurs most commonly in the supraspinatus tendon
  - Accounts for 7% of patients with shoulder pain
  - Self-limited but pain may be severe enough to warrant intervention such as percutaneous lavage

Imaging Features

- Normal tendon
  - Long axis—fibrillar, linear, and echogenic.
  - Short axis—speckled, ovoid, and echogenic (Figure 120.1)
- Tendinosis: thickened, hypoechoic, with or without loss of normal fibrillar pattern, may be diffuse or focal, with or without hyperemia on color/power Doppler imaging (Figure 120.2)
- Full-thickness tear: The tendon fibers are completely disrupted (Figure 120.3):
  - Hypoechoic to anechoic gap in tendon, extending from bursal to articular surface, which may be focal or involve the entire tendon
  - Echogenic hemorrhage may be present if acute.
  - Tendon stump may be retracted beneath the acromion if chronic.
  - May see the deltoid muscle directly contacting bone in chronic tears

Table 120.1. Protocol for Ultrasound Examination of the Shoulder

STRUCTURE	PATIENT POSITION	ASSESSMENT
Long head biceps tendon (LHBT)	Arm at side, elbow flexed, palm up	Assess in short and long axis from rotator interval proximally to pectoralis major junction distally
Subscapularis tendon	Arm at side, elbow flexed, shoulder externally rotated, palm up	Assess in short axis from cranial to caudal; assess in long axis from lateral to musculotendinous junction
Dynamic imaging	Arm at side, elbow flexed, palm up, externally and internally rotating at the shoulder	LHBT subluxation or dislocation, subcoracoid impingement
Supraspinatus (SST) and infraspinatus (IST) tendons	Modified Crass or Crass position	Start with the probe aligned with the long axis of the LHBT in the rotator interval, moving the probe posteriorly to image the SST and IST in long axis. Turn the probe perpendicularly to image the SST and IST in short axis from medial to lateral.
Acromioclavicular joint		
Subacromial-subdeltoid bursa, dynamic imaging	Transducer positioned in coronal oblique plane, at the lateral edge of the acromion, with the probe covering lateral acromion and humeral head; patient abducts arm	Evaluate bursa: thickness, fluid, hyperemia Subacromial impingement; pooling of bursal fluid beneath acromion, incomplete supraspinatus gliding underneath the acromion
Infraspinatus and teres minor tendons, spinoglenoid notch, posterior joint recess	Transducer positioned just below and parallel to the scapular spine. Be sure to image laterally through the distal IST footprint on the humeral head.	

- Granulation tissue of variable echogenicity may be present if tear is chronic.
- Massive rotator cuff tear: greater than 5 cm (involves multiple tendons; in the European classification, a massive tear is defined as involving 2 or more tendons)

- Partial-thickness tendon tear: anechoic or hypoechoic cleft extending through only a portion of the tendon (Figure 120.4)
  - Articular surface tear only extends to the articular aspect of the tendon.
  - Bursal surface tear only extends to the subacromial-subdeltoid bursal side of the tendon:

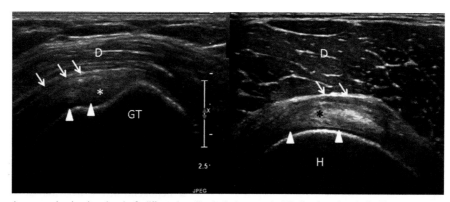

Figure 120.1. Normal supraspinatus tendon in 2 different patients. In long axis (*A*), the tendon is fibrillar and echogenic. The normal tendon (*asterisk*) inserts on the greater tuberosity of the humeral head (GT). Note the deltoid muscle (D) is echogenic because of fatty infiltration and atrophy. In short axis (*B*), the normal supraspinatus tendon (*asterisk*) is speckled and echogenic in appearance. The deltoid muscle (D) in this younger patient demonstrates a normal hypoechoic appearance with thin, echogenic internal septae. On both images, the hyaline cartilage is thin and hypoechoic (*arrowheads*). The subacromial-subdeltoid bursa, situated between the deltoid muscle and supraspinatus tendon, is thin, linear, and hypoechoic (*arrows*).

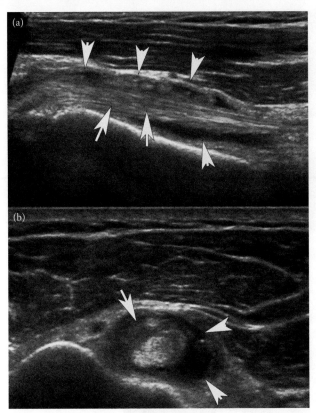

Figure 120.2. Long head of the biceps tendinosis and tenosynovitis. In long axis (*A*) and short axis (*B*), the tendon demonstrates focal hypoechogenicity (*arrows*) consistent with tendinosis. Fluid and synovial distention of the LHBT sheath (*arrowheads*) are consistent with tenosynovitis.

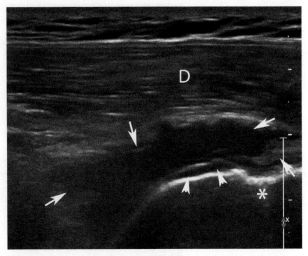

Figure 120.3. Full-thickness supraspinatus tendon tear. In this long-axis image, the supraspinatus tendon is torn and retracted so far beneath the acromion that the tendon stump is not seen. Hypoechoic fluid, echogenic synovium, and debris fill the tendon gap (*arrows*). Note the echogenic appearance of the hyaline cartilage surface (*arrowheads*), caused by the interface with the hypoechoic fluid, also known as the *cartilage interface sign*. Cortical irregularity (*asterisk*) of the greater tuberosity has been shown to correlate with supraspinatus tears. D = deltoid.

- Accompanied by volume loss and flattening at the bursal aspect of tendon
- If a tear extends from the bursal aspect into the footprint of the tendon, but does not contact the articular surface of the tendon, then it is considered a bursal-sided tear.
- Intrasubstance tear (2 subtypes)
  - Longitudinal/delaminating type associated with intramuscular cyst
  - Within the substance of the tendon footprint
  - Both subtypes not visible on arthroscopy
- *Rim-rent* tear is a specific partial-thickness tear subtype that extends from the anterior supraspinatus articular surface into the tendon footprint:
  - Associated with younger athletes and overhead-throwing sports
  - Also referred to as a PASTA (partial articular surface tendon avulsion) lesion
- Calcific tendinosis (tendinopathy) (2 different appearances on US)
  - Amorphous or cloudlike, with or without appreciable shadowing, associated with the resorptive (painful) phase (Figure 120.5)
  - Well-defined, ovoid, with shadowing structures
  - If calcifications become very large, they can impede abduction and cause secondary impingement on the rotator cuff.

Long Head of the Biceps Tendon

- Often associated with subscapularis and supraspinatus tendon pathology, subcoracoid impingement, and subacromial impingement
- If subscapularis is torn, the LHBT may dislocate medially into the joint.
- Tendinosis and longitudinal partial tearing are the most frequently seen LHBT pathologies, most commonly occurring in the rotator interval.
- Tenosynovitis is commonly seen in the LHBT sheath (see Figure 120.2):
  - Hypoechoic fluid or synovium within the tendon sheath with or without hyperemia on color/power Doppler imaging
    - Overuse and RA are common causes.
- Rupture commonly at the supraglenoid tubercle and biceps-labral anchor, or within the rotator interval
  - Associated with superior glenoid labral tear
  - If acute, fluid and hemorrhage usually extend distally into the musculotendinous junction.
  - If chronic, long head biceps muscle will become atrophic, with echogenic fatty infiltration

Subscapularis Tendon

- Isolated tear is unusual.
- Cranial fibers are most frequently torn.
- Associated with anterior shoulder dislocation, overuse, supraspinatus and LHBT injury, and subcoracoid impingement
- Concomitant tear of transverse humeral ligament allows LHBT to dislocate medially.

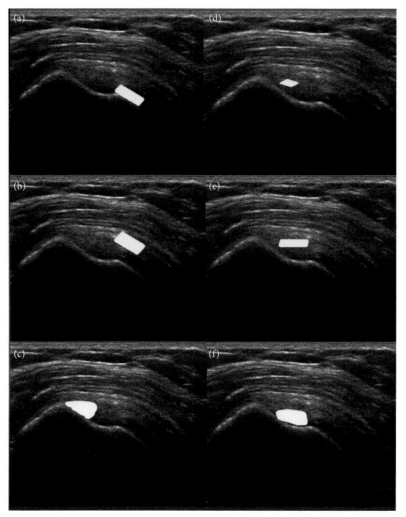

Figure 120.4. Schematic representation of partial-thickness rotator cuff tear subtypes. An articular-sided partial-thickness tear (*A*) involves only a portion of the affected tendon and the tear extends to the articular surface. A bursal-sided partial-thickness tear (*B*) involves only the bursal aspect of the tendon. A bursal-sided partial-thickness tear (*C*) in this example involves only the footprint of the tendon and does not contact the articular surface. This type of tear is often mistaken for a full-thickness tear. A partial-thickness intrasubstance tear occurring within the tendon footprint (*D*) may be difficult for arthroscopists to see. An intrasubstance, delaminating partial-thickness tear (*E*) extends longitudinally along the tendon fibers; this, too, may be difficult to detect on arthroscopy. A *rim-rent* partial-thickness tear (*F*) involves the articular surface of the tendon and extends into the tendon footprint.

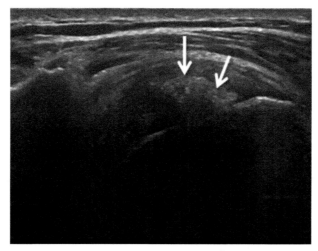

Figure 120.5. Calcific tendinosis. An amorphous, echogenic, shadowing calcification (*arrows*) is seen within the posterior supraspinatus extending into the anterior infraspinatus, in keeping with the resorptive phase of calcific tendinosis.

Supraspinatus Tendon

- Most commonly injured tendon in the shoulder and rotator cuff
- Commonly associated with injury to other cuff tendons
- Older patients, degenerative partial-thickness tears
  - Most commonly occur at the bursal surface of the posterior supraspinatus and often extend into the anterior fibers of the infraspinatus
  - Impingement by overlying subacromial spurs or by osteophytes of the AC joint
- Younger patients: overhead-throwing sports
  - Partial-thickness tears occur most commonly at the articular surface.
  - Rim-rent tears are most often at the anterior leading edge of the supraspinatus tendon, at the articular surface, with extension into the tendon footprint.
  - Partial-thickness bursal surface tears usually occur in the anterior leading edge of the supraspinatus.

Infraspinatus Tendon

- Full-thickness tears are usually associated with supraspinatus tear extension into infraspinatus.
- Partial-thickness articular surface tears associated with internal posterosuperior impingement, where posterior humeral head and posterior glenoid impinge on each other in shoulder abduction and external rotation
  - Associated with posterior superior labral tear

Teres Minor Tendon

- Rarely injured
- Tears associated with massive rotator cuff tears

Findings Associated with Rotator Cuff Tears

- Cortical irregularity at the greater tuberosity
  - Seen in patients older than 40 years, high correlation with partial-thickness articular and full-thickness supraspinatus tears
  - Considered a normal variant in the bare area subjacent to the infraspinatus tendon in patients of all ages
- *Cartilage interface* sign
  - Full-thickness and partial-thickness tears
  - Fluid in tendon gap is associated with posterior acoustical enhancement and causes the underlying hyaline cartilage to appear as linear and hyperechoic.
- Joint effusion
- *Sagging bursa* sign
  - Transducer pressure causes the echogenic peribursal fat to protrude into the rotator cuff tendon, causing the normally convex contour to become concave.
  - Sign of full-thickness or deep partial-thickness tendon tear
- Muscle atrophy
  - Chronic rotator cuff tears
  - Muscle is echogenic, diminished in volume
  - Poor prognostic indicator for rotator cuff repair

- Teres minor atrophy is common, frequently asymptomatic, and may be associated with quadrilateral space syndrome.
- Intramuscular cysts
  - Associated with full- and partial-thickness tears of the rotator cuff

Pitfalls in the Sonographic Evaluation of the Rotator Cuff

- Anisotropy—artifactual area of hypoechogenicity
  - Reposition probe so that beam is 90 degrees to tendon.
- In the setting of a full-thickness or massive rotator cuff tear, granulation tissue or bursal complex fluid extending into the tendon defect may be mistaken for an abnormal intact cuff:
  - Dynamic compression may help to differentiate intact abnormal cuff from debris and fluid.
- Normal overlap of posterior supraspinatus and anterior infraspinatus fibers may be mistaken for abnormality in the long axis:
  - Caused by anisotropy of the infraspinatus fibers overlapping supraspinatus fibers
  - Reposition probe to eliminate artifact.

Acromioclavicular Joint

As the AC joint is quite superficial in most people, OA and infection can usually be easily assessed with US. OA manifests with capsular hypertrophy, joint fluid and synovitis, osteophytes, and subchondral cysts. If the AC joint is infected, there is usually markedly thickened, hyperemic synovium on color/power Doppler imaging with complex fluid in the joint. US is useful to guide AC joint aspiration, which is easily performed from a lateral to medial approach, using the clavicle as a backstop. A common cause of a soft tissue mass in the area of the AC joint is fluid extending into the AC joint from a large rotator cuff tear, otherwise known as the *geyser sign*.

Subacromial Impingement

The subacromial arch is created by the coracoacromial ligament extending from the coracoid process to the acromion and the clavicle. Both the subacromial-subdeltoid bursa and the supraspinatus pass through the arch. The distal acromion and clavicle are prone to developing osteophytes at the AC joint and enthesophytes at the deltoid origin at the acromion, which then may impinge on the supraspinatus tendon. On dynamic abduction maneuvers, the patient will have pain and difficulty abducting the arm, and the subacromial-subdeltoid bursa may demonstrate bunching up or pooling of fluid on abduction.

Subacromial-Subdeltoid Bursa

The normal subacromial-subdeltoid (SASD) bursa appears as a thin, hypoechoic, linear structure deep to the echogenic fat plane subjacent to the deltoid and the acromion. SASD bursitis is seen as a localized anechoic to hypoechoic or complex fluid collection and synovial hypertrophy with or without

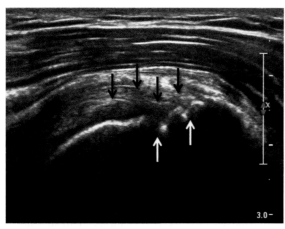

Figure 120.6. Postoperative rotator cuff. A long-axis US image demonstrates echogenic shadowing foci within the supraspinatus tendon (*black arrows*), consistent with suture material. The repaired tendon is anchored within 2 troughs in the greater tuberosity (*white arrows*).

hyperemia on color/power Doppler imaging. Common causes are acute or repetitive trauma, infection, RA, and gout. SASD bursitis may be sterile or septic.

Posterior Joint and Spinoglenoid Notch

Common causes of joint effusions in the shoulder include rotator cuff tears; trauma caused by fracture, dislocation, or ligament injury; infection; OA; and RA. Joint effusions are best seen in the posterior joint recess. This is best imaged by aligning the probe inferior to the scapular spine and scanning laterally until the glenohumeral joint is identified. Joint aspiration may also be performed in this location. A joint effusion will be compressible with transducer pressure, and swirling debris may be seen within the joint. Synovial hypertrophy may be present in the setting of inflammation or infection. Synovial hypertrophy has variable echogenicity and may have hyperemia on color/power Doppler imaging. It is distinguished from a complex joint effusion in that synovitis is not compressible, whereas a joint effusion is compressible but not hyperemic.

Postoperative Rotator Cuff

A rotator cuff repair can be identified on US by locating 1 or 2 troughs containing soft tissue anchors within the humeral head (Figure 120.6). The postoperative rotator cuff may frequently appear thin or hypoechoic compared to a normal cuff. Intratendinous sutures are seen as small echogenic foci within the tendon. Fluid is usually present near the SASD bursa.

One only needs to identify continuous intact fibers for the repair to be considered intact; the repair does not need to be "watertight."

Key Points

- US is extremely useful for the evaluation of the rotator cuff, LHBT, SASD bursa, and AC joint.
- US can accurately differentiate between full- and partial-thickness rotator cuff tears, differentiate the subtype of partial tear, and assess the degree of tendon involvement, with results equal to MRI.
- Dynamic examination allows the assessment of subacromial and subcoracoid impingement.
- US can image the postoperative rotator cuff without the limitations of metallic artifact commonly encountered with MRI.
- US is the test of choice for evaluation of suspected rotator cuff injury in patients older than 40 years.

Recommended Reading

Papatheodorou A, Ellinas P, Takis F, Tsanis A, Maris I, Batakis N. US of the shoulder: rotator cuff and non-rotator cuff disorders. *Radiographics.* 2006;26(1):e23.

References

1. de Jesus JO, Parker L, Frangos AJ, Nazarian LN. Accuracy of MRI, MR arthrography, and ultrasound in the diagnosis of rotator cuff tears: a meta-analysis. *AJR Am J Roentgenol.* 2009;192(6):1701–707.
2. Greis AC, Derrington SM, McAuliffe M. Evaluation and nonsurgical management of rotator cuff calcific tendinopathy. *Orthop Clin North Am.* 2015;46(2):293–302.
3. Jacobson JA, Lancaster S, Prasad A, van Holsbeeck MT, Craig JG, Kolowich P. Full-thickness and partial-thickness supraspinatus tendon tears: value of US signs in diagnosis. *Radiology.* 2004;230(1):234–42.
4. Kim HM, Dahiya N, Teffey SA, et al. Location and initiation of degenerative rotator cuff tears: an analysis of three hundred and sixty shoulders. *J Bone Joint Surg Am.* 2010;92(5):1088–96.
5. Papatheodorou A, Ellinas P, Takis F, Tsanis A, Maris I, Batakis N. US of the shoulder: rotator cuff and non-rotator cuff disorders. *Radiographics.* 2006;26(1):e23
6. Teefey SA, Rubin DA, Middleton WD, Hildeboldt CF, Leibold RA, Yamaguchi K. Detection and quantification of rotator cuff tears. Comparison of ultrasonographic, magnetic resonance imaging, and arthroscopic findings in seventy-one consecutive cases. *J Bone Joint Surg Am.* 2004;86-A(4):708–16.

CHAPTER 121

Ultrasound of the Elbow

Corrie M. Yablon

Background

Elbow injuries have increased in the past decade as larger numbers of adults and children are participating in overhead-throwing and racquet sports. Most elbow injuries are chronic and repetitive in nature. Common indications for US examination of the elbow are joint effusion, common extensor tendon and ligament pathology, olecranon bursitis, and peripheral nerve entrapment. The distal biceps tendon, triceps tendon, and common extensor and common flexor tendons are easily evaluated. Radial and ulnar collateral ligamentous injury can be imaged dynamically. US offers added advantages over MRI by providing higher resolution, portability, lower cost, ease of comparison to the contralateral asymptomatic side, and dynamic imaging capability. US is less useful for the evaluation of deep joint and primary bone pathology because the sound beam cannot penetrate bone.

Ultrasound Examination of the Elbow

- Defined whole-elbow protocol or a focused, symptom-based approach may be used.
- Examination may be performed with patient supine or seated with the arm resting on a table.
- High-frequency linear transducers of at least 12 MHz preferred.
- Anterior: anterior joint recess, distal biceps tendon, brachialis, median nerve
- Medial: common flexor tendon, UCL, ulnar nerve, medial joint
- Lateral: common extensor tendon, RCL, lateral joint, radial nerve
- Posterior: posterior joint recess, distal triceps tendon, olecranon bursa

Tendon Pathology

- Most useful to screen the elbow tendons in their long axes, and if abnormal, additional short-axis images may be obtained:
  - Distal biceps tendon is most commonly injured.
  - Triceps tendon is least commonly injured.
  - Most tendon injury in the elbow is caused by repetitive motion injury, which then causes tendon degeneration and may lead to rupture.
- Tendinosis
  - Mucoid degeneration of tendon; not inflammatory, so *tendinitis* is not appropriate term
- Partial-thickness tears

- Caused by overuse
- Usually treated conservatively
- Rupture
  - May occur because of acute trauma; chronic overuse; in systemic diseases such as RA, lupus, or diabetes; or with anabolic steroids
  - Tendon rupture will usually require surgery.

Common Extensor Tendon Injury

- Usually caused by chronic repetitive trauma due to varus stress of the elbow joint or because of repetitive wrist extension and supination, as occurs with the tennis backhand
- Frequently referred to as *lateral epicondylitis* or *tennis elbow* (Figure 121.1)
  - Term *epicondylitis* is inaccurate, as there is mucoid degeneration rather than inflammation.
  - Most commonly affects the extensor carpi radialis brevis origin at the lateral epicondyle
- Tendinosis and partial-thickness tears are most common, may also be seen with enthesophyte formation at the lateral epicondyle
  - Associated with RCL injury
  - With or without hyperemia on color Doppler imaging

Common Flexor Tendon Injury

- Overuse syndrome commonly occurs in golfers and in athletes who engage in overhead-throwing sports:
  - Chronic repetitive injury with valgus stress across elbow joint
- Frequently referred to as *medial epicondylitis* or as *golfer's elbow*
  - Term medial epicondylitis is inaccurate, as there is mucoid degeneration of the tendon, and no inflammation in the tendon itself.
  - Usually involves pronator teres and flexor carpi radialis at the medial epicondyle
- Tendinosis and partial-thickness tears are most frequent injury; full-thickness tears are less common:
  - May be associated with enthesophyte formation
  - Associated with injury to the underlying UCL

Triceps Tendon Injury

- Caused by repetitive, forceful extension

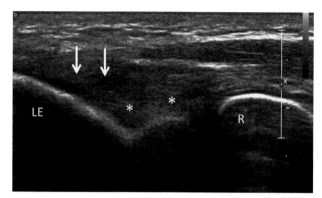

Figure 121.1. Lateral epicondylitis (epicondylosis) on the long-axis US image. The common extensor tendon origin at the lateral epicondyle (LE) of the distal humerus is heterogeneous in echotexture with a focal hypoechoic cleft (*arrows*) consistent with partial-thickness tear. *Asterisks* mark the underlying RCL. R = radial head.

- Partial-thickness tears most commonly occur in the superficial aspect of the tendon (lateral and long head triceps tendon insertions) while the deeper, medial head triceps insertion remains intact.
- Rupture may occur when there is forced flexion and the elbow is in extension:
  - Most commonly seen in weightlifters
  - May occur during fall on an outstretched hand or boxing
  - May be accompanied by avulsion of the olecranon process

Imaging Pearl
- Important to image the full width of the tendon in short axis. The long-axis assessment should extend from the olecranon proximally to the musculotendinous junction.

Distal Biceps Tendon Injury
- Usually occurs in the dominant arm with forced extension while the elbow is flexed against a load
- Younger patients: injury common during weightlifting
- Injury incidence increases with age.
- Rupture more common in male patients than female patients.
- Rupture usually accompanied by ecchymosis of anterior elbow and forearm
- Tendon frequently tears 1-2 cm proximal to the radial tuberosity, rather than from the radial tuberosity insertion (Figure 121.2).
- If biceps aponeurosis (lacertus fibrosus) remains intact, there may be little to no retraction of the tendon stump:
  - May see fluid layering over pronator muscle group
- If biceps aponeurosis is torn, then tendon may retract proximal to the elbow joint.
- If tendon is retracted, visible deformity or bulging of the biceps muscle may occur.
- Scanning from the biceps muscle belly distally, the retracted tendon stump will be visualized, surrounded by fluid or hematoma.
- If not retracted, then scanning should be extended to radial tuberosity to localize the site of tendon rupture.

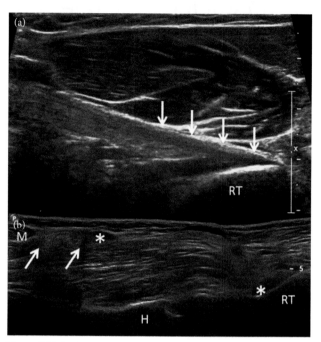

Figure 121.2. Distal biceps tendon rupture on the long-axis US images. Image (*A*) demonstrates a normal, intact distal biceps tendon (*arrows*) as a linear, fibrillar structure inserting on the radial tuberosity (RT). Image (*B*) shows a ruptured distal biceps tendon that is retracted into the upper arm. Note the associated echogenic hematoma (*arrows*). *Asterisks* mark the length of tendon retracted from the expected insertion on the RT. H = humerus; M = distal biceps muscle.

- Distal biceps tendon insertion may be very difficult to visualize in patients who are very muscular or obese.
- When not retracted, visualization may be made difficult by fluid in the bicipitoradial bursa, or by echogenic hemorrhage surrounding the distal tendon.

Imaging Pearls to Distinguish Full-Thickness from Partial-Thickness Distal Biceps Tears
- Important to visualize both long and short heads of the biceps tendon insertions on the radial tuberosity
- Short head inserts distally and medially to the long head on the radial tuberosity.
- Short head tears are more common than long head in partial-thickness tears.
- Dynamic imaging is useful to distinguish between full-thickness and partial-thickness tears.

Ligament Injury
- LCL and UCL are most commonly injured in overhead-throwing sports.
- Trauma and posterior elbow dislocation are less frequent causes of elbow ligament injury.

Imaging
- Normal ligament: fibrillar echotexture, similar to tendons, although more compact as their collagen fibers are more densely packed than tendons
- Sprain: ligament thickened and/or hypoechoic

- If injury is remote, ligament may be attenuated and lax in appearance.
- Partial-thickness tear: partial discontinuity of the ligament with concomitant thickening and hypoechoic appearance, with or without hyperemia on color/power Doppler imaging (Figure 121.3)
- Rupture or full-thickness tear: complete ligament discontinuity with intervening fluid, hemorrhage, or granulation tissue, depending on the age of the injury

Ulnar Collateral Ligament
- UCL function: stabilizes medial elbow joint in valgus stress
- UCL composed of anterior, posterior, and transverse bands
- Anterior band is most easily seen on US and is clinically the most important component.
- Injured by repetitive overhead-throwing motion, such as baseball pitching

Ulnar Collateral Ligament Imaging Pearls
- Elbow should be slightly flexed to bring the anterior band into the coronal plane.
- Probe should be placed over the medial epicondyle, aligned with the forearm.
- *Dynamic imaging* helps distinguish between partial- and full-thickness tears:
    - Especially when hemorrhage or granulation tissue are present
    - Valgus stress can be applied to the elbow in partial flexion to look for widening of the ulnotrochlear joint on the affected side compared to the asymptomatic side.
    - In asymptomatic pitchers, a difference of greater than 1.4 mm in the medial joint space of the pitching arm versus the nonpitching arm indicates ligamentous laxity.

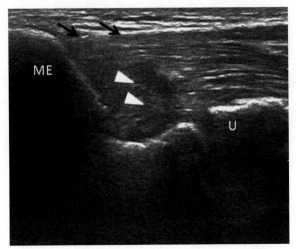

Figure 121.3. UCL tear on the long-axis US image. A partial-thickness tear of the UCL is demonstrated by hypoechoic cleft extending through the entire ligament (*arrowheads*). The overlying common flexor tendon (*arrows*) is intact. ME = medial epicondyle; U = ulna.

Lateral Collateral Ligament
- Composed of the RCL, the annular ligament, and the LUCL
- RCL inserts into the annular ligament.
- Annular ligament surrounds the radial head and inserts onto the ulna.
- RCL stabilizes the lateral elbow in varus stress.
- Injury occurs when varus stress with external rotation is applied to the elbow joint.
- LUCL extends from the lateral epicondyle to the supinator crest of the ulna and provides posterolateral stabilization of the elbow joint.

Imaging Pearl
- RCL is imaged with the proximal aspect of the probe on the lateral epicondyle and the distal aspect in line with the forearm.

Peripheral Nerves
- May be entrapped as they pass through osteofibrous tunnels
- Nerves composed of hypoechoic fascicles with intervening echogenic perineurium
- Short axis: speckled/*honeycomb* appearance
    - Most useful imaging plane to locate peripheral nerves
- Long axis: Nerves are striated, but more coarsely packed than tendons.
- Abnormal nerves are swollen and hypoechoic, usually proximal to area of entrapment:
    - If abnormal in short axis, long axis can demonstrate extent of the abnormality.
    - Hyperemia may be present on color/power Doppler examination.

Ulnar Nerve
- Injured by trauma, repetitive motion, ulnar nerve subluxation/dislocation
- Most common site of injury/entrapment is cubital tunnel:
    - Between medial epicondyle and olecranon process, beneath Osborne fascia and cubital tunnel retinaculum
    - Cubital tunnel syndrome—second most common entrapment neuropathy in the upper extremity after CTS

Imaging Pearls
- Static images assess the size and echotexture of the ulnar nerve:
    - Ulnar nerve cross-sectional area exceeding 9 mm^2 is abnormal.
- Dynamic imaging: transducer positioned over the medial epicondyle and the olecranon while elbow is flexed and extended
    - Ulnar nerve should remain positioned behind the medial epicondyle.
    - Flexion will usually elicit ulnar nerve subluxation or dislocation if present.

- On flexion, ulnar nerve will either subluxate or dislocate anterior to the posterior margin of the medial epicondyle.
- Medial head of triceps muscle may also subluxate with ulnar nerve (Figure 121.4):
  - *Snapping triceps syndrome*

Median Nerve

- May be entrapped at level of distal humerus by ligament of Struthers, a normal anatomical variant
  - Ligament of Struthers extends from the supracondylar process of the distal humerus to the medial epicondyle.
- May be entrapped in antecubital fossa by the 2 heads of the pronator teres muscle

Radial Nerve

- Deep branch of the radial nerve may become entrapped as it passes between the deep and superficial heads of the supinator muscle.
- Deep branch may also be compressed by the bicipitoradial bursa.

Joint Pathology

- Common causes: trauma, infection, OA, RA, crystal deposition disease

- Effusion is best seen in the posterior recess of elbow (Figure 121.5).
- Echogenic olecranon fat pad is displaced posteriorly by effusion.
- Effusion may be simple and anechoic to complex and echogenic.
- Effusions will be compressible with transducer pressure, and swirling debris may also be seen within the joint.
- Simple effusions should not be hyperemic.
- Hemarthrosis may be seen in trauma, hemophilia, or anticoagulation.
- Synovial hypertrophy may be present with inflammation or infection:
  - Variable echogenicity
  - With or without hyperemia on color/power Doppler imaging
  - A complex joint effusion with synovitis is not compressible, whereas a simple joint effusion is compressible and not hyperemic.
- Osteophytes are seen with OA:
  - Common at medial and lateral epicondyles, radial head, olecranon process

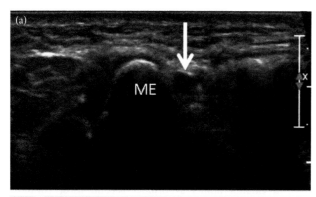

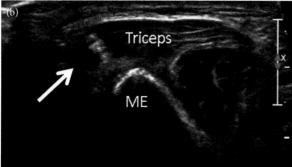

Figure 121.4. Ulnar nerve dislocation on the short-axis US images. Image (*A*) is obtained with the elbow in extension; the ulnar nerve (*arrow*) is normally situated posterior to the medial epicondyle (ME) of the distal humerus. Image (*B*), obtained with the elbow in flexion, shows the ulnar nerve (*arrow*) dislocated anterior to the ME along with the medial head of the triceps muscle consistent with "snapping triceps syndrome."

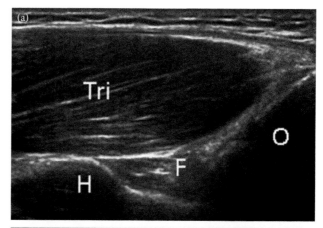

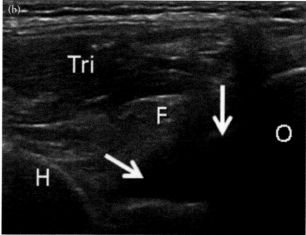

Figure 121.5. Elbow joint effusion on the long-axis US images. Image (*A*), demonstrates a normal elbow joint, imaged from the posterior aspect of the elbow at the distal humerus (H) and olecranon (O). Tri = triceps muscle; F = posterior fat pad. In image (*B*), a simple joint effusion appears anechoic (*arrows*) and displaces the posterior fat pad (F) posteriorly.

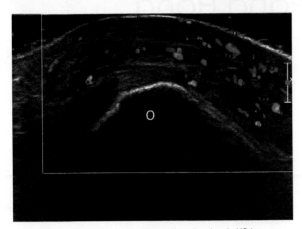

Figure 121.6. Olecranon bursitis on the short-axis US image. There is marked soft tissue swelling posterior to the olecranon process (O), with hyperemia on color Doppler imaging consistent with complex olecranon bursitis.

- Intraarticular bodies may be seen in OA or remote trauma:
  - Well-defined, echogenic, shadowing structures within the joint space

Olecranon Bursa

- Located superficial to olecranon process of ulna
- Normally collapsed, difficult to see
- Olecranon bursitis may be sterile or septic.
- Common causes of bursitis: acute/chronic trauma, infection, RA, gout
- Localized fluid collection about the posterior elbow at the olecranon
- Simple or complex fluid with internal septations
- Peripheral hyperemia on color/power Doppler imaging (Figure 121.6)
- Compressible with transducer pressure

Key Points

- US is extremely useful for the evaluation of elbow pain.
- US is helpful in assessing the degree of tendon and ligament injury and can differentiate between full-thickness and partial-thickness tears with dynamic imaging.
- US is frequently used in evaluation of peripheral nerve entrapment.
- Dynamic imaging can elicit transient ulnar nerve subluxation or dislocation from the cubital tunnel.
- Joint effusions and olecranon bursitis are easily assessed with US.

Recommended Reading

De Maeseneer M, Brigido MK, Antic M, et al. Ultrasound of the elbow with emphasis on detailed assessment of ligaments, tendons, and nerves. *Eur J Radiol*. 2015;84(4):671–81.

References

1. Bain GI, Durrant AW. Sports-related injuries of the biceps and triceps. *Clin Sports Med*. 2010;29(4):555–76.
2. De Maeseneer M, Brigido MK, Antic M, et al. Ultrasound of the elbow with emphasis on detailed assessment of ligaments, tendons, and nerves. *Eur J Radiol*. 2015;84(4):671–81.
3. Jacobson JA. *Fundamentals of Musculoskeletal Ultrasound*. 2nd ed. Philadelphia, PA: Elsevier; 2013.
4. Kandemir U, Fu FH, McMahon PJ. Elbow injuries. *Curr Opin Rheumatol*. 2002;14(2):160–67.
5. Lee KS, Rosas HG, Craig JG. Musculoskeletal ultrasound: elbow imaging and procedures. *Semin Musculoskelet Radiol*. 2010;14(4):449–60.
6. Nazarian LN, McShane JM, Ciccotti MG, et al. Dynamic US of the anterior band of the ulnar collateral ligament of the elbow in asymptomatic major league baseball pitchers. *Radiology*. 2003;227(1):149–54.

CHAPTER 122

Ultrasound of the Wrist and Hand

Corrie M. Yablon

Background

US is increasingly used to image the hand and wrist. US provides soft tissue resolution of tendons, ligaments, and peripheral nerves that is superior to MRI. US enables excellent visualization of the flexor and extensor tendons and is useful for the workup of hand and wrist pain in the settings of chronic overuse, acute trauma, rheumatologic diseases, or postoperative assessment. Dynamic assessment of tendon, ligament, and other soft tissue injuries of the joints can be performed. US is useful in the workup of common soft tissue masses about the hand and wrist.

Ultrasound Examination of the Wrist and Hand

Sonographic examination of the wrist and hand may be performed using a defined protocol or a focused, symptom-based approach. Several articles and books have been published detailing the technique of sonography of the wrist and hand, which is beyond the scope of this chapter. Briefly, the examination is best performed with the patient seated across from the examiner, with the forearm resting on a table. High-frequency linear transducers of at least 12 MHz should be used, but a small footprint 17- or 18-MHz transducer is preferable. Palmar structures examined include the flexor tendons, joints of the hand and wrist, annular pulleys, and the median and ulnar nerves. Dorsal structures examined include the extensor tendons, ulnar collateral ligament of the thumb, and extensor hoods including sagittal bands. Although it is beyond the scope of this chapter, the dorsal and volar bands of the scapholunate and lunotriquetral ligaments, the dorsal and volar extrinsic wrist ligaments, and to some extent, the TFC may also be assessed with US examination if the appropriate expertise is available.

Tendon Pathology

Tendinosis in the hand and wrist is usually caused by overuse. Partial-thickness tears are caused by overuse, trauma, or laceration. Tendon rupture occurs most frequently secondary to acute trauma or laceration; chronic overuse; systemic disease, such as RA, lupus, diabetes; or anabolic steroid use. Tendon rupture will usually require surgery, so it is important to distinguish between partial- and full-thickness tears.

Extensor Carpi Ulnaris Tendon Injury
- Associated with ulnar-sided wrist trauma/pain, RA

- Usually caused by chronic repetitive microtrauma
- Tendinosis and partial-thickness tears are most common.
- Usually there is some degree of normal subluxation of extensor carpi ulnaris (ECU) out of ulnar groove, however, subluxation greater than 50% out of ulnar groove is considered abnormal.

De Quervain Tenosynovitis
- Most common tendon injury in the wrist
- Affects the first extensor compartment: abductor pollicis longus and extensor pollicis brevis tendons
- Associated with chronic overuse, RA, pregnancy, new mothers (lifting newborn), predominant in female patients
- Tender to palpation, tendinosis, and tenosynovitis with or without hyperemia on color/power Doppler interrogation (Figure 122.1)
- Responds to conservative therapy

Other Tendon-Related Injuries
- Extensor and flexor tendons of digits and hand injured because of trauma/laceration
- *Boxer knuckle*: injury to the extensor hood (sagittal bands) at the MCP joint, causing subluxation of extensor tendon during flexion of digits
  - If only 1 of the sagittal bands is injured, the tendon subluxates away from the injured side. This appearance becomes more pronounced with MCP flexion.
- Flexor tendon annular pulley injury: usually A2 pulley in rock climbers (Figure 122.2, illustrated in Figure 106.25, in Chapter 106, "Internal Derangement of the Wrist and Hand")
  - Partial-thickness tears most frequent—thickened, hypoechoic pulley on US.
  - Full-thickness tear associated with *bowstringing* of flexor tendon (an abnormal gap between the flexor tendons and the adjacent phalanxes)
- *Trigger finger*: also known as *stenosing tenosynovitis*
  - Nodular thickening of the flexor tendon sheath, impeding normal glide of tendon (frequently involves A1 pulley)
  - May cause flexion contracture
- Dynamic US useful to assess tendon injury and integrity of postoperative repair

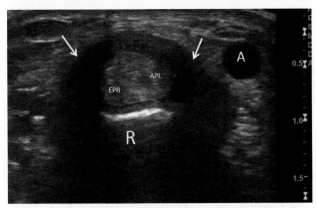

Figure 122.1. De Quervain tenosynovitis. Short-axis US image demonstrates mildly hypoechoic abductor pollicis longus (APL) and extensor pollicis brevis (EPB) tendons surrounded by hypoechoic fluid (*arrows*), consistent with tenosynovitis. R = distal radius; A = radial artery.

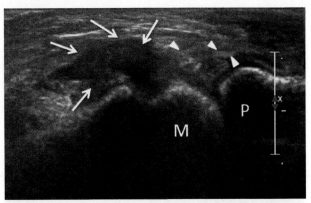

Figure 122.3. Stener lesion on the long-axis US image. A full-thickness tear is seen involving the UCL of the thumb, with retraction of the ligament stump (*arrows*) proximal to the thumb MCP joint, superficial to the adductor aponeurosis (*arrowheads*). M = thumb metacarpal, P = proximal phalanx.

Ligament Injury

- Intrinsic carpal ligaments and TFC can be identified on US, but MRI remains the gold standard for evaluation.
- Thumb ulnar collateral ligament injury at the MCP joint is the most common ligament injury in the hand:
  - Usually ruptures from the distal attachment at the proximal phalanx base
  - May be associated with avulsed fracture fragment
  - Dynamic imaging with valgus stress at the MCP joint shows ulnar-sided widening of the MCP joint when the UCL is injured.
  - Gentle flexion of the thumb interphalangeal (IP) joint can be used to identify normal movement in the adductor aponeurosis.

- Need to distinguish nondisplaced UCL tear (nonsurgical treatment) from displaced UCL tear/ Stener lesion (requires surgery)
  - Ligament stump displaced proximal to the adductor aponeurosis (Figure 122.3)
  - Dynamic imaging shows entrapment of the adductor aponeurosis at the UCL stump.

Peripheral Nerves

- May be entrapped as they pass through osteofibrous tunnels in the wrist
- Nerves are composed of hypoechoic fascicles with intervening echogenic perineurium.
- Short axis: speckled/*honeycomb* appearance
- Most useful imaging plane to locate peripheral nerves
- Long axis: nerves are striated, but more coarsely packed than tendons
- Abnormal nerves are swollen and hypoechoic, usually proximal to area of entrapment:
  - If abnormal in short axis, long axis can demonstrate extent of the abnormality.
  - Hyperemia may be present with color/power Doppler examination.

Median Nerve

- Most commonly injured nerve at the wrist
- May be entrapped in carpal tunnel
  - Carpal tunnel is located distal to wrist crease.
  - Flexor retinaculum forms the roof of carpal tunnel, extending from the scaphoid and trapezium on the radial side, to pisiform and hamate hook on ulnar side of wrist.

Imaging Pearl

- Take 2 cross-sectional measurements of the median nerve in short axis, at the level of the pronator quadratus just proximal to the carpal tunnel, and in the proximal carpal tunnel at level of the pisiform (Figure 122.4):

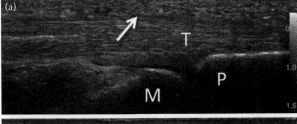

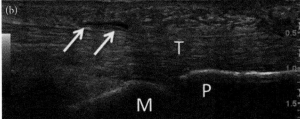

Figure 122.2. Annular pulley injury on the long axis US images. In image (*A*), a normal A1 pulley (*arrow*) is discernable as a paper-thin, linear trilaminar structure at the volar aspect of the third MCP joint. Image (*B*) demonstrates the contralateral symptomatic side, where the injured A1 pulley (*arrows*) is thickened and hypoechoic with a small amount of adjacent anechoic fluid. M = metacarpal head; P = proximal phalanx; T = flexor tendon.

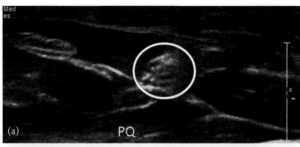

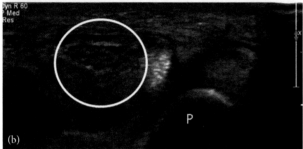

Figure 122.4. Carpal tunnel syndrome. (*A*) The median nerve is assessed in the short axis at the level of the pronator quadratus muscle (PQ) and then compared to the short-axis image at the level of the carpal tunnel (*B*). The cross-sectional area of the median nerve at the 2 locations is compared. In this case, the difference between the 2 areas is greater than 2 mm², consistent with carpal tunnel syndrome. The patient was symptomatic. P = pisiform.

- Greater than 2 mm² difference in cross-sectional area (nerve typically larger at the level of pisiform) is associated with carpal tunnel syndrome.
- Hyperemia may be present on color/power Doppler interrogation.
  - Correlate with symptoms—may be asymptomatic

Ulnar Nerve
- May be entrapped at the canal of Guyon between the pisiform, hamate hook, and ulnar artery
- Susceptible to injury in hamate hook fractures

Joint Pathology
- Common causes: trauma, overuse, RA and OA, gout, infection
- Joint effusions—simple versus complex
- Synovial hypertrophy may be present with inflammation or infection:
  - Variable echogenicity
  - With or without hyperemia on color/power Doppler imaging (power Doppler preferred)
  - Not compressible; distinguished from a complex joint effusion, which is compressible but not hyperemic
- Osteophytes seen with OA
  - Common at DIP, PIP, thumb carpometacarpal (CMC) joints
- Intraarticular bodies may be seen in OA or remote trauma
  - Well-defined, echogenic, shadowing structures within the joint space

- RA (see Chapter 127, "Ultrasound for Rheumatologic Diseases")
  - Associated with synovial hypertrophy, with or without hyperemia on color/power Doppler imaging (power Doppler preferred for detection of hyperemia)
  - Erosions in PIP, MCP, carpal and distal radioulnar joints
  - US can document response to therapy (ie, diminished hyperemia and synovium).

Common Soft Tissue Masses of the Wrist and Hand
- Ganglion cysts most common (Figure 122.5)
  - Frequently associated with scapholunate ligament injury
  - May occur anywhere in the wrist or hand
  - Lobulated or ovoid, hypoechoic to anechoic fluid collection, with or without internal septations
  - No internal color/power Doppler flow
  - Noncompressible with transducer pressure
  - Look for a *tail* connecting ganglion to joint.
- Dupuytren contracture (Figure 122.6)
  - Palpable nodular thickening of the palmar aponeurosis superficial to the flexor tendons that may lead to tendon contracture at the MCP or PIP joints
    - Hypoechoic nodule contiguous with the palmar aponeurosis
    - Dynamic flexion of the tendon can show impedance of normal tendon gliding by nodule.
- GCT of the tendon sheath
  - Also known as *localized PVNS*
  - Hypoechoic solid mass associated with a tendon sheath
  - Dynamic assessment shows tendon moving independently of mass.
  - Hyperemia may be present with color/power Doppler examination.

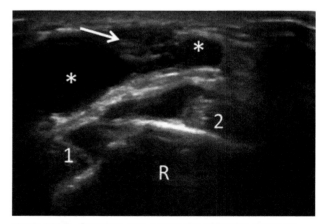

Figure 122.5. Ganglion cyst. A short-axis US image obtained at the distal radius shows a lobulated ganglion cyst (*asterisks*) that compresses an abnormally enlarged superficial branch of the radial nerve (*arrow*). Other images show the ganglion cyst arising from the tendon sheath of the first extensor compartment (1). There is a small amount of anechoic fluid in the second extensor compartment tendon (2) sheath. R = distal radius.

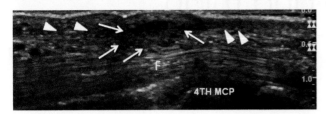

Figure 122.6. Dupuytren contracture. This patient felt a palpable nodule on the palmar aspect of his hand. Long-axis US in this location shows a lobulated hypoechoic nodule (*arrows*) in the superficial palmar tissues, contiguous with the palmar aponeurosis (*arrowheads*). Note this lesion does not contact the flexor tendon (F).

Key Points

- Use at least 12-MHz transducers for high-resolution US imaging of the wrist and hand.
- Dynamic imaging is useful to diagnose Stener lesion of the thumb UCL and to assess normal tendon translation in setting of injury or adjacent soft tissue mass.
- Median nerve entrapment at the carpal tunnel is associated with a greater than 2 mm^2 difference in the cross-sectional area between proximal and distal measurements.

- Joints can be assessed for effusions, erosions, synovial hypertrophy and hyperemia, and osteophytes.

Recommended Reading

Lee JC, Healy JC. Normal sonographic anatomy of the wrist and hand. *Radiographics.* 2005;25(6):1577–90.

Chiavaras MM, Jacobson JA, Yablon CM, Brigido MK, Girish G. Pitfalls in wrist and hand ultrasound. *AJR Am J Roentgenol.* 2014;203(3):531–40. doi:10.2214/AJR.14.12711. Review.

References

1. Klauser AS, Halpern EJ, De Zordo T, et al. Carpal tunnel syndrome assessment with US: value of additional cross-sectional area measurements of the median nerve in patients versus healthy volunteers. *Radiology.* 2009;250(1):171–77.
2. Lee JC, Healy JC. Normal sonographic anatomy of the wrist and hand. *Radiographics.* 2005;25(6):1577–90.
3. Martinoli C, Bianchi S, Nebiolo M, Derchi LE, Garcia JF. Sonographic evaluation of digital annular pulley tears. *Skeletal Radiol.* 2000;29(7):387–91.
4. Taljanovic MS, Melville DM, Gimber LH, et al. High-resolution US of rheumatologic diseases. *Radiographics.* 2015;35(7):2026–48.

CHAPTER 123

Ultrasound of the Hip and Thigh

Yoav Morag

Introduction

Although the depth of structures and large area of concern may limit the utility of US examination when evaluating the hip and thigh for some indications, US has proven itself as a very useful tool when applied for specific indications. The high spatial resolution coupled with patient guidance and the ability to perform a dynamic study allow for identification of subtle pathology or abnormal motion of different structures.

Technique and Positioning

US of the hip and thigh is typically performed with a linear high-frequency transducer (10 MHz or higher). Evaluation of deeper structures, such as the hamstring tendons and muscles, may be performed with a lower frequency convex transducer. Although the relatively deep location of many hip structures may be challenging, appropriate transducer selection and image optimization most of the time allows for adequate imaging. The patient is typically placed in the supine position, however, a prone position is needed for scanning posterior structures such as the hamstring origin and muscles as well as the sciatic nerve. Dynamic evaluation is needed to assess for abnormal motion of structures such as the iliopsoas tendon and ITB in cases of a *snapping hip*. Identification of pathology such as subtle hip joint distention may be aided by comparison to the contralateral side.

US examination may be focused on a specific structure, however, a comprehensive examination is preferred. When scanning the hip and thigh, it is convenient to divide the structures into anterior, medial, lateral, and posterior compartments (Table 123.1). Each compartment has anatomic landmarks that allow for proper positioning of the US transducer. Scanning is done in both short and long axes of the examined structures.

Anterior Compartment

The examination is performed with the patient supine and the hip in extension and slight external rotation. The transducer is held in an oblique sagittal orientation parallel to the femoral head–neck axis, allowing for identification of the echogenic contour of the femoral head and neck and of the anterior joint recess (Figure 123.1). The hip joint capsule, including the iliofemoral ligament, is identified as an overlying soft tissue layer, which appears hyperechoic if imaged in the perpendicular plane. Gentle rocking of the transducer may aid in cases where this layer appears hypoechoic because of anisotropy.

With the transducer in the oblique sagittal orientation parallel to the femoral head–neck axis, the thin anechoic cartilage layer may be seen superficial to the femoral head. The anterior superior labrum, a fibrocartilaginous structure attached to the acetabulum, can also be identified on US as a homogenous echogenic triangular structure bordering the anterior acetabulum.

With the transducer in the transverse plane just superior to the femoral head, the iliopsoas tendon is visualized superficial to the iliopectineal eminence.

US evaluation of the quadriceps muscle group is performed with the hip in extension. The examination is typically performed with a 10- to 17-MHz transducer, however, lower frequency transducers may be needed to evaluate deeper layers. The rectus femoris muscle arises proximally with 2 heads; the direct head originating from the anterior inferior iliac spine and an indirect head arising from the acetabular ridge. Scanning in the axial plane from the level of the anterior inferior iliac spine distally will allow identification of the fibrillar appearance of the direct head and the echogenic shadowing deep to the direct head representing the indirect head.

Medial Compartment

The medial compartment, which includes the adductor longus, brevis, and magnus muscles, as well as the gracilis muscle, is evaluated with the patient in the supine position, the thigh in external rotation, and the knee slightly flexed. The transducer is initially placed in the transverse plane at the pelvic brim, followed by scanning in the sagittal oblique plane parallel to the orientation of these muscles (Figure 123.2).

Lateral Compartment

US examination is performed in the lateral decubitus position with the symptomatic side facing up. The initial examination can be performed with a 10- to 12-MHz transducer, which may be replaced with a lower frequency transducer for the deeper structures. Although there is controversy regarding the anatomy of the greater trochanter, the 4 greater trochanter facets described by Pfirrmann et al serve as anatomic landmarks. Scanning in the transverse plane will allow identification of the gluteus minimus tendon attachment to the anterior facet, the broad attachment of the gluteus medius to the lateral facet, and a narrow attachment on the superolateral facet. This configuration has been likened to the rotator cuff tendons of the shoulder. Scanning in the oblique coronal plane parallel to the tendon will allow identification of the tendon fibers.

Table 123.1. Anterior, Lateral, Medial, and Posterior Compartments of the Hip and Thigh

COMPARTMENT	KEY STRUCTURES	COMMON PATHOLOGY
Hip		
Anterior	Anterior hip joint	Fluid, synovitis, labral tear
	Iliopsoas tendon	Iliopsoas bursitis, snapping iliopsoas tendon
	Rectus femoris origin	Tendinosis, tear
	Sartorius origin	Tendinosis
Lateral	Gluteus medius and minimus tendons	Gluteus medius and minimus tendinosis and tears, bursitis
	Iliotibial band	Snapping iliotibial band
Medial	Hip adductors	Adductor longus tendon tear
Posterior	Hamstring tendon origin	Hamstring tendon tears
	Sciatic nerve	
Thigh		
Anterior	Quadriceps muscles	Tears, hematomas
Posterior	Hamstring muscles	Tears, hematomas
	Sciatic nerve	

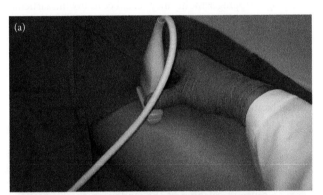

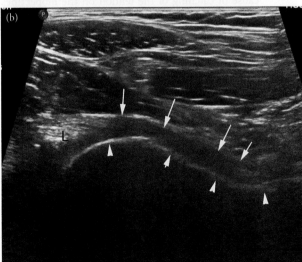

Figure 123.1. US of the anterior hip. (*A*) Positioning of the transducer for US scanning along the long axis of the anterior right femoral head neck. (*B*) Note collapsed normal anterior joint recess (*arrows*) superficial to the hyperechoic femoral cortex (*arrowheads*). L = acetabular labrum.

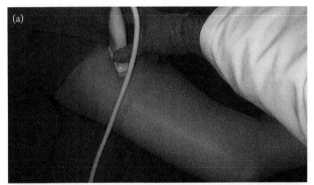

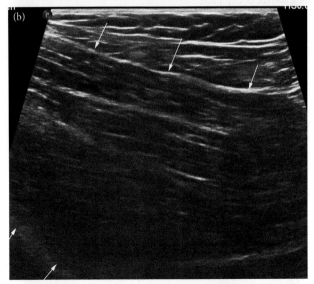

Figure 123.2. US of the medial hip/proximal thigh. (*A*) Positioning of the transducer in the sagittal oblique plane for US scanning along the medial aspect of the proximal thigh. (*B*) Note normal hypoechoic appearance of the adductor muscles (*arrows*) with hyperechoic muscular septa in the long axis.

Posterior Compartment

The gluteus maximus muscle is also evaluated in the short and long axes. US evaluation of the hamstring complex may be limited given the depth of these structures and the large area involved. The examination is performed with the patient in the prone position with the ischial tuberosity serving as an anatomic landmark. In the short axis, the semimembranosus tendon can be seen arising deep/anterior and separate from the conjoint tendon formed by the semitendinosus and long head biceps femoris tendons.

Pathology and Imaging Findings

Anterior Compartment

Joint Effusion and Synovitis

- A persistent hypoechoic appearance to the hip joint capsule and iliofemoral ligament on US examination may represent capsuloligamentous pathology. These structures should measure no more than 7 mm in thickness irrespective of the echogenicity.
- Distention and displacement of the joint capsule is indicative of anterior joint recess content such as fluid or synovial tissue.
- An anechoic layer deep to and displacing the capsule will represent joint fluid (Figure 123.3).
- A hypoechoic or echogenic layer deep to the capsule may represent synovial tissue, however, complex fluid may also have this appearance.
- Application of color/power Doppler or compression may at times allow the distinction between synovial tissue and joint fluid (Figure 123.4). The appearance of fluid is usually nonspecific, and if there is a clinical concern for infection, joint aspiration may be needed.

Acetabular Labral Tears

Labral tears can occur in the context of FAI syndromes, degenerative changes, and trauma among other etiologies and may be a source of hip pain.

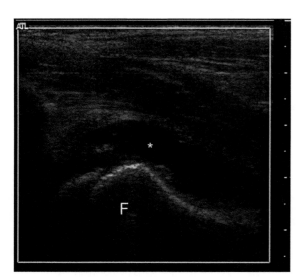

Figure 123.3. Hip joint effusion. Oblique long-axis (sagittal) color Doppler US image depicts anechoic hip joint fluid (*asterisk*) along the femoral head and neck (F).

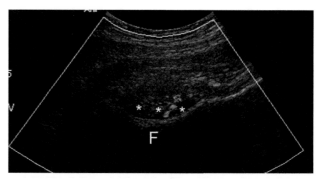

Figure 123.4. Hip synovitis. Oblique long-axis (sagittal) color Doppler US image depicts echogenic distention of the hip joint (*asterisks*) with accompanying hyperemia consistent with synovitis. F = femur neck.

- Anterior labral tears appear as hypoechoic clefts within the substance of the labrum on US examination.
- At times, the only indication of a labral tear will be a paralabral cyst adjacent to the labrum, which may appear as anechoic, hypoechoic, or hyperechoic multilobular lesions dependent on cyst complexity.

Snapping Hip

The iliopsoas muscle is an important hip flexor with iliopsoas tendon pathology a cause of anterior hip pain as well as hip *snapping*. Snapping of the hip may occur because of intraarticular etiology and external (lateral) and internal (medial) causes.

- Intraarticular causes of snapping include labral tears, intraarticular bodies, and synovial chondromatosis, whereas external causes include catching of the iliotibial tract or gluteus maximus muscle over the greater trochanter during hip flexion and extension.
- The most common cause of hip snapping is internal, by the iliopsoas tendon.
  - Snapping of the iliopsoas tendon often corresponds to sudden rapid medial to lateral or lateral to medial movement of the iliopsoas tendon. This can occur because of catching of the tendon on the iliopectineal eminence as it moves from a relative anterolateral position to a more posteromedial position, catching of the tendon on anterior paralabral cysts, or flipping of the tendon over the iliacus muscle during provocative maneuvers.

Iliopsoas Tendon and Bursa

- In degenerative tendinopathy, the iliopsoas tendon may appear hypoechoic, thickened with heterogeneous appearance, and with loss of the normal fibrillar echotexture.
- US also plays an important role in assessing the iliopsoas tendon following total hip arthroplasty as anteriorly protruding acetabular components may impinge on the overlying iliopsoas tendon.
- The iliopsoas bursa is located between the iliopsoas myotendinous junction/tendon and the hip joint capsule with a connection to the hip joint in 15% of the cases.
  - Bursal fluid accumulation may occur as a result of various etiologies including hip joint effusion and inflammatory arthropathies such as RA.

- Accumulation of large amounts of fluid may cause femoral nerve compression.
- The bursa can be identified on US if distended by fluid or echogenic synovial tissue (Figure 123.5).
- The iliopsoas bursa may be collapsed by transducer pressure unlike paralabral cysts, which may occur in close proximity.

Calcific Tendinosis

Calcium hydroxyapatite deposition in the periarticular tendons may be accompanied by an acute inflammatory reaction. The hip is one of the common locations for this pathology, and the acute severe pain may mimic other etiologies such as infection. Reported involved tendons about the hip include the rectus femoris, gluteal and iliopsoas tendons, among others.

- On focused US scanning over the area of pain, an echogenic cluster representing the focal deposition of calcium can be seen surrounding a typically hypoechoic thickened tendon with associated hyperemia (Figure 123.6).
- US-guided lavage of the calcifications can be performed if clinically indicated.

Quadriceps Muscle Group

The quadriceps femoris muscle group includes the rectus femoris, vastus medialis, vastus lateralis, and vastus intermedius muscles, which are powerful extensors of the knee. The rectus femoris, which is the most commonly injured muscle in this group, is also an extensor of the hip joint. Partial-thickness, full-thickness (but partial width), and complete (full-thickness, full-width) tendon tears can occur in the rectus femoris.

- Rectus femoris injuries include proximal tendon, myotendinous, and myofascial injury.
  - Myotendinous injury may occur along the indirect head central tendon or along the direct head anterior myotendinous junction.
  - In central myotendinous injury, fluid surrounding the central tendon may form a *bullseye* appearance (Figure 123.7), and the central tendon may appear

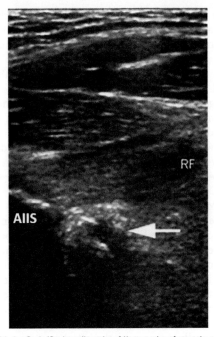

Figure 123.6. Calcific tendinosis of the rectus femoris origin. Long-axis (oblique sagittal) US image depicts echogenic calcifications (*arrow*) deep to the direct head of the rectus femoris tendon (RF) in a patient presenting with acute hip pain and RF calcific tendinosis. AIIS = anterior inferior iliac spine.

thick, ill-defined, and irregular when scanning in the axial plane.

- Intramuscular hematomas may also occur in the rectus femoris and have a varied US appearance corresponding to the age of the hematoma.
- Rectus femoris tears may be accompanied by retraction, which may form a palpable mass. US will identify the torn retracted muscle and exclude a neoplasm.

Medial Compartment
Muscle Injuries

The most commonly injured muscles in this compartment are the adductor longus and gracilis, usually involving the

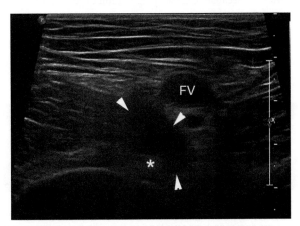

Figure 123.5. Iliopsoas bursitis. Short-axis (transverse) US image depicts anechoic fluid distention of the iliopsoas bursa (*arrowheads*) partially encompassing the iliopsoas tendon (*asterisk*). FV = femoral vessels.

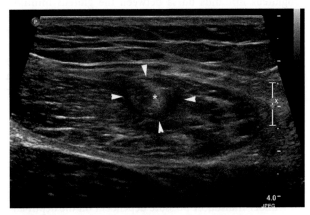

Figure 123.7. Injury of the rectus femoris myotendinous junction with *bullseye* appearance. Short-axis (transverse) US image depicts a rectus femoris central myotendinous injury with hypoechoic fluid (*arrowheads*) surrounding the central myotendinous junction (*asterisk*).

proximal tendon or myotendinous region. The mechanism is typically an acute or chronic sport-related injury typically with hip hyperabduction and abdominal wall hyperextension.

- US can identify tendinosis and partial- and full-thickness tears.
- A gap between the symphysis pubis and the tendon stump may be apparent on US in cases with complete tendon tears.
- However, US is not as sensitive as MRI in identifying low-grade or chronic injuries.

Lateral Compartment
Gluteal Musculature

Gluteal tendinopathy or greater trochanter pain syndrome is associated with lateral hip pain, which is exacerbated with weight bearing and with sleeping on the symptomatic side. The etiology of gluteal tendinopathy is thought to be multifactorial including repetitive microtrauma in the context of degeneration or certain athletic activities. The spectrum of gluteal tendinopathy includes tendinosis of varying degrees, partial-thickness tendon tears, and complete tendon tears, which typically occur near the attachment to the greater trochanter.

- On US, tendinosis will manifest as hypoechoic changes with loss of the fibrillar appearance of the tendon, with varying degrees of tendon swelling and heterogeneity.
- Tears will present as tendon thinning or well-defined anechoic clefts, which vary between partial-thickness tendon tears to complete (full-width, full-thickness) tears with or without retraction and surrounding fluid.
- A completely uncovered or *bald* facet indicates a full-thickness tendon tear.
- US can also identify calcifications within the tendon as well as accompanying bursal fluid.
- Prominent greater trochanteric cortical irregularity has been associated with gluteal tendinopathy. However, tendinosis or tendon calcifications may be asymptomatic.

Greater Trochanter Bursae

There are a number of bursae about the hip, including the subgluteus minimus bursa between the gluteus minimus tendon and the greater trochanter anterior facet, the subgluteus medius bursa between the gluteus medius tendon, and the greater trochanter lateral facet and the trochanteric bursa overlying the posterior facet deep to the gluteus maximus muscle (Figure 123.8). Additional bursa may be seen between the iliotibial tract and the greater trochanter.

- Bursal fluid or synovial tissue can be identified with US as anechoic or hypoechoic bursal distention with variable hyperemia on color/power Doppler interrogation in the area of focal pain.
- The examined bursa may or may not be compressible under transducer pressure dependent on the depth and on the content of the bursa.
- US examination may also provide guidance for bursal aspiration or steroid injection if clinically indicated.

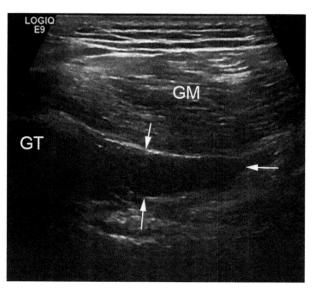

Figure 123.8. Greater trochanteric bursitis. Oblique long-axis (coronal) US image of the posterolateral hip depicts fluid-filled trochanteric bursa (*arrows*) deep to the gluteus maximus muscle (GM), superficial to the greater trochanter (GT).

Posterior Compartment
Hamstring Musculature

The hamstring muscle complex includes the long head biceps femoris, the semitendinosus, and the semimembranosus. The semitendinosus and long head biceps femoris typically form a conjoint tendon at the inferomedial aspect of the ischial tuberosity while the thick semimembranosus tendon arises from the superolateral aspect of the ischial tuberosity and courses superior and medial to the other hamstring tendons. Injury to the hamstring complex can occur as an acute event or because of chronic microtrauma. Acute injuries typically occur with knee and hip in extension during eccentric contraction. In the acute setting, the proximal hamstring complex is the most commonly injured muscle in the athlete, although the biceps femoris muscle is the most commonly injured of these 3 muscles. The most common site of injury varies according to age; in skeletally immature individuals, apophyseal avulsions occur. In young adults, injury typically occurs at the myotendinous junction, whereas proximal tendon tears are common in older individuals because of underlying tendon degeneration.

- The ability of US to detect hamstring injury varies according to the degree, depth, and chronicity of the injury.

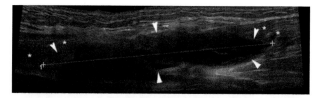

Figure 123.9. Retracted semimembranosus tendon tear. Extended FOV US image in the long axis (sagittal) depicts a full-thickness semimembranosus tendon tear with heterogeneous hematoma (*arrowheads*) between the retracted tendon stumps (*asterisks*) (measurement of the gap using digital calipers).

- Chronic tendinopathy may manifest as hypoechoic thickening with variable heterogeneity of the proximal tendon.
- Low-grade partial tears/strains that typically occur in younger adults at the myotendinous junction may be difficult to identify on US.
- More severe injury with progressive structural disruption of the myofibrils and accompanying hematomas and fluid will be more easily apparent on US.
- Isolated epimyseal injury can be identified on US as fluid along the muscle periphery and typically involves the distal biceps muscle.
- The greater the cross-sectional area of injured muscle has been associated with longer rehabilitation times and increased risk of re-tear in athletes.
- Tendon avulsions are relatively uncommon in adults and more frequently involve the conjoint tendon.
- Identification of tendon avulsions/full-thickness proximal tendon tears and quantifying the degree of tendon retraction are important factors when considering surgical intervention (Figure 123.9).
- The ability of US to identify injury to the hamstring complex decreases as fluid slowly resorbs in the subacute setting.
  - In the chronic setting, encasement of the nerve by scar from the hamstring complex injury may cause sciatic nerve swelling and loss of fascicular structure, which can be identified on US examination.

Key Points

- US is useful in evaluation of hip joint effusions, hip tendons, hip and thigh muscles, and hip bursae and is frequently used to guide aspirations and therapeutic injections.
- Dynamic US examination may identify the etiology of a snapping hip.
- The iliopsoas bursa may be collapsed by US transducer pressure unlike paralabral cysts.
- US is helpful in the diagnosis of calcific tendinosis of the hip tendons and may present with acute severe pain, clinically mimicking other etiologies such as infection.
- Central myotendinous injury of the rectus femoris may appear as a bullseye on transverse US scanning.
- A completely uncovered greater trochanter facet indicates a full-thickness gluteal tendon tear.
- The ability of US to identify injury to the hamstring complex is reduced as fluid slowly resorbs in the subacute setting.

Recommended Reading

Molini L, Precerutti M, Gervasio A, Draghi F, Bianchi S. Hip: Anatomy and US technique. *J Ultrasound.* 2011;14(2):99–108. doi:10.1016/j.jus.2011.03.004.

References

1. Beltran L, Ghazikhanian V, Padron M, Beltran J. The proximal hamstring muscle-tendon-bone unit: a review of the normal anatomy, biomechanics, and pathophysiology. *Eur J Radiol.* 2012;81(12):3772–79. doi:10.1016/j.ejrad.2011.03.099.
2. Blankenbaker DG, De Smet AA, Keene JS. Sonography of the iliopsoas tendon and injection of the iliopsoas bursa for diagnosis and management of the painful snapping hip. *Skeletal Radiol.* 2006;35(8):565–71. doi:10.1007/s00256-006-0084-6.
3. Connell DA, Bass C, Sykes CA, Young D, Edwards E. Sonographic evaluation of gluteus medius and minimus tendinopathy. *Eur Radiol.* 2003;13(6):1339–47. doi:10.1007/s00330-002-1740-4.
4. Jacobson JA, Khoury V, Brandon CJ. Ultrasound of the groin: techniques, pathology, and pitfalls. *AJR Am J Roentgenol.* 2015;205(3):513–23. doi:10.2214/AJR.15.14523.
5. Kong A, Van der Vliet A, Zadow S. MRI and US of gluteal tendinopathy in greater trochanteric pain syndrome. *Eur Radiol.* 2007;17(7):1772–83. doi:10.1007/s00330-006-0485-x.
6. Lutterbach-Penna RA, Kalume-Brigido M, Morag Y, Boon T, Jacobson JA, Fessell DP. Ultrasound of the thigh: focal, compartmental, or comprehensive examination? *AJR Am J Roentgenol.* 2014;203(5):1085–92. doi:10.2214/AJR.13.12286.
7. Martinoli C, Garello I, Marchetti A, et al. Hip ultrasound. *Eur J Radiol.* 2012;81(12):3824–31. doi:10.1016/j.ejrad.2011.03.102.
8. Molini L, Precerutti M, Gervasio A, Draghi F, Bianchi S. Hip: anatomy and US technique. *J Ultrasound.* 2011;14(2):99–108. doi:10.1016/j.jus.2011.03.004.
9. Pfirrmann CW, Chung CB, Theumann NH, Trudell DJ, Resnick D. Greater trochanter of the hip: attachment of the abductor mechanism and a complex of three bursae—MR imaging and MR bursography in cadavers and MR imaging in asymptomatic volunteers. *Radiology.* 2001;221(2):469–77. doi:10.1148/radiol.2211001634.
10. Robben SG, Lequin MH, Diepstraten AF, den Hollander JC, Entius CA, Meradji M. Anterior joint capsule of the normal hip and in children with transient synovitis: US study with anatomic and histologic correlation. *Radiology.* 1999;210(2):499–507. doi:10.1148/radiology.210.2.r99fe52499.
11. Steinert L, Zanetti M, Hodler J, Pfirrmann CW, Dora C, Saupe N. Are radiographic trochanteric surface irregularities associated with abductor tendon abnormalities? *Radiology.* 2010;257(3):754–63. doi:10.1148/radiol.10092183.

CHAPTER 124

Ultrasound of the Knee

Yoav Morag

Introduction

The knee is a gliding hinge joint with 6 degrees of freedom for rotation and translation. This complex function is made possible by the anatomy of the knee. The orientation and tightness of the knee stabilizers are affected by the position of the knee and by the forces applied by adjacent muscles.

The central structures in the knee, such as the menisci and cruciate ligaments, as well as the cartilage, are typically evaluated by MRI. However, US is highly suitable for evaluation of the peripheral/superficial structures of the knee given the high spatial resolution of this imaging modality and the ability to perform a dynamic study, as well as assess structures in different positions of the knee. As in US of other joints, the ability to perform a patient-guided examination as well as the ability to compare to the contralateral knee may allow for identification of subtle pathology.

Position and Technique

US examination of the knee is typically performed with a high-frequency linear transducer (12 MHz or higher). Deeper structures, as in the posterior knee may require lower frequency transducers. Anatomic landmarks are key and guide the examiner when evaluating the knee joint. Patient and knee position are modified throughout the examination according to the structure examined and include both supine and prone positions. Changes in knee position may also eliminate anisotropy, a common artifact when evaluating fibrillar structures. The examination may be modified according to the clinical query and dynamic maneuvers such as varus and valgus stress and compression. Color or power Doppler interrogation may be employed to evaluate for hyperemia. Evaluation of the different knee structures should be performed both in the short and long axes. The US probe should be positioned perpendicular to the examined ligaments and tendons in order to minimize anisotropy artifact.

When performing a complete US examination of the knee, it is helpful to divide the knee into 4 compartments: anterior, medial, lateral, and posterior (Table 124.1).

Anterior Compartment

The anterior compartment structures are evaluated in the supine position with the knee slightly flexed (20-30 degrees) to minimize anisotropy of the visualized tendons. The patella serves as a convenient bony landmark in this compartment.

The extensor mechanism of the knee includes soft tissue and osseous components. The quadriceps tendon is formed by convergence of the rectus femoris, vastus medialis, vastus lateralis, and vastus intermedius tendons inserting distally on the proximal pole as well as the lateral, medial, and dorsal surfaces of the patella. There are typically 3 layers to the quadriceps tendon although 1 to 5 layers have been described. The most superficial quadriceps tendon fibers arising from the rectus femoris continue superficial to the patella, forming the prepatellar quadriceps continuation. The patellar tendon is the distal continuation of the quadriceps tendon, extending beyond the inferior patellar pole to insert on the tibial tuberosity. The medial retinaculum provides medial stability to the patellofemoral articulation, with the MPFL being the most superior and substantial component of this structure.

Scanning in the transverse plane cranially from the superior pole of the patella allows identification of the quadriceps tendon (Figure 124.1). The fibrillar nature of the quadriceps tendon can be appreciated when rotating the transducer to the sagittal plane. The normal 3-layered structure of the quadriceps tendon is not always appreciated on US. The broad punctate patellar tendon will be identified when scanning in the transverse plane cranially from the tibial tuberosity or when scanning caudally from the inferior pole of the patella. When rotating the transducer to the sagittal plane, the fibrillar nature of this tendon will be seen. If the knee is not adequately flexed, artifactual hypoechoic changes caused by anisotropy may be identified along the quadriceps and patellar tendons. Slight waviness of the patellar tendon may be visualized when the knee is terminally extended. The MPFL can be identified with the transducer in the transverse plane placed between the superior half of the patella and the medial femoral epicondyle. On US examination, 1 to 3 MPFL layers may be visualized.

The anterior joint recesses and fat pads located deep to the quadriceps tendon can be identified when placing the transducer in the sagittal plane with the heel of the probe over the superior pole of the patella (Figure 124.2). Echogenic soft tissue superior to the patella and along the anterior femoral shaft represent the suprapatellar (quadriceps) and prefemoral fat pads, respectively. The synovial-lined suprapatellar recess is located between the fat pads and will be identified on US examination if distended with variable amounts of fluid or synovial tissue (Figure 124.2).

Medial Compartment

US examination of the medial compartment is typically performed in the supine position with the knee extended. Slight external knee rotation may allow better visualization of the posteromedial corner.

The femoral attachment of the MCL is near the medial femoral epicondyle (MFE), a small bony protuberance on the medial aspect of the distal femur. Scanning in the transverse

Table 124.1. Anterior, Lateral, Medial, and Posterior Compartments of the Knee

COMPARTMENT	KEY STRUCTURES	COMMON PATHOLOGY
Anterior	Extensor mechanism	Quadriceps and patellar tendon tears and tendinosis
		Bursitis
	Anterior joint recess	Joint fluid, synovitis, synovial proliferative disorders
Lateral	BFT, FCL, POP, ITB	ITB friction syndrome, tendon/ligament injury
Medial	MCL	Ligament injury
Posterior	SM-GM bursa	Baker cyst
Other	Peripheral menisci	Parameniscal cysts, meniscal tears

Abbreviations: BFT, biceps femoris tendon; FCL, fibular collateral ligament; MCL, medial collateral ligament; POP, popliteus tendon; SM-GM bursa, semimembranosus-gastrocnemius bursa.

plane along the medial aspect of the distal femur will allow identification of the MFE and the adjacent MCL and posterior oblique ligament (POL) origins. Rotating the transducer to the coronal plane will allow a longitudinal view of the MCL, including its superficial and deep components. The pes anserinus tendons can be identified coursing superficial to the distal MCL as the examiner moves the transducer caudally in the coronal plane.

The distal semimembranosus tendon has multiple attachments to the tibia and joint capsule, which can be identified on US. A bony groove at the posteromedial tibia serves as the attachment point for the direct arm of the semimembranosus tendon and is an important landmark when scanning in the sagittal plane.

Lateral Compartment

US examination of the lateral compartment is typically performed in the supine position with knee extension and with variable degrees of internal rotation to better visualize the more posterior structures.

The lateral supporting structures of the knee typically evaluated by US include the ITB, fibular collateral ligament (FCL) a.k.a. LCL proper, biceps femoris tendon (BFT), and the popliteus tendon.

The ITB attaches on the Gerdy tubercle, a bony prominence at the anterolateral tibia. US examination is performed in the coronal plane with the transducer heel placed over the Gerdy tubercle, allowing for visualization of the distal ITB.

The BFT will be visualized in the short axis when scanning in the transverse plane from the fibular head cranially. Rotating the transducer to the coronal plane while remaining centered on the BFT will depict the tendon in the long axis. In this position, angling the transducer anteriorly while anchoring the transducer heel on the distal BFT attachment will allow visualization of the FCL in the long axis. The broad fan-shaped femoral origin of the FCL is typically hypoechoic, which should not be considered pathologic. The interdigitation of the distal FCL between the 2 attachments of the BFT should not be misconstrued as BFT pathology as well. The femoral popliteal groove can be seen deep to the FCL femoral attachment and serves as a landmark for the popliteus tendon insertion. Given the curvilinear course of the popliteus tendon, hypoechoic changes related to anisotropy are typically present when imaging this tendon. When evaluating the lateral aspect of the knee, the examiner should also examine the common peroneal nerve that courses from the posterolateral aspect of the knee to the anterior aspect of the fibular head/neck.

Posterior Knee

US examination of the posterior compartment is typically performed in the prone position with the knee in extension. In larger knees, it is best to attempt to scan with a 12-MHz or higher frequency transducer and replace it with a lower

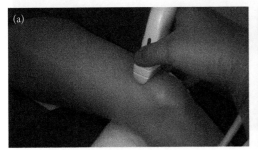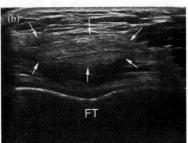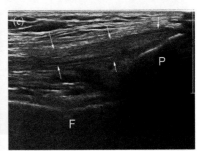

Figure 124.1. Normal quadriceps tendon. (*A*) Scanning in the short (transverse) plane cranial to the patella allows identification of (*B*) the quadriceps tendon (*arrows*) superficial to the femoral trochlea (FT). The fibrillar nature of the tendon (*arrows*) can be appreciated after rotating the transducer 90 degrees while centered over the long axis of the tendon (*C*). F = femur; P = patella.

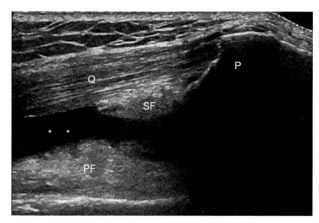

Figure 124.2. Suprapatellar joint effusion. Long;-axis (sagittal) US image depicts anechoic fluid distending the suprapatellar recess (*asterisks*) deep to the quadriceps tendon (Q) and suprapatellar fat pad (SF) and superficial to the prefemoral fat pad (PF). P = patella.

frequency transducer if images are suboptimal. An important anatomic landmark in the posterior knee is the medial head of the gastrocnemius muscle (GM)-semimembranosus tendon (SM) juxtaposition. Placing the transducer over the medial aspect of the calf will allow identification of the medial head of GM while scanning cranially to the GM-SM juxtaposition (Figure 124.3). Rocking the transducer in the transverse plane may allow easy identification of the fibrillar SM. Anisotropy of the fibers of the GM or SM frequently seen on transverse scanning should not be misinterpreted as a small Baker cyst.

Pathology and Imaging Findings

Anterior Compartment

Quadriceps and Patellar Tendons
Quadriceps and patellar tendon ruptures are less common than patellar fractures and typically occur in the context of chronic tendon degeneration associated with increasing age, repetitive

microtrauma, systemic diseases, and certain medications such as steroids. The most common indirect mechanism for quadriceps tendon injury is sudden quadriceps mechanism contraction with a flexed knee. Quadriceps tendon tears typically occur 1-2 cm proximal to the patellar attachment in the relatively avascular area of the tendon. Patellar tendon tears are less common than quadriceps tendon tears and typically occur in younger more active patients and involve the proximal portion of the tendon.

- Although complete rupture of the extensor mechanism can be diagnosed clinically, partial-thickness tendon tears may pose a diagnostic challenge, emphasizing the importance of US evaluation.
- Chronic quadriceps and patellar tendon degeneration may appear on US as diffuse or focal tendon thickening, loss of the fibrillary pattern, hypoechoic changes, or heterogeneous appearance to the tendon.
- Discontinuity of the fibrillar structure on US is consistent with a tendon tear, which may be a partial-thickness tear, focal full-thickness tear, or complete tendon tear (Figures 124.4 and 124.5).
  - Gentle passive flexion and extension of the knee may allow identification of the tendon stumps when the tendon gap is filled by soft tissue component/hematoma.
- Retinacular tears at the femoral or patellar attachments may occur following patellar dislocations and are also associated with patellar tendon tears.

Anterior Knee Bursae
There are a number of bursae along the extensor mechanism including the prepatellar bursa and the deep and superficial infrapatellar tendon bursae. These bursae may become distended with fluid or synovial tissue because of various etiologies including chronic overuse, trauma, inflammation, infection, and crystal deposition.

- A small amount of fluid may be identified in the deep infrapatellar bursa in asymptomatic knees on US.
- On US, the prepatellar bursa located superficial to the patella typically has a thick, irregular soft tissue rim with

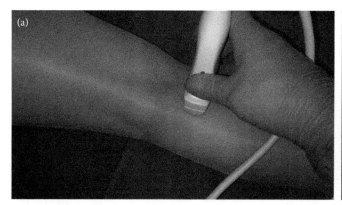

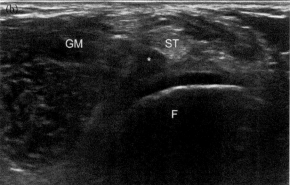

Figure 124.3. Normal structures at the posteromedial aspect of the knee. (*A*) Scanning in the short (transverse) plane over the medial calf toward the knee will allow identification (*B*) of the area of semimembranosus medial head of gastrocnemius juxtaposition. Anisotropy artifact in the semimembranosus (*asterisk*) should not be mistaken for a Baker cyst. ST = semitendinosus tendon; GM = medial head of gastrocnemius; F = femur.

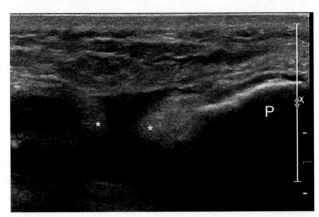

Figure 124.4. Full-thickness quadriceps tendon tear. Long-axis (sagittal) US image shows a full-thickness distal quadriceps tendon tear with proximal and distal tendon stumps (*asterisks*) and intervening anechoic fluid. P = patella.

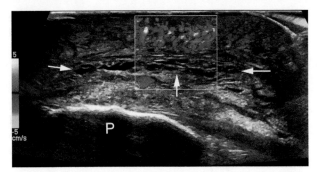

Figure 124.6. Prepatellar bursitis. Long-axis (sagittal) US image depicts prepatellar bursitis with central complex fluid (*arrows*) and surrounding hyperemic tissue. P = patella.

variable peripheral hyperemia and variable amounts of central fluid (Figure 124.6).

- Scanning should be performed with minimal probe pressure to allow for identification of the central fluid component.
- US cannot identify the etiology of the bursal distention/fluid.

Joint Fluid

- US can identify small amounts of joint fluid in the suprapatellar recesses (7-10 mL) as well as in the other joint recesses.
  - Scanning should be performed with only light transducer pressure so as not to displace the fluid.
- Distinguishing hypoechoic synovial tissue and complex joint fluid may be performed by applying transducer pressure causing fluid displacement or applying color/power Doppler in order to visualize blood flow present in active synovitis.
- Joint aspiration may be needed in order to differentiate between synovial tissue without discernible blood flow and complex joint fluid and in order to identify the etiology of the joint fluid.

Medial Compartment

The MCL and POL are the main static stabilizers to valgus stress on the knee. The MCL is the most commonly injured ligament of the knee. The mechanism of injury typically includes

an impact to the lateral aspect of the knee with the foot planted or external tibial rotation with the knee flexed.

- US can identify MCL grade 1 injuries as thickened and hypoechoic changes with intact fibers (Figure 124.7), grade 2 MCL injuries as partial disruption of some components of the MCL and grade 3 injuries as disruption of both superficial and deep components of the MCL.
- Gentle dynamic valgus stress testing can also be employed to assess for increased knee laxity.
- The pes anserinus bursa may be identified along the course of the distal pes anserinus tendons as an anechoic or hypoechoic unilocular or multilocular soft tissue structure, which may be accompanied by surrounding increased blood flow on color/power Doppler scanning.

Lateral Compartment
Iliotibial Band

ITB friction syndrome is an overuse syndrome presenting as lateral knee pain worse at initial knee flexion.

- Thickening of the ITB, adjacent edema, and focal pain with transducer pressure at the level of the lateral femoral condyle with possible bursal fluid distention on US are compatible with ITB friction syndrome.

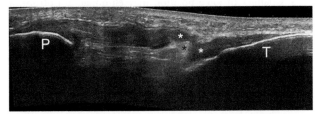

Figure 124.5. Full-thickness patellar tendon tear. Long-axis (sagittal) US image depicts patellar tendon rupture with proximal and distal stumps (*white asterisks*) and intervening fat (*black asterisk*). P = patella; T = tibial tuberosity.

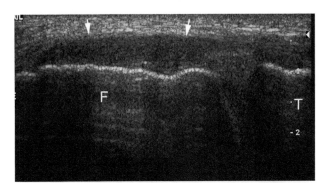

Figure 124.7. Grade 1 MCL sprain. Long-axis (coronal) US image depicts grade 1 sprain of the proximal MCL (*arrows*) with hypoechoic changes and swelling without ligamentous discontinuity. F = femur; T = tibia.

- Fluid in a normal joint recess may be seen deep to the distal ITB and should not be mistaken for a parameniscal cyst or ITB bursa.

Fibular Collateral Ligament, Biceps Femoris Tendon, and Popliteus Tendon

The FCL is a cordlike structure arising from the lateral femoral condyle, converging with the BFT, and inserting on the lateral fibular head. FCL injury may occur because of direct injury to the medial knee causing varus stress as well as hyperextension or noncontact injury.

The BFT is composed of 2 heads with distal tendinous, capsular, and aponeurotic attachments. The direct tendon fibers attach on the fibular head, medial and posterolateral to the FCL attachment. There is a variable tendinous anterior arm attaching to the lateral tibia and to an anterior aponeurosis. Biceps femoris injury has been reported in various sports, typically with hyperextension.

The popliteus tendon inserts on the popliteal groove at the posterolateral femur. The femoral attachment is rarely injured.

- On US, ligamentous and tendinous disruption can present as partial- or full-thickness disruption with or without retraction and waviness of the stumps (Figure 124.8).
- FCL waviness can be present with an intact ligament with knee flexion.
- It is important to accurately describe the type of LCL complex injury, including avulsion from the osseous attachment, pure ligamentous or tendon injury, or myotendinous junction injuries, as it may impact the type of treatment.
  - Dynamic assessment with gentle varus stress may also be employed to assess integrity of fibers.
  - Chronic partial-thickness injuries may show changes in tendon/ligament thickness with associated hypoechogenicity and loss of the fibrillar appearance.

Posterior Compartment
Baker Cyst

A common indication for US assessment of the posterior knee is to evaluate for the presence of a Baker cyst, which represents a distention of the semimembranosus–medial head of gastrocnemius bursa. A Baker cyst originates from a capsular recess on the posteromedial aspect of the knee. It extends in a soap-bubble configuration between the medial belly of the gastrocnemius (MG) muscle and the adjacent SMT/semitendinosus tendons. A necklike connection with the knee joint between the MG and ST is typically evident.

- Baker cysts may vary in size and complexity and may contain fluid, blood products, septations, loose bodies, and soft tissue components/synovial thickening (see Figure 118.18 in Chapter 118, "An Introduction to Musculoskeletal Ultrasound").
- Adjacent hypoechoic fluid about the Baker cyst may indicate leaking or rupture (Figure 124.9).

Menisci

There is ongoing controversy regarding the role of US in the evaluation of the menisci.

- US cannot assess the central components of the menisci.
- Heterogeneity and clefts involving the peripheral menisci as well as the presence of parameniscal cysts, which are associated with meniscal tears, can be identified by US.
- Parameniscal cysts may be unilocular/multilocular and hypoechoic/hyperechoic depending on the cyst complexity.
  - Parameniscal cysts may dissect far from the menisci, especially on the medial side of the knee, and visualization of the necklike extension to the meniscus is important for the correct diagnosis.

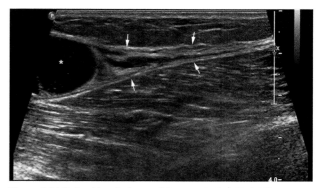

Figure 124.9. Leaking Baker cyst. Long-axis (sagittal) US image depicts a ruptured Baker cyst with linear hypoechoic fluid tracking along tissue planes (*arrows*) from its inferior aspect (*asterisk*).

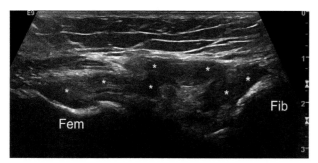

Figure 124.8. Full-thickness complete FCL tear. Long-axis (coronal) US image depicts complete rupture of the distal FCL with a wavy thickened proximal stump and a small displaced distal stump (*asterisks*). Fem = femur; Fib = fibula.

Key Points
- Changes in knee position may eliminate anisotropy, a common US artifact when evaluating fibrillar structures.
- Flexion of the knee may cause waviness of the FCL.
- Gentle dynamic assessment, such as flexion and extension and varus/valgus stress of the knee, may be helpful in evaluation of extensor tendon and collateral ligament integrity.
- Gastrocnemius anisotropy should not be mistaken for a small Baker cyst.
- The normal heterogeneous appearance of the proximal FCL and distal BFT should not be mistaken for tendinopathy.

■ Identification of the SM-GM necklike connection to the knee joint is key in correctly identifying a Baker cyst.

Recommended Reading

De Maeseneer M, Marcelis S, Boulet C, et al. Ultrasound of the knee with emphasis on the detailed anatomy of anterior, medial, and lateral structures. *Skeletal Radiol.* 2014;43(8):1025–39. doi:10.1007/s00256-014-1841-6.

References

1. Bonaldi VM, Chhem RK, Drolet R, Garcia P, Gallix B, Sarazin L. Iliotibial band friction syndrome: sonographic findings. *J Ultrasound Med.* 1998;17(4):257–60.
2. Craft JA, Kurzweil PR. Physical examination and imaging of medial collateral ligament and posteromedial corner of the knee. *Sports Med Arthrosc Rev.* 2015;23(2):e1–6. doi:10.1097/JSA.0000000000000066.
3. De Maeseneer M, Marcelis S, Boulet C, et al. Ultrasound of the knee with emphasis on the detailed anatomy of anterior, medial, and lateral structures. *Skeletal Radiol.* 2014;43(8):1025–39. doi:10.1007/s00256-014-1841-6.
4. Hirschmann MT, Muller W. Complex function of the knee joint: the current understanding of the knee. *Knee Surg Sports Tramatol Arthrosc.* 2015;23(10):2780–88. doi:10.1007/s00167-015-3619-3.
5. Ibounig T, Simons TA. Etiology, diagnosis and treatment of tendinous knee extensor mechanism injuries. *Scand J. Surg.* 2016;105(2):67–72. doi:10.1177/1457496915598761.
6. Kusma M, Seil R, Kohn D. Isolated avulsion of the biceps femoris insertion-injury patterns and treatment options: a case report and literature review. *Arch Orthop Trauma Surg.* 2007;127(9):777–80. doi:10.1007/s00402-006-0216-4.

CHAPTER 125

Ultrasound of the Calf, Ankle, and Foot

Yoav Morag

Introduction

US examination of the calf/lower leg, ankle, and foot is often performed in acute and chronic settings for various indications including muscle and tendon tears, ligamentous and retinacular injuries, joint effusions and synovitis, tenosynovitis, bursitis, plantar fascial injuries, and Morton neuroma. Dynamic US examination is useful in the evaluation of a *snapping ankle*, in particular, intermittent subluxations or dislocations of the peroneal tendons. A patient-guided approach allows the examiner to focus on the area of concern while the high spatial resolution of US and the superficial location of many of the evaluated structures in the ankle and foot allow identification of subtle pathology.

Technique and Positioning

US of the lower extremity distal to the knee is typically performed with high-frequency linear array transducers (12 MHz or higher). Deeper structures, as in the calf, may require lower frequency transducers, especially in the context of fatty infiltration of calf and shin muscles. A compact high-frequency (eg, 18 MHz) linear array transducer with a small footprint (*hockey stick*) may be helpful in certain instances as in evaluation for Morton neuroma or for an intermetatarsal bursal effusion. As in other MSK US examinations, all structures should be examined in both the short and long axes.

US evaluation of the calf, posterior ankle, and of the plantar fascia is performed in the prone position. The ankle and foot should be positioned hanging beyond the US stretcher margins to allow for plantar flexion and dorsiflexion of the foot when examining the Achilles tendon. Weight-bearing is often needed to identify transient muscle herniation. The posterior surface of the calcaneus serves as a convenient anatomic landmark. The short axis of the Achilles tendon will be visualized when scanning in the axial plane cranially from this landmark as a homogenous multipunctate structure with a convex posterior border and concave or flat anterior border. When rotating the transducer 90 degrees, echogenic contiguous Achilles tendon fibers will be visualized. At the distal attachment, the Achilles tendon may appear hypoechoic because of anisotropy, and the transducer should be gently rocked to differentiate between true pathology and this artifact. Dynamic evaluation of the tendon with gentle plantar and dorsiflexion of the foot or compression of the calf is performed to identify congruent motion of the whole Achilles tendon unit and exclude complete tendon rupture with hemorrhage, scar tissue, or fat filling the gap. Scanning cranially to evaluate the Achilles musculotendinous junction as well as the gastrocnemius and

soleus muscles and the plantaris tendon in the long and short axes is an integral part of US examination of the calf.

The plantar surface of the posterior calcaneal tuberosity serves as a landmark for identification of the plantar fascia. Scanning distally in the coronal plane will allow identification of the different components of the plantar fascia, especially of the central band, which is the thickest and strongest component. This structure should appear echogenic and homogenous and should measure 4 mm or less in maximal thickness at the calcaneal origin.

When scanning other structures of the ankle, it is helpful to divide these into 3 compartments: anterior, medial, and lateral (Table 125.1). Scanning is typically performed in the supine position. US evaluation of the tibiotalar joint is performed by scanning over the anterior ankle joint in the sagittal plane (Figure 125.1). The hypoechoic articular hyaline cartilage typically measures 1-2 mm in thickness and should not be mistaken for joint fluid. Scanning over the anterior ankle in the axial oblique plane will allow identification of the 3 extensor tendons from medial to lateral: tibialis anterior, extensor hallucis longus, and extensor digitorum tendons. The lateral and medial malleoli serve as anatomic landmarks for the lateral and medial compartments accordingly. Placing the transducer in the oblique axial plane posterior to the distal fibular shaft/lateral malleolus will allow identification of the peroneus longus and peroneus brevis tendons (Figure 125.2), which are closely apposed structures at this level with the peroneus brevis tendon closer to the lateral malleolus. While gradually angling the transducer into the oblique coronal plane, these tendons can be followed distally to the fanlike attachment of the peroneus brevis on the fifth metatarsal base/tuberosity and to the midfoot in the case of the peroneus longus tendon. An os peroneum, if present, resides in the peroneus longus tendon about the cuboid groove and has an appearance of a shadowing focus. The plantar aspect of the peroneus longus tendon with its attachment onto the first metatarsal base is examined in the prone position. Dynamic evaluation for peroneal tendon instability at the level of the lateral malleolus can be done by scanning during dorsiflexion and eversion of the foot. Examination of the peroneal tendons should also be completed in the long axis, scanning distally from the musculotendinous junction.

The lateral malleolus also serves as a convenient landmark for identifying the anterior talofibular ligament (ATFL), anterior tibiofibular ligament (AITFL), and the calcaneofibular ligament (CFL). By placing the transducer over a line connecting the lateral malleolus with the talus, the distal tibia, and the posterior calcaneus, these 3 ligaments can be identified accordingly. The CFL is also typically identified when evaluating

Table 125.1.

COMPARTMENT	KEY STRUCTURES	COMMON PATHOLOGY
Calf and heel	Achilles tendon, gastrocnemius and soleus muscles, plantaris tendon	Achilles tendinopathy, muscle injury, plantaris tendon injury
Plantar foot	Plantar fascia	Plantar fasciitis, plantar tears, plantar fibromatosis
Anterior ankle	Tibiotalar joint, anterior tendons,[a] peroneal nerves	Joint effusion, synovitis and intraarticular bodies, tibialis anterior tendinopathy
Medial ankle	Medial tendons,[b] tibial nerve, deltoid ligament	Posterior tibial tendinopathy/tear
Lateral ankle	Peroneus longus and brevis tendons	Peroneus brevis tendinopathy/tear, peroneal tendons instability
Forefoot	MTP joints, plantar plate, flexor and extensor tendons	Morton neuroma, intermetatarsal bursitis, plantar plate injury, joint effusion and synovitis

[a] Anterior tendons: tibialis anterior tendon, extensor hallucis longus tendon, extensor digitorum longus tendon.
[b] Medial tendons: posterior tibial tendon, flexor digitorum longus tendon, flexor hallucis longus tendon.

the peroneal tendons in the short axis posterior inferior to the lateral malleolus.

In a similar fashion, the medial malleolus serves as an anatomic landmark for the medial compartment. When scanning in the axial oblique plane at the level of the medial malleolus, the medial compartment structures can be identified from medial to lateral: posterior tibial tendon (PTT), flexor digitorum longus tendon (FDL), neurovascular bundle, and the flexor hallucis longus tendon (FHL). The PTT abuts the posterior aspect of the medial malleolus and is typically larger than FDL. Scanning distally will allow further evaluation of the tarsal tunnel as well as the PTT fanlike attachment on the navicular, cuneiforms, and metatarsal bases. On occasion, echogenic foci can be seen within the distal PTT corresponding to an os naviculare (accessory navicular). The FDL and FHL are typically scanned up to the midfoot area unless there is clinical concern regarding more distal tendon pathology. The examination should be completed by scanning these structures in the longitudinal fashion in an oblique sagittal plane. The deltoid ligament/MCL has superficial and deep components. Scanning in the coronal plane with the

transducer placed just inferior to the medial malleolus will allow identification of the deltoid ligament fibers just deep to the PTT and FDL tendons.

US examination of the forefoot is initially performed in the supine position with the plantar aspect of the foot dorsiflexed so that the sole of the foot faces the sonographer or in the prone position. The examination is performed at the level of the MTP joints with the ball of the foot serving as an anatomic landmark. The examination is initially performed in the sagittal plane for evaluation of the flexor tendon, the triangular plantar plates, and the MTP joints. Dynamic evaluation with passive flexion/extension of the toes is performed to demonstrate normal gliding motion of the tendons. The intermetatarsal space is then evaluated in the same plane while applying gentle pressure from the dorsal aspect of the forefoot. This maneuver widens the intermetatarsal space and allows for easier identification of Morton neuromas or bursitis. Scanning along the plantar aspect in the coronal plane/ short axis allows comparison between adjacent intermetatarsal spaces and easier identification of smaller masses or bursae. A sonographic Mulder sign may be elicited by applying gentle

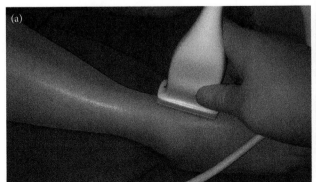
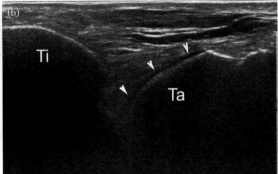

Figure 125.1. US of the anterior ankle. (*A*) Transducer positioning for scanning of the anterior ankle in sagittal plane. (*B*) Note hypoechoic talar dome (Ta) cartilage (*arrowheads*) without a tibiotalar joint effusion. Ti = tibia.

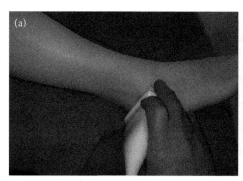
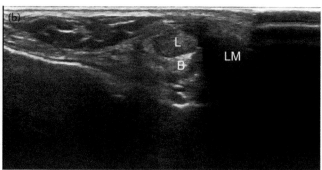

Figure 125.2. US of the lateral ankle. (*A*) Transducer positioning for scanning of the lateral ankle in axial oblique plane. (*B*) Note closely opposed peroneus longus (L) and peroneus brevis (B) tendons abutting the lateral malleolus (LM).

compression of the forefoot at the metatarsal head level (metatarsal squeeze test) while slowly releasing pressure on the transducer. US examination of the forefoot is completed by scanning the dorsal aspect of the forefoot in the sagittal and coronal planes and evaluation of the dorsal MTP joints and extensor tendons.

Pathology and Imaging Findings

Achilles Tendon

Although the Achilles tendon is the strongest tendon in the body, it is also the most commonly torn tendon of the ankle. The spectrum of disease includes paratenonitis, tendinosis, and tendon tears. The relatively hypovascular midportion of the Achilles tendon, approximately 2-6 cm proximal to the calcaneal insertion (watershed), is most prone to tendon pathology.

- On US examination, tendinosis is characterized by tendon thickening, hypoechogenicity, and tendon heterogeneity.
- Achilles tendon tears may be partial or full thickness (Figure 125.3).

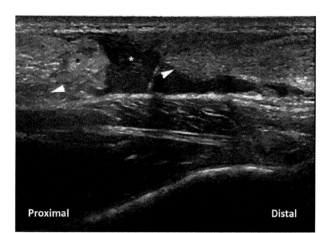

Figure 125.3. Achilles tendon rupture. Long-axis (sagittal) US image depicts a complete Achilles tendon tear with proximal and distal tendons stumps (*arrowheads*) and with fluid (*white asterisk*) and soft tissue (*black asterisk*) filing the gap between the stumps.

- The tendon gap may be filled by fluid, hemorrhage, debris, scar, or herniation of the Kager fat pad.
- The location of the tear, as well as the size of the gap as measured in different degrees of ankle flexion, will impact treatment selection.
- Scanning in the long axis with plantar flexion of the foot will approximate the tendon stumps.
- Paratenonitis represents inflammation accompanied with edema at the posterior, lateral, and medial aspect of the Achilles tendon.
- Fluid distention of the retrocalcaneal or retro-Achilles bursae may also accompany Achilles tendon pathology.

Tennis Leg Injury

Achilles tendon tears may be accompanied by plantaris tendon tears. Injury to the medial head of the gastrocnemius muscle (a.k.a. *tennis leg injury*) is not uncommon and may be isolated or accompanied with other injuries such as soleus muscle and Achilles tendon tears. The injury varies from muscle strain to partial or complete tears, which typically occur at the musculotendinous junction. The patient will often be able to pinpoint the area of injury.

- Muscle strain may have a normal US appearance or may show focal or diffuse increased echogenicity.
- Musculotendinous tears present as a spectrum from blunting of the muscle fibers to frank detachment of the muscle fibers with an intervening anechoic/hypoechoic fluid filled cleft along the musculotendinous junction of the medial head of gastrocnemius and soleus aponeurosis (Figure 125.4).

Plantar Fascia

The plantar fascia is a connective tissue structure that plays an important role in maintaining the longitudinal arch of the foot and is composed of medial, central, and lateral cords, of which the central bundle is the most important. Plantar fasciitis (also termed *fasciopathy*) is a common cause of inferior heel pain and typically occurs at the calcaneal origin because of repetitive trauma and microtears.

- On US, hypoechoic changes with loss of the echogenic fibrillar structure, heterogeneity, and thickening of the fascia (>4 mm) are consistent with plantar fasciitis (Figure 125.5).

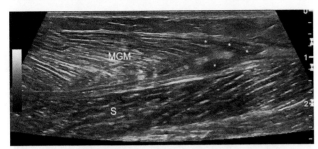

Figure 125.4. Acute tennis leg injury. Long-axis (sagittal) US image depicts partial avulsion of the medial head gastrocnemius muscle (MGM) from soleus aponeurosis. Note blunted MGM muscle fibers surrounded by fluid and hematoma (*asterisks*). S = soleus muscle.

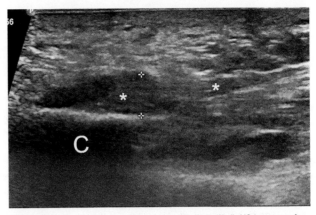

Figure 125.5. Plantar fasciitis. Long-axis (sagittal) US image of the plantar fascia (*asterisks*) depicts hypoechoic changes and thickening (digital caliper measurement) of the plantar fascia origin consistent with plantar fasciitis. C = calcaneus.

- Increased blood flow/hyperemia may also be present with color/power Doppler imaging.
- Injury to the plantar fascia following an acute traumatic event may appear similar to plantar fasciitis on US, however this occurs typically 2-3 cm distal to the calcaneal origin.
- Plantar fibromatosis, a rare benign fibroproliferative disorder of the plantar fascia, typically presents with fusiform hypoechoic or isoechoic soft tissue nodules intimately associated with the plantar fascia (Figure 125.6).
  - Intrinsic vascularity on color/power Doppler examination may be present.
  - Plantar fibromatosis often involves the distal two-thirds of the fascia.
  - US is an optimal examination for identifying additional small nonpalpable nodules or nodules in the contralateral foot, which occur in the context of plantar fibromatosis.

Anterior Ankle
Tibiotalar Joint Effusion
- Ankle joint effusion on US appears as anechoic or hypoechoic distention of the tibiotalar joint and will be compressible to varying degrees with transducer pressure (Figure 125.7).

- Small amounts of joint fluid may be seen in asymptomatic ankles, although aspiration may be needed to identify the etiology of abnormal tibiotalar joint effusions.
- Additionally, echogenic intraarticular bodies and synovitis may be identified on US examination.

Tibialis Anterior Tendon
- The anterior tibialis tendon (ATT), which mainly attaches onto the medial cuneiform bone, provides 80% of the dorsiflexion power of the ankle but is rarely injured given the straight course of the tendon and minimal mechanical demands placed on it (Figure 125.8).
  - Fluid about the distal 1-2 cm of this tendon is almost always considered pathologic.

Lateral Ankle
Peroneal Tendons
The peroneal tendons pronate and evert the foot. The peroneus brevis tendon is positioned between the peroneus longus tendon and lateral malleolus and thus susceptible to degenerative tears. Peroneus brevis longitudinal split tears are the most common and are typically seen in athletes and elderly. These tears may be associated with lateral ligamentous injuries,

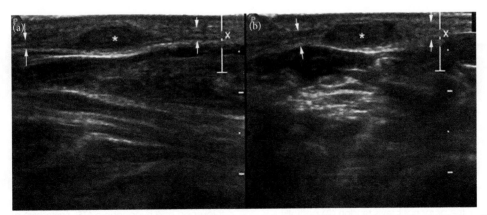

Figure 125.6. Plantar fibroma. (*A*) Long-axis (sagittal) and (B) short-axis (coronal) US images depict a hypoechoic soft tissue nodule (*asterisk*) loosely associated with the plantar fascia (*arrows*) consistent with a plantar fibroma.

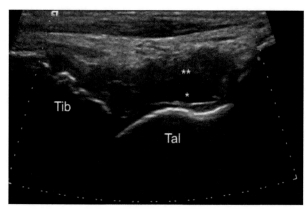

Figure 125.7. Ankle joint effusion with synovitis. Long-axis (sagittal) US image depicts distention of the tibiotalar joint with anechoic fluid (*asterisk*) and hypoechoic synovial proliferation (*double asterisk*) with accompanying blood flow (mild hyperemia) in the synovial component on color Doppler imaging. Tal = talus; Tib = tibia.

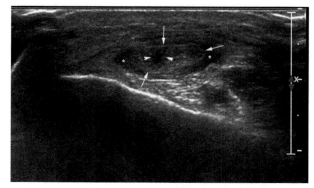

Figure 125.8. Intrasubstance tear and tenosynovitis of the tibialis anterior tendon. Short-axis (transverse) US image depicts an intrasubstance tear (*arrowheads*) of the anterior tibial tendon (*arrows*) with a circumferential hypoechoic soft tissue rim (*asterisks*) consistent with tenosynovitis.

crowding in the retromalleolar groove and superior peroneal retinacular injuries.

- Peroneus brevis split tears can be visualized by US as longitudinal hypoechoic clefts, and the peroneus longus tendon may be displaced into the peroneus brevis tendon defect (Figure 125.9).
  - Two distinct peroneus brevis hemi-tendons are formed, which may rejoin distally.
  - This is usually preceded by comma-shaped elongation of the peroneus brevis tendon in short axis consistent with interstitial tearing (boomerang sign), typically within the retromalleolar groove.
- Loss of the normal positioning of the peroneal tendons at the lateral malleolus/retromalleolar groove will occur with subluxation/dislocation of the tendons in the context of superior peroneal retinacular injury.
  - This instability includes the transient intrasheath subluxation and may be apparent only with dynamic US evaluation with ankle dorsiflexion and eversion.
- Although less common, peroneus longus tendon tears typically occur about the peroneal tubercle and cuboid groove and may be associated with proximal retraction or fracture of an os peroneum.

Anterior Talofibular Ligament

The ATFL belongs to the LCL complex, is the most vulnerable among the ankle ligaments, and may be the only torn ligament in 70% of lateral ankle sprains.

- US examination can identify ligamentous thickening and hypoechoic changes consistent with stretch injury/sprain without disruption (grade 1 injury).
  - Partial or complete disruptions of the ligament (grades 2 and 3 injuries respectively) may be difficult to distinguish clinically from one another and are characterized by an associated hypoechoic cleft involving a part of or the entire ligament thickness (Figure 125.10).

Medial Ankle

Posterior Tibial, Flexor Digitorum Longus, and Flexor Hallucis Longus Tendons

The PTT is the most commonly injured among the medial ankle tendons. PTT pathology is a frequent cause of medial ankle pain and swelling and a potential cause of progressive flatfoot deformity. Shear stress can cause transverse tendon tears in the area between the medial malleolus and navicular attachment site, and acute rupture can also occur.

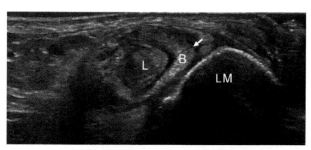

Figure 125.9. Peroneus brevis longitudinal split tear. Short-axis (transverse) US image depicts an early longitudinal split tear (*arrow*) of the peroneus brevis tendon (B) partially encompassing the peroneus longus tendon (L). LM = lateral malleolus.

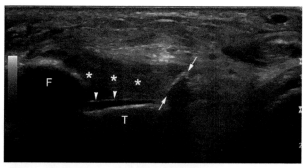

Figure 125.10. ATFL tear. Long-axis (sagittal) US image depicts a thickened and hypoechoic ATFL (*asterisks*) attached to an echogenic avulsed ossific fragment (*arrows*). Note hypoechoic hyaline articular cartilage (*arrowheads*). F = fibula; T = talus.

- Fluid and synovial thickening in the PTT sheath are consistent with tenosynovitis that may be accompanied with variable degrees of hyperemia on color/power Doppler imaging.
- Tendinosis is characterized by tendon thickening with variable degrees of hypoechogenicity and hyperemia.
- Tendon disruption can be identified on US, and split tears show longitudinal hypoechoic intrasubstance clefts.
- FDL and FHL tendons are less commonly injured compared to the PTT.

Tarsal Tunnel Syndrome and Deltoid Ligament
Tarsal tunnel syndrome is caused by entrapment of the tibial nerve/nerve branches within the tarsal tunnel.

- US can identify space-occupying lesions in the tarsal tunnel, such as ganglion cysts, as well as changes in tibial nerve morphology.

The deltoid ligament is rarely injured compared to the LCL complex.

Forefoot
Morton Neuroma
Morton neuroma represents focal nonneoplastic soft tissue enlargement of the plantar digital nerve with variable degree of perineural fibrosis, local vascular proliferation, edema of the endoneurium, and axonal degeneration. It is a common cause of interdigital pain, most frequently located in the third intermetatarsal web space, although it may involve other web spaces or more than 1 web space.

- Patient-guided US examination may point to the region of pathology.
  - Identification of the lesion may be enhanced by pressure on the opposing surfaces of the forefoot while scanning and by performing a sonographic Mulder technique, with plantar popping of the lesion that is sometimes accompanied with an audible click.
  - Typically, Morton neuromas are located in the pathway of the digital plantar nerves at the plantar aspect of the intermetatarsal head web space, just plantar to the intermetatarsal ligament but sometimes may extend dorsally and/or have a bilobed appearance.
- Intermetatarsal bursitis, which may occur in conjunction with Morton neuroma, may also cause interdigital pain but is typically compressible unlike Morton neuroma.

Plantar Plate
The fibrocartilaginous plantar plate located on the plantar aspect of the MTP joints provides support for the metatarsal head.

- The second MTP joint is the most common site for plantar plate injury and US can identify plantar plate tears.
  - These injuries most commonly occur laterally and can mimic Morton neuroma clinically.

Key Points
- US examination is frequently used in evaluations of muscle, tendon, and ligamentous injuries in the calf, ankle, and foot.
- Dynamic US is key when evaluating for Achilles tendon integrity, peroneal tendon dislocation, and Morton neuroma.
- The central bundle is the strongest and thickest component of the plantar fascia and should measure 4 mm or less in maximal thickness at the calcaneal origin.
- Peroneus brevis pathology typically occurs at the level of the lateral malleolus and includes tendinosis, tenosynovitis, partial tears, longitudinal split tears, and complete tendon ruptures.
- Peroneus longus tendon tears are less common compared to peroneus brevis and typically occur about the peroneal tubercle and cuboid groove.
- The PTT is the most commonly injured tendon at the medial aspect of the ankle, which can be readily evaluated with US.
- Intermetatarsal bursae will be collapsible under transducer pressure unlike Morton neuromas.

Recommended Reading
Allison SJ, Nazarian LN. Musculoskeletal ultrasound: evaluation of ankle tendons and ligaments. *AJR Am J Roentgenol.* 2010;194(6):W514. doi:10.2214/AJR.09.4067.

References
1. Allison SJ, Nazarian LN. Musculoskeletal ultrasound: evaluation of ankle tendons and ligaments. *AJR Am J Roentgenol.* 2010;194(6):W514. doi:10.2214/AJR.09.4067.
2. Cho KH. Ultrasound of the foot and ankle. *Ultrasound Clin.* 2012;7(4):487–503. http://dx.doi.org/10.1016/j.cult.2012.08.004.
3. Lee JC, Healy J. Sonography of lower limb muscle injury. *AJR Am J Roentgenol.* 2004;182(2):341–51. doi:10.2214/ajr.182.2.1820341.
4. Sconfienza LM, Orlandi D, Lacelli F, Serafini G, Silvestri E. Dynamic high-resolution US of ankle and midfoot ligaments: normal anatomic structure and imaging technique. *Radiographics.* 2015;35(1):164–78. doi:10.1148/rg.351130139. Review.
5. Torriani M, Kattapuram SV. Technical innovation. Dynamic sonography of the forefoot: the sonographic Mulder sign. *AJR Am J Roentgenol.* 2003;180(4):1121–23. doi:10.2214/ajr.180.4.1801121.

CHAPTER 126

Ultrasound of the Peripheral Nerves

Carlo Martinoli, Sonia Airaldi, and Federico Zaottini

Introduction

Nerve pathology may cause chronic pain and disability. Although the evaluation of neuropathies primarily relies on clinical examination and electrophysiology, diagnostic imaging is increasingly used as a complement to help define the site and cause of nerve dysfunction and to exclude other pathologic conditions underlying the patient's symptoms.

Normal Nerves and Scanning Technique

US can directly image nerves and reveal a specific fascicular echotexture.

- On the long-axis US images, nerves appear as elongated structures with alternating hypoechoic and hyperechoic bands (Figure 126.1A). On short-axis images, they show a stippled (honeycomb-like) appearance because of many small hypoechoic rounded foci embedded in a hyperechoic background (Figure 126.1B). The hypoechoic areas correspond to fascicles, whereas the echogenic tissue is due to the interfascicular and outer epineurium.
- US examination starts by scanning nerves in short axis. Once the nerve of interest is identified based on anatomical landmarks, the probe is swept proximally and distally, using the so-called elevator technique, to rapidly screen long nerve segments, looking for any abnormality affecting it and its surroundings. Long-axis planes are complementary and used if an abnormality is found.

Compressive Neuropathies

Based on US assessment, nerve compressive syndromes can be divided in 3 classes:

- *Class 1*—large nerves (eg, median, ulnar, peroneal, tibial, etc)
  - US evaluation requires midrange equipment and probe frequency range up to 13 MHz. Diagnosis is based on pattern recognition analysis and, for the carpal and cubital tunnels, calculation of the nerve cross-sectional area (CSA).
- *Class 2*—small nerves (eg, posterior and anterior interosseous, musculocutaneous, sural, distal divisional branches of large nerves, etc)
  - High-end equipment and probe frequency range up to 18 MHz is required. Diagnosis is based on pattern recognition analysis and calculation of the nerve

diameter because CSA measurements cannot be applied (nerve size too small).
- *Class 3*—large (eg, the femoral and sciatic in their intrapelvic course) and small (eg, the deep peroneal) nerves that are poorly visible or nondetectable with US because of a deep course or intervening bone
  - For motor/mixed nerves, the US diagnosis is based on indirect evaluation of muscles.
  - US detection of denervation is based on loss of bulk and hyperechoic appearance of the affected muscles.
  - US is not as accurate as MRI to differentiate the process of early denervation related to intramuscular extracellular edema from fatty atrophy.
- Regardless of the entrapment site, the US signs of compressive neuropathy are stereotypical. They include nerve flattening at the compression point and nerve swelling proximal or (less commonly) distal to it. The transition between swollen and flattened segments is abrupt and referred to as the *notch sign* (Figure 126.2).
- For quantification of findings, the most relevant measure is the nerve CSA (for class 1 nerves) or the maximum nerve diameter (for class 2 nerves). The CSA should be sampled at the site where the nerve is maximally enlarged and histopathologic changes are most severe.
- In the early phases of compression, intraneural edema and venous congestion are the main factors leading to the nerve enlargement. A positive correlation exists between nerve CSA and severity of electromyography (EMG) findings.
- In severe/longstanding compressions, the nerve echotexture may appear massively hypoechoic with loss of the fascicular pattern, which is caused by swelling of the fascicles and reduced echogenicity of the epineurium (Figure 126.2). Irreversible intraneural fibrosis may occur. Different from early disease, nerves with fibrotic changes remain swollen after decompressive surgery and have poor functional improvement.

Polyneuropathies

Inherited Disorders

- *Charcot-Marie-Tooth disease* includes demyelinating (CMT-1) and axonal (CMT-2) forms. Marked generalized fascicular enlargement reflecting *onion bulb* Schwann cell hypertrophy because of attempted remyelination typifies CMT-1A. Axonal forms (CMT-2) are more heterogeneous and show mild nerve enlargement.

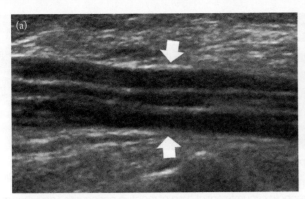
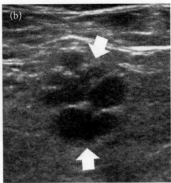

Figure 126.1. US appearance of normal nerves. Longitudinal (*A*) and transverse (*B*) 12-5 MHz US images of the tibial nerve at the proximal leg. (*A*) The nerve (*arrows*) is composed of multiple hypoechoic parallel linear areas separated by hyperechoic bands. (*B*) The nerve (*arrows*) is characterized by rounded hypoechoic areas in a homogeneous hyperechoic background.

- *Hereditary neuropathy with liability to pressure palsy* (HNPP) is a congenital disorder characterized by segmental demyelination and tomaculous or *sausage-shaped* myelin sheath swelling. US may show multifocal nerve enlargement (tomacula) following trivial trauma.

Immune-Mediated (Dysimmune) Polyneuropathies

- In *chronic inflammatory demyelinating polyradiculoneuropathy* (CIDP), US reveals segmental nerve abnormalities where conduction blocks are identified at electrophysiology. Fascicles may alternate with thickened and thinned segments (Figure 126.3*A*).
- In *acute inflammatory demyelinating polyradiculoneuropathy* (AIDP or Guillain-Barré syndrome), US is able to detect focal changes in nerve/fascicle thickness in early disease when electrophysiology is still negative. US shows reduced fascicular swelling during treatment before neurophysiological improvement appears.
- In *multifocal motor neuropathy* (MMN), US can detect multifocal nerve swellings.

Leprosy (Hansen disease)

- Leprosy is a multifaceted infectious disease caused by *Mycobacterium leprae* in which skin and nerves in

the extremities are specifically involved. It is the most common treatable cause of neuropathy worldwide.

- US can reveal markedly swollen nerves with loss of the fascicular echotexture and thickened epineurium (Figure 126.3*B*). Acute neuritic phases may be predicted by intense intraneural hyperemia at Doppler imaging, the so-called nerve inferno, a sign suggesting rapid progression of nerve damage and the need for immediate immunosuppressive therapy with corticosteroids (Figure 126.3*C*).

Nerve Injuries

Penetrating trauma, stretching, and contusion are the mechanisms of nerve injuries.

Penetrating Injuries

- In complete nerve transection, stump (terminal) neuromas develop as oval hypoechoic masses in continuity with the edges of the severed nerve. Detection of terminal neuromas may help to map the location of the nerve ends, which may be displaced and retracted away from the site of injury (Figure 126.4*A*).
  - Surgical repair after nerve injury involves excision of the neuroma; the gap length, therefore, should include the end-to-end distance plus the neuroma length.

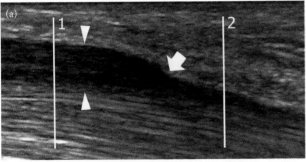
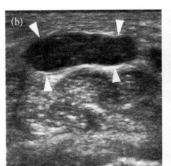
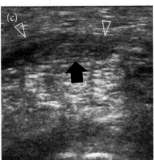

Figure 126.2. Compressive neuropathy. (*A*) Longitudinal 17-5 MHz US image of the median nerve at wrist in a patient with CTS shows abrupt change (*arrow*) of the nerve shape at the proximal boundary of the flexor retinaculum and swelling (*arrowheads*) of the nerve proximal to it. (*B*) Transverse image at the level 1 indicated in (*A*) shows markedly enlarged median nerve (*arrowheads*), which appears uniformly hypoechoic. (*C*) Transverse image at the level 2 indicated in (*A*) shows reduced size of the median nerve within the distal carpal tunnel (*arrow*) with convex appearance of the flexor retinaculum (*arrowheads*).

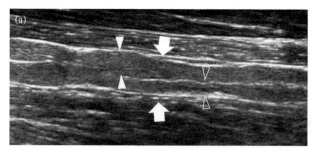
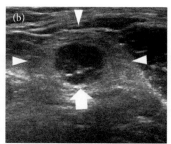
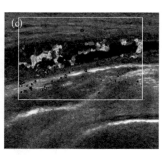

Figure 126.3. Polyneuropathies: (*A*) CIDP and (*B, C*) leprosy. (*A*) Longitudinal 12-5 MHz US image of the median nerve (*arrows*) at the middle forearm shows hyperechoic fascicles characterized by alternating thinned (*void arrowheads*) and thicker (*white arrowheads*) segments consistent with CIDP. (*B*) Transverse 12-5 MHz US image of the common peroneal nerve at the knee shows a swollen nerve (*arrow*) with abnormal fascicles surrounded by a hyperechoic circumferential area of reactive perineuritis (*arrowheads*) in a patient with leprosy. (*C*) Longitudinal 12-5 MHz color Doppler US image reveals intense intraneural hyperemia reflecting acute reversal reaction (immunologically mediated episode of acute or subacute inflammation that affects a subset of leprosy patients and remains a major cause of nerve damage).

■ In partial nerve tears, US can estimate the percentage of injured and preserved fascicles. A spindle neuroma may develop in continuity with the injured nerve. US is unable to assess the status of the fascicles within the neuroma and cannot predict outcome and recovery time (Figure 126.4*B*).

Stretching Injuries

■ Stretching injuries typically occur following sprain or strain injuries. In significant trauma without laceration, a fusiform hypoechoic swelling with loss of the fascicular echotexture can reflect a developing spindle neuroma and is related to intraneural fibrosis in a nondisrupted nerve trunk. An oblique course and the presence of fixation points make nerves vulnerable to stretching injuries. These lesions also occur where nerves pierce fascial planes.

Contusion Trauma

■ Contusion trauma most often occurs where nerves run closely apposed to bony surfaces (eg, superficial bony prominences, spurs, osteophytes) and are vulnerable to external pressure. Contusion leads to segmental nerve thickening with swollen fascicles and thickened epineurium. Similar findings occur in ulnar nerve instability at the elbow (friction neuritis).

Nerve Tumors and Tumorlike Lesions

Neurogenic Histotypes

■ Benign peripheral nerve sheath tumors include 2 main forms: schwannoma (also known as *neurinoma* or *neurilemmoma*) and neurofibroma.

■ The US diagnosis basically relies on detection of a soft tissue mass in continuity with a nerve at its proximal and distal poles. This feature may not be seen in cases of tumors arising from nerves that are too small and distal nerve branches. A rim of fat, the *split fat sign*, suggesting an origin of the mass in the intermuscular space about the neurovascular bundle is another finding associated with these lesions.

■ Some differential features have been reported between schwannomas and neurofibromas. Schwannomas are eccentric ovoid masses, whereas neurofibromas encase the fascicles of the parent nerve developing in a fusiform shape (Figure 126.5*A*). Neurofibromas may show a *target sign*, consisting of a hyperechoic (fibrous) core and a hypoechoic (myxomatous tissue) rim.

■ Plexiform neurofibromas are pathognomonic for type 1 neurofibromatosis (NF-1). They usually involve a long nerve segment and its branches with tortuous expansion, and their gross appearance has been described as a *bag of worms* (Figure 126.5*B*).

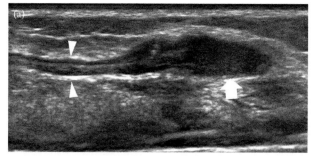
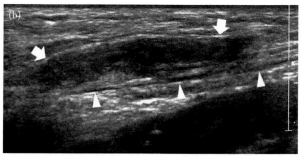

Figure 126.4. Nerve injuries. (*A*) Complete nerve transection following penetrating trauma. Longitudinal 17-5 MHz US image of the posterior leg demonstrates a stump neuroma (*arrow*) in continuity with the proximal sural nerve end (*arrowheads*). (*B*) Partial nerve tear by a penetrating wound. Longitudinal 17-5 MHz US image of the forearm shows a traumatic neuroma (*arrows*) within the substance of the ulnar nerve (*arrowheads*). The neuroma develops from the superficial injured fascicles, whereas the deep fascicles are unaffected.

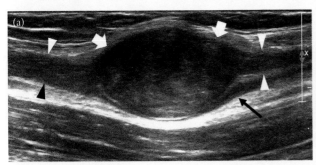 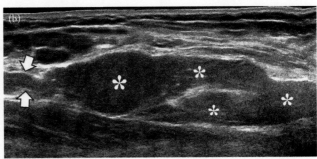

Figure 126.5. Nerve tumors. (*A*) Schwannoma of the median nerve at the middle third of the arm. Longitudinal 12-5 MHz US image depicts the tumor as an oval homogeneous hypoechoic mass (*white arrows*) in continuity with 1 thickened fascicle (*arrowheads*) of the median nerve. Note some spared fascicles (*black arrow*) displaced at the periphery of the mass. (*B*) Plexiform neurofibromas in a patient with type 1 neurofibromatosis. Longitudinal 12-5 MHz US image of the median nerve (*arrows*) at the middle forearm demonstrates multiple elongated masses (*asterisks*) arising from adjacent nerve fascicles. This appearance has been described as a "bag of worms."

■ Malignant forms tend to be larger (>5 cm) than benign histotypes and often appear as inhomogeneous hypoechoic masses with calcifications, areas of internal bleeding and necrosis, and indistinct margins as a result of their infiltrative growth. Despite these differences, a clear separation between benign and malignant forms is frequently unfeasible with US.

Nonneurogenic Intraneural Masses

■ Nonneural nerve sheath masses (eg, lipomas, paragangliomas, hemangiomas, lymphomas, extrinsic neoplasms, and ganglion cysts) may either originate, infiltrate, or adhere to a nerve.

■ *Fibrolipomatous hamartoma* is a developmental tumorlike nerve disorder related to accumulation of mature fat and fibroblasts in the epineurium that often presents at birth or during early childhood. The US appearance of fibrolipomatous hamartoma reflects its histopathology with increased epineurial fat surrounding slightly enlarged fascicles.

■ *Intraneural ganglia* appear as elongated cystic masses contained within the nerve sheath and most commonly affect the common peroneal nerve. The pathogenesis is related to penetration of joint fluid into the nerve trunk through a small articular (capsular) branch. The fluid extends along the articular branch through small capsular fenestrations and, after exiting the joint, it progresses upstream to reach the main nerve trunk. Intraneural ganglia do not have a fibrous/synovial lining.

■ In complete nerve transection, stump (terminal) neuromas develop as oval hypoechoic masses in continuity with the edges of the severed nerve. Detection of terminal neuromas may help to map the location of the nerve ends, which may be displaced and retracted away from the site of injury.

Recommended Reading

Brown JM, Yablon CM, Morag Y, Brandon CJ, Jacobson JA. US of the peripheral nerves of the upper extremity: a landmark approach. *Radiographics*. 2016;36(2):452–63. doi:10.1148/rg.2016150088. Review.

Yablon CM, Hammer MR, Morag Y, Brandon CJ, Fessell DP, Jacobson JA. US of the peripheral nerves of the lower extremity: a landmark approach. *Radiographics*. 2016;36(2):464–78. doi:10.1148/rg.2016150120. Review.

References

1. Abreu E, Aubert S, Wavreille G, et al. Peripheral nerve tumors and tumor-like neurogenic lesions. *Eur J Radiol*. 2013;82:38–50.
2. Chiou HJ, Chou YH, Chiou SY, et al. Peripheral nerve lesions: role of high-resolution US. *Radiographics*. 2003;23:E15.
3. Duncan I, Sullivan P, Lomas F. Sonography in the diagnosis of carpal tunnel syndrome. *AJR Am J Roentgenol*. 1999;173:681–84.
4. Hobson-Webb LD, Padua L, Martinoli C. Ultrasonography in the diagnosis of peripheral nerve disease. *Expert Opin Med Diagn*. 2012;6:457–71.
5. Kermarrec E, Demondion X, Khalil, et al. Ultrasound and magnetic resonance imaging of the peripheral nerves: current techniques, promising directions, and open issues. *Semin Musculoskelet Radiol*. 2010;14:463–72.
6. Martinoli C, Bianchi S, Gandolfo N, et al. US of nerve entrapments in osteofibrous tunnels of the upper and lower limbs. *Radiographics*. 2000;20:199–217.
7. Martinoli C, Bianchi S, Pugliese F, et al. Sonography of entrapment neuropathies in the upper limb (wrist excluded). *J Clin Ultrasound*. 2004;32:438–50.

Key Points

■ US can directly image nerves and reveals a specific fascicular echotexture.

■ On the long-axis US images, nerves appear as elongated structures with alternating hypoechoic and hyperechoic bands, whereas on the short-axis images, they show a stippled (honeycomb-like) appearance.

■ Regardless of the entrapment site, the US signs of compressive neuropathy include nerve flattening at the compression point and nerve swelling proximal or (less commonly) distal to it.

8. Murphey MD, Smith WS, Smith SE, et al. Imaging of musculo-skeletal neurogenic tumors: radiologic-pathologic correlation. *Radiographics.* 1999;19(5):1253–80.

9. Silvestri E, Martinoli C, Derchi LE, et al. Echotexture of peripheral nerves: correlation between US and histologic findings and criteria to differentiate tendons. *Radiology.* 1995;197(1):291–96.

10. Spinner RJ, Atkinson JL, Tiel RL. Peroneal intraneural ganglia: the importance of the articular branch. A unifying theory. *J Neurosurg.* 2003;99(2):330–43.

11. Zaidman CM, Al-Lozi M, Pestronk A. Peripheral nerve size in normals and patients with polyneuropathy: an ultrasound study. *Muscle Nerve.* 2009;40(6):960–66.

CHAPTER 127

Ultrasound of the Rheumatologic Diseases

Robert Lopez-Ben

Introduction

The term *rheumatologic disease* encompasses a plethora of multisystem autoimmune disorders that can affect the MSK system to varying degrees of severity. Imaging, including radiography as well as cross-sectional modalities, such as MRI and US, has an important role in clinical practice in the initial diagnosis and assessment of disease activity of many of these diseases. This chapter will focus on the role of US in the diagnosis and disease activity assessment of RA, seronegative arthritides (psoriatic and reactive), and crystal deposition diseases (ie, gout and CPPD arthropathy).

Disease severity for many of these conditions can be variable, but can lead to fixed joint deformities and significant disabilities and morbidities. Several studies have established that early treatment with antiinflammatory and disease-modifying antirheumatic agents (DMARDs) may decrease joint damage and lead to improved functional outcomes in patients with RA. Some of the newer antiinflammatory drugs targeting specific components of the inflammatory cascade, such as antitumor necrosis factor agents or interleukin inhibitors, are highly effective, but also expensive and can be associated with serious side effects. Hence, there is an increased importance in establishing accurate diagnosis and assessing therapeutic response as well as disease course during treatment.

Cross-sectional imaging techniques, such as MRI and US, have traditionally been used in these patients to evaluate for complications of chronic inflammation such as tendon tears, entrapment neuropathies, or secondary joint infections. In comparison to CT, MRI, and US, radiography has low sensitivity for detection of bone erosions. Yet, it remains the most commonly used imaging modality in clinical practice for detecting erosions in RA. However, erosions detected with US and MRI become apparent on radiography in most RA cases within 1-2 years. Along with MRI, US is being used to directly evaluate the synovial inflammation, as well as assessing erosive osseous disease. It has been reported to be particularly useful in detecting erosions in patients in the early stages of disease. MRI, unlike US, can assess for BME, which may be a prognostic indicator of erosive disease; however, US is a more economical modality and lends itself to assessing multiple joints more quickly.

Patient and Transducer Positioning

Given the typical involvement of the hands and feet early in inflammatory arthritis, US of the joints commonly targeted by these diseases is typically performed. Higher frequency (ie, 10 MHz or greater) linear transducers with small footprints are used in order to increase anatomic resolution when imaging these small parts.

For RA, evaluation of the MCP and PIP joints of the hands, as well as the wrist joints, is performed as this disease has a predilection for symmetrical involvement of these joints. In order to expedite the performance time of the examination, and given the joint-specific disease predilections, some practitioners will scan the second through fifth MCP joints and the second and third PIP joints of the hand, as well as the wrists. Scanning the MTP joints of the feet, as well as the ankle joints, can increase the diagnostic yield for synovial inflammation and erosive disease burden when patients are symptomatic in these areas.

The MCP and PIP joints, as well as the MTP joints, are scanned circumferentially when possible, with special attention to both the palmar/plantar and dorsal aspects of both joints. These joints have palmar/plantar and dorsal joint recesses that are best seen when there is a joint effusion (Figure 127.1) or synovitis. Synovitis will be identified earliest in the dorsal synovial recess of the MCP or MTP joints and the palmar synovial recess of the PIP joints. A slight depression on the dorsal aspect of the distal metacarpal can be seen in approximately 33% of normal second, third, and fifth MCP joints, less than 2 mm in depth (Figure 127.2). This should not be confused with a bone erosion. The wrist and ankle joints are scanned circumferentially, with attention to the 6 extensor tendon compartments dorsally and the flexor tendons volarly in the wrist, the flexor tendons medially, the extensor tendons anteriorly, and the peroneal tendons laterally in the ankle for the presence of tenosynovitis (Figure 127.3).

In patients with psoriatic arthritis, scanning of the DIP joints of the hands is also performed, given their increased involvement in this disease. In patients with reactive arthritis, the lower extremity joints (feet, ankles, knees) are commonly involved and hence imaged, with attention to the entheses of major tendon attachments such as the Achilles and patellar tendons. In patients with suspected gout, evaluation of the first MTP joints of the feet, as well as the tarsometatarsal and midfoot dorsal joint recesses, can be performed to assess for common areas of crystal deposition.

Synovial hyperemia is a marker of synovial inflammation. Power or color Doppler interrogation can help identify synovial or entheseal vascularity. Power Doppler has traditionally been more sensitive than color Doppler in assessing blood flow within small vessels, with accuracy comparable to contrast-enhanced MRI. When using color or power Doppler, it is important to minimize transducer pressure on the joint as the signal from the small synovial

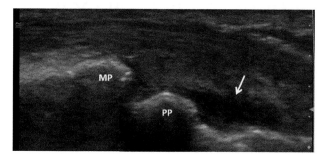

Figure 127.1. Distension of the palmar joint recess. Long-axis grayscale US image of the fifth PIP joint shows distension of palmar joint recess from a joint effusion (*arrow*) in a patient with psoriatic arthritis. PP = proximal phalanx; MP = middle phalanx.

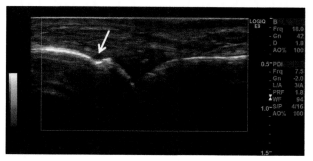

Figure 127.2. Normal dorsal depression at the metacarpal head. Long-axis power Doppler US image of right index finger MCP joint shows normal dorsal depression (*arrow*) without significant joint effusion or hyperemia.

vessels can be obliterated with excessive overlying pressure. Motion/flash and edge artifacts should not be confused with increased synovial blood flow. The Doppler color gain setting is optimized by setting its baseline just above the level of noise to increase sensitivity, but there should be no signal within normal cortical bone. Intraarticular Doppler signal is usually not seen in normal joints, especially in the MCP and PIP joints, although low levels of Doppler signal may be seen in patients with osteoarthritis. Several European studies have shown that sonographic microbubble contrast agents can improve visualization of synovial vascular Doppler signal in less superficial joints, such as the sacroiliac or hip joints, and help in differentiating active versus inactive synovitis. These agents are currently not approved by the U.S. Food and Drug Administration for examination of joints.

Imaging Findings of Common Rheumatologic Diseases

Rheumatoid Arthritis

Evaluation of symptomatic and target joints for synovitis and erosions is performed. The presence and extent of synovitis is a prognostic indicator of future bone damage. Erosive changes can occur within the first 6 months in aggressive RA, which indicates a poor prognosis. When compared to radiography, 6.5 times as many erosions can be identified by US in patients with early RA.

- Synovitis can be visualized on US as thickened, hypoechoic, noncompressible intraarticular tissue with increased Doppler signal (as opposed to joint effusions, which are compressible and do not have increased Doppler signal) (Figure 127.4).
- Increased synovial vascularity correlates with disease activity and can be used to determine treatment response.
- The EULAR/OMERACT (European League Against Rheumatism/Outcome Measures in Rheumatoid Arthritis Clinical Trials) semiquantitative grading of synovial power Doppler signal is commonly used: 0 = no intraarticular Doppler signal; 1 = single signal; 2 = moderate signal from confluent vessels; and 3 = severe signal with greater than 50% of the imaged synovial tissue with visualized vessels.
- Erosions are defined on US as an irregular discontinuity of the articular margin bone cortex in 2 perpendicular planes, greater than 2 mm in depth (Figure 127.5).
- Proposed transverse diameter criteria for erosion size categorization are small = <2 mm; moderate = 2-4 mm; and large = >4 mm. They have increased through transmission when they contain hypoechoic pannus within them.

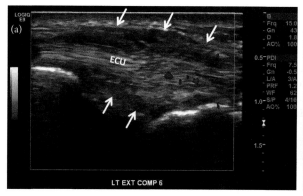
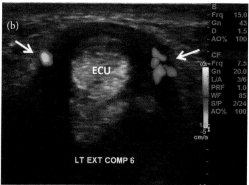

Figure 127.3. Extensor carpi ulnaris (ECU) tenosynovitis in RA patient. (A) Long-axis power Doppler US image and (B) short-axis color Doppler US image of the dorsal ulnar aspect of the wrist shows distension of the ECU tendon sheath with hypoechoic tenosynovitis and increased power Doppler signal related to hyperemia (*arrows*).

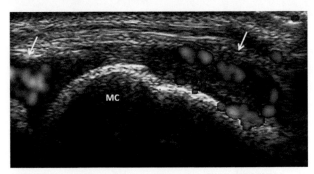

Figure 127.4. Grade 3 Doppler synovitis. Long-axis power Doppler US image of the right index finger MCP joint in RA patient shows grade 3 Doppler synovitis involving greater than 50% of the imaged synovial tissue (*arrows*). MC = metacarpal head.

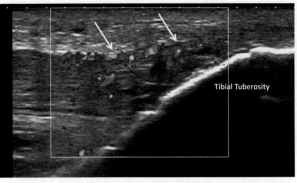

Figure 127.6. Enthesitis in reactive arthritis. Long-axis color Doppler US image of the left patellar tendon insertion to the tibial tuberosity in a patient with reactive arthritis shows marked hyperemia with increased intratendinous signal (*arrows*).

■ If the patient complains of foot pain, examining the MTP joints may be helpful as 10-15% of patients at clinical presentation will have erosions detected in the feet but not the hands.

Psoriatic and Reactive Arthritis

Patients with these types of inflammatory arthritis will have synovitis and erosive changes, similar to RA, but with asymmetric and different target joint involvement (DIP joints), as well as evidence of entheseal inflammation, the latter with secondary periarticular reactive bone formation.

■ Evaluation of commonly involved entheses, such as the Achilles tendon calcaneal insertion in the hindfoot, or quadriceps and patellar tendon attachments in the knee, can show focal swelling and hypoechogenicity, as well as increased intratendinous and peritendinous Doppler signal, in patients with psoriatic and reactive arthritis (Figure 127.6).

■ When evaluating the small joints of the hands with US in a patient with undifferentiated inflammatory arthritis, psoriatic arthritis may show more adjacent tendon inflammation and increased Doppler signal at the joint capsule enthesis (Figure 126.7), features that may help in differentiating from RA.

■ *Sausage-digit* dactylitis is a frequent clinical manifestation of these diseases, and US can help in identifying the underlying flexor tendon tenosynovitis (Figure 127.8).

Gout and Calcium Pyrophosphate Dihydrate Deposition Disease Arthropathy

■ As can be seen with the inflammatory arthritides, US can also show erosive changes in crystal deposition diseases, and these tend to appear deeper, have more well-defined margins, and frequently, less adjacent synovial hyperemia by Doppler criteria when compared with RA.

■ Distended hypoechoic synovial tissue can have a *snowstorm* appearance with US caused by numerous hyperechoic stippled crystal aggregates (Figure 127.9).

■ In tophaceous gout, intraarticular or paraarticular tophi will have a similar inhomogeneous echogenic appearance (Figure 127.10), at times surrounded by a thin hypoechoic rim or halo. There may be an adjacent erosion present when intraarticular (Figure 127.11), especially when involving the MTP joints.

■ US can also help identify the intraarticular hyaline cartilage deposition of monosodium urate (MSU) and CPPD crystals. MSU crystals will deposit on the surface of the cartilage, creating an echogenic thick double-contour

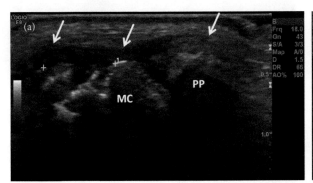

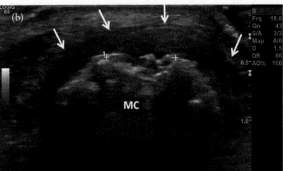

Figure 127.5. Large osseous erosion in RA patient. (*A*) Long-axis and (*B*) short-axis grayscale US images of the fifth MCP joint show increased synovial fluid complex (*arrows*) and a large irregular osseous erosion at the dorsal ulnar aspect of the metacarpal head (*between calipers*). MC = metacarpal head; PP = proximal phalanx.

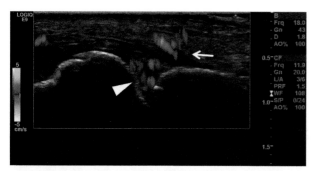

Figure 127.7. Enthesitis in psoriatic arthritis. Long-axis color Doppler US image of the medial aspect of the great toe MTP joint shows marked hyperemia within the joint consistent with active synovitis (*arrowhead*) with additional hyperemia at the distal capsular attachment site related to enthesitis (*arrow*).

sign (Figure 127.12). It is important not to confuse this appearance with the normal thin echogenic contour of the articular cartilage interface with synovial fluid.

- Chondrocalcinosis from deposited CPPD crystals will aggregate in the middle layer of the hyaline cartilage and appear as echogenic punctate or linear foci within the cartilage, paralleling the bone contour.
- CPPD crystals can also be identified on US as punctate echogenic foci within fibrocartilage structures, such as the menisci in the knee or the TFC in the wrist, or in the synovium (Figures 127.13 and 127.14); the latter can also occur with gout.
- CPPD intraarticular crystal aggregates may cause intraarticular *snowstorm* appearance similar to gout.

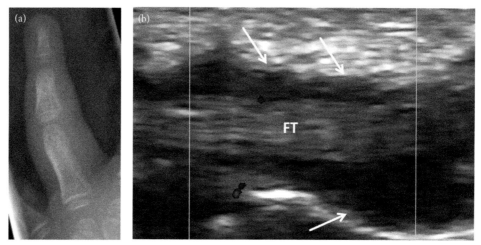

Figure 127.8. Sausage digit in a 4-year-old patient with juvenile psoriatic arthritis. (*A*) AP radiograph of the left ring finger shows diffuse soft tissue swelling. (*B*) Long-axis power Doppler US image in the same patient at the volar aspect of the proximal phalanx shows tenosynovitis with a distended common flexor tendon (FT) sheath (*arrows*) and mild hyperemia.

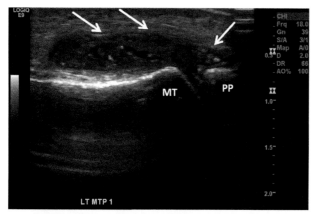

Figure 127.9. Intraarticular gouty crystals (*snowstorm*). Long-axis US image of the dorsal aspect of the great to MTP joint shows heterogeneous joint effusion with multiple small echogenic foci consistent with uric acid crystals (*arrows*), which were mobile with transducer pressure creating *snowstorm* appearance. MT = metatarsal head; PP = proximal phalanx.

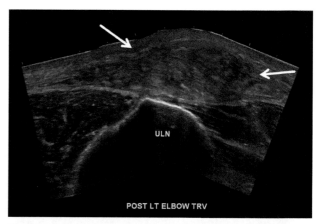

Figure 127.10. Tophaceous gout at the elbow. Short-axis extended FOV US image of the posterior aspect of the proximal ulna (uln) shows marked heterogeneous echogenic distension of the olecranon bursa consistent olecranon bursitis with tophaceous gout (*arrows*).

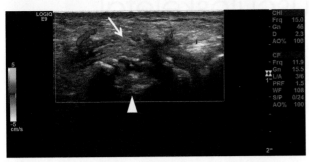

Figure 127.11. Intraarticular gouty tophus with associated osseous erosion. Long-axis color Doppler US image of the dorsal radial aspect of the third MCP joint shows heterogeneous joint effusion with small hyperechoic foci related to uric acid crystals and an echogenic intraarticular tophus (*arrow*) with associated large osseous erosion in the third metacarpal head (*arrowhead*).

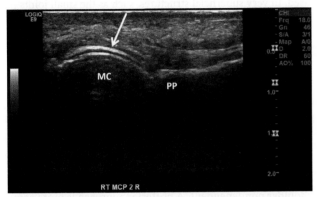

Figure 127.12. Double-contour cartilage sign in gout patient. Long-axis US image of the dorsal radial aspect of the right second MCP joint (same patient as in Figure 127.11) shows echogenic double-contour cartilage sign from monosodium urate crystal deposition on surface of hyaline cartilage (*arrow*). MC = metacarpal head; PP = proximal phalanx.

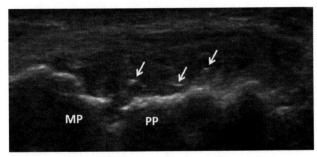

Figure 127.13. CPPD arthropathy. Long-axis grayscale US image of the middle finger PIP joint shows punctate echogenic foci (*arrows*) within the distended dorsal synovial recesses consistent with intraarticular crystal aggregates. PP = proximal phalanx; MP = middle phalanx.

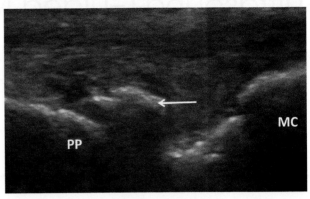

Figure 127.14. CPPD arthropathy. Long-axis grayscale US image of the middle finger MCP joint shows echogenic linear intraarticular foci (*arrow*) overlying the base of the proximal phalanx with posterior acoustic shadowing consistent with conglomerate CPPD crystal aggregation.

- When examining the patient, knowledge of target joints involved in the different rheumatologic diseases can help differentiate these conditions and direct the US examination.
- Doppler signal within a swollen, hypoechoic enthesis can be identified in psoriatic and reactive arthritis.
- US can help identify tophi and intraarticular crystal deposition.

Recommended Reading

Taljanovic MS, Melville DM, Gimber LH, et al. High-resolution US of rheumatologic diseases. *Radiographics*. 2015;35: 2026–48.

References

1. Wakefield RJ, Balint PV, Szkudlarek M, et al. Musculoskeletal ultrasound including definitions for ultrasonographic pathology. *J Rheumatol*. 2005;32:2485–87.
2. Farrant JM, O'Connor PJ, Grainger AJ. Advanced imaging in rheumatoid arthritis. Part 1: synovitis. *Skeletal Radiol*. 2007;36:269–70.
3. Farrant JM, O'Connor PJ, Grainger AJ. Advanced imaging in rheumatoid arthritis. Part 2: erosions. *Skeletal Radiol*. 2007;36:381–89.
4. Wakefield RJ, Gibbon WW, Conaghan PG, et al. The value of sonography in the detection of bone erosions in patients with rheumatoid arthritis. A comparison with conventional radiography. *Arthritis Rheum*. 2000;43(12):2762–70.
5. Thiele RG, Schlesinger N. Diagnosis of gout by ultrasound. *Rheumatology*. 2007;46:1116–21.
6. De Avila Fernandes E, Kubota ES, Sandim GB, Mitraud SA, Ferrari AJ, Fernandes AR. Ultrasound features of tophi in chronic tophaceous gout. *Skeletal Radiol*. 2011;40:309–15.
7. O'Connor PJ. Crystal deposition disease and psoriatic arthritis. *Semin Musculoskelet Radiol*. 2013;17:74–79.
8. Balint PV, Kane D, Wilson H, McInnes IB, Sturrock RD. Ultrasonography of entheseal insertions in the lower limb in spondyloarthropathy. *Ann Rheum Dis*. 2002;61:905–10.
9. Gutierrez M, Filippucci E, Salaffi F, Di Geso L, Grassi W. Differential diagnosis between rheumatoid arthritis and psoriatic arthritis: the value of ultrasound findings at metacarpophalangeal joints level. *Ann Rheum Dis*. 2011;70:1111–14.

Key Points

- US can identify synovial inflammation (synovitis) and may identify radiographically occult erosions in rheumatologic diseases.
- Intraarticular Doppler signal is a marker of active synovitis and can help differentiate synovial hypoechogenicity from a joint effusion.
- Erosions are defined on US as irregular discontinuities of the articular margin bone cortex in 2 perpendicular planes, greater than 2 mm in depth.

CHAPTER 128

Ultrasound-Guided Musculoskeletal Procedures

Robert Lopez-Ben

Introduction

US can be used to guide a variety of MSK interventions, but the most common indications are joint (Figures 128.1 and 128.2), bursal (Figure 128.3), peritendinous/intramuscular aspirations (Figure 128.4) and therapeutic injections (Figure 128.5), and soft tissue biopsies (Figure 128.6). An exhaustive review of all US-guided MSK interventions (including its use for soft tissue biopsies, tumor ablation guidance, and peripheral nerve root blocks among some of the many uses) is beyond the scope of this chapter. Many of these procedures can be guided with fluoroscopy or CT, however, US can provide a faster way to guide some of these procedures without the use of ionizing radiation. This chapter will focus on general principles of using US for some of these common indications, with some practical information for their performances.

Before any planned intervention, informed consent is obtained with the procedure explained to the patient. The more commonly encountered or serious complications of needle procedures are discussed, including but not limited to bleeding, infection, allergic reactions, and potential peripheral nerve injury, if applicable. A complete US examination of the area, including interrogation with color/power Doppler, is performed to assess for adjacent neurovascular structures to be avoided. The choice of transducers to be used will depend mostly on the specific anatomic considerations for the particular intervention. Superficial structures targeted for intervention are best visualized with high-frequency linear transducers (10 MHz or higher), such that the US beam is as close to perpendicular with the needle path using a small footprint transducer, in order to provide adequate real-time visualization of the needle path and target. For deeper structures, such as the hip, especially in obese patients, lower frequency curvilinear probes can provide better penetration of the sound beam and better visualization of the needle, especially when the needle must be placed at a steep angle.

Sterile technique is paramount, with sterile coupling gel and transducer probe covers routinely preferred. In some tight anatomic spaces, such as in the small joints of the hands and feet, a probe cover may be too cumbersome to use, so sterilization of the transducer probe with betadine and/or alcohol preparations can be used.

A freehand technique is typically used, preferentially parallel to the long axis of the transducer, allowing continuous visualization of the needle tip during the procedure. When accessing deeper structures with a steeper oblique path to the target, a needle guide attached to the transducer can also be used. In very superficial structures, such as the small joints of the feet and hands, the needle path must sometimes be near perpendicular to the long axis of transducer probe and may not be able to be visualized in its entirety, but short-axis imaging of the needle path can be used in these cases to check the depth of the needle.

Patient and Transducer Positioning

Shoulder Joint and Subacromial-Subdeltoid Bursa

A lateral decubitus position is preferred, with the targeted shoulder nondependent. A posterior approach is more commonly used. In many patients, a standard 1.5-inch 25-gauge needle may reach the upper joint, but sometimes a longer 22-gauge spinal needle may have to be used to access the joint. With the patient's hand over the contralateral shoulder, an axial image of the posterior shoulder should identify the humeral head, posterior labrum and glenoid, joint capsule, and overlying rotator cuff muscles. Using either a lateral or medial approach, the needle is directed toward the junction of the humeral head and posterior labrum (Figure 128.1). Once the needle is positioned underneath the joint capsule at the most medial aspect of the posterior humeral head, a small test injection of local anesthetic should be free of resistance.

If the subacromial-subdeltoid bursa is targeted, the needle tip is placed within the hypoechoic interface between echogenic fat planes just deep to the deltoid muscle and immediately superficial to the bursal surface of the rotator cuff tendons. The subacromial-subdeltoid bursa may also be injected using the anterior approach with the patient in semirecumbent position on the US stretcher.

Elbow Joint

A posterior lateral approach is most commonly used, with the elbow flexed, with the puncture performed to the side of the triceps tendon. A posterior medial approach is not favored because of the location of the ulnar nerve at the cubital tunnel. The probe can be positioned axial or longitudinal with regard to the joint, and the needle is directed into the posterior joint space at the olecranon recess of the posterior humerus, immediately deep to the echogenic posterior fat pad (Figure 128.2).

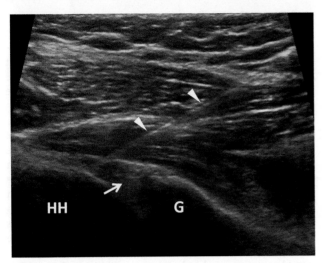

Figure 128.1. Transverse US image of the posterior right shoulder in a patient undergoing US-guided joint injection of contrast for MR arthrography. A 22-gauge spinal needle (*arrowheads*) has been placed from a medial approach through the deltoid muscle and infraspinatus tendon into the glenohumeral joint, immediately lateral to the posterior superior labrum (*arrow*). G = glenoid; HH = humeral head.

Hip Joint, Greater Trochanteric Bursa, and Iliopsoas Bursa

The hip joint is usually accessed via a longitudinal approach parallel to the long axis of the femoral neck. The femoral neurovascular structures are identified, and the needle path is planned lateral to these. The needle is directed superiorly to the concavity underneath the joint capsule at the junction of the anterior femoral neck and head. In thin patients, a transverse approach can be used with the needle placed via an anterolateral path into the femoral neck/head junction.

Greater trochanteric pain syndrome, usually caused by insertional tendinopathy of the gluteus medius tendon, is a common condition referred for injection of local anesthetic and corticosteroid. When injecting the trochanteric bursa, the patient is usually placed in a lateral decubitus position with the hips and knees flexed. The transducer is positioned transverse to the long axis of the femur. The injection is performed with a 22-gauge spinal needle directed from a posterior to anterior approach. The injectate is placed in the peritendinous soft tissues at the location of the greater trochanteric bursa.

Iliopsoas bursa injection is performed with the patient in supine position, using a freehand technique, and lower frequency curvilinear or linear probes, with transducer selection depending on factors such as body habitus and geometry. Injections are performed using the anterior lateral approach at the level of the joint line (iliopectineal eminence) with a 22- or 20-gauge spinal needle aiming for the lateral aspect of the tendon (Figure 128.3).

Knee Joint

The joint is best accessed when the patient flexes the knee (a small pillow behind the knee can be used to support this position with the patient supine), and the approach is anterior. In patients with a joint effusion, the suprapatellar recess can be visualized directly underneath the quadriceps tendon at the superior patellar border and can be accessed via a longitudinal or transverse approach, with the needle puncture site medial or lateral to the quadriceps tendon. Alternatively, especially when little to no joint effusion is present to visualize the suprapatellar recess, the lateral or medial patellofemoral joint recess can be targeted with the probe placed transversely between the patellar lateral or medial border and the adjacent femoral condyle.

Ankle Joint

With the patient supine, the anterior tibiotalar joint is evaluated in a longitudinal direction. The location of the dorsalis pedis artery and extensor tendons is noted and a path avoiding these structures is planned. The needle is usually placed from an inferior approach in a sagittal plane into the joint. Alternatively, the anterior lateral or medial tibiotalar joint recess can be approached via a transverse approach, with care taken to avoid the anterior talofibular ligament if the lateral approach is used.

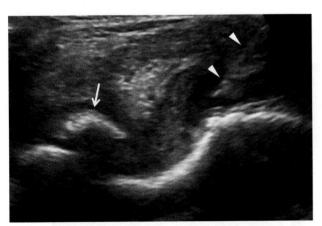

Figure 128.2. Transverse US image of the posterior right elbow in a patient with RA referred for intraarticular injection of corticosteroid. A 22-gauge needle (*arrowheads*) has been placed into the posterior lateral olecranon recess of the elbow joint at the level of the distal humerus. Note an incidental small intraarticular osteochondral body medially (*arrow*).

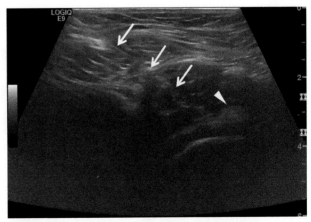

Figure 128.3. US-guided iliopsoas bursal injection. Transverse US image of the anterior aspect of the hip joint at the level of the superior acetabulum shows a 20-gauge spinal needle (*arrows*) placed along the lateral aspect of the iliopsoas tendon (*arrowhead*) for bursal injection.

Common Musculoskeletal Ultrasound-Guided Interventions

Joint Aspirations and Injections

Using the specific anatomic considerations previously described, US is commonly used for joint injections and arthrocentesis. Joint injections of contrast can be performed under US guidance prior to CT or MR arthrography as an alternative to standard fluoroscopic guidance. For both contrast and local corticosteroid injections, 22-gauge needles are commonly used. For arthrocentesis, larger gauge needles (20 or 18 gauge) are typically used in order to effectively and potentially aspirate more viscous fluid, especially in the setting of suspected infection. Similarly, 20- and 18-gauge needles are typically used for viscosupplementation injections for treatment of degenerative joint disease (ie, hyaluronic acid formulations with their higher viscosity).

Articular, bursal, or peritendinous/tenosynovial injections of a mixture of corticosteroids and local anesthetic are commonly performed for their analgesic and antiinflammatory effects, especially in the setting of severe inflammatory arthritis or end-stage degenerative joint disease. Because the corticosteroid preparations are very echogenic due to increased specular reflectors, the location of the injection material can be readily identified during real-time US. It is important to recognize that local skin atrophy and depigmentation can occur when corticosteroids are placed subcutaneously. Methylprednisolone acetate (Depo-Medrol) is less prone to skin atrophy than triamcinolone acetonide (Kenalog), so the former is the preferred formulation when injecting superficial joints. Local anesthetic agents can be chondrotoxic in large amounts, so moderation in the amount of anesthetic injected and use of ropivacaine as opposed to bupivacaine hydrochloride is suggested to diminish this risk when injecting into joints. The volume of injectate will vary depending on the joint size and can range from less than 1 mL in the small joints of the hand to 5 mL in larger joints such as the hip or knee. A common mixture administered is 1 mL of 40 mg of triamcinolone or methylprednisolone with 2 mL of 0.5% preservative-free bupivacaine. When injecting larger joints, some prefer to use 80 mg of corticosteroid.

Soft Tissue Fluid Collections

Aspiration of MSK abscesses can be safely performed with US guidance with 18-gauge needles. Using Seldinger technique and serial tract dilatation, sonographic placement of pigtail drainage catheters to gravity drainage within the abscess cavity, ranging in size from 8 to 16 French, can be performed.

Aspirations of intramuscular (Figure 128.4) or intermuscular hematomas in the setting of muscle tears are sometimes requested in the high-level athlete to expedite healing response by approximating the tissue ends. This can be performed with an 18-gauge needle. Strict aseptic technique is warranted because of the potential risk for infection if contaminating the hematoma cavity. Depending on the extent and timing of clot formation, there is variable success in the aspiration of these collections. When scanning the area prior to the intervention, the presence of multiple internal septations and lack of compressibility with overlying transducer pressure may correlate with decreased success in hematoma evacuation. Pressure bandages can be applied after hematoma evacuation to try to prevent reaccumulation. Lower grade muscle strains without hematoma can also have variable recovery, and there are case series suggesting that US-guided injections of local anesthetic and corticosteroid (2-4 mg of water-soluble dexamethasone sodium phosphate mixed with 3-4 cc of 0.5% bupivacaine) at the myotendinous injury site can quicken return to play. More recently, use of platelet-rich plasma (PRP) injection (usually 5 mL injectate volume) has been popularized (Figure 128.5) because of the potential risk of myotendinous weakening by corticosteroids. Of note, the efficacy of these interventions is debated in the literature.

US-guided percutaneous aspiration of ganglion cysts is sometimes performed when the cysts are symptomatic because of pressure on adjacent neurovascular structures. Because of the viscosity of their internal contents, an 18-gauge needle is commonly used. Injecting a small amount of saline or lidocaine into the cyst may be of help in aspirating the more gelatinous collections. A small amount of local corticosteroid can be injected after aspiration, although it is controversial if this helps decrease cyst recurrence. If the ganglion cyst recurs

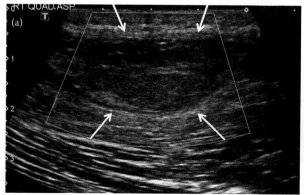
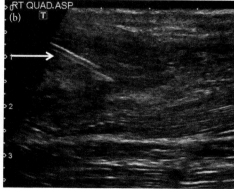

Figure 128.4. US-guided intramuscular hematoma evacuation. (*A*) Long-axis color Doppler US image of the right anterior thigh in a football player shows a quadriceps muscle hematoma (*arrows*) that developed after blunt trauma. (*B*) Long-axis US image of the same region shows placement of an 18-gauge needle (*arrow*) into a hematoma and partial evacuation/aspiration.

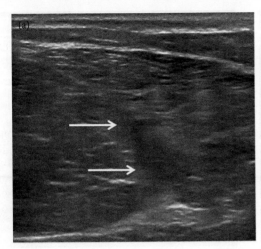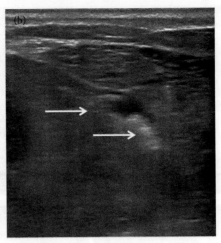

Figure 128.5. PRP injection into a muscle tear. (*A*) Transverse US image of the posterior thigh in a professional football player shows a grade 2 tear (*arrows*) of the semimembranosus muscle. (*B*) Transverse US image of the same region obtained after PRP injection shows echogenic deposition of injectate within the previously seen tear (*arrows*).

after initial treatment, subsequent aspirations are of decreased benefit.

Intratendinous Interventions

Calcific Tendinosis

Calcium hydroxyapatite crystal deposition can occur in multiple tendons and peritendinous locations, but most commonly presents with rotator cuff symptomatology when located near the greater tuberosity insertion. Although its course is usually self-limiting, US-guided aspiration and lavage is an effective, minimally invasive technique when symptoms have not improved with conservative treatment. Three phases in the calcific stage of this disease can be recognized. The formative and resting phases tend to have discrete, well-circumscribed borders with strong posterior acoustic shadowing. Aspiration can be difficult in these

phases. The resorptive phase is usually more symptomatic, will have less posterior acoustic shadowing on US, and is usually more amenable to aspiration.

Either a 1- or a 2-needle technique can be performed. Needle size can vary from 22 to 18 gauge. With a 2-needle technique, 1 syringe is used for pulsed lavage and the other for aspiration. When a single-needle technique is performed, a single puncture into the calcification is performed (Figure 128.7*A*), usually with a 20-gauge needle attached to a 12-mL syringe filled with 1% lidocaine or saline. It is important to inject into the calcification initially (Figure 128.7*B*), avoiding aspiration in order for the needle tip not to clog. Short intermittent pulsed injections of lidocaine or saline into the calcification are performed, and a cloudy calcium suspension will usually be seen to return into the syringe when the plunger is released. The syringe should be positioned so the dependent calcium will accumulate in the syringe and not the hub of the needle. After

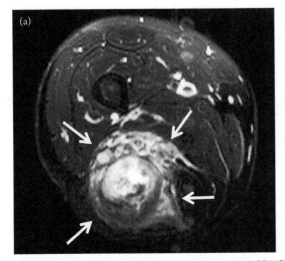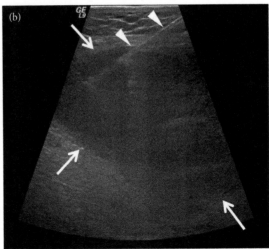

Figure 128.6. US-guided biopsy of a soft tissue sarcoma. (*A*) T2W FS MR image of the thigh shows a heterogeneous soft tissue sarcoma in the posterior muscle compartment (*arrows*). (*B*) Transverse US image of the same region shows a biopsy needle (*arrowheads*) at the periphery of the posterior thigh sarcoma (*arrows*).

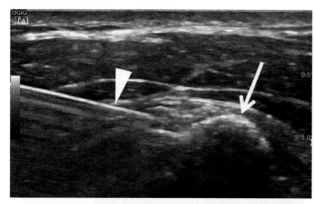

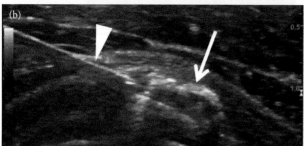

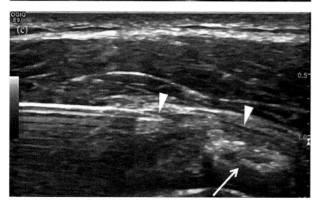

Figure 128.7. Calcific tendinosis lavage with subsequent steroid injection into the subacromial-subdeltoid bursa. (*A*) Transverse US image of the shoulder shows placement of a 20-gauge needle (*arrowhead*) into the supraspinatus tendon calcification (*arrow*). (*B*) Transverse US image of the same region obtained during calcium lavage shows a needle (*arrowhead*) and saline within the calcification (*arrow*). (*C*) Transverse US image of the anterior aspect of the shoulder in the same patient obtained during subsequent steroid injection into the subacromial-subdeltoid bursa shows a 25-gauge needle within the partially distended bursa (*arrowheads*) with adjacent echogenic steroid injectate. Note lavaged supraspinatus tendon calcification (*arrow*) containing residual small amount of fluid.

several minutes of this lavage, US visualization will show a decrease in the calcium intratendon deposition. The needle is then positioned into the subacromial-subdeltoid bursa and a bursal injection of local corticosteroid (Figure 128.7*C*) is performed to prevent post procedure inflammatory bursitis. If the calcium deposit is not in a phase amenable to aspiration, performing multiple punctures of the calcium with the needle tip may help stimulate later resorption of the calcium.

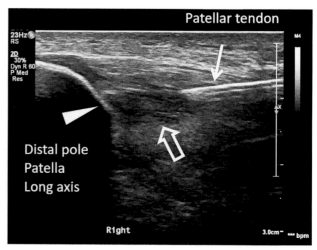

Figure 128.8. Dry-needling of the proximal patellar tendon. Longitudinal US image of the anterior knee shows an 18-gauge needle (*arrow*) extending into the thickened hypoechoic proximal patellar tendon (*open arrow*). During the procedure, the needle is inserted parallel to the patellar tendon fibers. Ten to twenty passes are made through the affected area (*open arrow*) and inferior patellar pole periosteum (*arrowhead*). Courtesy of Marina Obradov MD.

Degenerative Noncalcific Tendon Injections
Intratendinous injection of corticosteroid is contraindicated because of the increased risk of tendon rupture with load bearing in experimental models. Peritendinous corticosteroid injections should thus be performed with caution, especially in the lower extremities.

Several US-guided techniques including dry-needling (Figure 128.8); percutaneous tenotomy; and injections including prolotherapy (dextrose solutions), autologous blood, and more recently, PRP injections, have been used to stimulate healing pathways in overuse injuries/degenerative tendinosis, including but not limited to Achilles tendinosis in the ankle, infrapatellar tendinosis in the knee, and lateral and medial epicondylosis in the elbow. A combination of US repeated needling of the affected area of the tendon with small-gauge needles, with subsequent injection of the preceding chosen treatment, is usually performed. Postprocedure pain can be treated with analgesics, with avoidance of NSAID medications as these may blunt the desired inflammatory reaction. Given the potential delayed risk for tendon rupture, decreased tendon loading is recommended, including the use of crutches after lower extremity tendon intervention, especially in the setting of Achilles tendinosis.

Key Points
- US is commonly used to guide aspirations of joints and soft tissue collections and to direct injections of local corticosteroids or other therapeutics.
- Before any planned intervention, a complete US evaluation of the MSK anatomic structures to be targeted is performed, with attention placed to the position of neurovascular structures to be avoided by the needle path.

- High-frequency linear transducers are preferred when targeting superficial MSK structures.
- Knowledge of individual joint anatomy is essential in planning US needle approach.
- Intratendinous injection of corticosteroid is contraindicated.

Recommended Reading

Louis, LJ. Musculoskeletal ultrasound intervention: principles and advances. *Radiol Clin North Am.* 2008;46(3):515–33.

References

1. Aina R, Cardinal E, Bureau NJ, et al. Calcific shoulder tendonitis: treatment with modified US-guided fine needle technique. *Radiology.* 2001;221:455–61.

2. Cardinal E, Beauregard CG, Chem RK. Interventional musculoskeletal ultrasound. *Semin Musculoskeletal Radiol.* 1997;1:311–18.

3. Dave RB, Steven KJ, Shivaram GM, McAdams TR, Dillingham MF, Beaulieu F. Ultrasound-guided musculoskeletal interventions in American football: 18 years of experience. *AJR Am J Roentgenol.* 2014;203:W674–83.

4. Fessell DP, Jacobson JA, Craig J, et al. Using sonography to reveal and aspirate joint effusions. *AJR Am J Roentgenol.* 2000;174:1353–62.

5. Hansford BG, Stacy GS. Musculoskeletal aspiration procedures. *Semin Intervent Radiol.* 2012;29:270–85.

6. Joines MM, Motamedi K, Seeger LL, DiFiori JP. Musculoskeletal interventional ultrasound. *Semin Musculoskelet Radiol.* 2007;11:192–98.

7. Lee KS. Platelet-rich plasma injection. *Semin Musculoskelet Radiol.* 2013;17:91–98.

Appendix 1

Commonly Used Abbreviations

Imran M. Omar

A number of abbreviations are used in musculoskeletal radiology to succinctly discuss a variety of imaging techniques and pathologies. The following list includes many of the most commonly used abbreviations in musculoskeletal radiology, and many of them have been used throughout this book.

2D	two-dimensional		FIESTA	*Fast Imaging Employing Steady-state Acquisition*
3D	three-dimensional		FOV	field-of-view
ABC	aneurysmal bone cyst		FS	fat-suppressed/fat-saturated
ABER	abduction/external rotation		FSE	fast spin echo
AC	acromioclavicular		GCT	giant cell tumor
ACL	anterior cruciate ligament		Gd	gadolinium/gadolinium-based contrast agent
ACR	American College of Radiology		GLAD	glenolabral articular disruption
ALL	anterior longitudinal ligament		GRE	gradient recalled echo
ALPSA	anterior labroligamentous periosteal sleeve avulsion		HAGL	humeral avulsion of the inferior glenohumeral ligament
AP	anterior-posterior		HOA	hypertrophic osteoarthropathy
AS	ankylosing spondylitis		HPOA	hypertrophic pulmonary osteoarthropathy
bSSFP	*balanced Steady-State Free Precession*		IFI	ischiofemoral impingement
BFH	benign fibrous histiocytoma		IGHL	inferior glenohumeral ligament
BID	bilateral interfacetal dislocation		ITB	iliotibial band
BME	bone marrow edema		IV	intravenous
CMF	chondromyxoid fibroma		LCH	Langerhans cell histiocytosis
CPPD	calcium pyrophosphate deposition		LCL	lateral collateral ligament (also called *fibular collateral ligament* in the knee)
CRMO	chronic recurrent multifocal osteomyelitis			
CRP	C-reactive protein		LM	lateral meniscus
CT	computed tomography		LSMFT	liposclerosing myxofibrous tumor
CTA	computed tomography arthrography		LT	ligamentum teres
CTS	carpal tunnel syndrome		LTL	lunotriquetral ligament
CUBE	3D fast spin echo sequence (produced by General Electric)		LUCL	lateral ulnar collateral ligament
			MCL	medial collateral ligament
DDH	developmental dysplasia of the hip		MCP	metacarpophalangeal
DEFT	*Driven Equilibrium Fourier Transform*		MFH	malignant fibrous histiocytoma
DESS	*Double Echo Steady State*		MGHL	middle glenohumeral ligament
DIP	distal interphalangeal		MHE	multiple hereditary exostosis
DISH	diffuse idiopathic skeletal hyperostosis		MM	medial meniscus
DISI	dorsal intercalary segmental instability		MO	myositis ossificans
DOMS	delayed-onset muscle soreness		MPFL	medial patellofemoral ligament
DTI	diffusion tensor imaging		MRA	magnetic resonance arthrography
DXA	dual x-ray absorptiometry		MRI	magnetic resonance imaging
EG	eosinophilic granulomatosis		MSK	musculoskeletal
EHE	epithelioid hemangioendothelioma		MTP	metatarsophalangeal
ESR	erythrocyte sedimentation rate		NFS	nonfat-suppressed/nonfat-saturated
FAI	femoroacetabular impingement		NOF	nonossifying fibroma
FCL	fibular collateral ligament		NSAID	nonsteroidal antiinflammatory drug
FD	fibrous dysplasia		OA	osteoarthritis
FFE	fast field echo		OCL	osteochondral lesions

ON	osteonecrosis
OPLL	ossification of the posterior longitudinal ligament
ORIF	open reduction/internal fixation
PA	posterior-anterior
PCL	posterior cruciate ligament
PDW	proton density weighted
PET	positron emission tomography
PET/CT	hybrid positron emission tomography/computed tomography
PIP	proximal interphalangeal
PLC	posterior ligamentous complex
PLL	posterior longitudinal ligament
PLRI	posterolateral rotatory instability
PNET	primitive neuroectodermal tumor
PNST	peripheral nerve sheath tumor
POEMS	syndrome of polyneuropathy, organomegaly, endocrinopathy, monoclonal gammopathy and skin findings
POLPSA	posterior labroligamentous periosteal sleeve avulsion
PVNS	pigmented villonodular synovitis
RA	rheumatoid arthritis
RCL	radial collateral ligament
RFA	radiofrequency ablation
RIS	radiation-induced sarcoma
RMO	regional migratory osteoporosis
RT	radiation therapy
SAPHO	syndrome of synovitis, acne, pustulosis, hyperostosis and osteitis
SCFE	slipped capital femoral epiphysis
SCL	scapholunate ligament

SE	spin echo
SGHL	superior glenohumeral ligament
SI	sacroiliac
SIF	subchondral insufficiency fracture
SLAC	scapholunate advanced collapse
SLAP	superior labral tear anterior-posterior
SLE	systemic lupus erythematosus
SNAC	scaphoid nonunion advanced collapse
SNR	signal-to-noise ratio
SPACE	*Sampling Perfection with Application optimized Contrasts using different flip angle Evolution*
STIR	short tau inversion recovery
TE	echo time
T1W/T1WI	T1-weighted/T1-weighted imaging
T2W/T2WI	T2-weighted/T2-weighted imaging
TFC	triangular fibrocartilage
TFCC	triangular fibrocartilage complex
TLICS	thoracolumbar injury and severity classification scale
TLSO	thoracolumbar spinal orthotic
TOH	transient osteoporosis of the hip
TR	repetition time
TrueFISP	true *Fast Imaging with Steady-state Precession*
TT-TG	tibial tuberosity/trochlear-groove distance
UCL	ulnar collateral ligament
UID	unilateral interfacetal dislocation
US	ultrasound
VISTA	*Volume Isotropic Turbo spin echo Acquisition*
VMO	vastus medialis obliquus muscle
WHO	World Health Organization

Appendix 2

Contraindications to Magnetic Resonance Imaging

Imran M. Omar

Introduction

The powerful magnetic fields used in MRI can interfere with the function of many implantable devices that perform critical functions, such as pacemakers and central nervous system stimulating devices. In some instances, the magnetic field can either lead to localized thermal damage or migration of metallic structures. Additionally, the metals in some devices can lead to susceptibility artifacts that can greatly corrupt MR images despite optimal imaging techniques, making them nondiagnostic. The following is a list of contraindications for MRI. Because many device manufacturers have recognized that MRI can be beneficial to the patients receiving these implants, they have started to make devices that are MRI compatible under particular circumstances. Thus, some of the contraindications currently listed as absolute are or may become relative contraindications in the future, and it is important to check with specific device manufacturers whether a specific device is MRI compatible and for what conditions it is approved (eg, field strength) prior to putting patients into an MRI scanner. Finally, for devices that are approved for MRI, it is often best to use alternative imaging strategies that can reasonably answer a specific question before turning to MRI. For example, in patients with suspected rotator cuff tendon tears, US is an excellent technique and can be attempted first. However, if the clinical concern is for labral tear, MRI may still be the first-line imaging modality because it is by far the best technique available.

Absolute Contraindications

- Cardiac pacemaker or defibrillator device—many newer devices are approved for MRI under specific circumstances. The compatibility should be checked with the device manufacturer, and the patients should be approved by a cardiologist and monitored during the study.
- Aneurysm clip
- Deep brain stimulator device
- Cochlear implant
- Metallic foreign bodies in eye
- Drug infusion device

Relative Contraindications

- Surgical clips
- Recently placed metallic implants
- Bone or nerve stimulator devices
- Abdominal aortic aneurysm stent/grafts
- Claustrophobic patients
- Inability to lie still (eg, patients in pain, pediatric patients, elderly patients). These patients may require analgesia or sedation and monitoring during scan.

Index